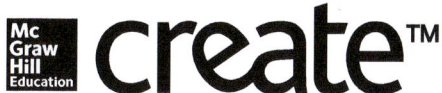

301.05 A512a 2020 v.1
Magill, Kevin R.
Taking sides: clashing views in United States History

Taking Sides: Clashing Views in United States History, Volume 1: The Colonial Period to Reconstruction, 18/e

Kevin Magill and Tony Talbert

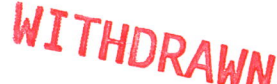

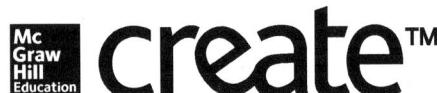

http://create.mheducation.com

Copyright 2020 by McGraw-Hill Education. All rights reserved. Printed in the United States of America. Except as permitted under the United States Copyright Act of 1976, no part of this publication may be reproduced or distributed in any form or by any means, or stored in a database or retrieval system, without prior written permission of the publisher.

This McGraw-Hill Create text may include materials submitted to McGraw-Hill for publication by the instructor of this course. The instructor is solely responsible for the editorial content of such materials. Instructors retain copyright of these additional materials.

ISBN-10: 1260497321   ISBN-13: 9781260497328

1 2 3 4 5 6 QVS 23 22 21 20 19

Contents

- i. Detailed Table of Contents 1
- ii. Preface by Magill and Talbert 7
- iii. Introduction by Magill and Talbert 11

Unit 1 17

1. Colonial Society by Magill and Talbert 18
    - 1.1. Is America Exceptional? by Magill and Talbert 19
    - 1.2. Did the Core Values in Colonial Ideology Lead to Conflict with Native Americans and U.S. Imperialism? by Magill and Talbert 34
    - 1.3. Was the Pequot War Largely a Product of Native American Aggression? by Magill and Talbert 74
    - 1.4. Was the Colonial Period a "Golden Age" for Women in America? by Magill and Talbert 90
    - 1.5. Was Encephalitis Responsible for the Salem Witchcraft Hysteria? by Magill and Talbert 106
    - 1.6. Should the Great Awakening Be Understood Primarily Through Religious Evangelicalism? by Magill and Talbert 124
    - 1.7. Was the American Revolution "Common Sense"? by Magill and Talbert 147

Unit 2 169

2. Revolution and the New Nation by Magill and Talbert 170
    - 2.1. Did the Founding Fathers Create a Democratic System that Would Attend to the Problems of a Democracy? by Magill and Talbert 171
    - 2.2. Was the Second Amendment Designed to Protect an Individual's Right to Own Guns? by Magill and Talbert 190
    - 2.3. Was Alexander Hamilton an Economic Genius? by Magill and Talbert 212
    - 2.4. Were Jackson's Anti-Politics and Nationalism Beneficial for Increased Democratic Participation? by Magill and Talbert 233

Unit 3 259

3. Antebellum America by Magill and Talbert 260
    - 3.1. Did Educational Opportunities for Women in the New Nation Expand Their Participation in Antebellum Society? by Magill and Talbert 261
    - 3.2. Was Antebellum Temperance Reform Driven by Theological Doctrine? by Magill and Talbert 283
    - 3.3. Was the Mexican War an Exercise in American Imperialism? by Magill and Talbert 308
    - 3.4. Was John Brown an Irrational Terrorist? by Magill and Talbert 324

Unit 4 339

4. Conflict and Resolution by Magill and Talbert 340
    - 4.1. Was the Civil War Fought Over Slavery? by Magill and Talbert 341

4.2. Are Historians Wrong to Consider the War Between the States a "Total War"? by Magill and Talbert 357
4.3. Did African American Slaves Exercise Religious Autonomy? by Magill and Talbert 375
4.4. Was Abraham Lincoln America's Greatest President? by Magill and Talbert 394
4.5. Did Reconstruction Fail as a Result of Racism? by Magill and Talbert 410

Detailed Table of Contents

Unit 1: Colonial Society

Issue: Is America Exceptional?
YES: Seymour Martin Lipset, from "Still the Exceptional Nation?" *The Wilson Quarterly* (2000)
NO: Godfrey Hodgson, from "The Corruption of the Best," Yale University Press (2010)

Seymour Martin Lipset (1922–2006) argues that the United States remains uniquely exceptional for a number of reasons. First the United States relies upon less taxation and social welfare, second it is uniquely influenced by Protestantism, third its people benefit from a higher rate of social mobility than in other first world nations. Godfrey Hodgson suggests the "myth of American exceptionalism" is just that- a myth. He believes that people focus too much on American uniqueness and ignore the international influence, historical processes, and ideologies that have developed American values.

Issue: Did the Core Values in Colonial Ideology Lead to Conflict with Native Americans and U.S. Imperialism?
YES: Maureen Konkle, from "Indigenous Ownership and the Emergence of U.S. Liberal Imperialism," *American Indian Quarterly* (2008)
NO: Jessica R. Stern, from, "A Key into *The Bloudy Tenent of Persecution*: Roger Williams, the Pequot War, and the Origins of Toleration in America," *Early American Studies* (2011)

Maureen Konkle argues that the ideology of colonialism has allowed discourses to develop that have been fundamental to the project of U.S. imperialism. She suggests that marginalizing narratives, particularly of Indigenous Peoples, have contributed to the justification U.S. aggression, conflict, and genocide. Konkle lastly implies that these colonizing narratives continue to exist and affect our ideology today, though less overt than they once were. Jessica Stern believes that careful examination of Roger Williams arguments suggests that religion never justified violence and that Native Americans and Christians shared a moral code. She suggests first that, rather than critique colonial ideology we should consider that individuals are prone to misunderstand foreign people and ideas and should therefore not be trusted to judge outsiders. Second, she suggests that civil peace relies on locating similarities between people and tolerating differences.

Issue: Was the Pequot War Largely a Product of Native American Aggression?
YES: Steven T. Katz, from "The Pequot War Reconsidered," *The New England Quarterly* (1991)
NO: Alfred A. Cave, from "The Pequot War and the Mythology of the Frontier," University of Massachusetts Press (1996)

Steven Katz believes the Pequots conducted a series of aggressive raids, ambushes, and murders in the 1630. He suggests the Pequot Indians attempted to destroy the European Colonies after the two sides failed in their negotiations. Katz further believes that the colonists conducted a defensive war in support of their New England settlements, which was justified in protecting themselves from Pequot aggression. Alfred A. Cave believes the Pequot War started because Puritanical leaders were able to convince settlers that the Indigenous Americans were Satanic. This European colonial perception led them to clash with the Pequots believing they needed to eliminate Indigenous autonomy, intimidate their population and controlling the land and recourses.

Issue: Was the Colonial Period a "Golden Age" for Women in America?
YES: Gloria L. Main, from "Gender, Work, and Wages in Colonial New England," *William and Mary Quarterly* (1994)
NO: Cornelia Hughes Dayton, from "Women Before the Bar," University of North Carolina Press (1995)

Gloria Main highlights that more New England women entered the paid work force, received higher wages, and saw increased recognition for their labors following the Seven Years War. She believes because women were more highly valued for their labor and that labor was relatively scarce in the early colonial period, that they received higher wages and economic autonomy. Cornelia Hughes Dayton challenges the "golden age" thesis, arguing that women were being used for their labor and that improvements in their condition benefited the patriarchy. She argues that increased access to county courts for women in seventeenth-century was negated as new rules and practices were implemented in the eighteenth century. The changes strengthen patriarchal authority and reversed many of the gains that had been made.

Issue: Was Encephalitis Responsible for the Salem Witchcraft Hysteria?
YES: Laurie Winn Carlson, from "A Fever in Salem: A New Interpretation of the New England Witch Trials," Ivan R. Dee (1999)
NO: Lyle Koehler, from "The Salem Village Cataclysm: Origins and Impact of a Witch Hunt, 1689-92," University of Illinois Press (1980)

Laurie Winn Carlson suggests that witchcraft hysteria occurred because of the Colonist's physical and neurological responses to an unrecognized outbreak of encephalitis. She suggests the outbreak affected people's physical and neurological behaviors causing them to act hysterically. Lyle Koehler points out that most of the Witchcraft accusers were women and likely seeking to overcome their own feelings of personal powerlessness by speaking out in a patriarchal and oppressive world. These women relished the sense of power they received from the community's attention to their allegations- allegations that were designed to conquer the supernatural forces around them.

Issue: Should the Great Awakening Be Understood Primarily through Religious Evangelicalism?
YES: Thomas S. Kidd, from "The Great Awakening: The Roots of Evangelical Christianity in Colonial America," Yale University Press (2007)
NO: David A. Varel, from "The Historiography of the Second Great Awakening and the Problem of Historical Causation, 1945-2005," *Madison Historical Review* (2011)

Thomas S. Kidd believes that a Great Awakening occurred because influential preachers engineered divinely inspired revivals in the mid-eighteenth century causing an evangelical movement that spread across the colonies, changing the nature of Christianity. David A. Varel tracks the historiography of the Second Great Awakening and suggests that historian need to consider more that evangelicalism. He believes that factors such as: social control, democratization, and denominational concentration present a problem in determining historical causation. He therefore suggests that the Second Great Awakening should be understood through the many intersectional aspects that helped create this evangelical movement. He additionally notes, though it was a national phenomena, the Second Great Awakening greatly varied in its local and regional manifestations and should not be understood solely through its most famous preachers.

Issue: Was the American Revolution "Common Sense"?
YES: Thomas Paine, from *Common Sense, Jan. 1776, Introduction, Pt. III-IV*, Primary Source Collection, www.americainclass.org (1776)
NO: Rev. Charles Inglis, from *A Loyalist Rebuttal to Common Sense, 1776*, Primary Source Collection, www.americainclass.org (1776)

Thomas Paine's 1775 pamphlet titled *Common Sense* presents the author's case for independence from Britain. Written in common vernacular and widely read, *Common Sense* is considered to be the most influential text of the Revolutionary period. It remains the all-time best selling American title to this day. In this piece, Paine makes a fiery case for American independence by concentrating on moral and political arguments related to advocating for independence. His argument begins with general and theoretical reflections about government and religion. Paine then applies these intellectual traditions to the colonial situation. Charles Inglis's 1776 *The Deceiver Unmasked; Or, Loyalty and Interest United: In Answer to a Pamphlet Entitled Common Sense* is the author's rebuttal to Thomas Paine's *Common Sense*. Written to consolidate the support of American Loyalists, Inglis makes a case for American reconciliation with Britain. His response to *Common Sense* is a repudiation of Paine's revolutionary ideas and a call for an English cultural revival in her colonies. Inglis's argument suggests Paine is naive to think that a new government would be less tyrannical than England.

Unit 2: Revolution and the New Nation

Issue: Did the Founding Fathers Create a Democratic System That Would Adequately Attend to the Problems of a Democracy?
YES: James Madison, from "Federalist No. 10," *The Federalist Papers No. 10* (1787)
NO: Aristotle, from "Politics Book VI: A Treatise on Government," J.M. Dent & Sons (1912)

In *Terms of The Senate 26 June*, Madison suggests the major problem with a new democratic system would be that it would require an egalitarian society. He believed those citizens without means would vote for policies that would lead to the redistribution of land and capital. Madison saw this as a problem, believing the country needed to be controlled by a certain class of men. In *Politics*, Aristotle also described inequality as a major problem in a democratic system.

Taking the opposite approach to Madison, Aristotle argues a democratic society should be concerned with removing tyranny and oligarchy so communities of free and equal men are able to access its systems. He them believed that citizens could democratically work toward the common good for all in the society.

Issue: Was the Second Amendment Designed to Protect an Individual's Right to Own Guns?
YES: William W. Van Alstyne, from "The Second Amendment and the Personal Right to Arms," *Duke Law Journal* (1994)
NO: Lawrence Delbert Cress, from "A Well-Regulated Militia: The Origins and Meaning of the Second Amendment," The Library of Virginia (1987)

William W. Van Alstyne contends that those who adhere to the belief that the Second Amendment to the U.S. Constitution protects an individual's right to own firearms is as historically and legally secure as those liberties guaranteed to individuals within the First Amendment to the U.S. Constitution. Van Alstyne therefore asserts that judicial and legislative mechanisms of interpretation of Second Amendment liberties have been put in place and to date those interpretations lean toward the protection of individual rights to gun ownership. Lawrence Delbert Cress suggests that the Second Amendment refers to gun ownership for only to those participating in the "well-regulated militia," whose job it was to protect citizens from a tyrannical national government and other domestic incursions.

Issue: Was Alexander Hamilton an Economic Genius?
YES: Donald F. Swanson and Andrew P. Trout, from "Alexander Hamilton's Economic Policies After Two Centuries," *New York History* (1991)
NO: Edward Peter Stringham, from "Hamilton's Legacy and the Great Man Theory of Financial History," *Independent Review* (2017)

Donald F. Swanson and Andrew P. Trout contend that Alexander Hamilton's historic legacy is too often mischaracterized as one of financial interest alone. Swanson and Trout argue that Hamilton's legacy as America's greatest financial genius must encompass his commitment to supporting the development of a multi-institutional national system of governance that addressed both political and financial realities of the time. Hamilton's genius is founded in equal parts risk-taker and strategic pragmatist when enacting fiscal and philosophical policies that established America's national government on firm pathway to international prominence. Edward Peter Stringham argues against applying the "genius" (i.e., great man theory of history) to Alexander Hamilton, as has been done in the Hamilton musical, suggesting that Hamilton's primary philosophy was not grounded in a commitment to multi-institutional nationalism but primarily in developing a centralized economic system that should also not be solely credited to Hamilton but instead to the countless people who worked behind the scenes to make the historical and modern United States economy possible.

Issue: Were Jackson's Anti-Politics and Nationalism Beneficial for Increased Democratic Participation?
YES: Kori N. Schake, from "Trump and the 'New Nationalism:' It's Not New at All," *Hoover Digest* (2017)
NO: Donald Ratcliffe, from "The Right to Vote and the Rise of Democracy, 1787-1828," *Journal of the Early Republic* (2013)

Kori N. Schake suggests that Andrew Jackson and Donald Trump both champion a populist style, which did and will strengthened American democracy by "activating antibodies in opposition to [their] policies, mobilizing the civic powers that undergird our democracy into greater activism." She offers comparisons in the presidential approaches of both men suggesting that their elections represent the US people's routine disenfranchisement with the governmental status quo. Donald Ratcliffe argues that despite the fact that it is often understood as a golden age for democracy the Jacksonian Era was not a social revolution. He claims, "suffrage had significantly expanded" in the "United States [and it] had, in many ways, become a functioning democracy long before 1815." However, he contends that the Jackson presidency affected the radial ideology of the Democratic Party.

Unit 3: Antebellum America

Issue: Did Improved Educational Opportunities for Women in the New Nation Significantly Expand Their Participation in Antebellum Society?
YES: Mary Kelley, from "Learning to Stand and Speak: Women, Education, and Public Life in America's Republic," University of North Carolina Press (2006)
NO: Lucia McMahon, from "Between Cupid and Minerva" and "Education, Equality, or Difference," Cornell University Press (2012)

Mary Kelley describes how expanding educational opportunities encouraged women to redefine themselves by opening doors to careers beyond the domestic sphere, economic self-support, and public participation in civil society that transformed their understanding of the rights of citizenship in the post-revolutionary and antebellum United States. Lucia McMahon concludes that the unprecedented access to education afforded women in the early national period fostered recognition of women's intellectual capacity, but she argues that most educated women confronted a limited range of opportunities in a society that remained largely committed to a social and political order rooted in notions of sexual difference and male hierarchy.

Issue: Was Antebellum Temperance Reform Driven by Theological Doctrine?
YES: Laura A. Schmidt, from "'A Battle Not Man's but God's': Origins of the American Temperance Crusade in the Struggle for Religious Authority," *Journal of Studies on Alcohol* (1995)
NO: John J. Rumbarger, from "The Social and Ideological Origins of Drink Reform, 1800-1836," State University of New York Press (1989)

Laura A. Schmidt argues that the temperance movement was developed primarily to offer clergymen a solution to those who contested their authority in a time of social transformation. Many believed religious salvation occurred through the suppression of vice, which allowed the clergymen an additional avenue to: win souls to God, guard collective salvation, and petition the government to promote religious obedience. John J. Rumbarger believes Temperance was directed by men of power who "defined, directed, and controlled" the movement to feed the expansionist tendencies of the American economy by encouraging a more productive and reliable workforce.

Issue: Was the Mexican War an Exercise in American Imperialism?
YES: Ramón Eduardo Ruiz, from "Manifest Destiny and the Mexican War," Dorsey Press (1988)
NO: Norman A. Graebner, from "The Mexican War: A Study in Causation," *Pacific Historical Review* (1980)

Ramón Eduardo Ruiz believes that the Unites States demonstrated their imperialist tendencies by aggressively pursuing and waging war against Mexico in an effort to conquer and take her northern territories. Ruiz suggests that Mexico was never able to recover from this incursion. Norman A. Graebner suggests that the United States indeed adopted aggressive foreign policies designed to secure territory. However he argues that President Polk was not interested in war. Instead he suggests that the intention of his policies was to force Mexico to sell New Mexico and California to the United States and to recognize the legitimacy of the annexation of Texas.

Issue: Was John Brown an Irrational Terrorist?
YES: James N. Gilbert, from "A Behavioral Analysis of John Brown: Martyr or Terrorist?" Ohio University Press (2005)
NO: Scott John Hammond, from "John Brown as Founder: America's Violent Confrontation with Its First Principles," Ohio University Press (2005)

James N. Gilbert believes that the actions of John Brown are a textbook definition of terrorism in modern society. Brown believed the United States was going to be incapable of the social reform needed to abolish slavery and therefore saw it as his responsibility to use violence to achieve that goal. Gilbert also discusses Brown's belief that adherence to a higher power was his justification for his acts of terror. Scott John Hammond instead believes that John Brown was committed to higher moral and political goals including the basic principals of human freedom, political equality, and legal egalitarianism. Therefore, he was not a terrorist, but a citizen committed to the ideals set forth by the founding fathers.

Unit 4: Conflict and Resolution

Issue: Was the Civil War Fought Over Slavery?
YES: Charles B. Dew, from "Apostles of Disunion: Southern Secession Commissioners and the Causes of the Civil War," University of Virginia Press (2001)
NO: Gary W. Gallagher, from "The Union War," Harvard University Press (2012)

Charles B. Dew presents documentation, which suggests that a number of white southerners attempted to gain support for secession in the southern states by arguing for the need to preserve slavery and white supremacy as social norms. Dew suggests that these appeals demonstrate the primary motive for secession. Gary W. Gallagher, analyzes the letters of white northern soldiers during the Civil War which suggest the common soldier cared little about slavery as an institution. Further, many of the letters were open hostility toward the idea that the union would African American troops. In other words, Gallagher believes the main motivation of these troops was saving the Union and not the abolition of slavery.

Issue: Are Historians Wrong to Consider the War Between the States a "Total War"?
YES: Mark E. Neely, Jr., from "Was the Civil War a Total War?" *Civil War History* (2004)
NO: James M. McPherson, from "From Limited War to Total War, 1861-1865," *Magazine of the Missouri Historical Society* (1992)

Mark E. Neely convincingly asserts that the U.S. Civil War was not a "total war" based upon three factors. First, President Lincoln's continued insistence that Union generals made a distinction between combatants and non-combatants in the exercise of the war (though Grant and Sherman openly disagreed). Second, Lincoln's continued willingness to negotiate relatively lenient terms of peace that instead of demanding unconditional surrender offered Confederate leaders the opportunity of enter into discussions as long as they accepted the full restoration of the Union and the abandonment of slavery. And third, Neely contents that the U.S. Civil War did in fact have limitations and codes of conduct, which means it was not in fact a total war. He even cites the work of Brian Bond who argues that a true total war is unattainable. In stark contrast, Jame M. McPherson asserts that whether the notion of "total war" was the official policy Lincoln and his generals it was exactly that which was accomplished through the destruction of the southern states' economies, the dismantling of the symbiotic state-based Confederacy, and the complete abolition of a system of slavery that served as both the philosophical and cultural zeitgeist of the Confederacy. Simply put, McPherson argues that "total war" was indeed the outcome with the extensive destruction of Southern civilian populations and the south's economy as a whole.

Issue: Did African American Slaves Exercise Religious Autonomy?
YES: Albert J. Raboteau, from "Slave Autonomy and Religion," *Journal of Religious Thought* (1982)
NO: John B. Boles, from "Masters & Slaves in the House of the Lord: Race and Religion in the American South, 1740–1870," University Press of Kentucky (1988)

Albert J. Raboteau asserts that the exercise of religion among African American slaves in the 19th century United States allowed for the development of a cohesive organization founded within a common lived experience. Through the development of an autonomous religious culture African American slaves formed a philosophical and pragmatic bond of interests that resulted in the pursuit of freedom from oppression. John B. Boles counters the notion of the segregated congregational religious experience among Anglos and African American slaves in the southern region of the United States during the 19th century. While Boles acknowledges the importance of religious customs and organizational structures within the enslaved African American population he asserts that Anglos and African Americans shared a common religious experience both in philosophy (interpretation of Christian text) and practice (attendance in worship services).

Issue: Was Abraham Lincoln America's Greatest President?
YES: Phillip Shaw Paludan, from "The Presidency of Abraham Lincoln," University Press of Kansas (1994)
NO: Melvin E. Bradford, from "Remembering Who We Are: Observations of a Southern Conservative," University of Georgia Press (1985)

Phillip Shaw Paluden offers a portrait of greatness in his description of Abraham Lincoln who was first and foremost deeply committed to the process of the American "political-constitutional system." Paluden primary thesis asserting Lincoln's status as America's greatest President is rooted in the notion that "Lincoln was not either a constitutionalist or an egalitarian" in his commitment to preserving the Union and ending slavery. Instead, Lincoln's ideological devotion to the notion that "Constitutional government" and full equality were not simply complementary but codependent. Therefore, Lincoln's greatness lied in his commitment to the "process" and fully expected that both equality and the union would survive. In contrast Melvin E. Bradford seeks to challenge what he calls the "myth of the American Messiah." Bradford contends that indeed Lincoln was at the heart of many of the changes that were brought about during the era and simply put would never have come to pass if not for Lincoln pushing them forward (e.g., emancipation of African American enslaved peoples, increased powers of federalism, eventual ratification of Reconstruction Amendments after Lincoln's death, etc.). While many would consider this a sign of Lincoln's greatness Bradford argues that it is an example of "Lincoln's dishonesty and obfuscation" of the nation's constitutional principles as established by the Founding Father's commitment to republican principles. Moreover, Bradford argues that Lincoln's failure as a U.S. President is evidenced by his overstep of authority as granted by Article II of the U.S. Constitution and his setting in motion the rise of the "imperial Presidency" which is what the Founding Fathers intended to prevent.

Issue: Did Reconstruction Fail as a Result of Racism?
YES: Lisa J. McLeod, from "Transubstantiation of Andrew Johnson: White Epistemic Failure in Du Bois' Black Reconstruction," *Phylon* (2014)
NO: Adam Fairclough, from "Was the Grant of Black Suffrage a Political Error? Reconsidering the Views of John W. Burgess, William A. Dunning, and Eric Foner on Congressional Reconstruction," *Journal of the Historical Society* (2012)

Lisa J. McLeod discusses WEB DuBois's *Black Reconstruction* to highlight White people's epistemic and moral failure in the Post-Civil War era. President Johnson went from poor White farmer to champion of the plantation owner. McLeod suggests that the failed legacy of Reconstruction continues to affect social institutions and White consciousness today. Adam Fairclough believes that policy regarding the integration of African Americans into the political process ensured reconstruction would be unsuccessful. He suggests that more radical policy and a political revolution would have been required for an effective Reconstruction.

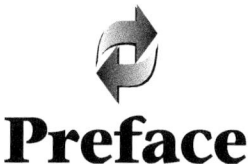

Preface

For over two decades Dr. Larry Madaras and Dr. James M. SoRelle have served as the lead authors and editors of the *Taking Sides: Clashing Views in United States History* series. During these 20+ years, Drs. Madaras and SoRelle have crafted what is undeniably one of the most influential learning and teaching texts adopted in history, social studies, and American Studies classrooms across the United States and worldwide. In 2018, Dr. Madaras and Dr. SoRelle have entrusted this seminal series to two new authors and editors to continue the tradition of excellence in history education. We are honored to accept this opportunity to follow in the footsteps of our mentors, our colleagues, our friends. Thank you Larry and Jim for your examples of scholarship that allow us to not only follow the path you have cleared for us but also instilling in us the confidence to emulate your example of forging new pathways of critical inquiry in history education.

Our academic and professional theory and practice have been significantly influenced the belief that the study of history, and all humanities and social sciences, is most powerful and transformative when it is meaningful, active, challenging, integrative and value-based (NCSS, 2016). For these reasons, we have designed and organized this 18th edition of *Taking Sides: Clashing Views in United States History* in a way that will engage both the teacher and learner in a participatory process of academic and civic discourse. Each of the primary and secondary documents found in the four units of this text have been carefully selected to provide all readers the opportunity to develop a depth and breadth of insights that will facilitate what Blevins, Salinas, and Talbert identify as *critical historical inquiry* (Blevins, Salinas, & Talbert, 2015). Inherent in the act of *critical historical inquiry* are the powerful and transformative teaching and learning behaviors of asking probing questions, thinking critically and reflectively, making reasoned inferences based upon data, and developing reasoned explanations and interpretations of events and issues in the past and present" (Singleton & Giese, 1999, p. 148).

As you immerse yourself in this text we encourage you the teacher and learner to not simply read the exemplary primary and secondary documents offered to you but to also incorporate the learning outcomes, the critical thinking and reflection questions, and the common ground summaries into your lesson and study plans. Taken as a whole, this 18th edition of *Taking Sides* will provide the teacher and learner the opportunity to critique historical and contemporary texts not only as academic historians but also as critical minded citizens committed to the Jeffersonian ideal that democracy is intrinsically dependent on a citizenry that is educated, informed, and active with concern of civic, might we also add, critical issues. Inside the pages you will discover a diversity of narratives that at time will collide with traditional interpretations of historical events and texts. It is our hope that your history classrooms will become "the places where the contending voices in the debate over what history means, or should mean, in a democracy come together" (Blevins et al., 2015; Stearns, Seixas, & Wineburg, 2000).

Book Organization

This 18th edition of *Taking Sides: Clashing Views in United States History* continues the organizational format of presenting critical historical issues and their accompanying pairs of primary and secondary documents and essays in a chronologically thematic structure that facilitates the inclusion of the whole text into any United States history, social studies, and even American Studies survey courses. The 20 critical historical issues presexnted in this 18th edition offer an Introduction, which provides a summary of the content and context that follows in the contrasting views represented in the carefully selected primary and secondary documents and essays. This edition, like the one before it, continues the expanded focus on *alternative perspectives* and *diverse voices* that are applicable to the issues, problems, and questions posed in the text. It is our intent to offer you the reader the opportunity to engage in critical historical inquiry as a means of encountering the complexity and nuances of the historical issues that cannot be addressed in a simple Yes/No response. The teacher- and student-focused *Learning Outcomes* have been designed to both guide and engage all readers in a well-focused scope and sequence of content knowledge that will inform both the learning and teaching process. To better contextualize the origins of the contrasting primary and secondary documents and essays we have provided a brief biographical sketch of each of the authors.

Following the contrasting primary/secondary documents and essay selections, there are several features that are designed to generate further understanding through critical historical inquiry of the topical issues. First, the feature entitled *Critical Thinking and Reflection* is comprised of several probing questions that are designed to stimulate challenging and integrative dialogue related to the learning outcomes and the dueling perspectives found in the documents and essays. The second feature, *Is There Common Ground?*, encourages the teacher and the student to think more deeply about the issue by highlighting areas of consensus that the contributors share on the topic being debated as well as alternative perspectives within the debate as offered by we the editors. Third, *Additional Resources* is a feature that offers a brief list of important books and/or journal articles relating to the issue. In addition to text-based resources, we have provided updated Internet sites (URLs) to aid in further exploration of the historical topics being debated and to extend the diversity of voices that better facilitate critical historical inquiry.

Acknowledgments

"I look upon ourselves as partners in all of this, and that each of us contributes and does what he can do best." Dr. Jonas Salk reminds us of the significant impact of collaborative endeavors when individuals graciously share their gifts and talents for the benefit of the whole. Indeed the synergy of many contributors has led to the successful completion of this 18th edition of *Taking Sides: Clashing Views in United States History*. As we have previously acknowledged, but once is certainly not enough, we are truly grateful to Dr. Larry Madaras and Dr. Jim SoRelle for sharing their wisdom and wit as scholars who modeled in the pages they wrote and classes they taught the values of powerful and transformative history that is meaningful, active, challenging, integrative, and value-based. The cornerstone of the *Taking Sides: Clashing Views in United States History* is Jill Meloy, senior product developer for McGraw-Hill Create®/CLS, and the entire staff of McGraw-Hill Education. Jill entrusted in us to continue the tradition of excellence that this seminal series has established over the last three plus decades. We are sincerely grateful for Jill's professional guidance, patient encouragement, and persistent humor.

Special thanks to our colleagues Victoria A. Davis, Dr. H. Scottie Johnson, Justin Kruger, Chris G. Lemley, and Dr. Neil G. Shanks whose contributions to this edition provided a diversity of voices that enriched the analysis of the 20 historical topics presented. Finally, we are endearingly grateful to our wives Dr. Sandra A. Talbert and Elizabeth Harrelson–Magill for their constructive feedback as they listened to us compose multiple drafts, their constant encouragement as deadlines approached, and their caring and creative spirits shared unconditionally. Dr. Magill would like to thank Dr. Talbert for his diligence, brilliance, mentorship, and most of all his friendship. He is forever grateful for his brother. In turn, Dr. Talbert shares his abiding admiration for Dr. Magill who as a scholar embodies the mind of Thoreau seeking truth amidst confusion and the heart of Emerson never failing to look for the best in others or give the best of himself. And now we turn the page to write the next chapter.

Kevin R. Magill
Tony L. Talbert
Baylor University

Editors of This Volume

Kevin R. Magill is an assistant professor of Secondary and Social Studies Education at Baylor University. Dr. Magill received PhD in Social Studies Education from The University of Texas at Austin and holds Masters Degrees in Education and Public Administration from The University of California, Davis, and California State University, Stanislaus, respectively. He also earned a BA in Communication Studies while attending California State University, Stanislaus. Dr. Magill's research explores two areas, first, how social studies teachers understand the relationship between teaching and civics and how their own ontologies and ideologies inform their pedagogical practices. Second, he considers how and when teachers help social studies students utilize cultural knowledge and critical inquiry to do the authentic work of civics. Dr. Magill's most recent scholarly works include "The primacy of relation: Social studies teachers and the praxis of critical pedagogy" with Professor Cinthia Salinas and "Critically civic teacher perception, posture and pedagogy: Negating civic archetypes" published in *Theory and Research in Social Education* and *The Journal of Social Studies Research*, respectively. He also published a coedited book with Professor Arturo Rodriguez recently called, *Imagining Education: Beyond the Logic of Global Neoliberal Capitalism*. Prior to his work in the academy, Dr. Magill was a middle and high school teacher in public and private schools in Seaside, Vacaville, and Sacramento, California where he taught Social Studies, English Language Arts, and Opportunity/Intervention.

Tony L. Talbert is associate dean for Strategic Initiatives and Professor of Social/Cultural Studies Education and Qualitative Research in the School of Education at Baylor University. He received a BA in History and Political Science from Stephen F. Austin State University in 1986, an MA in American Studies from Baylor University in 1991, and an Ed.D. in Social/Cultural Studies and Qualitative Research from the University of Houston in 1998. Dr. Talbert refers to his field of research and teaching as Education as Democracy which integrates social and cultural studies education into a focused discipline of qualitative inquiry examining school and community stakeholder empowerment through activist engagement in political, economic, and social issues. Dr. Talbert's thirty-two (32) years of experience as an educator has allowed him to serve as a public high school teacher, education specialist and consultant for the Texas Education Agency, Professor, Associate Dean, Department Chair, and Graduate Program Director at such institutions as Sam Houston State University, Mississippi State University, The University of Houston, and Baylor University. Over his career in academia, Dr. Talbert has published over forty (40) peer-reviewed journal articles and book chapters, presented more than eighty (80) peer-reviewed and invited research presentations, collaboratively obtained in excess of $2.8 million in funded research, served as the chair and methodologist for dozens of masters and doctoral theses and dissertations, coeditor of two academic journals, chair of several special interest groups for national professional organizations and a popular invited speaker and consultant for education organizations and conferences, private corporations, and government entities where he has showcased his creative teaching, research, and public activism seminars. In 2013, Dr. Talbert decided that it had been far too long since he had been fully immersed in the real world of teaching. After a 20-year absence from the public school classroom, he returned to a local high school where he taught world history to 166 10th-grade students. His experiences have been captured in both academic journal and popular press articles and will be the subject of a book in the future. Dr. Talbert was named as the recipient of the 2014 McGraw-Hill Distinguished Scholar Award for his contributions to qualitative research in the field of education.

References

Blevins, B., Salinas, C., & Talbert, TL (2015). Critical historical thinking: Enacting the voice of the other in the social studies curriculum and classroom. In C. S. White (Ed.), *Critical qualitative research for social education*. Charlotte, NC: IAP Information Age Publishing.

Epstein, T. (2009). *Interpreting national history: Race, identity, and pedagogy in classrooms and communities*. New York: Routledge.

National Council for the Social Studies—NCSS. (2016). *A vision of powerful teaching and learning in the social studies*. Retrieved from https://www.socialstudies.org/publications/socialeducation/may-june2016/vision-of-powerful-teaching-and-learning-in-social-studies

Singleton, L., & Giese, J. (1999). Using online primary sources with students. *The Social Studies, 90*(4), 148–151.

Academic Advisory Board Members

Members of the Academic Advisory Board are instrumental in the final selection of articles for Taking Sides books. Their review of articles for content, level, and appropriateness provides critical direction to the editors and staff. We think that you will find their careful consideration reflected in this volume.

Stanley Adamiak
University of Central Oklahoma

Robert Alderson
Georgia Perimeter College

Kevin Caldwell
Blue Ridge Community College

Jianyue Chen
Northeast Lakeview College

Anthony Conley
Ivy Tech Community College, Northeast

John L. Daly
SUNY Brockport

Richard M. Filipink
Western Illinois University

Stephen Gibson
Allegany College of Maryland

Henry H. Goldman
Longview Community College

Kevin R. C. Gutzman
Western Connecticut State University

Timothy Hack
Salem Community College

Aimee Harris-Johnson
El Paso Community College

Stephen Katz
Community College of Philadelphia

Gary McElhany
Southwestern Assemblies of God University

Brian Miller
Emporia State University

Carey M. Roberts
Liberty University

Karl Rodabaugh
Winston-Salem State University

Tracy Shilcutt
Abilene Christian University

Elizabeth Speed
University of Texas—El Paso

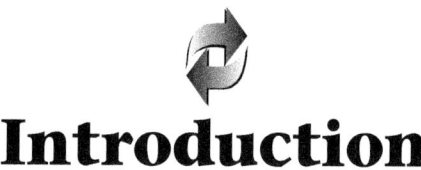

Introduction

We learn from history that we learn nothing from history

~ George Bernard Shaw.

At risk of alienating devotees of the eminent Mr. Shaw we must take issue with this notion that our unique species that occupy this planet have not and do not learn from history. Granted we can point to specific points in time when individuals and even entire nations have seemingly ignored the lessons that history has taught us. We certainly can note egregious examples of human's inhumanity toward other humans and nonhuman species. There's no doubt that we are able to analyze moments in human history when foolhardy decisions were made despite the best evidence of history directing an opposite decision as the best choice. Most assuredly the annals of history, be they documented from the oral, written, and dare I say *virtual augmented* traditions, convey a story of humanity replete with bad choices, dumb ideas, blind allegiance, and enumerable travesties of justice in the face of lessons of history failed to be learned.

Even despite this most prolific body of evidence that seems to support Mr. Shaw's assertion it is evident to the student and scholar of history that humans do learn from the lessons of the past and perhaps even cherish the archiving and telling of these lessons to current and future generations. Perhaps it is not that we fail to learn from history but instead we too often fail to act on this knowledge thereby changing the course of our individual and collective actions. Perhaps too it is that we assume the prepackaged information presented us is beyond reproach, or that opinions are facts. However, it is this essential choice of acting on or ignoring what we've learned from the lessons of history that seems to best characterize the human experience. Whether history repeats itself or rhymes seems to come down to our approach as humans to the dilemma of addressing our own Gordian Knot. Do we simply accept the tangled fibers of a knot that make up our collective history as hopelessly intractable? Do we take bold action in cutting the knot from its entangled state and in doing so violate time honored traditions, customs, and mores? Do we pause to reflect on the lessons of the past as contextualized within the realities of the present as a guide to our future actions involving the preservation, the elimination, or perhaps the reconsideration of whether the knot is indeed a dilemma or an opportunity?

It is this hope, perhaps belief, in the capacity of humans to engage in critically reflective dialogue that inspire we as authors and editors of this *Taking Sides*: Clashing Views in United States *History*, Volume 1, Edition 18 to offer to you the reader opportunities to consider a diverse array of theories, conjectures, and even emboldened opinions shared through the collected writings of persons who have lived and studied the historic dilemmas offered in this text. Throughout this text you will discover the voices of those who lived amidst these dilemmas in America's distant past as presented through primary documents. You will also find contained within the units of this text the secondary seminal and more contemporary sources that offer insights from a vicarious interpretation of the dilemmas characterized in the 20 issues that comprise this book.

Conceptual Framework: Polticial–Economic–Religious–Social–Intellectual–Area (PERSIA)

In previous editions of the *Taking Sides: Clashing Views in United States History*, Dr. Larry Madaras and Dr. James M. SoRelle have applied the three predominant schools of American history as the interpretive lenses for both the organization and analysis of the issues and competing scholarly views presented. Drs. Madaras' and SoRelle's classical application of the *Progressive School*, the *Neoconservative, or Consensus School*, and the *New Left School* of historical interpretive frameworks provided a depth and breadth of perspectives that we the new editors of this *Taking Sides* series have benefited from in our own academic and professional development over the last 17 years. The brilliant vision for the *Taking Sides* series cast by Drs. Madaras and SoRelle has certainly be honored in this new edition but with a slightly different twist that incorporates a theoretical and organizational framework borrowed from the field of Social Studies Education (i.e., history, geography, civics and government, culture and society, and economics).

As scholars within Social Studies Education, we believe that the complexity of the issues presented in this text require an overarching framework that integrates academic disciplines that originate from both the liberal arts and social sciences. Social Studies Education, both in theory and practice, provides opportunities to explore issues and ideas, problems and solutions through interconnected and often overlapping fields of study. From history to sociology, political science to economics, the encompassing study of geography, and perhaps a half-dozen supporting disciplines (i.e., anthropology, archeology, law, philosophy, psychology, and theology), the comprehensive and indeed complex field of Social Studies Education provides the ideal academic landscape with which to explore the fascinating issues offered in this edition of the highly successful *Taking Sides: Clashing Views in United States History* series.

To assist the reader in better understanding the conceptual and organizational structure in which this text was developed, it is important to introduce the concept of PERSIA. More precisely, the acronym PERSIA which is applied as a graphic organizer that structures the general knowledge of the academic disciplines that comprise Social Studies Education into six thematic areas. So, what are the six thematic areas that comprise the conceptual framework that is PERSIA?

- Political influences and concerns (e.g., issues of power, authority, governance, civic ideals, and practices as manifest in the rise of dominant individual leaders and governing institutions.);
- Economic influences and concerns (e.g., issues of production, distribution, and consumption as evidenced by the development of agrarian, industrial, and technological systems of exchange and investment.);
- Religious influences and concerns (e.g., issues of individual and group beliefs and practices as they influence cultural and institutional norms and deviations.);
- Social influences and concerns (e.g., issues of individuals, groups, institutions and how they influence and are influenced by the multiple variables of identity development and the subsequent cultural formations that evolve from these individual, group, and institutional identities.);
- Intellectual influences and concerns (e.g., issues of science, technology, arts, philosophy, and the interdependent nature of human intellectual evolution emanating from local innovations to global phenomenon.); and
- Area/geographical influences and concerns (e.g., issues of people, places, and environments as framed within the spatial concepts of geography and interpreted through the cultural lenses that guide the interpretive exploration between human beings, the environment, and the global interdependence of people and their limited resources).

The unifying thread that binds these six thematic areas of PERSIA is the assertion that to fully understand human history one must acquire the skills of historical inquiry, analysis, and synthesis to recognize the ever-present impact of time, continuity, and change as evidenced through the values, beliefs, cultures, and institutions that comprise the storied legacies of women and men past and present. Simply put, the study of history reveals the worst of our human species and how Shaw's indictment of our seemingly inability to *learn from our past* dooms us to repeat these errors ad infinitum. And yet we also recognize that the study of history weaves beautiful tales of the best of our human species and how even in the midst of war, civil unrest, and the scourges of racism, bigotry, and intolerance we as people find hope in the promise of a future because we share an interdependent past in what Ralph Waldo Emerson describes as ". . . man is a bundle of relations, a knot of roots, whose flower and fruitage is the world."

Throughout the text the reader will experience the explicit representation of historical knowledge (i.e., *Progressive, Neo-Conservative/Consensus,* and *New Left* schools) and skills (i.e., historical inquiry, analysis, and synthesis) while also encountering the implicit presence of PERSIA's six thematic areas as represented in the 20 carefully selected and articulated issues of PERSIA-related historical importance.

History is certainly about the past, but it is also about the present, and the future. Our new introductions pose questions related to these unresolved questions within the contemporary moment. We consider how and why history has been interpreted in particular ways and attempt to reveal implications for acting as stewards of our democracy. Metaphorically speaking, understanding the essential nature of the Gordian Knot begins with its examination. Through study we might think beyond the structures that regulate one's thinking about it. Solving its mythological puzzle requires unique analysis, thinking past what has been given, and acting to transform the ways it has existed. We suggest the intellectually curious can similarly unlock the secrets of US history through shared inquiry. New analysis can lead us to new interpretation for social analysis and transformation. However, this task requires our active historical learning, critical historical inquiry, and authentic acting. We therefore ask the reader to consider what we have presented and then to conduct their own deep dive into these issues so you will further reveal the social, intellectual, political, economical, spiritual, cultural, and intersectional aspects of historical relation. We hope you proceed by seeking new information that will nuance author interpretations and support your agency as a historical informed social actor.

Upon first appearance the organization of this text appears to adhere to a linear chronological structure that presents the opportunity for the reader to develop a cause and effect understanding of historical events. Yet, with closer examination one begins to recognize that the six thematic areas of PERSIA provide a breadth of interdependence among the topics presented, while the sources chosen to represent these contrasting views on the topics offer a depth of historiographical interpretation that challenge the linear view of history with an entwined narrative. Indeed the cause and effect phenomenon within history is always in play. Or as is oft misquoted and wrongly attributed to Mark Twain, "History doesn't repeat itself but it often rhymes." More on the Twain quote at the end of this introduction.

The following "rhyming" organizational structure of this text has been developed to present to you the reader 20 historical topics as presented through the lens of 40 significant historians, theorists, authors, and even a handful of pundits, patriots, philosophers, politicians, and pamphleteers. The clashing views articulated through both primary and secondary documents offer an intriguing analysis and interpretation of historical events that continue to resonate as significant issues to be considered and debated by each of us in our contemporary lives.

Colonial Society

Many of the historical questions in this unit speak to the ideological fabric of the U.S. ethos. This was a time in which Americans could not reasonably imagine what would lay ahead. Detailed within these debates presented by Maureen Konkle, Jessica R. Stern, Steven T. Katz, Alfred A. Cave et al. are the realities of how the southern Colonies were established as a joint stock company looking for gold, while the New England Colonies were principally founded by Puritans tying to separate themselves from what they saw as a corrupt Church of England. Each of these aims might be understood as miserable failures—or in hindsight, successful beyond their wildest dreams. New England did not become the perfect Biblical Society of the colonist's dreams, but what emerged, as debated by Thomas S. Kidd and David A. Varel, is the most powerful nation in human history—a nation dedicated, in many ways, to the Protestant values and ethics established in the Colonial era. Similarly, the Southern Colonies did not find gold, though they toiled in this pursuit for many years beyond what is logical based on a delusional myth. However, the society that emerged worked both within and apart from the emerging economic systems to establish themselves as a unique Colonies that were able to take economic agency from their European roots. Each of the colonies was also driven by myth and dilution that helped them achieve amazing things, such as a new nation with relative freedom for some, but also established the conditions by which snake oil salesmen, misunderstandings, war, and political abuse would thrive. Authors in this unit such as Seymour Martin Lipset and Godfrey Hodgsen have considered the ideas of American exceptionality, colonial ideology, social change, religion, revolution, and the ways we perceive the "other." These prominent ideas are present in the questions historians such as Gloria L. Main Cornelia Hughes Dayton, Laurie Winn Carlson, and Lyle Koehler have posed concerning exploring this unique period. This epoch saw Americans contend with religious immigration, forced immigration and enslavement, disease and death, cultural interactions, economic imperialism, and war. Though these topics and dispositions did not begin or end in this epoch, colonial conversations have established the framework for what the United States is and has become as evidenced by the prophetic contrasting views offered by none other than Thomas Paine and Rev. Charles Inglis. Indeed, the historical residue of this time still informs how we exist. We still struggle to work through many of the historical question of this period. Study of this era can no doubt inform the ways we consider our contemporary condition as we continue to become who we desire to be as a nation.

Revolution and the New Nation

The historical questions in this unit of the volume speak to the political, economic, and social systems that emerged from the ideologies of the colonial period and became inextricable aspects of the democratic fabric of the United States. Equity, freedom, capitalism, and, nationalism all played a historical role in the new nation, its foundation, and its evolution. Although the new nation emerged with great promise inspired by Enlightenment ideals, those ideals were quickly overshadowed by pernicious traditions of bias and bigotry ensuring democracy would not truly be realized for the common man and women. Uniquely contrasted in this unity are the ideas of James Madison (Federalist No. 10) and Aristotle (Politics: Book VI) who offer perspectives that situate our comparisons and contrasts of the antecedents and subsequent ideas and ideals that formed and preserved a nation and its people. As the matters of establishing and sustaining a new nation took precedence over ideals of justice and equality we see in the contrasting views of historians Donald F. Swansonk, Andrew P. Trout, Kori N. Schake, Donald Ratclifffe, and economist Edward Peter Stringham how it became apparent that the Revolution was likely as much about developing an economic sphere of influence as it was about creating a democratic nation. Through the diverse interpretive lenses that compare and contrast contemporary interpretation of the decisions that were made in the past the authors in this epoch examine the complexities of the topics in ways not often considered in US History classes and curriculum. For example, what is the purpose of our political system—democracy or economic protectionism? What is the spirit of the Second Amendment? Did the economic legacy of Hamilton lead us on a path toward neoliberalism and was he this great man of history? What is the relationship between nationalism and reinvigorating our democracy? Each of these questions posed by characters of history in days gone by reverberate today in the debates taking place among contemporary actors in the halls of governments and the aisles of supermarkets across America.

Antebellum America

How do we distinguish between a terrorist and a freedom fighter? When do we label an action imperialistic or nationalistic? What are the criteria for determining when social justice activists become members of a meddling mob? Implicit, and at times explicit, are questions that emerge from the spirited debates presented by the authors of the documents in this unit. The young American nation began to wrestle with a deeper understanding of herself and her citizens while elected and would be leaders continued to make choices that would establish an American presence in global affairs for the foreseeable future. As the political and economic policies and practices of the United States were asserted more frequently on the international stage, we see the perspicuous emergence of the notion of American Exceptionalism as evidenced through the vast land acquisitions and cultural appropriations that occurred with such events and edicts as the Louisiana Purchase, the War of 1812, and the Monroe Doctrine. Debated throughout this unit are the risks and rewards of the free exercise of US imperialism that saw the size of the nation double in a matter of decades (Ramón Eduardo Ruiz and Norman A. Graebner, Manifest Destiny and the Mexican American War). In the midst of what appeared to be a meteoric expansion of American ascendency were the pernicious cracks in the very ideals that would serve as the foundation for the so-called American Exceptionalism. Access to equality of opportunities for human rights, citizenship, education, and well-being are debated by James N. Gilbert, Scott John Hammond, Mary Kelly, Lucia McMahon, Laura A. Schmidt, and John J. Rumbarger. Inherent in these debates are the cause and effect triggers that lure us into believing in the linear repetitive phenomenological interpretation of history. Yet upon closer examination we are able to see through the writings of the authors selected for this unit's topics of debate that there is not so much a linearity of cause and effect relationships among the issues presented but perhaps multiple branches, some twisting others turning back onto themselves. It is through this closer examination of the nuances of the issues presented that we begin to see the emerge milieu of PERSIA themes that provide a fascinating juxtaposition of traditional positivist historic cause and effect (linear-repetitive) versus a nontraditional post-positivist correlation and choice (multidirectional-rhyming) interpretation of clashing views in the U.S. history.

Conflict and Resolution

In 2015, author and activist Jim Wallis joined journalist and television commentator Roland Martin to discuss Wallis' book, *America's Original Sin: Racism, White Privilege and the Bridge to a New America*. While the transcripts from this interview could easily serve as the introduction to this unit's focus of topics for debate, it is essential that we not be lured into a singularity of topical focus that obscures the multiple antecedent (cause) and subsequent (effect) variables that should be considered as factors in the issues surrounding this tumultuous period in American history. As previously noted, each unit of this text offers examples of American history teetering on the head of pin sometimes tilting toward the ideals that point to our exceptional character as a nation of diverse people groups while at other times turning quickly toward dark realities of human behavior that undermines the legitimacy of the foundational value claims that make up the American narrative. Wallis is indeed correct that the historic issues of this era in U.S. history speak to a "deliberate dehumanizing and debasing of African-Americans" (J. Wallis, personal communication, January 28, 2016).

It is with this sentiment that we present to you the interdependent complexities of historic issues that do not shy away from acknowledging the realities that U.S. economic successes, past and present, and indeed U.S. political and social institutional failings are directly attributable to the enslavement of millions of African and African American women, children, and men prior to and during this period in history. Embedded in the topics for debate offered by Charles B. Dew, Gary W. Gallagher (slavery and warfare), Mark E. Neely, James M. McPherson (carnage and total war) are glimpses of the economic transitions that followed this period which established the conditions for a hybrid market economy where free market values are espoused as virtuous while simultaneously being violated in practice by monied and power interests who benefited from enslaved, indentured, and inequitably cast men, women, and children brought to and born on these American shores. As both northern and southern regions of the United States experienced a pre–Civil War agrarian and industrialization boom and the northern United States reaped the economic benefits of a post–Civil War southern confederacy collapse, a hybrid-ideology of economic, political, and social free-market capitalism and American Exceptionalism continued to thrive. It is important that the reader recognizes that Phillip Shaw Paludan's and Melvin E. Bradford's debate on the Abraham Lincoln's greatness or mediocrity is an extension of the conversation offered by Lisa J. McLeod and Adam Fairclough who examine the root causes of the failure of post–Civil War economic, political, and social reconstruction. For within these two topics of debate, like a Charlie Mingus *quodlibet,* the historic rhythmic counterpoint to the undeniably exceptional American narrative are the glaring exceptions to the American values of equity of opportunity for all people of the United States.

Whether we turn our ear to the tune of Reconstruction era promises of freedom and equality that were never realized due to the evolving definition of slavery as manifest in Jim Crow legislation and exploitation or listen to the equally resonate melody of the new waves of immigration that fed both the factory system and the nativist system of discrimination, the legacy of this historic musical score informs our contemporary PERSIA-focused ideological discussions and rhetorical reasoning. Lest we end the discussion of this unit of the text on a sour note, we offer to you a topic of debate that embodies the truly exceptional American experience as discussed by Albert J. Raboteau and John B. Boles who examine the resilient and defiant spirit of humanity as evidenced in African American slaves exercise of religious autonomy amidst relentless persecution.

Conclusion

Issue by issue, topic upon topic this volume of *Taking Sides: Clashing Views in United States History* presents to you the reader 40 diverse voices that confront our nation's brightest and darkest choices in history. In a matter of speaking, we offer to you the reader our own *Gordian Knot* as we challenge you to confront these historic choices though made in centuries past were ultimately made on your behalf in this present day. Holocaust survivor and Nobel Laureate Elie Wiesel reminds us that "Without memory, there is no culture. Without memory, there would be no civilization, no society, no future" (Wiesel, 2008). Even the casual reader of the important issues raised in the contrasting interpretations of historical ideas and events presented in this book will recognize the *rhyming* presence of prominent PERSIA contemporary matters of debate that fill the pages of blogs and books and the sound bytes of cable news and coffee talk throughout 21st-century America. Indeed, we must remember so we do not repeat. Or, as promised early in this introduction we return to Mr. Twain as we offer a more precise representation of his quote that challenges the assertion that *history repeats itself* with a typically Twainian twist, *History never repeats itself, but the Kaleidoscopic combinations of the pictured present often seem to be constructed out of the broken fragments of antique legends.* It is our hope that throughout this text we have offered to you the reader an array of lenses that allow you to develop a clearer focus on the diverse, indeed perhaps fragmented, perspectives that comprise the interpretation of clashing views in United States history.

Kevin R. Magill
Tony L. Talbert
Baylor University

References

Wallis J. (2016, January 28). Interview by R. Martin [Video recording]. NewsOne Now, Roland Martin. One Digital Archives, New York City, New York.

Wiesel, E. (2014). *God is God because He remembers*. In J. Allison, D. Gediman, & National Public Radio (Eds.), *This I believe II: More personal philosophies of remarkable men and women.* New York: Macmillan.

Unit 1

UNIT

Colonial Society

*T*he exploration and settlement of the Western Hemisphere took place in a global context of migration, empire-building, and national rivalries. Europeans who settled in North America encountered various circumstances that reinforced their localist sensibilities by limiting their contacts across colonial lines, but over time they recognized much that they had in common with one another and that set them apart from their native homelands. For many, this experience led them to insist upon the uniqueness of American society.

The ethnic identity of these European colonists affected their relations with Native Americans as well as with each other. These contacts ranged from cordiality to conflict and differed by time and place. The opportunities for success that presented themselves to individual residents often varied by gender, ethnicity, and race.

Religion, too, impacted life in colonial America in both the seventeenth and eighteenth centuries. Some, though not all, colonists migrated specifically for religious purposes, but not all of these migrants shared the same religious precepts. Consequently, religion occasionally produced tensions that affected the society and interpersonal relations in profound ways.

Many of the historical questions in this unit speak to the ideological fabric of the United States ethos. This was a time in which Americans could not reasonably imagine what would lay ahead. Detailed within these debates presented by Maureen Konkle, Jessica R. Stern, Steven T. Katz, Alfred A. Cave et al. are the realities of how the southern Colonies were established as a joint stock company looking for gold, while the New England Colonies were principally founded by Puritans tying to separate themselves from what they saw as a corrupt Church of England. Each of these aims might be understood as miserable failures—or in hindsight, successful beyond their wildest dreams. New England did not become the perfect Biblical Society of the colonist's dreams, but what emerged, as debated by Thomas S. Kidd and David A. Varel, is the most powerful nation in human history—a nation dedicated, in many ways, to the Protestant values and ethics established in the Colonial era. Similarly, the Southern Colonies did not find gold, though they toiled in this pursuit for many years beyond what is logical based on a delusional myth. However, the society that emerged worked both within and apart from the emerging economic systems to establish themselves as a unique Colonies that were able to take economic agency from their European roots. Each of the colonies was also driven by myth and dilution that helped them achieve amazing things, such as a new nation with relative freedom for some, but also established the conditions by which snake oil salesmen, misunderstandings, war, and political abuse would thrive. Authors in this unit such as Seymour Martin Lipset and Godfrey Hodgsen have considered the ideas of American exceptionality, colonial ideology, social change, religion, revolution, and the ways we perceive the "other." These prominent ideas are present in the questions historians such as Gloria L. Main Cornelia Hughes Dayton, Laurie Winn Carlson, and Lyle Koehler have posed concerning exploring this unique period. This epoch saw Americans contend with religious immigration, forced immigration and enslavement, disease and death, cultural interactions, economic imperialism, and war. Though these topics and dispositions did not begin or end in this epoch, colonial conversations have established the framework for what the United States is and has become as evidenced by the prophetic contrasting views offered by none other than Thomas Paine and Rev. Charles Inglis. Indeed, the historical residue of this time still informs how we exist. We still struggle to work through many of the historical question of this period. Study of this era can no doubt inform the ways we consider our contemporary condition as we continue to become who we desire to be as a nation.

ISSUE

Selected, Edited, and with Issue Framing Material by:
Kevin R. Magill and Tony L. Talbert, *Baylor University*

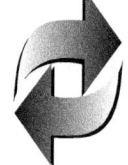

Is America Exceptional?

YES: **Seymour Martin Lipset**, from "Still the Exceptional Nation?" *The Wilson Quarterly* (2000)

NO: **Godfrey Hodgson**, from "The Corruption of the Best," Yale University Press (2010)

Learning Outcomes

After reading this issue, you will be able to:

- Define what is meant by the term "American exceptionalism."
- Understand that American exceptionalism possesses both positive and negative characteristics.
- Discuss the characteristics that set the United States apart from the rest of the developed nations in the world.
- Consider the global context of the American historical experience.

ISSUE SUMMARY

YES: Seymour Martin Lipset (1922–2006) claims that the United States remains an "outlier" nation in that it is much less welfare-oriented, the federal government taxes and spends less, Americans are more heavily influenced by Protestant Christianity, and Americans benefit from a higher rate of mobility into elite positions than is the case in other developed nations.

NO: Godfrey Hodgson suggests the "myth of American exceptionalism" is just that–a myth. He believes that people focus too much on American uniqueness and ignore the international influence, historical process, and ideologies that have developed American values.

In 1994, Speaker of the House of Representatives Newt Gingrich told members of the Heritage Foundation that it was time to "reassert American exceptionalism." The message was clear: the United States had lost those qualities that distinguished it from other nations around the world. Indeed, Gingrich was merely recognizing what a number of social scientists and historians had been saying for the past 20 years—that the concept of American exceptionalism had diminished as U.S. claims to preeminence in global affairs had dwindled. It seemed that publisher Henry Luce's 1941 prophecy that the twentieth century would be "The American Century" was in jeopardy.

While Alexis de Tocqueville is frequently credited with originating the concept of American exceptionalism in his classic *Democracy in America* (1835), the idea predates the French aristocrat's arrival in the United States by two centuries. John Winthrop's lay sermon, "A Modell of Christian Charity," delivered to the Puritan passengers aboard the *Arbella* bound for Massachusetts Bay Colony in 1630, was probably the earliest reference to America (or a small portion thereof) having a distinctive, special mission to play on the world stage. Drawing upon the Sermon on the Mount, Winthrop explained the importance of establishing a pure Christian commonwealth in the New World. "For we must be as a city upon a hill," he intoned. "The eyes of all people are upon us." A secularized version of this mission was presented in 1776 with the publication of Thomas Paine's famous Revolutionary-era pamphlet *Common Sense*. Following the creation of the United States, Thomas Jefferson, Noah Webster, and other prominent citizens of the new nation voiced the belief that the country possessed a number of characteristics that set it apart from corrupt and decaying Europe.

While Tocqueville identified the twin components of democracy and equality as the basis for American distinctiveness, it was an American historian, Frederick Jackson Turner, who captured the attention of scholars and students by associating the unique qualities of national character in the United States with the frontier experience. Turner first presented this argument at the annual meeting of the American Historical Association in 1893 in a paper entitled "The Significance of the Frontier in American History." The Turner thesis remained a hot topic of historical discussion for three-quarters of a century as Turnerians and anti-Turnerians debated the details of the impact of the frontier on American life.

An important extension of the Turner thesis is offered in David M. Potter, *People of Plenty: Economic Abundance and the American Character* (University of Chicago Press, 1954), which identifies another factor contributing to the distinctive American character. Michael Kammen, in *People of Paradox: An Inquiry Concerning the Origins of American Civilization* (Alfred A. Knopf, 1972), argues that American distinctiveness is derived from the contradiction produced by a culture created from an interaction of Old and New World patterns. Students interested in pursuing these questions of culture and character should consult Michael McGiffert, ed., *The Character of Americans: A Book of Readings*, rev. ed. (Dorsey Press, 1970).

The issue of exceptionalism is also at the heart of discussions of the nature of American culture carried on by historians interested in the Old World and New World roots of the American people and the society they created beginning in the seventeenth century. Just how new and different was that early American culture? How much did it depart from the cultural heritage of those tens of thousands of immigrants who arrived in England's North American colonies prior to the American Revolution? Opposing historical perspectives can be found in Gary Nash's *Red, White, and Black: The Peoples of Early America*, 3d ed. (Prentice Hall, 1992), which emphasizes the need to appreciate the numerous non-English and non-European elements of American culture, and David Hackett Fischer's *Albion's Seed: Four British Folkways in America* (Oxford University Press, 1989), which suggests that there is a distinctly British tone in American culture and society.

For more than 50 years Seymour Martin Lipset provided a broad-based defense of the concept of American exceptionalism in a number of scholarly works. The most important of these included *Agrarian Socialism* (University of California Press, 1950; rev. and expanded ed., 1971); *The First New Nation: The United States in Historical and Comparative Perspective* (Basic Books, 1963); and *American Exceptionalism: A Double-Edged Sword* (W. W. Norton, 1996). Support for Lipset's interpretation can be found in Daniel Boorstin, *The Genius of American Politics* (University of Chicago Press, 1953); Louis Hartz, *The Liberal Tradition in America* (Harcourt, Brace & World, 1955); and the essays collected in Byron Shafer, ed., *Is America Different? A New Look at American Exceptionalism* (Oxford University Press, 1991). Critics of the exceptionalism model are represented in Laurence Veysey, "The Autonomy of American History Reconsidered," *American Quarterly* (Fall 1979); and William C. Spengemann, *A Mirror for Americanists: Reflections on the Idea of American Literature* (University Press of New England, 1989). Michael Kammen's "The Problem of American Exceptionalism: A Reconsideration," *American Quarterly* (March 1993), presents a valuable summary of both sides of the debate.

Is the United States different in fundamental ways from other nations? Has its historical development produced distinctive institutions and citizens? Is it legitimate to focus upon certain characteristics that may appear to separate the United States from other nations at a time when more emphasis is being placed upon global integration? These are some of the questions generated by the following selections.

In the first selection, Seymour Martin Lipset reaffirms the notion of American exceptionalism while claiming that the United States is not as exceptional politically as it once was. Drawing upon the statistical evidence of the social scientist's polling and survey techniques, Lipset argues that the United States is set apart from developed European nations by being less committed to the welfare state, spending and taxing much less than European governments, and maintaining a stronger commitment to religious faith. On the darker side, the U.S. possesses a higher proportion of nonvoters, the highest crime rate and prison population, and a greater maldistribution of income than its European counterparts.

English-born Godfrey Hodgson recognizes certain unique characteristics of colonial British North America and the early United States but claims that much of what was exceptional about early America had faded in the post–Civil War environment of industrialization and urbanization. He criticizes the presentation of U.S. history as a "patriotic commemoration" which largely ignores the extent to which America was shaped by vast international historical processes.

YES

Seymour Martin Lipset

Still the Exceptional Nation?

Was Karl Marx right? More than 100 years ago, he declared in *Capital* that "the country that is the most developed shows to the less developed the image of their future," and his early followers had little doubt that the United States was that most developed harbinger country. "Americans will be the first to usher in a Socialist republic," declared the German Social Democrat August Bebel in 1907—even though the American Socialist Party was faring miserably at the polls while his own party held many seats in the Reichstag. Only after the Russian Revolution in 1917 did the Left and its liberal sympathizers begin to look elsewhere for a vision of the future. Now Europe set the standard and America followed—all too sluggishly, in the minds of many.

How could the world's most advanced capitalist society also be the most impervious to the socialist idea? Even the Great Depression failed to alter its course—America's minuscule Socialist and Communist parties emerged from the 1930s with even less support than they had enjoyed at the beginning of the decade. The American experience cast doubt on the inner logic of historical materialism, the essential Marxist doctrine which holds that the shape of a nation's culture and politics is determined by underlying economic and technological forces. The question engaged the attention of many socialists, as well as Lenin and Trotsky; Stalin attended a special commission of the Communist International on "the American Question."

What was a source of perplexity to some was, of course, a source of pride to others. To scholars, it was a phenomenon in need of explanation. Out of this puzzlement came the rebirth of the idea of "American exceptionalism," a concept first developed by Alexis de Tocqueville in *Democracy in America* (1835–40). The young Frenchman wrote that the United States, the lone successful democracy of his time, differed from all the European nations in lacking a feudal past and in being more socially egalitarian, more meritocratic, more individualistic, more rights-oriented, and more religious. These American tendencies were reinforced by the country's religious commitment to the "nonconformist," largely congregationally organized Protestant sects, which emphasized the individual's personal relationship with God, a relationship that was not mediated by state-supported, hierarchically organized churches of the kind that prevailed in Europe.

In 19th-century America, the ideology of the American Revolution was transformed into an all-encompassing liberalism stressing liberty, antistatism, and individualism. In Europe, a dominant conservativism was wedded to the state—it was conservatives such as Britain's Benjamin Disraeli, for example, who invented the welfare state—and it naturally gave birth to state-centered opposition, social democracy. Because its liberal ideology stifled the emergence of a state-centered opposition, the United States became an anomaly.

Today, however, the United States once again finds itself the apparent image of the future. Not only is it the world's sole superpower and its economic colossus, but it seems to be pointing the way toward the political future. The American political system, long considered an aberration because its two main parties embrace liberal capitalism, now looks like the model for the developed world.

Nothing symbolizes this change more dramatically than the political pep rally cum summit meeting that brought four social democratic heads of government to Washington in April 1999 under the auspices of America's centrist Democratic Leadership Council. Britain's Tony Blair, Germany's Gerhard Schröder, the Netherlands' Wim Kok, and Italy's Massimo D'Alema did not come to press the cause of democratic socialism on their backward cousins across the Atlantic. They wanted to join with Democrat Bill Clinton in affirming what they called the Third Way. And they have done so more than once, meeting most recently in Florence last November, where they were joined by Brazil's Fernando Henrique Cardoso. These putative social democratic leaders, as *Washington Post* columnist E. J. Dionne notes, "accept capitalism as a given, but promise to do something about its inequalities and

---

Lipset, Seymour Martin. "Still the Exceptional Nation?" From The Wilson Quarterly, 2000, pp. 31–36, 40–45 (edited). Copyright ©2000 by Martin Seymour Lipset. Reprinted by permission of his wife, Sydnee Lipset.

uncertainties. They talk not of 'socialism' but of 'community,' not of 'collectivism' but of 'solidarity.'" They sound, in other words, very much like America's New Democrats.

All of this suggests that Marx may have been right: the development of an economically and technologically advanced society follows a certain logic, and the United States shows where that logic leads—even if it is not to socialism. But if this is true, will it make sense any longer to speak of American exceptionalism? Will the political cultures of other advanced societies increasingly converge with that of the United States?

The change in the character of Europe's political parties largely reflects the remaking of Europe's economic and class structures along American lines. The European emphasis on *stände,* or fixed, explicitly hierarchical social classes rooted in a feudal and monarchical past, is increasingly a thing of the past. Growing economic productivity is opening access to everything from clothes, cars, and other consumer goods to advanced schooling, powerfully muting the "lifestyle" differences, including accents and dress, that traditionally separated Europe's social classes. The new economic order has been accompanied by demographic shifts, notably a drastic decline in birthrates and an extension of life spans, that have confronted all the developed nations with a common dilemma: raise taxes significantly to pay for more social security, health care, welfare, and other expensive government services, or find ways to cut spending.

The United States has led the economic transformation, shifting sharply away from the old industrial economy built on manual labor, a process that was especially agonizing during the 1970s and '80s. The old economy of General Motors, U.S. Steel, and Standard Oil has given way to the economy of Microsoft, Citigroup—and McDonald's. The proportion of workers employed in manufacturing dropped from 26 percent in 1960 to 16 percent in 1996. In the United Kingdom, manufacturing employment declined from 36 percent of the total to 19 percent, a pattern that prevails from Sweden (with a drop from 32 to 19 percent) to Australia (from 26 to 13.5 percent).

The Old World societies are also following the American lead away from class awareness and organization. Union membership, for example, is declining almost everywhere. Between 1985 and 1995, the proportion of the American labor force carrying a union card fell by 21 percent. Today, only 14 percent of all employed Americans—and only 10 percent of those in the private sector—belong to unions. The proportional losses in France and Britain have been even greater, 37 percent and 28 percent, respectively. In Germany, the decline is a more modest 18 percent.

During the post–World War II era, the distribution of income and occupational skills in Europe has reshaped itself to fit American contours. It has changed from something best illustrated by a pyramidal shape, enlarging toward the bottom, to one better illustrated by a diamond, widest in the middle. The traditional working class, in other words, is shrinking. The middle class is growing, creating solidly bourgeois societies in Europe. Political parties on the left now have little choice but to appeal more to the growing middle strata than to their traditional constituencies, industrial workers and the poor.

Call it what you will—"postindustrial society," "postmaterialism," or the "scientific-technological revolution"—the changing cultures of the emerging societies closely fit the Marxian causal model. The political and cultural "superstructures" are determined, as sociologist Daniel Bell has noted, by the technological structures and the distribution of economic classes.

Many of the trends that Marx anticipated, especially a steady increase in the size of the industrial proletariat, have not occurred. Throughout the industrialized world, job growth is concentrated in the technological and service occupations. College enrollments have swelled, and the degree-bearing population has grown enormously. Alain Touraine, a leading French sociologist and leftist intellectual, writes: "If property was the criterion of membership in the former dominant class, the new dominant class is defined by knowledge and a certain level of education."

With their roots in the university and the scientific and technological worlds, and with a heavy representation in the public sector, the professions, and the industries spawned by computers, the new workers have developed their own distinctive values. Political scientist Ronald Inglehart of the University of Michigan, pointing as well to the influence of a half-century of affluence, argues that these changes have spawned a new set of "postmaterialist" values. An affluent, better-educated citizenry has shifted its political attention away from bread-and-butter economic issues to new concerns: the environment, health, the quality of education, the culture, equality for women and minorities, the extension of democratization and freedom at home and abroad, and last, but far from least, the definition of a more permissive (and highly controversial) morality.

The United States has also been in the forefront of the postmaterialist new politics, quickly exporting the latest concerns of Berkeley, Madison, and other university towns to Paris and Berlin. It gave birth to all the major successful modern movements for egalitarian social change and for improving the quality of life—feminism, environmentalism, civil rights for minorities, and gay rights—just as it did the democratic revolutions of the 19th century. Writing in 1971, as the new politics was beginning to emerge, the French political analyst Jean-François Revel observed in *Without Marx or Jesus* that the "revolutionary stirrings have had their origin in the United States." The Continent's "dissenters . . . are the disciples of the American movements." . . .

The United States clearly is no longer as exceptional politically as it once was. Its political life—dominated by two procapitalist political parties and defined by traditional, moralistic, sectarian religion, classical liberalism (laissez faire), and environmentalist and other post-materialist tendencies—is setting a model for other developed countries. The convergence has even stripped the United States of its past monopoly on populist politics, the traditional outlet of the discontented and dispossessed in a country without a working-class political party. . . .

Yet for all that, the United States remains exceptional in other important ways. It is still an outlier at one end of many international indicators of behavior and values. It is still much less statist and welfare oriented, and its governments (federal and state) tax and spend much less in proportionate terms than European governments. It is the most religious country in Christendom, the only one still strongly influenced by the moralistic and individualistic ethos of Protestant sectarianism. It has higher rates of mobility into elite positions than any other nation. It combines exceptional levels of productivity, income, and wealth with exceptionally low levels of taxation and social spending, and equally exceptional levels of income inequality and poverty.

The United States remains well ahead of other large developed countries in per capita income, retaining the lead it has held since the second half of the 19th century. In 1997, U.S. per capita income (measured in terms of purchasing power parity) was $28,740. Switzerland was the only developed country to come close, at $26,320, while Norway ($23,940), Japan ($23,400), and Denmark ($22,740) followed. At the same time, the United States boasts the lowest rate of unemployment in the developed world, about four percent, while Europe has some 20 million out of work, or more than 10 percent of the labor force. Poverty, currently the condition of 13.7 percent of Americans, is more widespread than in Europe, though rates are dropping. (Among African Americans, the poverty rate dropped to 29 percent in 1995, passing below 30 percent for the first time in the nation's history. Today it stands at 28.4 percent.)

The United States is the only Western country in which government extracts less than 30 percent of the gross domestic product in taxes—it took 28.5 percent in 1996. Spending on social welfare is correspondingly low. One has to go outside the Western world to find societies with a smaller state. The Japanese tax take was a tenth of a percent lower, but among the remaining member states of the Organization for Economic Cooperation and Development (OECD), only Turkey (25.4 percent), South Korea (23.2 percent), and Mexico (16.3 percent) have lower taxation levels.

American exceptionalism is distinctly double-edged. The United States is not as egalitarian in economic terms as the rest of the developed world. It has the highest proportion of nonvoters in national elections, as well the highest rates of violent crime and the biggest prison population (in per capita terms). Thanks to its meritocratic orientation, it is among the leaders in the unequal distribution of income. Gauged by the Gini coefficient, the social scientist's standard measure of income inequality, the U.S. score of 37.5 is almost 10 percent higher than that of the next closest country (Britain) among the Western democracies, and far above Sweden's 22.2. To put it in simpler terms, the richest 20 percent of Americans have incomes about nine times greater than the poorest 20 percent, while in Japan and Germany the affluent enjoy incomes only four and six times greater, respectively.

Yet because individualism and meritocratic ideals are so deeply ingrained in them, Americans are much less troubled by such differences than Europeans. According to a 1990 study, Americans are more likely to believe that there should be "greater incentives for individual effort," rather than that "incomes should be made more equal." Proportionately fewer Americans (56 percent) agree that "income differences are too large," as compared with Europeans (whose positive responses range from 66 to 86 percent). In a survey reported in 1995, people in six countries were asked: "How would you prefer to be paid—on a fixed salary . . . or mostly on an incentive basis which will allow you to earn more if you accomplished a lot, but may result in less earnings if you don't accomplish enough?" A majority of Americans (53 percent) opted for the incentive plan; the survey's British, French, Spanish, and German respondents chose a fixed salary by margins ranging from 65 to 72 percent.

A 1996 survey shows that a policy that reduces income disparities is supported by less than one-third (28 percent) of Americans, while positive responses elsewhere range from 42 percent in Austria to 82 percent in Italy. The British fall in the middle at 63 percent.

Americans are more likely than Europeans to agree that "large income differences are needed for the country's prosperity." Nearly one-third of Americans surveyed in 1987 justify inequality this way, as compared with an average of 23 percent among seven European countries (Great Britain, Austria, West Germany, Italy, Hungary, Switzerland, and the Netherlands). A 1992 review of American public opinion data over 50 years reports: "Surveys since the 1930s have shown that the explicit idea of income redistributing elicits very limited enthusiasm among the American public. . . . Redistributive fervor was not much apparent even in [the] depression era. Most Americans appear content with the distributional effects of private markets."

The historian Richard Hofstadter wrote that the 1930s introduced a "social democratic tinge" into the United States for the first time in its history. The Great Depression brought a strong emphasis on planning, on the welfare state, on the role of the government as a major regulatory actor, and even on redistribution of income. The great crisis challenged the historic American national commitment to the assumptions of classical liberalism and laissez faire, spawning, among other things, New Deal-inspired policies and a growth in trade union strength. These trends, however, have gradually inverted in the reasonably prosperous half-century since the end of World War II. The tinge—which never approached the full flush of Europe—has faded.

Despite the European Left's embrace of the free market, European governments are still, by American standards, very deeply involved in the economy and society. The differences stem in part from historical identities and values, in part from institutions that have been established over the last century. Once in place, government policies are defended by those who benefit from them, even as they continue to shape expectations about what government can do. The major European countries provided important social services long before the United States, which did not enact pension, unemployment, or industrial accident insurance until the 1930s. It is the only developed nation that does not have a government-supported, comprehensive medical system, and it is one of the few that do not provide child support to all families.

Today, Americans are still more opposed than Europeans to government involvement in economic affairs, whether through wage and price controls, publicly funded job creation, or the length of the work week. Nor are they favorably disposed toward government regulation in other realms, such as seat belt laws. Only 23 percent of Americans believe it is government's responsibility "to take care of very poor people who can't take care of themselves," according to a 1998 study by the late public opinion expert Everett Carll Ladd. They are less disposed than Europeans to believe that the state is obligated to supply a job for everyone who wants one, to provide a decent standard of living for the unemployed, or to guarantee a basic income.

The value differences between the United States and Europe are also reflected in attitudes toward social mobility and personal achievement. Americans are more likely than Europeans to see personal effort, hard work, ambition, education, and ability as more important for getting ahead in life than social background. Confronted with the proposition that "what you achieve depends largely on your family background" in a 1990 survey, only 31 percent of Americans agreed, compared with 53 percent of the British, 51 percent of the Austrians, and 63 percent of the Italians. Asked to choose between hard work and "luck and connections" as the most likely route to a better life, 44 percent of Americans pointed to hard work. Only 24 percent of the most like-minded European group, the British, agreed.

The American commitment to meritocracy is also reflected in the fact that Americans are more disposed than Europeans to favor increased spending on education. (And Americans tend to oppose offering help as a "handout" in the form of outright government grants to students, which Europeans back, preferring instead student loans.) Given that education is seen as the key to upward mobility, it is not surprising that the United States has spent proportionally much more public money on education than Europe, while Europe has devoted much more to welfare. The United States has led the world in providing the kinds of general education needed to get ahead. Since the early 19th century, it has been first in the proportion of citizens graduating from public elementary school, then high school, and more recently in the percentages attending college and receiving postgraduate training.

The other developed countries are now rapidly closing the education gap, however. College entry rates increased by more than 25 percent in 16 OECD countries between 1990 and '96, while the rate in the United States remained about the same. This change and others in education suggest that American-style individualism and ambition have spread to the point where the United States cannot be considered exceptional in these respects.

Does it still make sense to speak of the United States as the exceptional nation? As social democratic parties the world over shift toward the free market, the differences between the United States and other Western democracies may continue to narrow. Yet deeply rooted institutions and values do not easily lose their influence. The Western democracies may now all fit the liberal mold, but liberalism, too, has its divides. Europe still tends toward the economically egalitarian side, with a penchant for active government; Americans prefer a competitive, individualist society with equality of opportunity and effective but weak government.

There is no reason, moreover, to believe that we have seen the end of change—much less the "end of history." For all its rewards, the free market is not a source of great inspiration. Capitalism does not pledge to eliminate poverty, racism, sexism, pollution, or war. It does not even promise great material rewards to all. Neoconservative thinker Irving Kristol echoes a long line of capitalism's defenders when he allows that it offers "the least romantic conception of a public order that the human mind has ever conceived."

It is hard to believe that the West's now-contented young will not some day hunger again for the "exalted notions" that Aristotle described more than 2,000 years ago. Yet when they do, America will still have an ideological vision, the individualist, achievement-oriented American Creed, with which to motivate its young to challenge reality. The evolving social vision of Europe will necessarily hearken back to the very different ideals of the French Revolution and social democracy.

One does not have to peer far into the future to see that the contest between the forces of change and the defenders of the status quo is not over. In the formerly communist countries of Europe, left and liberal advocates of the free market and democracy confront conservative defenders of the power of state bureaucracies. Elsewhere in Europe, Green parties press the cause of environmentalism and other postmaterialist concerns. And nobody can predict what forces may be put into play by future events, from economic crisis to the rise of China. New movements and ideologies will appear and old ones will be revived. Economic hardship may bolster communitarian efforts to relegitimate the state's role in attacking social, sexual, and racial inequalities.

Even looking only at what is already in view, the United States still stands out. For instance, in every one of the 13 richest countries in the European Union, Green parties are represented in the national parliament or the country's delegation to the European Parliament. Greens have recently participated in ruling government coalitions in Belgium, Finland, France, Germany, and Italy. Only the United States lacks even a minimally effective Green party. One of the great puzzles of the 20th century was posed by the title of German sociologist Werner Sombart's 1906 book, *Why Is There No Socialism in the United States?* The puzzle of the next century may be, Why is there no Green party in the United States?

SEYMOUR MARTIN LIPSET (1922–2006) was the Hazel Professor of Public Policy and Sociology in the Institute of Public Policy at George Mason University. A senior fellow of the Hoover Institution at Stanford University and a senior scholar of the Wilstein Institute for Jewish Policy, his publications include *American Exceptionalism: A Double-Edged Sword* (W. W. Norton, 1995) and *Jews and the American Scene*, coauthored with Earl Raab (Harvard University Press, 1995).

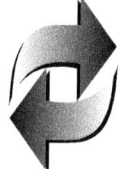

Godfrey Hodgson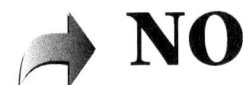

The Corruption of the Best

I have criticized American exceptionalism, sometimes sharply, on several different grounds. I first argued that the history of the United States ought to be seen as only one part of a broader history, not as the teleological preparation of a present and future perfection; as history, that is, and not as patriotic commemoration.

That history has not exclusively been the product of Puritan religion or the frontier, or any other purely American influences. On the contrary, it has been shaped by vast international historical processes, from the expansion of Europe and the African slave trade, through the Reformation and the Enlightenment, the global competition between the European powers, especially Britain and France, and the industrial revolution. America's development was greatly affected by two world wars, the Depression of the 1930s, and the Cold War. It has continued in the context of the rise of a global economy, first in the early years of the twentieth century and then, after the interruptions of the "short twentieth century," in the past few decades.

Of course there were events and processes that were specific to the United States. They included mass immigration, the frontier, slavery, and the minting of an American political ideology. Their part in shaping the modern nation should never be underestimated. Yet nor should they be exaggerated at the expense of the wider processes that affected the world as a whole. Indeed, the first three of those four cardinal factors in American history also affected the development of many other nations. Historians, in other words, should not cherry-pick what was unique in the American experience and ignore its historical context. And there is an important reason for this. If Americans are brought up in their education, and encouraged by their leaders, to believe that they are a unique and special people, that will affect the way they behave toward the rest of the world, over which they now have so much influence and so much power.

I have suggested that in the early decades after the Revolution, in part as a result of developments in the colonial period, American society truly was more exceptional than it has subsequently become. That exceptionalism consisted in a relatively greater achievement of both freedom and equality, at least for white males, than was to be found elsewhere. The development of freedom and equality in America was always, however, more limited, more constrained, and more under attack than patriotic myth would sometimes have us believe.

After the Civil War, I have maintained, at the very time when the myth of the unique democratic influence of the frontier was coming into existence, America was in many ways becoming less exceptional. That was in part because the United States was beginning to experience the consequences of the industrial revolution, of unregulated capitalism, and of urbanization, in the same way that these forces were already affecting the British Isles and western and central Europe. In some respects, no doubt, the United States had greater resources for resisting or deflecting those dangerous consequences. But by the 1880s, to contrast a Europe enslaved by poverty with a land of opportunity inhabited by "people of plenty" was historically inaccurate. After the abolition of slavery, in fact, American politics were more and more about the "social question": about poverty, inequality, injustice—exactly the matters that were concerning writers, social reformers, and political leaders in Europe. On the one hand, the period brought the development, for the first time on American soil, of what was called in Europe a "proletariat." On the other, in what Mark Twain called the Gilded Age, America bred, on a far larger scale than ever before, a class of plutocrats whose wealth gave them social and political power. So far from being the mother of capitalism, as is sometimes suggested, the United States, though always a capitalist country, came later than several European countries to fully developed industrial capitalism.

America was also becoming less exceptional in reality (though not necessarily less exceptionalist in rhetoric) precisely because—largely unnoticed or at least unappreciated in the United States—Europe, too, was going through an Age of Liberalism. Mid-nineteenth-century Europe was the world of John Stuart Mill and William Ewart Gladstone. Greater freedom, equality, and democracy were aspired to, and—albeit imperfectly—achieved. This was admittedly more painful in Europe, because of the strength of established powers, vested interests, and traditions. But then it was not that easy in America, either. You could say that America was becoming less exceptional because Europeans, or many of them, were adopting American values. But those values had in any case long been European values too for most Europeans.

Many of the historical realities that had once made Europe appear so different from America were disappearing or at least were under attack in late-nineteenth-century and early-twentieth-century Europe. Absolute monarchy had been displaced by constitutional monarchy in Britain, Holland, and Scandinavia. The power of aristocracy was being crippled, not least by the effects of imported American foodstuffs on agricultural rents. Empire was dividing the politics of the imperial powers from 1900 on, the time of the Boer War, and by the second decade of the twentieth century two of the three major political parties in Britain, the Liberals and Labour, were already committed to decolonization in the long term. Americans, and especially American conservatives, have a high opinion of Winston Churchill. British people remember that in the 1930s he was one of the rather few British politicians who strenuously opposed independence for India.

In the twentieth century, America was exceptional not so much for a commitment to democratic ideals but for two other reasons. For one thing, the United States became exceptionally rich, partly because of its natural and human resources, but also because, unlike its European rivals, it was not devastated and impoverished but was enriched by two world wars. At first, and especially in the generation immediately after World War II, that wealth was widely and generously spread. Inequality declined sharply in America during and immediately after World War II. But the "glorious thirty years" after 1945 were a time of rapidly increasing prosperity, far more widely distributed than ever before, in Western Europe and in Japan as well. Workers in automobile plants in Britain and Germany, France and Italy, like auto workers in the United States, were improving their standard of living, buying their own homes, seeing their children go to college, helped by powerful trade unions. More recently, in America and in Europe, economic growth has been disproportionately appropriated by the very rich, both by those who have inherited and by those who have earned their good fortune for themselves. But the differences in the standard of living between America and the rest of the developed world are now differences of degree, not, as they had been before the 1960s, differences of kind.

Once, American incomes were something Europeans could only dream of. Now, in Western Europe at least, it is a question of whether the American average income is reached next year or the year after.

In the 1930s and 1940s the United States also escaped the political disaster of fascism, and indeed played an important, though not (as exceptionalists sometimes imply) the only, role in destroying fascist and Nazi rule. The fact that fascism never seriously threatened the American political system (or, for that matter, the political systems in Britain, the British dominions, or Scandinavia) reflects the strength of the democratic tradition and the political skill of President Roosevelt, as well as the robust common sense of most Americans. Yet even in America some fascist tendencies and quasi-fascist movements appeared.

Untouched by foreign invasion, the American economy boomed in both world wars, at the very time when America's rivals were in their greatest difficulties. The United States "did well" out of the two world wars. After 1945 it was natural for American exceptionalism to be seen in large measure as the consequence of exceptional economic success and military power, not to mention the Faustian power of nuclear weapons and the ability to deliver them almost everywhere at will. So in the 1950s the current version of exceptionalism was a new blend of the moral exceptionalism of Roosevelt's fight for the Four Freedoms and pride in economic recovery, material progress, and military power. A good example is the book by David Potter, *People of Plenty*. "In every aspect of economic welfare," Potter wrote, "the national differentials between the United States and other countries are immense." The United States, he said, had 7 percent of the world's population and 42 percent of the world's income. The equivalent figures today show that the U.S. gross national product is $13.2 trillion out of a world GNP of $48 trillion, or about 27 percent (slightly less than the European Union's share of $14.5 trillion), and the U.S. population, though much larger at about 300 million, is only 4.5 percent of the world's estimated population of 6.6 billion people, a lower proportion than fifty years earlier. The average American in 1949, Potter stated, consumed 3,186 calories, "unquestionably the highest nutritional standard in the world." Half a century later, few would equate calorie consumption with nutritional standards. Moreover, Potter claimed, the high American standard of living was the result much less of natural resources than of the "economic efficiency of all kinds of Americans." The phrase now evokes a gentle smile. Potter's book, like many works of the 1950s, was explicitly devoted to disproving "zany" Marxist or socialist ideas. Many similar books written in the 1950s—for example, works by Max Lerner or Daniel Boorstin—were predicated on similar assumptions of incomparable American material superiority in areas where today the American advantage is comparatively slight and sometimes depends on what precise method of comparison is used.

In recent decades this second, material exceptionalism, now less clear, has helped to breed or to strengthen a third, missionary exceptionalism. This is the belief that it is the destiny, some say the God-given destiny, of the United States to spread the benefits of its democratic system and of its specific version of capitalism to as many other countries as possible. This view is not wholly new. Seeds of it can be seen in early Protestant religion. It played a part in the patriotic rhetoric of the new Republic, in tile confidence of the champions of Manifest Destiny that theirs was an "empire of liberty," and in the belief system of many American leaders, including especially Woodrow Wilson but also, in different ways, Theodore Roosevelt, Franklin D. Roosevelt, Harry Truman, and John F. Kennedy.

One specific new element in the American belief system, from the last quarter of the twentieth century, was the elevation of American capitalism, alongside American freedom and American democracy, in the pantheon of American exceptionalism. Of course, America has been the home of capitalism from the start, though not its only home. There was a fascinating episode in the earliest years of the Pilgrims' struggle to survive in Plymouth Colony, described in William Bradford's classic account. At first the Pilgrims intended to hold all land and wealth in common. But when the young colony was desperately worried about the shortage of food, the governor, Bradford, "with the advice of the chiefest among them," assigned land as property to each family. This experience, Bradford comments, "may well evince the vanity of that conceit of Plato's and other ancients applauded by some of later times; that the taking away of property and bringing in community [meaning communism or at least common ownership] into a commonwealth would make them happy and flourishing, *as if they were wiser than God.*"

Although ideas of communal ownership of property were to be found in the sixteenth and seventeenth century—for example, among the Anabaptists in sixteenth-century Westphalia, Moravia, and Bohemia and the seventeenth-century Levellers and Diggers in England—capitalism was closely associated with Protestantism, in Holland and Germany as well as in Britain and New England, as has been argued by great modern historians, including Max Weber and R.H. Tawney. If modern capitalism was largely developed in Holland and Britain in the sixteenth and seventeenth centuries, and carried across the Atlantic by Protestant colonists, capitalism itself is as old as civilization. Its fundamental ideas, such as the idea of investing in the hope of future profit, are as old as agriculture, and the part played by markets in setting prices can be traced back at least as far as the earliest towns in the Near East. It is true that at certain times and in certain places—for example, in the ancient river valley civilizations, when economic behavior and prices were regulated by royal authority, and in the European Middle Ages, when usury was prohibited by the church—capitalism was subordinated to temporal or spiritual authority. But capitalism existed long before the United States of America.

Economic historians distinguish a series of successive phases in the development of capitalism, for example, petty capitalism, mercantile capitalism, industrial capitalism, and finance capitalism. None of these can be said to have developed exclusively or even mainly in the United States. It is true, however, that in the twentieth century many European societies reacted to economic crisis by adopting one or another version of socialism. Even in the United States, from 1933 to the 1970s, the federal government embraced a form of social democracy, though control of enterprise was exercised not mainly by state ownership but by state regulation. In Western Europe, as well as in the former British dominions and in Latin America, though various "socialist" devices, including public ownership, were more widespread than in the United States, the economic system was still one variant or another of capitalism, more or less regulated. (Sometimes it was described as a "mixed economy.") It is possible therefore to speak of the United States as having led the way in the propagation of neoliberal ideas in the late twentieth century, but misleading to suggest that capitalism as such is in any way an American invention.

In the past thirty years or so, however, and especially after the presidency of Ronald Reagan, an exceptionalist philosophy has been more confidently enunciated and more openly accepted as the basis for American foreign policy. This missionary spirit has come in two variants. One is the gentler and more consensual version, as preached and practiced by the Clinton administration. Its leaders acknowledged that they were followers of Woodrow Wilson, and that they inherited his desire to bring the benefits of American democracy to the world. But they wanted to do so, as far as possible, only to the extent that others wanted those benefits. They were keen that America should be the leader. But they interpreted that to mean that others were eager to be led. They wanted to act out their beliefs, so far as possible, with the agreement of as many other nations as possible. This, too, had been the instinct, or at least the practice, of the previous Republican administration of George H. W. Bush.

At least as long ago as the debates in the early Cold War years over the National Security Act, and over NSC-68 and the sharp consequent increases in defense budgets, there had been those, the "hawks," who were impatient of restraint. They saw the nation as being virtually at war with communism. They resented the occasional reluctance of allies to endorse American interests or to go along with American initiatives. They called for maximum military readiness and brushed aside those who warned of the dangers of transforming America into a "garrison state" or a "national security state." Surprisingly, perhaps, it was not when the danger of communism was at its height, but when it had to all intents and purposes disappeared in the early 1990s, that the partisans of aggressive, unilateral missionary policies finally triumphed.

I have argued, as many others have now done, that these policies have been disastrous, not only for the damage they have inflicted on the domestic American economy or even for America's reputation in the world, but also for any realistic prospect of achieving their own goals. There can be little doubt that the prospects of spreading American ideals of democracy have weakened, not improved, especially in the Middle East, since the invasion of Iraq in 2003. Survey data from late 2007 suggest that roughly two-thirds to three-quarters of the world's population disapprove of the American invasion and occupation of Iraq. The prospects of American democracy would be seriously damaged by an attack on Iran or even by a nod and a wink to an Israeli attack on Iran. Nor has the prosperity of the United States been enhanced by the new aggressive foreign policy. An America on bad terms with its suppliers of energy, raw materials, cheap manufactured goods, migrants, and credit is not going to be a stronger America, especially if its finite resources have been dissipated in incompetently planned military adventures. Finally, the domestic regime that accompanies conservative foreign policy seems unlikely to strengthen the society in the long term. An America, for example, in which the richest 1 percent were piling up ever greater fortunes, and chief executives of corporations earned many hundreds of times more than their average employee, while half the population could not afford to buy a home or go to the doctor, would not be a stronger America, however spectacular the fortunes accumulated by a few....

From the beginning, one legitimate and positive component of American national pride has been the idea that the United States had unique qualities as a society and a special destiny as a nation. That conviction has been a powerful motivating incentive. It has caused Americans on the whole to set themselves high standards, especially in their public life. If they sometimes supposed that their standards were higher than anyone else's, that may not have been altogether a bad thing. If it set an example for other nations to emulate, so much the better.

At different times in the past, exceptionalism has admittedly taken the objectionable shape of a pompous and intolerant "Americanism," or even "100 percent Americanism." This was the stuff of blowhard Fourth of July oratory in every generation. It took the form of the odious prejudices of nineteenth-century Nativists and of the second Klan of the 1920s, with its bigoted hatred of Catholics and Jews as well as African Americans.

This was the soil in which the Red-baiting and witch-hunting of the 1950s grew. One of my students recently showed me a strip cartoon booklet circulated to schools in 1950 by the service organization Lions International. It recited a propaganda version of "history" in which cavemen, ancient Egyptians, and Spartans were portrayed as slaves. It contrasted the Spartans, directly compared to Russians, with the freedom-loving Athenians, though of course there was slavery in Athens as well as in Sparta. Americans were portrayed as uniquely brave soldiers for freedom, explicitly contrasted with British "socialism." As this cockamamie version of world history went on, to be told to the children, it was made clear that Americans were in danger of being enslaved... by taxation.

There is no means of telling how widespread such propaganda about American history was in the early Cold War years. It was certainly not far to seek. Nor perhaps should it be taken too seriously. Some of George Bush's admirers at the 2004 convention carried posters asking how they were to shoot liberals if their guns were taken from them, but everyone knew that that was only a joke in bad taste, not the portent of an American fascism.

The American exceptionalism I am describing is quite different from such coarse prejudice. It has been on the whole a tradition that stresses the superiority of America and Americans, not the inferiority of anyone else. That may be irritating to those of us who are not Americans, but it is generously meant. George W. Bush may not have taken the trouble to find out whether the people of Iraq were pleased to have him impose his conception of democracy on them, but at least it was liberty, not slavery, that he thought he was offering.

The corruption of the best, says the old Latin tag, is the worst. My thesis is not that American exceptionalist thought is intrinsically corrupting or that it was destructive in the past, but that what has been essentially a liberating set of beliefs has been corrupted over the past thirty years or so by hubris and self-interest into what is now a dangerous basis for national policy and for the international system.

Even in the times when its overall thrust was beneficent, the exceptionalist narrative of American history left out half the story. The history of the migration to America, I have suggested, could not be understood in isolation from the conditions and the political and religious beliefs of Europe at the time, certainly not by simply contrasting an American commitment to "liberty" with the presumably servile cultures of every one else. The religious faith of New England was not antithetical to European Christianity; it was one variant of the Protestant faith shared by Ulstermen and Swedes, Afrikaners and Prussians. The impulses that pushed Europeans to migrate to the United States were not wholly different from the motives of those who settled in Canada, or Australia, or the Argentine, or from those of the Russians who broke the black soils of the Ukraine, or even of the settlers from all over Europe who mined the gold and diamonds of South Africa.

Even in the twentieth century, at least the first two-thirds of it, if the American experience was more fortunate than that of other countries, still life in the United States was always influenced and conditioned by what was happening everywhere else. The United States was hardly untouched by the breakdown of the European diplomatic system in 1914 and of the world economic system in 1929, by the invention of the internal combustion engine in Germany in the 1890s or of radio by an Italian working in England, or by the work of nuclear physicists in Cambridge or Berlin in the 1920s. . . .

For more than two centuries Americans have been motivated to set themselves the highest public standards, both in the conduct of their own affairs and in their dealings with the rest of the world, by a national ideology. The essentials of that system of belief concerned such values as liberty, the political sovereignty of the people, equality before the law, and the paramount rule of constitutional law. From the beginning, that national ideology contained both exceptionalist and universalist elements. "The cause of America," said Tom Paine, "is in a great measure the cause of all mankind." The victory of the Union, said Abraham Lincoln, was "the last, best hope of earth." The emancipation of the slaves, he meant, would guarantee the freedom of all Americans. So the United States would be an example to the world. Some Americans in the nineteenth century believed that the "empire of liberty" would inevitably "overspread" at least the whole of North America and perhaps Central America and the Caribbean, and even the whole of the Americas as far as Tierra del Fuego. But public holiday rhetoric aside, there was no idea then that the United States either could or should bring freedom to the entire world. To this day, even the most messianic neo-Wilsonians have allowed their universalist ambitions to be checked by realism. It is one thing to invade Grenada, Lebanon, or at a stretch Iraq. No one is speaking of bringing democracy, by shock and awe, to nations with millions of soldiers and nuclear weapons, such as Russia, India, or China.

It was not until the twentieth century that this combination of exceptionalism with at least a theoretical universalism—a belief, that is, that the United States has a special destiny to bring freedom to the Americas, brought to bear on the idea that the United States could be an example of freedom to the world—began to take on the characteristics of a program. . . .

Underlying the whole story was a fabric of assumptions that were indeed predicated on a new, aggressive interpretation of the exceptionalist creed. The United States, it was said, would act as it saw fit. It neither needed nor wanted international agreement, approval, or cooperation. Those in the world who dissented in any way from the wrath to come were, by administration officials, not to mention their loyal journalists, ignored, or insulted, or derided.

So long as the world was threatened by dictators, first by fascist dictators, then by communists, the world was happy to accept American leadership. It helped that for decades that leadership was exerted in a spirit of generosity and comity. In those days, many around the world who were not Americans found it easy to share the ideals of the traditional American exceptionalist creed, among them freedom, democracy, and popular sovereignty. But in those days, such ideals were not presented in bluntly exceptionalist terms. Now the common ideals of what had come to be known as "the free world" were claimed as the private property of Americans.

To the world, however, freedom cannot mean military occupation. Democracy cannot mean a world's political decisions made behind closed doors in Washington. Popular sovereignty, as an ideal for the world, cannot be reduced to the wishes of the electorate in one country, still less to the instincts of an elite "within the Beltway" that seemed increasingly isolated from the rest of America. Prosperity, for the world, cannot mean the monopoly of the planet's resources by a few hundred corporations and a handful of financial enterprises.

Nothing is more passionately to be hoped for than that the American government will once again hold before it the values that inspired Jefferson and Madison, Lincoln and Roosevelt. Nothing is more heartily to be wished than that the American people should once again see itself, not as a master race whose primacy is owed to the shock and awe inspired by terrifying weaponry, but once again, freely and generously, as first among equals.

Such a change in the face America shows to the world will not come, of course, until Americans have shown once again, as they have so often done in the past, that they will not allow their generous instincts and sound values to be travestied by charlatans and bullies. Until American democracy girds itself to recapture the political system and reasserts its healthiest instincts, the United States is not likely to recapture the admiration and affection the American people earned by their achievements over the first two centuries of their national history. . . .

The point at which the principles of American democracy are reduced to mere boasting and bullying, justified by a cynical "realism," is the point at which the practice of American democracy, at home as well as abroad, is in mortal danger. It is also the point at which the best of the exceptionalism in the American tradition has been corrupted into the worst. We can only hope that mortal danger will be avoided.

The late **GODFREY HODGSON** was an English journalist and former Director of the Reuters Foundation Programme at Oxford University. The author of eleven books, most of them on some aspect of United States history, he served as the Washington bureau chief for *The Observer* and was the foreign editor for the *Independent*.

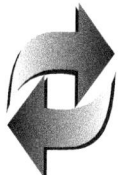

EXPLORING THE ISSUE

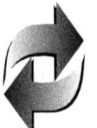

Is America Exceptional?

Critical Thinking and Reflection

1. How does Seymour Martin Lipset define "American exceptionalism"? Why does he believe that the United States is still different from the rest of the world?
2. According to Alexis de Tocqueville, how did the United States of the 1830s differ from all European nations?
3. According to Lipset, how does the United States today still differ from other nations?
4. According to Godfrey Hodgson, what qualities of the United States that are often described as unique are characteristics shared with other nations around the world?
5. According to Hodgson, what factors have contributed to a decline in the notion of American exceptionalism?

Is There Common Ground?

What do people mean when they talk about American exceptionalism? Most scholars approach this term from the perspective that the United States is in certain ways different from other nations. In other words, the United States is an exception to the rule when examining particular national characteristics; in Seymour Martin Lipset's terms, America is an "outlier" when compared to other countries, especially developed European nations to which it is frequently compared. And as Lipset suggests, those identifiable characteristics that set the United States apart from other nations, give it a unique quality, can be either positive or negative traits.

Many Americans, including political leaders ranging from John F. Kennedy to Newt Gingrich to Ronald Reagan to Barack Obama, have employed this term in something of a patriotic fashion and assumed that those features that presumably set the United States apart from other nations are, by definition, good things. They are prone to think of the United States as a model nation, not only set apart from others but also set above. From this vantage point, America is exceptional in the sense that it is superior to other nations, and there is an assumption that other countries should want to emulate the United States.

Critics of the use of this term approach their arguments from a variety of perspectives. Some disapprove because they consider the idea of American exceptionalism to be an expression of arrogance. Others, on the other hand, insist that the problem is that the United States is not different in many of the ways attributed to it. After all, they point out, the United States and its institutions grew out of Western European political and intellectual traditions shared with many other countries today. Generations of Americans, for example, have insisted that American national traditions and character were inherited from England or Germany or even the Celtic areas of Europe. Godfrey Hodgson recognizes that in an earlier time—the colonial era and early national period, in particular—Americans were more justified in claiming a uniqueness. After the Civil War, however, Hodgson believes that the United States became more like other industrializing nations in Europe. Lipset and others, according to Hodgson, miss the point that the United States is a nation among nations whose entire history has operated in a global context, whether individual Americans liked that or not.

Additional Resources

Thomas Bender, *A Nation Among Nations: America's Place in World History* (Hill & Wang, 2006)

Michael Ignatieff, ed., *American Exceptionalism and Human Rights* (Princeton University Press, 2005)

Deborah L. Madsen, *American Exceptionalism* (University Press of Mississippi, 1998)

David Noble, *Death of a Nation: American Culture and the End of Exceptionalism* (Cambridge University Press, 2002)

Sylvia Soderlind and James Taylor Carson, eds., *American Exceptionalisms: From Winthrop to Winfrey* (State University of New York Press, 2012)

Internet References . . .

The Alexis de Tocqueville Tour

www.tocqueville.org

Frederick Jackson Turner

nationalhumanitiescenter.org/pds/gilded/empire/text1/turner.pdf

Institute for the Study of Civic Values

http://www.sustainable.org/creating-community/civic-engagement/535-institute-for-the-study-of-civic-values-iscv-

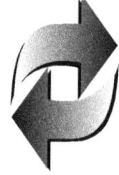

ISSUE

Selected, Edited, and with Issue Framing Material by:
Kevin R. Magill and Tony L. Talbert, *Baylor University*

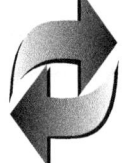

Did the Core Values in Colonial Ideology Lead to Conflict with Native Americans and U.S. Imperialism?

YES: Maureen Konkle, from "Indigenous Ownership and the Emergence of U.S. Liberal Imperialism," *American Indian Quarterly* (2008)

NO: Jessica R. Stern, from "A Key into The Bloudy Tenent of Persecution: Roger Williams, the Pequot War, and the Origins of Toleration in America," *Early American Studies* (2011)

Learning Outcomes

After reading this issue, you will be able to:

- Know and understand the reasons behind/for Henry Knox's development of a colonial policy based on liberal imperialism.
- Understand the role of the Scottish Enlightenment in the 18th century shifting U.S. views on Indigenous land ownership.
- Identify and understand the principal issues of U.S. imperialism toward Indigenous Peoples and how colonial views of land ownership changed over time.
- Explain the shift in thinking of Roger Williams toward Indigenous Peoples post-Pequot War.
- Understand the colonial arguments used to tout the superiority of White Christian settlers over Indigenous Peoples.

ISSUE SUMMARY

YES: Maureen Konkle argues that the Ideology of colonialism has allowed discourses to develop that have been fundamental to the project of U.S. imperialism. She suggests that marginalizing narratives, particularly of Indigenous Peoples, have contributed to the justification of U.S. aggression, conflict, and genocide. Konkle lastly implies that these colonizing narratives continue to exist affecting our Ideology today, but that they are less overt than they once were.

NO: Jessica Stern believes that careful examination of Roger Williams arguments suggests that religion never justified violence and that Native Americans and Christians shared a moral code. She suggests first that, rather than critique colonial Ideology, we should consider that individuals are prone to misunderstand foreign people and ideas and should therefore not be trusted to judge outsiders. Second, she suggests that civil peace relies on locating similarities between people and tolerating differences.

Issue Framing with Justin Kruger

The numerous interactions between European Colonists and Indigenous Americans differed by time, place, and group. Therefore, it is difficult for historians to identify consistent patterns of behavior through which we can uniformly consider colonial Ideology. Similarly, the ideologies of European colonists—Spanish, French, Dutch, and English—informed the ways they approached the various Indigenous tribes and one another, within what they understood to be the New World—a term which itself reveals Colonial Ideology. Given these realities, historical questions examining the relationship between the two groups have differed. Focusing on the English settlers, some scholars suggest that they followed a conscious, concerted effort to exterminate the Indigenous people for economic gain in efforts to establish a permanent home in the wilderness. Others suggest sporadic clashes that occurred between the groups demonstrate hostilities between both groups. However, there is no question Colonists were responsible for the decline of the Indigenous American population—a fact made clear when we consider that the population fell as much as 95 percent in the first century following Columbus's arrival. To be fair, though much of this decline can be attributed to violent encounters with Europeans, as historian William McNeill has suggests, the main weapon that overwhelmed Indigenous peoples in the Americas was the Europeans' breath, which transmitted disease germs for which most American Indians had no immunities. Large-scale intergroup violence erupted in Virginia in the 1620s, the 1640s, and the 1670s when disputes between Spain, France, and England forced Indigenous Americans to take sides. Tribes largely allied with France against England.

Speaking generally, relations between Indigenous Americans and Anglo-European colonists were challenged from the very beginning because these were two very different cultures and with very different ideologies. Early interactions resulted in inaccurate perceptions, misunderstandings, and failed expectations. Largely, the European response to their new neighbors was grounded in beliefs of divine providence and cultural superiority. Interestingly, the English Colonists depended on the generosity and wilderness techniques of the Indigenous Peoples as they struggled early in their colonization. However, after they established themselves, significant disagreements with their neighbors increased tensions, particularly about how the environment should be used. The ideologies became relational when for example, Indigenous subsistence farming, collided with Colonial desire to develop a market economy.

Maureen Konkle writes that by the early 1800s the US relationship with the Indigenous Peoples was now understood as a "conflict between savagery and civilization," a concept that would be used as the basis for further taking Indigenous lands. Drawing on the writings of the Scottish Enlightenment, the colonists positioned the Indigenous People as a backward and rudimentary civilization. Similarly, John Locke's agriculturalist theory further made a case for legitimizing theft of land. This scholarship played a role in developing colonial Ideology allowing racism, greed, and conflict to precede justice.

Naturally, Indigenous Peoples in the Northeastern U.S. had their own ideas for the land they had inhabited for centuries and would not easily relinquish or sell claims to their land. During the 17th century, Native ownership was a principle that divided colonists and the British. The British, at this time, did not offer Native American land recognition, but Colonists adhered to what they called natural law, meaning Indigenous occupied land had to be purchased. This concept lasted into the early 18th century until Colonial population growth and the desire for more land began to erode support for natural law. By the late 1790s, land speculators further challenged and attempted to dismantle laws that supported Indigenous land rights. However, secretary of War Henry Knox asserted that the U.S. relationship with Indigenous Peoples needed to be built upon peaceful foundations. Thomas Jefferson publicly supported this idea, but privately worked to ensure that the young country would expand its land holdings.

By the early 1800s, many nullified Indigenous land rights by claiming that territory needed cultivation to be described as land in this way. At this point, Colonial thought centered on the socially constructed idea that Indigenous Peoples were unable to own land or develop workable governments. It was from this perspective, Konkle argues that the United States adopted a policy of liberal imperialism. The Ideology of benevolent imperialism was one where "the colonized would cooperate" (the same justification was used by the British during their rule in India). She suggests that such thinking promised freedom while cultivating subjugation. The United States used the promise of citizenship to gain support from Indigenous groups then the United States simply took land from noncitizens and systematically denied Indigenous people equal rights as citizens. Simultaneously, US imperialists asserted that violence was inevitable as an unfortunate reality of advancing "society." These ideologies created an antipodal relationship between the United States and Indigenous Populations, a relationship made to resemble the benevolent father and child (an idea expressed by Supreme Court Chief Justice John Marshall in *Cherokee Nation v. Georgia* under the idea of "pupilage"). Subsequently, court cases further erased Indigenous land rights. Drawing on Mills' notion of a racial contract, Konkle posits that the United States engaged in thinking that ignored social realities in favor of a focus on the benefits proffered to whites. The colonial Ideology proved vital for a group looking to legitimize genocide and theft. Colonists demonstrated their propensity for examining and removing the stories of Indigenous Peoples (i.e., their histories, geographies, politics, and traditions) as a means of dehumanization to justify their imperial Ideology.

While Konkle explains that the Colonist belief in God caused them to see their ideological vision for a Christian civilization as divine right, Jessica Stern's focuses her historical inquiry on Roger Williams instead, a man well-known for his beliefs on religious tolerance. Stern examines the role of Williams as a mediator between northeast colonial settlers and Indigenous tribes such as the Pequot, Narragansett, and Mohegan. Prior to the Pequot War/Massacre, Stern argues that Williams was in line with Puritan ideal of religious purity and understood the Pequot as "devil's agents." In the aftermath of the massacre, however, first as an information gatherer and then mediator with the Indigenous groups, he began to believe in toleration—for which he is now most well-known.

In *The Bloudy Tenent of Persecution*, Williams describes the Indigenous People as an exemplar model for peaceful civil society, noting specifically, that peace in civil society is not tied to Christian beliefs. After being kicked out of England, Williams had come to the colonies as a prototypical Puritan that believed in religious purity and the conversion of non-Puritans, but he changed his philosophy. Post-Pequot War, Williams became increasingly disillusioned with religious uniformity as a prerequisite for a peaceful civil society which led Williams to develop his thinking on shared moral codes and their possibilities for peace. In writing between 1636 and 1640, Williams outlined his ideas for religious toleration, suggesting that complete cross-cultural/religious understandings and conversions were not possible. Instead he argued for toleration, noting that people tend to misunderstand that with which they are unfamiliar. At the same time, Williams noted the indiscriminate and perpetual violence being leveraged at all Indigenous Peoples. To his eyes, the colonists appeared unwilling to see the Indigenous people as anything other than enemies. Williams became disillusioned with justifications for conflict and argued that many calls for religious uniformity were unnecessary for civil peace. Instead he suggested that groups could share a moral code, and that state-enforced religion itself could lead to conflict (i.e., the Pequot War/Massacre). He cited a number of different civil societies of Native Americans who had developed societies where people and goods were respected. Williams sometimes disagreed with Indigenous thinking but nevertheless appreciated the "coherence of the Native American reasoning and the nature of their sense of justice."

In his role as mediator, Williams tried to show the humanity of Indigenous Peoples by translating their actions into cultural terms that could be understood by the colonists. In his writing, Williams took on their ideas of warfare and the desire for religious orthodoxy to attempt to break down the ideologies of colonial superiority. The impulse of war, he argued, was similar for both the colonists and Indigenous Peoples, but the ways they enacted them were starkly different. Williams wrote on the fallibility of cultural fixity in which people know and believe that what they are doing is the right and only way (i.e., property rights and systems of morality). He continued to critique that Indigenous Peoples would be punished when they did not follow Christian law and argued that Indigenous societies demonstrated that a peaceful civil society not dependent on Christ.

So what then are the tenants of Colonial Ideology? And did these ideologies lead to conflicts with the Indigenous people of North America? The authors of these texts suggest take opposing perspectives which differently situate Ideology in discussing the relationship between colonist and Indigenous Peoples. Perhaps, examination of Colonial Ideology following the French and Indian War can provide insight into the evolution of these ideologies as they relate to other relations. English Colonists actively worked to cultivate a War with England following the Proclamation of 1763 because the English forbade them from moving into the Ohio River Valley. This historical cause perhaps best demonstrates how U.S. American Ideology led to a war related to furthering economic interests. The Revolutionary War was not only a way to become self-determined politically but also a way to claim the valuable land west of the Appalachian watershed. We can, perhaps, see these actions as an extension of Colonial imperialism related to the Indigenous people. However, one could argue that the colonial Ideology still exists today as inextricable aspects of U.S. political thought, U.S. foreign policy, and U.S. justification for war. Consider the Iraqi War and the dehumanization associated with imperial and "savior" (religious and democratic messages) rhetoric as defense for U.S. treaty breaking, economic and geographical expansion. The ideologically informed imperialist model prepares citizens for invasion has unfolded from the colonial Ideology. Consider the framing of the following incidents that led to ideological perceptions following the colonial epoch—the explosion of the USS Maine, the sinking of the Lusitania, the threat of communism, and Iraqi weapons of mass destruction—Were these all ways to rally the U.S. population to war by cultivating imperialist Ideology? Were and are Americans fearful of other cultures or do they find reasons to fulfill their divine imperial right or are both true? These authors help reveal the nature of colonial Ideology through their historical analysis.

YES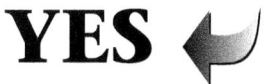

Maureen Konkle

Indigenous Ownership and the Emergence of U.S. Liberal Imperialism

"Westward the Star of Empire takes its way," and whenever that Empire is held by the white man, nothing is safe or unmolested or enduring against his avidity for gain.

    Maris Bryant Pierce, *Address on the Present Conditions and Prospects of the Aboriginal Inhabitants of North America, with Particular Reference to the Seneca Nation* (1839)

Writers on U.S. imperialism have been trying to establish not only what it is but why it's so peculiar—or how it is like but unlike other modern European imperialisms.[1] The continent is one obvious thing that makes it different, but, more specifically, it's how the conflict with the indigenous people who were and are on the continent produced a certain kind of imperialism and imperial ideology that makes it different. That imperial ideology is peculiarly abstract. Scholars have remarked upon the powerful—and frustrating, for analysis—abstractions of U.S. imperialism. Or, as historian William Appleman Williams put it, in the United States, empire is absent from explicit recognition but permeates U.S. society as a "way of life."[2] The idea of empire itself is completely naturalized (thus the way of life) but also utterly depoliticized (thus the difficulty of recognizing it as a historical process comparable to others). By the 1830s, the nation itself was understood as the site of an abstract world-historical conflict between savagery and civilization, a conflict in which civilization must and would prevail because God willed it and the continent required it. As the result of the inevitable forces of human history, imperial violence was not under anyone's control and not anyone's fault. Every dead Indian, real and imagined, told that story over and over again.

The conflict with indigenous people produced an imperial ideology that required a significant degree of abstraction because of the nature of relations with indigenous people. In North America Europeans set out to claim land they didn't know that was occupied by people they couldn't control. To make alliances, establish boundaries, and acquire land they made legal agreements, including treaties, that recognized indigenous ownership of land and therefore of political autonomy. After the formation of the United States that recognition, well established in North American legal and political practice, became a signifier of U.S. moral and political superiority. When indigenous nations resisted selling land, recognition became a problem for expansionists, who then needed to neutralize indigenous ownership but in such a way that it could be reconciled with the dominant political ideology. To do this they turned to an emerging narrative of a world-historical conflict between civilization and savagery in the United States itself in which indigenous people, as savage hunters, by definition couldn't own property and therefore didn't form governments. The purpose of this essay is to show that the construct of "savagism and civilization" in U.S. culture has a political context—the necessity of denying the principle of indigenous ownership—and a political effect—the positing of an imperial ideology, the primary claim of which was that imperialism didn't exist as a historical process but was rather the unfolding of God's will. The figure of the Indian was the linchpin of the imagined conflict between savagery and civilization, embodying that imperialist narrative. The figure wasn't just a product of blind racial prejudice or ethnocentric cultural misunderstanding, it stripped away history, geography, political life, and traditions from indigenous people to produce an abstraction that demonstrated that they didn't and couldn't own land and form legitimate governments.

The relations between indigenous people and the United States, historically and in the present, are the relations of liberal imperialism—that imperialism that presents itself as benevolent and civilizing, if only the colonized would cooperate and be properly raised up. In literary and historical scholarship, the term "liberal imperialism" usually describes British imperial history, particularly in late-eighteenth- and early-nineteenth-century

---

"Indigenous Ownership and the Emergence of U.S. Liberal Imperialism" by Maureen Konkle, is reproduced from *American Indian Quarterly* with permission from the University of Nebraska Press. Copyright ©2008.

India, and is at present a term political neoconservatives endorse as a positive description of hypothetical U.S. global hegemony.[3] Historically, liberal imperialism figured the colonized as backward children who had to be properly educated to enjoy (eventually, theoretically) property, individual rights, and citizenship. British intellectuals and government officials believed imperial power in India to be "simply the instrument required to align a deviant and recalcitrant history with the appropriate future," historian Uday Singh Mehta writes.[4] This required a paternalistic authority over the colonized and programs of education and reform focused on a hypothetical future in which the colonized would be brought up to speed civilizationally. In British India, colonial subjects were considered to be in a state of "tutelage"; in the United States, via Supreme Court Chief Justice John Marshall in *Cherokee Nation v. Georgia*, the equivalent concept was "pupilage," or, more broadly, the idea of the Indian as ward of a benevolent Great Father. The trick of liberal imperialism is that it promises freedom and delivers subordination, as its "evangelistic" reforming of the colonized, Mehta points out, goes on forever.[5] Furthermore, in the United States, the claims of civilizing Indians, of offering them citizenship, were a principal means of divesting indigenous people of land and political autonomy as well as of justifying the imperial relationship itself. Citizenship was a product of imperialism, not of benevolence.

I'm not taking issue in this essay with the substance of much of the scholarship on the representation of Indians, the idea of savagism and civilization, or the history of relations with indigenous people but rather with a prevailing assumption of the moral rectitude of the political "inclusion" of indigenous people as U.S. citizens and a relative lack of interest in indigenous political struggles for autonomy, historically and in the present day. The current dominant version of the history of Indians in the United States narrates as something like this: Europeans ethnocentrically did not believe that Indians used their land properly and therefore felt justified in taking it; but they sincerely wanted to help Indians become civilized, after which (they promised) Indians could become citizens. The important aspects of this narrative are Euro-Americans' regrettable ethnocentrism—they couldn't help themselves—and their sincerity. Even when they were bad, for the most part they meant well. The proof of their meaning well is the fact of indigenous citizenship in the United States. (What indigenous people thought of U.S. citizenship, whether or not they wanted it [usually not], and, if they did want it, what they meant to do with it are rarely addressed.) If past actions of the United States and its (non-indigenous) citizens must be condemned, the implication is that, at present, citizenship and cultural recognition and appreciation have resolved the principal problems of U.S. colonization. The "inclusion" of indigenous people in the U.S. body politic can be represented as a moral victory for the United States, an instance of the nation living up to its professed values, albeit belatedly. This might be called the liberal consensus on Indians, and it's entirely a product of nineteenth-century liberal imperialism.[6]

In much of the recent work discussing the history of U.S. imperialism, academic and otherwise, indigenous people barely register. If they appear, they are often treated as a done deal, a moot point; writers invoke tragedy and move on. This is also a product of an imperial ideology that conceives of its own history as world history and construes its own violence as unfortunate but inevitable, and indeed required, for progress to occur. The erasure of indigenous ownership and therefore of indigenous political society as such is the foundation of U.S. imperialism and imperial ideology. I want to sketch that point out here, I hope for further discussion.

Problems in Early U.S. Imperialism

Indigenous people owned their land and meant to keep it, at least enough of it, and when they made this point to Euro-Americans in the late eighteenth century, they invoked their diverse traditions but also colonial history. That they owned their land outright was a widely recognized and even basic principle in colonial North America. Then, in the early years of the United States, the recognition of indigenous ownership became a means for political elites to establish U.S. moral and political superiority, distinguishing it from British tyranny and indeed the practices of any other nation in the world. In contrast, in attempting to evade indigenous ownership and get more land more easily, expansionists were driving the political and cultural redefinition of indigenous people and their relationship to land. The problem was that the political elite couldn't readily jettison indigenous ownership when it was associated with the new state's exceptionalist claims.

In his recent book *How the Indians Lost Their Land: Law and Power on the Frontier* (2005), legal historian Stuart Banner maintains that seventeenth-century English settlers, who found "preexisting [systems] of property rights everywhere they went" in North America, relied in their relations with indigenous people on existing natural law theory, which held that occupancy determined property in land, and therefore indigenous land had to be purchased. This practice persisted through the late eighteenth century. English settlers recognized indigenous ownership not from altruistic or egalitarian motivations but for practical reasons having to do with the instability of land policies and ongoing power struggles. Colonial governments regulated land purchases through licenses, which were relatively easy to acquire, but this formality, Banner writes, "did not cause the English to think of Indian land title as a lesser form of ownership than English title," since "all landowners . . . faced a variety of restrictions on what they could do with their land."[7] The Royal Proclamation of 1763 recognized indigenous ownership, establishing the Crown as the sole authority for treating with Indian nations; it outlawed land speculation and set a boundary between the colonies and the Indian nations of the West. (The proclamation remains an important factor in Canadian-Aboriginal relations.)[8] After an initial effort in the immediate postrevolutionary period to assert that the British surrender transferred title to indigenous land to the United States, U.S. policy was to recognize the autonomy of indigenous people, purchase their land only with their consent, and make efforts to "civilize" them so that they might someday become incorporated into the United States. At that moment, Indians weren't necessarily doomed to disappear.

But as Euro-Americans clamored for more land, the principle of indigenous ownership began to be eroded, mainly in relation to the issue of preemption rights. Previous to the Revolution, Europeans understood the right of preemption to mean that only the European nation claiming interest in a particular territory had the right, in relation to other European nations, to buy land from indigenous people in that territory. It did not confer ownership or title but was rather something like a declaration of interest that European nations mutually recognized among themselves.[9] During the Revolution and especially afterward, preemption rights began to be redefined. States began selling preemption rights to land speculators, which meant that the purchaser had the first opportunity to buy the land when the government secured the title to the land from indigenous people. In the face of this transformation of preemption, in 1790, Congress passed the first of the Indian trade and intercourse acts, which, returning to British colonial policy, established the federal government as the sole authority for purchasing land from indigenous people who owned their land outright.

Those who had already secured preemption rights then sought to preserve their claims legally. One of the earliest cases brought was *Marshall v. Clark* (the Marshall involved was John Marshall's father), in which the court held that the state legislature could grant preemption rights to indigenous land but that the grantee took the risk upon himself as to what would happen to the land in the future (i.e., whether indigenous people would sell or not); courts in Tennessee and Pennsylvania later found the same.[10] The effect of these cases was to normalize and even expand this postrevolutionary redefinition of preemption rights. Despite the federal government's continued emphasis on indigenous ownership, lawyers and land speculators "began to think of the preemption right as the fee simple title, and the Indians' present right of possession as a kind of tenancy that would last as long as the Indians remained on the land," and, furthermore, that this had always been the case.[11]

If the principle of indigenous ownership continued to be eroded outside of government, inside government recognition of ownership was necessary for both strategic and ideological reasons. Secretary of War Henry Knox's 1789 report to Congress—the first session of the first Congress—is often pointed to as a succinct account of early U.S. Indian policy. In a review of relations with indigenous nations on U.S. borders, he wrote:

> The Indians being the prior occupants, possess the right of the soil. It cannot be taken from them unless by their free consent, or by the right of conquest in case of a just war. To dispossess them on any other principle, would be a gross violation of the fundamental laws of nature, and of that distributive justice which is the glory of a nation.[12]

That the United States would or could remove the Indians by force, Knox argued, was unlikely, given the state of U.S. finances and the desirability of keeping peace on the frontier. Indeed, he continued, Congress's initial belief that Britain's surrender gave it "the fee of all the Indians lands, within the limits of the United States," as contradicted by its own actions. Indigenous people rejected the idea, and then Congress was forced to accommodate them. For example, Knox pointed out, "it is manifest, from the representations of the confederated Indians at the Huron Village, in December 1786, that they entertained a different opinion, and that they were the only rightful proprietors of the soil," a position to which the United States acceded when it appropriated money to buy the land in question. Knox wrote that while states had authority for the disposition of land within their boundaries, only the federal government could have authority for relations with indigenous nations, and they "ought to be considered as foreign nations."[13]

Knox argued that a conciliatory system of making treaties with indigenous people would be a much better, and cheaper, means of "managing . . . the Indians, and attaching them to the United States" than "a system of coercion and oppression." Not only would it be more expensive, but "the blood and injustice" of it "would stain the character of the nation . . . beyond all pecuniary calculation." Knox placed heavy emphasis on U.S. "character" or legitimacy, contrasting the United States with Britain (which didn't have much character, in his opinion) and observing that "the obligations of policy, humanity, and justice, together with that respect every nation sacredly owes its own reputation, unite in requiring a noble, liberal, and disinterested administration of Indian affairs."[14] This was not entirely magnanimous: at that moment, the United States didn't have much choice but to recognize indigenous ownership. Knox and U.S. officials made a virtue out of necessity, incorporating recognition of indigenous ownership into their exceptionalist understanding of the United States.

Knox outlined a policy of nascent liberal imperialism—nascent in the sense that the United States didn't yet have overwhelming control of relations with indigenous nations. He positioned the United States as benevolent reformer and indigenous people as in need of civilizing. He assumed that, the superiority of the U.S. political system being obvious, indigenous people would surely cooperate. Ownership was the problem, however; it meant that indigenous people were still free to do what they wanted, including not sell. The difficulties that this conflict between politics and ideology presented to Euro-Americans can be seen in two well-known "private letters" from Jefferson to two of his Indian agents, both written in 1803.

Jefferson insisted on indigenous ownership, although his keenness for expansion put a great deal of pressure on the idea. Historians have agreed that he was bent on continental expansion with an apparent ruthlessness that seems difficult to reconcile with his political idealism.[15] While they tend to cling to the idea that Jefferson's professed benevolence toward indigenous people, though paternalistic, was sincere, historians have clearly established the manipulation, coercion, and aggression, couched in that benevolence, that characterized relations with indigenous people during his presidency but also in the early national period generally. Missionaries and U.S. officials were quite conscious of the ways in which they could break down indigenous polities in order to coerce indigenous people into selling land—they thought about it, tried different strategies, and gave each other advice on the topic.[16] This was long-standing practice about which Jefferson was certainly conscious. Anthony F. C. Wallace points out that in the manuscript of *Notes on the State of Virginia* (1787), in a passage in which Jefferson insisted that land had been purchased from Virginia Indians "in the most unexceptionable form," after the word "purchased" Jefferson "added, and then crossed out, the qualification: 'It is true that these purchases were sometimes made with the price in one hand and the sword in the other.'"[17] In 1803, Jefferson famously advised William Henry Harrison, his agent in Indiana Territory, to entrap indigenous people in debt to U.S.-run trading houses, "because we observe that when . . . debts get beyond what individuals can pay, they become willing to lop them off by a cession of lands."[18]

Jefferson told his agent in the south, Benjamin Hawkins, that U.S. citizenship for indigenous people was his ultimate objective: "Incorporating themselves with us as citizens of the U.S., this is what the natural progress of things will of course bring on, and it will be better to promote than retard it."[19] He advised Hawkins to keep quiet about this, however:

> It is possible, perhaps probable, that this idea may be so novel as that it might shock the Indians, were it even hinted to them. Of course, you will keep it for your own reflection; but, convinced of its soundness, I feel it consistent to pure morality to lead them toward it, to familiarize them to the idea that it is for their interest to cede lands at times to the United States, and for us to procure gratifications to our citizens, from time to time, by new acquisitions of land.[20]

Citizenship required ceding land; that was the point. Theoretically, the United States would legally acquire indigenous land with minimal trouble if Indians would volunteer to be citizens or, failing that, could somehow be coerced into it, and the imperial control of land could be reconciled without difficulty to the U.S. "character" that so concerned Knox. Indigenous resistance ruined this orderly vision. In the face of this resistance, Jefferson's appeal to the abstract realm of "pure morality" or, in the previously cited letter to Harrison, "pure humanity," reinforced the moral superiority and legitimacy of the United States and its officials while justifying coercion.

The apparent conflict between Jefferson's benevolence on the one hand and ruthlessness on the other has sometimes caused historians to reach for psychological explanations for his policies as well as his behavior.[21] It's also characteristic of much of the commentary on Jefferson and other figures considered "sympathetic" to Indians for scholars to ponder the sincerity of their benevolence, as if relations with indigenous people were only a matter of individual feeling and the point is to determine who was genuine and who was not. Paternalism was the mode of liberal imperialism, and professions of benevolence and sympathy primarily reinforced the point of Euro-Americans' moral superiority and legitimacy. Jefferson's problem was that he couldn't quite yet disengage recognition of indigenous ownership from the idea of that moral superiority. His effusions of benevolence for Indians, sincere or not, were rather more like a measure of his frustration. Forced to hang on to the principle of indigenous ownership and faced with indigenous resistance to selling, the only thing he could do, in practice, was to insist on how very much he loved his Indian brothers and wanted them to become one with the United States—while undermining them politically every chance he could get. Liberal imperialism didn't become coherent until the problem of indigenous ownership was successfully cleared away, in the society generally and in the political system in particular.

Property and Savages

By the early nineteenth century, the idea that indigenous people were exclusively hunters—who therefore, according to European law, couldn't claim possession of land over which they merely roamed—and, moreover, always had been hunters was common.[22] The idea of the Indian as exclusively a hunter was part of a larger narrative of savagism and civilization, the emergence of which Roy Harvey Pearce marks in the 1770s, with the formation of the United States. He attributes the rise of this grand, abstract narrative of civilization's conflict with and conquest of savagery in the United States in part to the influence of Scottish Enlightenment historiography, which provided the four stages theory of human history.[23] If Enlightenment history posited progress through the stages of human society from savagery to the culmination of European mercantile civilization, the Euro-American version of that history read the existence of indigenous people in North America as a kind of usurping of that order that had to be righted, where the beginning and the end of human society were locked in a battle for the future. Further, while Enlightenment history provided the frame for a narrative in which the defeat of the past by the future *must* occur, its incorporation of the agriculturalist theory of property provided the means of denying the principle of indigenous ownership. This theory is set out by John Locke in his *Second Treatise of Government* (1690), in which he defined indigenous North Americans as the exemplar of the savage in the state of nature, where property and government by definition didn't exist. This theory didn't affect North American practices in the eighteenth century, but it did gain authority over that time and permeated discussion about indigenous people by the end of the century, including in historiography. By the early nineteenth century, the theory of property that defined indigenous people as incapable of owning land and the grand narrative of savagery and civilization that contained it provided the means of redefining indigenous people as hunter-savages with no claim to ownership of land.

While U.S. historians widely acknowledge the agriculturalist theory of property in discussions of North American colonization, they haven't had much to say about the theory's colonial North American history.[24] Scholars in political philosophy and British colonial history have discussed that context at length, however, such that what historian David Armitage calls the "'colonial' reading of Locke's political theory" is well established.[25] Locke was, famously, secretary to Lord Shaftesbury and the lords proprietor of Carolina colony and wrote the *Fundamental Constitutions of Carolina* in 1669. He had a fairly extensive knowledge of the colonies and their operation, amassing a substantial collection of books on the topics of America and colonization and regularly questioning English settlers about their experiences. He also wrote extensively on the theory and administration of the American colonies.[26] In working out his theory of property, Locke implicitly and explicitly used a North American colonial setting, where indigenous people served as the embodiment of man in the state of nature.

In chapter 5 of the *Second Treatise*, Locke's professed object was to justify taking land without the consent of those who were on it: "I shall endeavour to shew, how Men might come to have a *property* in several parts of that which God gave to Mankind in common, and that without any express Compact of all the Commoners," he wrote in the opening paragraph. He then introduced "the wild *Indian*" as the inhabitant of the state of nature, where the products of nature were the common possession of all, "as [fruits and beasts] are produced by the spontaneous hand of Nature," a phrase that would be associated forever afterward with indigenous people in North America. Natural man had a property in whatever he could take from the spontaneous hand of nature in order to subsist, and natural law held that he could take as long as "there is enough, and as good left in common for others." Labor, but specifically commercial agriculture, established property in land, which led to written laws and, ultimately, government. The consent of the commoners for enclosure of commonly held land in the state of nature was not required, first, because God "commanded [man] to subdue the Earth, i.e., improve it for the benefit of Life," and, second, because "there was still enough, and as good left." Indeed, "he that leaves as much as another can make use of, does as good as take nothing at all." Those who protested such an arrangement were disputing God's will. There was "no room for Controversie about the Title, nor for Incroachment on the Right of others," Locke maintained, because "it was useless as well to carve himself too much, or take more than he needed."[27]

The quarreling and disputation Locke invoked draws one back to the historical context. With regard to the "good enough" qualification, James Tully points out that Locke had to insist that indigenous people/natural men would not be adversely affected by the taking of their supposedly vacant land, because if they were affected, he would have had to find some means of incorporating their consent into his theory.[28] His theory depended on the erasure of indigenous ownership and political society in the first instance, despite the fact that, as Tully notes, he would have been well aware that indigenous people formed political societies.[29] "As Families increased, and Industry inlarged their Stocks, their *Possessions inlarged* with the need of them," Locke wrote, "They incorporated, settled themselves together, and built Cities, and then, by consent, they came in time, to set out the *bounds of their distinct Territories*, and agree on limits between them and their Neighbours, and by Laws within themselves, settled the *Properties* of those of the same society." Indians did none of this: as they didn't desire to engage in commercial agriculture, they didn't need written laws or money, and they didn't form governments. The spontaneous hand of nature was all they needed or wanted, and they didn't therefore own any land. This doomed them to an inferiority of their own making. Because Indians refused to engage in commercial agriculture, they "have not one hundredth part of the Conveniencies we enjoy: and a King of a large and fruitful territory there feeds, lodges, and is clad worse than a day labourer in *England*."[30] But once civilized Europeans properly used the land, Locke maintained, everyone, including Indians, benefited.

Mehta points out that the notion of the consent of the governed—a government founded on "rational, individual self-interest"—deterritorialized government so that political society had no connection to history or geography. Since land had no meaning until labor was applied to it, it was "waste," according to Locke, and thus, Mehta writes, "worthless in its materiality and inert in its sentimental force," an idea that was a distinct departure from prevailing ideas about land in Europe.[31] Locke can be seen to be theoretically cleaning up the messy colonial relations in which it was his business to be involved. Confronted with indigenous people whose control of land and rules and practices, desires and demands had to be accommodated, despite their being not European and not Christian, imagining a state in which they had no political organization and made no demands and had no claims must have been quite attractive as a thought experiment.

During the eighteenth century, the agriculturalist theory of property circulated through Locke's interpreters, who included legal and political philosophers such as William Blackstone and Emeric de Vattel, prominent clergymen in the British North American colonies, as well as British historian William Robertson, an important figure in the Scottish Enlightenment whose *History of America* (1777) was the key account of North American indigenous people through the mid-nineteenth century.[32] Indians constituted the "rudest" form of human society, Robertson wrote, one that served as a living embodiment of "the infancy of social life." Indians had an "abhorrence of labour natural to the savage state," practicing an agriculture that was "neither extensive nor laborious" and meant only to supplement hunting and fishing. Indians didn't dominate nature, as God commanded, nor did they distinguish themselves much from animals, not enough to domesticate them: "They seem not to have been conscious of the superiority of their nature, and suffered all the animal creation to retain its liberty, without establishing their own authority over any one species." Indians resembled beasts of prey "both in occupation and in genius." "Being strangers to property," Robertson observed, "they are unacquainted with what is the great object of laws and policy, as well as the chief motive which induced mankind to establish the various arrangements of regular government."[33]

The confluence of the agriculturalist theory of property and the four stages account of human history can be seen in Hugh Henry Brackenridge's *Law Miscellanies* (1814), a compendium of commentaries on Blackstone, Pennsylvania law, and a variety of other legal topics. A justice of the Pennsylvania Supreme Court, better known today as the author of the satirical novel *Modern Chivalry* (1815), Brackenridge demonstrates how Robertson's conception of savagery, which allowed for some indigenous agriculture, came to be conceived as a purely hunter state, without agriculture of any kind, the better to be opposed to civilization. He also heightened the moral judgment to be made against indigenous people for refusing to engage in commercial agriculture to the same purpose. Brackenridge maintained that, in hunters, "the powers of genius are inactive, the arts and sciences remain unknown, and man continues to be an animal differing in nothing but in shape from the beasts of prey that roam upon the mountain." Hunters were "not human" because their "way of life" violated God's dictate that man should "till the ground." Furthermore, "common reason has discovered that . . . it must be most agreeable to the Creator that the earth be stored with inhabitants; and that in order to this end, a way of life be chosen in which individuals or particular nations may subsist with the least extent of territory." Indians being merely savage hunters in a state of nature, they could "therefore have but small pretence to a soil which they have never cultivated," though they might claim "those spots of ground where their wigwams have been planted, and . . . so much of the soil around them as may be necessary to produce grain to support them." He allowed that "perhaps they may have some priority of right to occupy a different country, should it be their choice to change the situation where former circumstances may have placed them."[34]

Any concession on the point was mainly owing to U.S. beneficence, however. Indians had no permanent claim to land, because when Europeans arrived, as in Locke, it was uncultivated "waste."

> The continent of North America may therefore on the first discovery of the coast, by any civilized European nation, be considered as, the greater part of it, a vacant country and liable to become the property of those who should take the trouble to possess it. Nevertheless, I do not mean to justify the waging an unnecessary war against the natives, or the extirpation of them altogether; but yet I would justify encroachment on the territory claimed by them, until they are reduced to smaller bounds, and under the necessity of changing their unpolished and ferocious state of life, for fixed habitations and the arts of agriculture. At the same time, I think it still advisable to purchase from them, if it may be done conveniently; because it is a dictate of humanity to decline insisting on the full extent of any claim of property, if it may involve the shedding of the blood of those, who though sunk beneath the dignity of human nature, yet bear the name and are seen in the shape of men.[35]

Enlightenment history allowed Brackenridge and others to redefine indigenous people in North America as those who were hunter-savages in the state of nature and who therefore couldn't, by definition, own property. And, though Brackenridge gutted the actual meaning of indigenous ownership, he retained the mechanism, the apparently scrupulously fair purchase of land, that made U.S. actions legally and morally defensible, at least to Euro-Americans. From this perspective, treaties were only formalities, since the United States already owned the land, but they also necessarily reasserted U.S. paternalism for and benevolence toward backward Indians as well as the moral superiority of the United States for having made treaties in the first place. For some among the U.S. intelligentsia, at least, indigenous ownership had been successfully contained by the early nineteenth century. The last step was to make that containment legal.

Institutionalizing the Erasure of Indigenous Ownership

The legalization came with *Johnson and Graham's Lessee v. William McIntosh* (1823), which declared indigenous people savage hunters, not landowners, making them the equivalent of tenants merely occupying their own land at the whim of the United States.[36] The case is the foundation of U.S. property law, the first case law students learn today. It's also one of the few cases of U.S. law to have had an international impact during the nineteenth century in the British colonies on the point that "native people had lost their lands by conquest."[37] It was cited as recently in the 1980s in Australian and Canadian courts for the same purpose.[38] Interestingly, then, along with the colonial history of the theory of property, it turns out that the English colonization of North America contributed some of the most substantial justifications for global European imperialism in the modern era.

In *Johnson v. McIntosh*, John Marshall redefined the existing doctrine of discovery such that, when representatives of European countries set foot on North American soil, they automatically owned all of it, as Brackenridge argued in 1814, because indigenous people were savages who had been subjected to conquest. Occupancy no longer determined ownership, as it had for British colonists; it was a temporary state indigenous people inhabited until the United States claimed its land. This was a radical change in the law, and, according to recent archival research on the case by legal historian Lindsay G. Robertson, Marshall didn't intend to make that radical change. Rather, he wished to protect preemption rights purchased by Virginians after the Revolutionary War in which he had a personal interest and that were not directly at issue in the case. After seeing what he had wrought, Lindsay Robertson argues, Marshall attempted to negate *Johnson* in his subsequent *Cherokee Nation* cases, *Cherokee Nation v. Georgia* (1831) and *Worcester v. Georgia* (1832), where he specifically endorsed the principle of indigenous ownership and political autonomy as recognized in treaties made with Indian nations.[39] Nevertheless, *Johnson* was the justification that Georgia and other states used to dispossess the Cherokees and other southern nations, and after Marshall's death in 1835 Jackson appointed Supreme Court justices succeeded in overturning *Worcester* in five cases decided between 1836 and 1841.[40] *Johnson v. McIntosh* institutionalized a liberal imperialism peculiar to the United States, intentionally or not.

Lindsay Robertson tells the exceedingly convoluted backstory of the *Johnson* decision, and in essence, he writes, it was a "collusive" case manufactured by land speculators on both sides to secure title to land grants (involving millions of acres) made during the Revolution in the Ohio Valley that were plainly illegal under the Proclamation of 1763.[41] While the case was initiated in the late eighteenth century, when Marshall wrote his decision in 1823 he changed the time frame involved to the postrevolutionary period in order to encompass the preemption rights that interested him personally. Then, in order to evade the problem of indigenous ownership, he grafted the new imperial narrative of savagery and civilization onto a legal history that, both Banner and Lindsay Robertson agree, was almost wholly invented.

Using an extended passage from his own history of North America to shore up his argument, Marshall asserted that European nations not only had the title to indigenous land but that they had always granted that land to settlers, while indigenous people still had possession and that the individual states had inherited that authority. The problem with this was, Lindsay Robertson points out, that Marshall based his argument on a reading of the significance of colonial charters to which he did not have access, citing only secondary sources consisting of an array of eighteenth-century histories of the United States, including William Robertson's *History of America*.[42] Banner describes Marshall's reading of the colonial charters and his historiography in general as "flat wrong."[43] But Marshall was plain in his argument: discovery established the "power to grant the soil, while yet in possession of the natives"; furthermore, "these grants have been understood by all, to convey a title to the grantees, subject only to the Indian right of occupancy," a right that Marshall was at that moment inventing but that he insisted had been universally recognized from the moment of the European discovery of America.[44] In this Marshall practiced what legal historian David E. Wilkins calls "retrohistory," a particular habit of the U.S. Supreme Court with respect to indigenous people, where the Court "*retroactively* [generates] an interpretation of historical events that contradicts the actual occurrence."[45]

Thereafter in his opinion Marshall sought to justify himself, and the paragraph where he turned from assertion to justification begins as follows:

> We will not enter into the controversy, whether agriculturalists, merchants, and manufacturers have a right on abstract principles, to expel hunters from the territory they possess, or to contract their limits. Conquest gives a title which the Courts of the conqueror cannot deny, whatever the private and speculative opinions of individuals may be, respecting the justice of the claim which has been successfully asserted.[46]

To start off, Marshall explicitly rejected the agriculturalist theory of property. His use of "conquest" has struck legal scholars as odd, however. Banner notes that this was the first instance in which Marshall used the word "conquest" and that it can't be explained. "Conquest was even less accurate than discovery as a theory denying Indians ownership of their land," he writes, noting also that invoking conquest allowed Marshall to distance himself from his own decision, which he "seem[ed] to have found a little distasteful."[47] Lindsay Robertson concurs, observing that in Marshall's telling "the Court was powerless to deny the adopted policy" to the point where "we were the victims of our colonial inheritance."[48]

Or world history. Marshall insisted that Indians were "fierce savages" locked in violent conflict with civilized Europeans, and there was no incorporating them as they were, as previous empires had incorporated populations subjected to conquest because Indians were so different and an anomaly in history—a prevalent theme in U.S. imperial discourse.[49] The notion of conquest is less inexplicable if you view Marshall's arguments through the emerging U.S. imperial ideology. If savagery and civilization were locked in conflict in the United States, the only possible, and inevitable, outcome was civilization's conquest of savagery. In 1789, Henry Knox wrote that there were two legitimate ways to get indigenous land: purchase or conquest. One might imagine that for Knox "conquest" was a concrete thing; he was a military man, after all, and had just led troops through a revolution. Conquest as he understood it was not possible in North America. But by 1823, because of the problems that purchasing indigenous land presented (i.e., indigenous people resisted selling), "conquest" had become an abstraction that would be put into service justifying concrete actions of the type Knox warned against, and it was implied as soon as Marshall invoked the idea of savagery. This mythological conquest allowed Marshall to deny indigenous ownership without explicitly relying on the radical notion that "agriculturalists . . . have a right . . . to expel hunters." But once he introduced the narrative of savagery in conflict with civilization, the agriculturalist theory of property that it had absorbed came along with it, even if Marshall tried—not very forcefully—to deny that he was arguing anything remotely controversial.

The idea that in the United States, *because* of the United States, civilization must and would effect a conquest of savagery was the principal discursive means by which indigenous ownership and therefore political society were erased in the period. But that erasure wasn't automatic or immediate; the point still had to be made, at least early on in the maturing of U.S. imperial ideology, in the late 1820s and early 1830s. The contention over the grand narrative of savagery and civilization's validity can be seen in two conflicting positions on Cherokee removal taken in the pages of the *North American Review* in 1830 by Jeremiah Evarts, an advisor to and defender of the Cherokees, and by Lewis Cass, then territorial governor of Michigan and soon to be Andrew Jackson's secretary of war.

In January 1830, Cass argued for removal using *Johnson* as his rationale, drawing out the immediate political implications of the savage versus civilized narrative. He argued that, as savages and hunters, Indians were the earliest form of human society; therefore, they couldn't possibly exist in contact with the highest form of human society without becoming corrupt, and the humane thing to do was to remove indigenous people from contact with civilization to some place where missionaries could work on them in isolation. This was the Jacksonians' standard argument. The fact that Indians wouldn't cooperate, no matter how benevolent Euro-Americans were, complicated Cass's plans for their improvement. "As civilization shed her light on them, why were they blind to its beams?" he asked. It was a mystery. They "resisted . . . every effort to meliorate their situation, or to introduce among them the most common arts of life," he wrote; they remained morally and intellectually "stationary."[50] Clearly, their resistance was a character flaw. While Cass was moving toward but was not quite yet at a biological explanation of difference that would soon become dominant in the United States, he relied principally on William Robertson's discussion of Indian character for his assertions.[51]

Following Marshall in *Johnson*, Cass argued that it had always been the case that Europeans claimed title to all North American land on first seeing it. If European governments claimed title to indigenous land on first sight, Cass wrote, "some peculiar circumstances must have existed to vindicate a claim, at first sight revolting to the common justice of mankind." Like Marshall, Cass introduced a new reading of North American colonial history, and it seems to have made him a little uneasy. And, as in Marshall's *Johnson* decision, the peculiarity was all owing to Indians' status as savages. They were hunters who merely roamed over their land, to which agriculturalists had a superior claim because everyone acknowledged that God willed Christians to dominate and subdue the earth, and Indians clearly did not, and therefore Europeans rightfully claimed Indian land. "There can be no doubt," Cass insisted, but "that the Creator intended the earth should be reclaimed from a state of nature and cultivated; that the human race should spread over it, procuring from it the means of comfortable subsistence, and of increase and improvement."[52]

There was plenty of doubt about this story, however. In October 1830, Jeremiah Evarts, a lawyer and secretary of the American Board of Commissioners for Foreign Missions, answered Cass with the Cherokees' argument that Marshall's discovery doctrine was based on historical untruths, that Britain and the United States had unmistakably recognized indigenous ownership and autonomy, and that the narrative of inevitable conflict between savage and civilized was absurd in light of historical facts.

> On the subject of the rights of the American aborigines, there has been much loose reasoning, and some quite as loose morality. It will be found, however, that respectable writers have more frequently been led into error by stating extravagant cases, and raising imaginary difficulties, than by examining the foundation of title to lands, or by looking at facts, as they took place on the settlement of this country.[53]

The first thing Evarts did was reject the idea that Europeans had a superior title to land "partly on the ground of superior civilization, and partly because they were common in the habit of using land for tillage, which was not generally done by the original inhabitants of America." He observed that Europeans had a right to claim unoccupied land but nothing more and asked, "How is it conceivable, that the mere discovery of a country should give the discoverers a title paramount to the title of the natives, whose ancestors had been in possession from time immemorial?" "The mere statement of the case shows the inherent absurdity of a claim, which has been so often made, that many people seem to think it reasonable," he continued.[54]

At the very least, the controversy demonstrates that indigenous ownership and its implications were widely recognized in the United States and that the idea, argued by Brackenridge and by Marshall in *Johnson* and held to be a fact by many contemporary scholars, that Euro-Americans always believed that Indians were hunters and therefore had no real claim to their own land is just not true. This was an argument that had to be made in the face of vigorous opposition from those who were unconvinced by the grand narratives put forward to support such claims—although perhaps "argument" is too strong a word because, as Evarts himself pointed out, the narrative only had to be endlessly repeated by those who benefited from it for it to appear to be true. He went on, in great detail, to argue that indigenous people had occupied the land, that their autonomy had been recognized in numerous treaties made by the United States and its imperial predecessors, and that the only moral and legal position for the United States was to recognize indigenous ownership and autonomy. Evidently, this essay had its influence on John Marshall, who made some of the same points in *Worcester v. Georgia* and who in that decision seems to have advocated a return to recognition of indigenous ownership as a means of establishing U.S. legitimacy. But that wasn't enough to stop the "blood and injustice" of imperial expansion or the power of the imperial ideology that fueled it.

Benevolence and Delusion

Indigenous ownership was the problem that faced U.S. imperialism at the turn of the eighteenth century, and it was complicated by how U.S. nationalist discourse incorporated the recognition of indigenous ownership as a signifier of moral and political superiority. The solution, as outlined here, was to redefine indigenous people as those who couldn't own land or form legitimate governments because they were savages. If recognizing indigenous ownership established a relationship of rough equality between the United States and indigenous nations, the new relationship was one of political oppression, but oppression masked by imperial benevolence. Accordingly, the proof of U.S. moral and political superiority was no longer recognition of ownership but the benevolence and paternal care expressed for Indians as backward children. Imperial benevolence and its many cultural forms—picturesque representations of ideal (dead) indigenous people, effusions of sympathy at their sad (inevitable) fate—were essential to this system of political oppression and violence.

Benevolence not only justified but construed as morally superior imperial violence—it was only doing what was right for the poor benighted Indians. It also gave colonial–imperial subjects a positive means of understanding their own place in the system. If any indigenous person embodied savagery, every Euro-American embodied civilization, and to really be civilized required *feeling* properly, benevolently, toward those poor benighted Indians. This doesn't mean that everyone did, of course, although an orientation toward benevolence would seem to be the case, especially with political and cultural elites. Having a population that could learn to feel better about itself for having the right feelings would also seem to be much more effective in the normalization of imperialism than just hating Indians as racially other. The imperial ideology that erased (because it had to) indigenous ownership and political society tied Euro-American subjectivity itself to that erasure at a very basic level. Americans were civilized, not savages, and the salient point about savages was that they didn't and couldn't own land.

The philosopher Charles Mills proposes a "racial contract" as a mirror to the theoretical social contract, arguing that as the social contract describes a society founded on consent, the racial contract describes a society founded on exclusion (and within this paradigm the remedy for indigenous people is not inclusion but recognition). As a part of his analysis he posits an "epistemology of ignorance": "One has to learn to see the world wrongly," he writes, "but with the assurance that this set of mistaken perceptions will be validated by white epistemic authority, whether religious or secular." To live in a racial polity, white individuals must learn to misinterpret what they experience, so that, in the case of indigenous people, every indigenous person, every event, everything associated with them must be understood in light of this narrative of savagery and civilization. "Part of what it means to be constructed as 'white' is a cognitive model that precludes self-transparency and genuine understanding of social realities," Mills continues. "White signatories [of the racial contract] will live in an invented delusional world, a racial fantasyland."[55] It *is* an "invented delusional world" in the nineteenth-century United States: consider the bizarre nature of actually believing that savagery and civilization—abstractions—were battling it out in the United States itself, and that, in some way, you yourself were a part of this battle, and that every indigenous person whom you might in some way encounter embodied this world-historical phenomenon and indeed was a walking abstraction—proof, one way or another, that conquest was at hand. On the face of it, anyway, this seems rather more complex than straightforward racial exclusion if only because it implicates all of human history and the United States itself as the culmination of human history. It's a bit breathtaking—breathtakingly insane—when you think about it. At least from those who've left a record, it's clear that this is the way that many people in the United States in the nineteenth century thought, as a matter of course, without self-consciousness, about themselves and their country. The point is, they *had* to.

The expressions of benevolence or sympathy for or sentimental representations of Indians, no matter how "sincere" they may appear to be, are never not ultimately about political oppression and violence. To put it another way, expressions of benevolence are never *only* expressions of individual feeling; they are always part of a larger system of thought. The fact that many scholars still often read benevolence, sympathy, and sentiment directed at indigenous people as merely individual is only an effect of the depoliticizing of indigenous people in U.S. imperialist thought. Indigenous people have understood how this system worked and have been describing it more or less from the moment they started writing in English. Toward the end of his *Eulogy on King Philip* (1836), William Apess mocked Andrew Jackson:

> You see, my red children, that our fathers carried on this scheme of getting your lands for our use, and we have now become rich and powerful; and we have a right to do with you just as we please; we claim to be your fathers. And we think we shall do you a great favor, my dear sons and daughters, to drive you out, to get you away out of the reach of our civilized people, who are cheating you, for we have no law to reach them, we cannot protect you although you be our children. So it is no use, you need not cry, you must go, even if the lions devour you, for we promised the land you have somebody else long ago, perhaps 20 or 30 years; and we did it without your consent, it is true. But this has been the way our fathers first brought us up, and it is hard to depart from it; therefore, you shall have no protection from us.[56]

His analysis was somewhat compressed, but Apess pretty much covered the principal issues in U.S. imperialism: the redefinition of preemption; the erasure of indigenous consent and autonomy; the insistence that it was all inevitable, no one's fault, and all for everyone's good besides; and finally, the maddeningly cloying professions of paternal benevolence in which such violence was delivered.

The abstractions of U.S. imperial discourse allow it to operate particularly insidiously, as William Appleman Williams pointed out, and imperial delusion persists. The narrative of civilization's conquest of savagery has come in handy, for example, when the U.S. government has wanted to justify taking land or resources from some other sovereign nation around the world without its consent. Since government has no inherent connection to land, history, or tradition, the universalized U.S. conception of democracy—the current analogue of "civilization"—can be projected onto any place. "Democracy" can then be metaphorically or sometimes literally dropped onto another sovereign nation, and if those who are dropped upon protest, then they must not be morally fit for this most perfect form of government. If the people have reason, then they will acquiesce to this benevolent introduction of civilization; if they don't, as Locke himself put it, then they "may be destroyed as a *Lyon* or a *Tyger*, one of those wild Savage Beasts, with whom Men can have no Society nor Security."[57] This narrative makes sense to Euro-Americans because it is part of their imperial heritage. It's an absurd and dangerous way of thinking, but it's normal for Euro-Americans, and it became normal because of the history of imperial relations with indigenous people in North America.

Notes

1. For example, see Linda Colley, "Imperial Trauma: The Powerlessness of the Powerful Part 1," *Common Knowledge* 11, no. 2 (2005): 198–214; Bernard Porter, *Empire and Superempire: Britain, America, and the World* (New Haven, CT: Yale University Press, 2006); and Neil Smith, *The Endgame of Globalization* (New York: Routledge, 2005).

2. William Appleman Williams, *Empire as a Way of Life* (New York: Oxford University Press, 1980).

3. See the critique of contemporary advocates of liberal imperialism, such as Niall Ferguson, in Chalmers Johnson, *Nemesis: The Last Days of the American Republic* (New York: Metropolitan Books, 2006), 71–89. Writers on the history of liberalism often remark that the term "liberalism" itself dates from the early nineteenth century and was applied retroactively. They also point out that liberalism and imperialism are "mutually constitutive" (David Armitage, "John Locke, Carolina, and the *Two Treatises of Government*," *Political Theory* 32, no. 5 [2004]: 602), or, as Uday Singh Mehta puts it, "the urge to [imperialism] is *internal*" to liberalism (*Liberalism and Empire: A Study in Nineteenth-Century British Liberal Thought* [Chicago: University of Chicago Press, 1999], 20).

4. Mehta, *Liberalism and Empire*, 30–31.

5. Ibid.

6. For recent works discussing U.S. imperialism that either reiterate the liberal consensus on Indians or leave out indigenous history altogether see Walter Nugent, "The American Habit of Empire, and the Cases of Polk and Bush," *Western Historical Quarterly* 38, no. 1, http://www.historycooperative.org/journals/whq/38.1/nugent.html, accessed April 21, 2007; Sandra M. Gustafson, "Histories of Democracy and Empire," *American Quarterly* 59, no. 1 (2007): 107–33; Thomas Bender, *A Nation among Nations: America's Place in World History* (New York: Hill and Wang, 2006); and Charles S.

Maier, *Among Empires: American Ascendancy and Its Predecessors* (Cambridge, MA: Harvard University Press, 2005). This is just a small sampling.

7. Stuart Banner, *How the Indians Lost Their Land: Law and Power on the Frontier* (Cambridge, MA: Harvard University Press, 2005), 20, 43, 29.
8. See Dale Turner, *This Is Not a Peace Pipe: Towards a Critical Indigenous Philosophy* (Toronto: University of Toronto Press, 2006).
9. Lindsay G. Robertson, *Conquest by Law: How the Discovery of America Dispossessed Indigenous People of Their Lands* (Oxford: Oxford University Press, 2005), 99–100.
10. *Marshall v. Clark*, Va. S. Ct. (1791).
11. Banner, *How the Indians Lost Their Land*, 163.
12. U.S. Senate, *Report from Henry Knox, Secretary of War, to the President of the United States, Relating to the Several Indian Tribes*, 1st Cong., 1st sess., August 7, 1789, 13.
13. U.S. Senate, *Report*, 13, 53.
14. Ibid.
15. See Robert M. Owens, "Jeffersonian Benevolence on the Ground: The Indian Land Cession Treaties of William Henry Harrison," *Journal of the Early Republic* 22 (Fall 2002): 405–35.
16. Bernard Sheehan, *Seeds of Extinction: Jeffersonian Philanthropy and the American Indian* (New York: W. W. Norton, 1974), 165–66.
17. Anthony F. C. Wallace, *Jefferson and the Indians: The Tragic Fate of the First Americans* (Cambridge, MA: Harvard University Press, 1999), 23–24.
18. Thomas Jefferson to William Henry Harrison, February 27, 1803, in *Political Writings*, ed. Joyce Appleby and Terrence Ball (Cambridge: Cambridge University Press, 1999), 525.
19. Thomas Jefferson to Benjamin Hawkins, February 18, 1803, in *Political Writings*, ed. Appleby and Ball, 522.
20. Ibid.
21. See, for example, Peter Onuf, *Jefferson's Empire: The Language of American Nationhood* (Charlottesville: University of Virginia Press, 2000), especially chapter 1; and Jeffrey Ostler, *The Plains Sioux and U.S. Colonialism from Lewis and Clark to Wounded Knee* (Cambridge: Cambridge University Press, 2004), 13–15.
22. Banner, *How the Indians Lost Their Land*, 152, 168. Banner cites both Arneil and Tully but dismisses their arguments; he seems to think they are arguing that Locke's theory of property was the legal norm in the British North American colonies, which they are not (47–48). Banner consciously narrows his focus to property alone and resists addressing the political valence of relations between indigenous people and Euro-Americans, which leads to his regular musing on how it was that a particular Euro-American writer could deny the history of indigenous ownership when it was a clearly established legal principle at the time.
23. Roy Harvey Pearce, *Savagism and Civilization: A Study of the Indian and the American Mind* (Berkeley: University of California Press, 1988), 4, 89, 91.
24. Barbara Arneil, *John Locke and America: The Defence of English Colonialism* (Oxford: Clarendon Press, 1996), 15–16.
25. Armitage, "John Locke," 603.
26. James Tully, "Rediscovering America: The Two Treatises and Aboriginal Rights," in *An Approach to Political Philosophy: Locke in Contexts* (London: Cambridge University Press, 1993), 140–41, 145–48; Bhikhu Parekh, "Liberalism and Colonialism: A Critique of Locke and Mill," in *The Decolonization of the Imagination: Culture, Knowledge, and Power*, ed. Jan Nederveen Pieterse and Bhikhu Parekh (London: Zed Books, 1995), 83.
27. John Locke, *Two Treatises of Government*, ed. Peter Laslett (Cambridge: Cambridge University Press, 2000), 286, 288, 291, 302.
28. James Tully, *Strange Multiplicity: Constitutionalism in an Age of Diversity* (Cambridge: Cambridge University Press, 1995), 74.
29. Tully, "Rediscovering America," 149–51. See also Vicki Hsueh, "Giving Orders: Theory and Practice in the Fundamental Constitutions of Carolina," *Journal of the History of Ideas* 63, no. 3 (2002): 425–47.
30. Locke, *Two Treatises*, 295, 296–97.
31. Mehta, *Liberalism and Empire*, 120, 125, 126.
32. Arneil, *John Locke and America*, 182–83; Pearce, *Savagism and Civilization*, 82–91.
33. William Robertson, *The History of America* (Edinburgh: Stirling & Slade, 1819), 51, 115, 121, 127–29.
34. Hugh Henry Brackenridge, *Law Miscellanies: An Introduction to the Study of Law* (Philadelphia: P. Byrne, 1814), 124, 125.

35. Brackenridge, *Law Miscellanies*, 125.
36. Sidney L. Harring, *White Man's Law: Native People in Nineteenth-Century Canadian Jurisprudence* (Toronto: Published for the Osgoode Society for Canadian Legal History by the University of Toronto Press, 1998), 89.
37. *Johnson and Graham's Lessee v. William McIntosh*, 21 U.S. (8 Wheat.) 543 (1823).
38. Robertson, *Conquest by Law*, 144.
39. *Cherokee Nation v. Georgia*, 30 U.S. (5 Pet.) 1 (1831); *Worcester v. Georgia*, 31 U.S. (6 Ret.) 515 (1832); Robertson, *Conquest by Law*, xi–xii.
40. Banner, *How the Indians Lost Their Land*, 188.
41. Early on, Robertson writes, the plaintiffs attempted to use a forged British document that supposedly allowed individuals or nongovernmental groups to buy land from indigenous people: the document they forged pertained to India, and the plaintiffs merely added an *n* (*Conquest by Law*, 4).
42. Robertson, *Conquest by Law*, 100–101.
43. Banner, *How the Indians Lost Their Land*, 183.
44. *Johnson v. McIntosh*, 574.
45. David E. Wilkins, *American Indian Sovereignty and the U.S. Supreme Court: The Masking of Justice* (Austin: University of Texas Press, 1997), 303.
46. *Johnson v. McIntosh*, 588.
47. Banner, *How the Indians Lost Their Land*, 185, 186.
48. Robertson, *Conquest by Law*, 112–13.
49. *Johnson v. McIntosh*, 590.
50. Lewis Cass, review of *Documents and Proceedings Relating to the Formation and Progress of a Board in the City of New York, for the Emigration, Preservation, and Improvements of the Aborigines of America*, North American Review 30, no. 66 (1830): 72.
51. See Reginald Horsman, *Race and Manifest Destiny: The Origins of American Racial Anglo-Saxonism* (Cambridge, MA: Harvard University Press, 1981); and James Brewer Stewart, "SHA Roundtable: Racial Modernity," *Journal of the Early Republic* 18, no. 2 (1998): 181–237.
52. Cass, review, 76, 77.
53. Jeremiah Evarts, review of *Speeches on the Indian Bill*, North American Review 31, no. 69 (1830): 397.
54. Evarts, review, 397.
55. Charles W. Mills, *The Racial Contract* (Ithaca, NY: Cornell University Press, 1997), 18.
56. William Apess, *Eulogy on King Philip*, in *On Our Own Ground: The Writings of William Apess, a Pequot*, ed. and introduction by Barry O'Connell (Amherst: University of Massachusetts Press, 1997), 307. The most recent edition of the standard *Norton Anthology of American Literature* describes Apess as a "tragic figure" who felt "betrayed" by U.S. "culture" ("William Apess," *Norton Literature Online*, http://wwwv2.wwnorton.com/college/english/naal7/contents/B/authors/apess.asp, accessed December 3, 2007).
57. Locke, *Two Treatises*, 274. See also Parekh, "Liberalism and Colonialism," 88; Tully, "Rediscovering America," 143–45.

MAUREEN KONKLE is an associate professor at the University of Missouri in the English Department. Her research focuses on Native Studies and American Literature. Specifically, Dr. Konkle specializes in nineteenth-century Native writing.

Jessica R. Stern

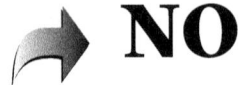

A Key into *The Bloudy Tenent of Persecution*

Roger Williams, the Pequot War, and the Origins of Toleration in America

> *We often read of his influence on the Indians. I cannot recall a suggestion, on the other hand, that the Indians might have been good for Roger Williams.*
> —J. Lewis Giddings,
> "The Indians and Roger Williams"

War is often a site where competing groups draw concrete lines between themselves and their foes, articulating preexisting conceptions of their identities and, as the war progresses, locating new characteristics that set themselves apart from their enemies. In colonial New England, scholars have argued, settlers asserted their difference from, and dominion over, New England's Native American population during the Pequot War (1637–1638) and King Philip's War (1675–1676). In her influential work, *The Name of War: King Philip's War and the Origins of American Identity*, Jill Lepore revealed that the Puritan elite used language and narrative to cast themselves as a civilized and law-abiding people, as opposed to their Native American enemies and Spanish colonial competitors.[1] More recently, scholars have turned their attention to the earlier Pequot War arguing that New England settlers established long-lasting symbolic and physical methods of domination over both combatant and noncombatant Native Americans.[2] The New Engenders' brutality during the Pequot War, which some scholars categorize as genocidal, was predicated on the Puritans' belief in a divine narrative that cast the settlers as defenders of Christianity and the unconverted Native Americans as the devil's instruments.[3] In this scenario, the New Englanders had to defeat the Pequot Indians, who were the natural enemies of Christianity, in order to establish a godly colony.[4] The settlers embraced violence with religious fervor. The Pequot War was a watershed event; Native Americans lost any chance of being accepted, as equals, into white Christian society.[5]

This article posits that the Pequot War and its aftermath affected another colonist, Roger Williams, in a dramatically different way.[6] At the beginning of the war, Williams conflated Pequot actions with unholy superstition, espousing views that were similar to those of his Puritan neighbors. The war convinced Williams, however, that religion never justified violence, and that Native Americans and Europeans shared a moral code. Williams spent the remainder of his life arguing that people of various religions could join together in civil society and that "the sword of the Lord" was spiritual in nature and should never be used for civil or physical ends. Williams provides a case study for historians who are increasingly asking how lived experience affected the debate on religious toleration. In an early modern European world, where the accommodation of different cultures and religions often led to ritualized violence, Williams provides an example of an individual who questioned claims about religious exclusivity after living in a culturally pluralistic environment.[7]

As I demonstrate in this article, not only did Williams become committed to achieving peace through toleration during the war but he also developed a number of rhetorical strategies and dispute-resolution methods that he later replicated in his writings on peace in pluralistic societies. Williams fully articulated his argument against religious violence and his manual for peaceful coexistence in the two pamphlets he published following the war: an ethnographic language guide to the Narragansett Indians titled *A Key into the Language of America* (1643), and a plea for religious toleration titled *The Bloudy Tenent of Persecution* (1644).

Despite the fact that these two works were published within 10 months of each other,[8] few scholars have examined the relationship between Williams's ethnographic and

---

Stern, Jessica R., "A Key into the Bloudy Tenent of Persecution: Roger Williams, the Pequot War, and the Origins of Toleration in America," *Early American Studies*. Copyright ©2011 The McNeil Center for Early American Studies. Used with permission of University of Pennsylvania Press.

tolerationist thought. Much of the existing work that does discuss *A Key* and *The Bloudy Tenent* in tandem suggests that Williams's religious ideas determined his discussion of Native American culture, rather than viewing the two bodies of thought as being in dialogue with each other.[9] Increasingly, scholars are suggesting that the Narragansetts directly influenced Williams's larger body of thought. The philosopher Scott L. Pratt, the pioneer of this stance, forcefully argues that Williams integrated Narragansett ideas about interaction, pluralism, community, and growth into his ideas of religious toleration. But most scholars who mention, tentatively, that Williams's intellectual development must owe something to the Native Americans have yet to offer a systematic argument about the linkages. Patricia Rubertone, an anthropologist, writes, "It is tempting to say that they were 'only' Indians and therefore did not warrant consideration equal to that of others whose lives intersected Williams's. Yet it seems that they were as instrumental in shaping the course of Williams's life in seventeenth-century New England as he was in representing them to later generations of European Americans." Rubertone's groundbreaking work, however, is focused on the Narragansetts and *A Key*; an analysis of Williams's tolerationist ideas is outside its purview. The philosopher Martha Nussbaum, who offers a wide-ranging examination of liberty of conscience in America, writes about his interactions with the Narragansetts, "Williams's experience of finding integrity, dignity, and goodness outside the parameters of orthodoxy surely shaped his evolving view of conscience." But Nussbaum's decision to examine only Williams's tolerationist texts and not his writings about Native Americans makes her (correct, I would argue) hunch suggestive and deserving of further inquiry.[10]

This article contributes to this emerging field of study by suggesting that the letters that Williams wrote during the Pequot War and its aftermath provide a body of sources we can use to understand how he pieced together an argument for toleration while living among the Native Americans. Tracing Williams's developing thought during the Pequot War reveals that his ideas about religious freedom were products of his experiences in America, and in particular his reflections on Native American and English settler interactions. This argument offers an alternative to the standard view of Williams as a man who was dedicated to the cause of liberty of conscience from the time he landed in Massachusetts Bay in 1631, a vision that is largely the effect of scholars using Williams's mature (post-1643) writings to understand the sparsely documented stances he took while in Massachusetts Bay (1631–1635). Though his contemporaries viewed him as ever transforming, and even volatile, this image depicts him as static.

The upstreaming method is also problematic because historians have shown that before 1640 there was nary a voice in England that argued against a magistrate's right to punish religious transgressions, which makes suspect the argument that Williams's ideas for toleration were intact before that time.[11] Therefore, we should look for indications of Williams's developing thought during his life in America and take advantage of the letters he wrote from 1636 to 1640.

An analysis of those letters demonstrates that two positions in Williams's argument for religious and cultural toleration grew out of his experiences as a mediator during and after the Pequot War: first, complete cross-cultural and cross-religious understanding, assimilation, and conversion were unattainable; second, civil peace relied on transcending these cultural and religious differences by locating preexisting universal similarities. His first conviction resulted from his witnessing the settlers' indiscriminate and brutal treatment of the neighboring Native Americans during and after the Pequot War. The settlers, Williams came to believe, simply did not have the capacity to determine which Native Americans were friends and which were foes, and they had no qualms about wrongfully convicting and abusing innocent Native Americans in the name of Christianity. This distrust in people's ability to judge one another accurately underlies a key argument in *The Bloudy Tenent of Persecution*, that civil authorities could not be trusted to judge one's spiritual state accurately, and thus should not have the power to persecute one for one's religious beliefs or practices. Williams's second conviction about universal moral similarities originated from the time he spent living with the Narragansetts and the work he performed after the Pequot War to protect New England Native American groups and individuals from the colonists' abuses. He would protect these Native Americans by explaining to Massachusetts Bay officials that they had a fully developed sense of morality that was indistinguishable from that of Christian Europeans and thus could be trusted as neighbors. This claim dominates *A Key to the Language of America*. In *The Bloudy Tenent*, this point is crucial to Williams's argument for religious toleration because it allows him to make the case that all individuals can be trusted to live in society without being forced to convert. In fact, for Williams, peace relies on building a society around these shared moral convictions, and not around Christianity.

The first part of this article argues that while living in Massachusetts Bay, Williams was animated by ecclesiological arguments regarding church purity, which encouraged him to express the radical separatist ideas that led to his expulsion. Shortly after Williams fled to Providence,

Massachusetts Bay officials asked him to work on their behalf to prevent the Narragansetts from aligning themselves with the Pequots in what became the Pequot War. The second part analyzes Williams's involvement in the war and its aftermath, identifying the development of his dedication to, and strategy for achieving, peace. The final section analyzes *A Key to the Language of America* and *The Bloudy Tenent of Persecution*, uncovering the arguments that had their genesis in Williams's Pequot War letters.

***

Roger Williams was not always preoccupied with civil peace and the appropriate role of religion in civil government. He was an ever-evolving figure with a willingness to follow his "tender Conscience" wherever it guided him.[12] Those closest to him were at times taken aback by the "newfound practices" he charged into.[13] His decision to move from England, where he was working as a chaplain for a Puritan-leaning family, to America was no exception. Like many of the Puritans who arrived in New England in the late 1620s and 1630s, Williams was fleeing the policies of William Laud, who was appointed bishop of London in 1628 and archbishop of Canterbury in 1633. Religious nonconformists, who refused to lecture from the official Prayer Book, wear a hood and surplice and conform to other ecclesiological practices that many deemed popish were subject to fines, imprisonment, and even physical torture.[14] Williams had turned down a "new England call" in 1629 but, after a startling illness in late 1630, which he probably interpreted as a divine message, he boarded a New England–bound boat, later explaining that his "conscience was persuaded against the national church and ceremonies, and bishops."[15]

Williams arrived in Boston less than a year after John Winthrop and his followers had landed with a patent to establish the Massachusetts Bay Colony. New England was a young region, and though most inhabitants agreed that the Anglican Church needed to be reformed, there was little consensus on doctrine, liturgy, or whether the New England churches should separate from the Anglican Church.[16] Williams, whom Plymouth Governor William Bradford described as "a man godly and zealous, having many precious parts but very unsettled in judgement," spent his time in Massachusetts Bay refining his beliefs about church purity.[17] More than once Williams's unfolding "singular opinions," and his habit of attempting "to impose them upon others," put him at odds with church members, which forced him to move constantly between Boston, Plymouth, and Salem, until the Massachusetts Bay General Court eventually ordered his expulsion back to England, which he escaped by fleeing south and founding Providence.[18]

Though Williams created controversy because of some of his ideas about proper conduct within the church, such as insisting that women wear veils, he was most focused on ensuring that the church was composed only of visible saints who did not have communion with corrupt churches. He was critical of the Church of England, which was indiscriminate in its membership, and the Boston Church, which posited that individuals could progress toward salvation and remain in the church.[19] Williams believed, like Congregationalist Puritans, that all members of the church, including the ministers, were spiritual equals who kept the church in balance; thus, one unregenerate member could jeopardize the spiritual well-being of the entire church.[20] Williams monitored the New England churches to ensure that church elders and ministers respected this equality and did not seize control of the church away from the church members. He harshly chastised elders at the Church of Boston when they failed to share a letter from the Church of Salem with the "whole bodie" of the church.[21]

Committed to these beliefs about church member equality and purity, Williams stood with separatist Puritans who demanded that church members sever their relationships with the tainted Church of England and refrain from mingling spiritually with the unregenerate.[22] Williams argued that "if a person uncleane by a dead body, touch holy things, those holy things become unclean unto him." Likewise, "Ordinances practiced by persons polluted through spirituall deadnesse and filthinesse of Communion, they become uncleane unto them, and are prophaned by them."[23] His criticisms of Massachusetts Bay policies reflected this conviction that if a civil authority required the unregenerate to enact certain religious practices, then the true believers would be contaminated in the process. The four positions that ultimately led the Massachusetts General Court to banish Williams stemmed from this conviction. First, Williams demanded that all New England churches separate from the impure Church of England, and further that no church members pray with a member of the Anglican Church or listen to an Anglican minister while visiting England.[24] Second, he claimed that the term *Christendom*, which included the wicked under a religious heading, was a fallacious construction that was harmful to the true believers; thus, England could not claim title to Native American land on the basis that it was a Christendom.[25] Third, Williams argued that magistrates could not enforce the first table of the commandments, specifically the observance of the Sabbath.[26] This insistence followed from his belief that compelling the unregenerate to attend services would undermine and defile the church.²⁷ And finally, Williams maintained that "a magistrate ought not to tender an oath to an unregenerate man, for that he thereby have communion with a wicked man in the worship of God, and cause him to take the name of God in vain."²⁸

Though Williams's criticisms of the colony had civil implications, his concern was squarely with religious purity, a point made by John Cotton, who convinced the General Court that Williams was best dealt with by the Boston ministers.²⁹ In his first letter to John Cotton, written two weeks after his departure from Massachusetts Bay, Williams remained focused solely on the topic of church pollution and separation, breathing not a word about the separation of church and state or liberty of conscience.³⁰ We can see in the pre-1636 Williams a desire to limit the authority of the government over religious matters, but we would be wrong to assume that his ideas about religious toleration, as they would appear in *The Bloudy Tenent* in 1644, were fully formed at this time. Could Williams have developed a robust theory of religious toleration on the basis of his fear that civil compulsion would corrupt standing churches? Yes, of course. Other tolerationists did just that.³¹ But ultimately, that ecclesiological argument did not animate *The Bloudy Tenent*. As Martha Nussbaum convincingly demonstrates, in his published writings on religious toleration (all written after 1643), Williams was not concerned about the corruption of the church that might ensue if the state was given religious authority;³² yet this was his primary concern when he lived in the Bay colony. Williams may have, in the words of Edmund Morgan, "reached his conclusion [about religious liberty] in some intuitive way before he had fully articulated the premises that underlay it," but the intervening seven years, and particularly the Pequot War, would provide Williams with justifications for, and elaborations on, what was in 1635 a defense of religious liberty rooted exclusively in ecclesiology.³³ Always one to speak in metaphors, Williams claimed in 1652, when sketching the history that led him to his beliefs about religious toleration, that his travels had been "directed by a naked Indian boy."³⁴

In October 1635, Massachusetts Bay magistrates lost patience with Williams and ordered him to leave the colony within six weeks. He fled, first into Narragansett Indian territory, and then to the land he obtained from the Narragansetts, which would become Providence and later Rhode Island. Williams had become acquainted with New England Native American groups before his banishment. While living in Plymouth and Salem, he made a living through trade, following in the footsteps of his father, who was a merchant in London.³⁵ He also ventured into neighboring towns to immerse himself in Algonquian, later describing a "Constant Zealous desire to dive into the Natives Language."³⁶ This interest in Algonquian was twofold, springing both from a desire to convert the Native Americans (a goal he eventually abandoned) and from a genuine interest in systems of language, which Williams demonstrated as a child when he mastered multiple languages and became an early adopter of shorthand.³⁷ He studied Native American culture and religion attentively and, in 1635, was able to provide examples of customs that bore resemblance to those of Judaism for the English Puritan minister Thomas Thorowgood to include in his book *Jewes in America*.³⁸

Williams was not driven by a deep respect for Native American culture.³⁹ He described drawing on a reserve of God-given patience to endure lodging "with them in their filthy Smoakie holes" while in Plymouth and Salem.⁴⁰ He slowly acclimated to their culture, but he rarely felt comfortable among them. He referred to their wooden beds as cold and their child-rearing practices as overindulgent, and he included the phrase "Mechemócut: *it stincks*" in a dialogue in *A Key* about their supper.⁴¹ Williams would eventually come to view their government as just as valid as European governments, but he would continue, as he stated in 1668, to "abhor most of their Customes," which were "Barbarous."⁴²

During his first year living "remote from others of our Countriemen amongst the Barbarous in this towne of New Providence," Williams found himself in the middle of what threatened to be a war between New England and the surrounding Native Americans.⁴³ Worsening frontier conditions, which pitted Connecticut settlers against the Pequot Indians, led Massachusetts Bay officials to ask Williams for his assistance (his fluency in Algonquian and familiarity with the New England natives were apparently common knowledge in New England). A series of accidental murders, unsatisfactory atonements, and increased English settlement near Pequot territory strained relations to the point where Massachusetts Bay and Connecticut colonists made preparations to march an army against the Pequots.⁴⁴ In the midst of these preparations, Boston Governor Henry Vane and the Massachusetts Bay General Council pled with Williams to use his "utmost and Speediest Endeavours" to break an emerging pan-Indian alliance by convincing the Narragansett and Mohegan Indians to ally themselves with the English. In 1670, Williams recounted the urgency and dedication with which he completed Boston's request, recalling that "the Lo. [Lord] helped me immediately to put my Life into my hand, and Scarce acquainting my Wife to ship my selfe all alone in a poore Canow, and to Cut through (a stormie Wind 30 mile in great Seas, every minute in hazard of Life) to the Sachims howse."[45] Throughout the war he worked closely with the Narragansetts to secure their alliance and to gain information about the Pequot Indians' military plans. Williams's proximity to the Narragansett territories gave him a personal incentive to intervene. He admitted to feeling ill at ease during his initial year in Providence, which he described as being "in the midst of these dens of Lyons."[46] Sir Henry Vane warned Williams to beware, for if the Narragansetts did not comply with Massachusetts' demands, Williams would find himself in harm's way.[47]

Williams's urgency was also due to the fact that he, like his Puritan contemporaries, initially believed that the Pequots were more than military adversaries; they were the devil's agents. In his first war letter, written at the time of military preparations, Williams informed John Winthrop that although the Pequots knew the settlers were preparing for war, they found comfort in their belief "that a witch amongst them will sinck the pinnaces by diving under water and making holes, etc." He hoped that "their dreames through the mercie of [the] Lord shall Vanish, and the Devill and his Lying Sorcerers shall be Confounded."[48] He replaced all Pequot rationality with superstition, designating them Satan's pawns rather than an autonomous people. At this point, Williams did not characterize their military tactics in civil rather than religious terms.[49]

As the war progressed, Williams unraveled religion from civil society. In conjunction with this shift, Williams revised his writing style to correspond with his evolving role as intermediary. In his early letters, his allegiance was solidly with New England. Christopher Felker, who has analyzed the legal dimensions of Williams's thought, characterizes Williams as Winthrop's legal adviser, or agent, in these early 1637 letters.[50] Williams revealed a detachment from both the Pequot enemies and his Narragansett informants. His terse catalog of intelligence information was devoid of the cultural exploration that characterized his later work. In a typical letter, Williams reported that the Narragansett leader Miantonomi, who offered to attack a group of Pequots without English assistance, "will put 40 or 50, or more as the Vessell will stow. He will put in Vitailes [victuals] himselfe for his men. He will direct the pinnace to the places and in the night land his men."[51] Williams secured English goods for the Narragansetts, who supplied him with information. He did not partake in bargaining himself, but rather traded information and goods from one side to the other. This position of carrier engendered a spy mentality, Williams transported information to be used for foreign purposes. Williams did not concentrate on these differences, as he did in his later letters and writings, but focused rather on the objects that were in his possession, whether information or goods.

While Williams was acting as an alliance builder and intelligence carrier, he was intimately involved in devising the New Englanders' battle plans, a fact that conflicts with his later role as peace advocate. Using information he gleaned from the Narragansetts, Williams advised Sir Henry Vane and John Winthrop about the expected length of the war (to do execution to purpose on the Pequots, will require not two or three days and away, but a riding by it and following of the work to and again the space of three weeks or a month); where the Pequots would shelter their women, children, and elderly (a marvellous great and secure swamp, which they called Ohomowauke); and from where the colonists should deploy (Nayantaquit) and keep their munitions (Aquednetick, called by us Rode-Island). The famous drawing included in Captain John Underhill's account of the attack at Fort Mystic closely resembles the advice Williams passed from the Narragansetts to Vane and Winthrop about how best to attack a Pequot fort: attack at night, so the soldiers could easily enter the Pequot homes "and do what execution they please," and lay an ambush between the fort and the nearby swamp "to prevent their flight."[52]

Days after the attack on Fort Mystic, Williams was keeping track of the movements of Native American troops as they ran from, and toward, the remaining Pequot warriors. On June 2, he recommended that the Connecticut soldiers under Captain Patrick "pursue Sasacous [a Pequot leader] in all his Motions" and that additional troops "stop for a day or 2." He apologized briefly for taking over the war plans, breaking into his orders to explain, "I conceaved (with submission) that it might save the Countrey no small charge and hazard and losse timely to advertize and give Intelligence."[53] Williams was adamant that New England defeat the Pequots quickly and decisively. When Williams heard that Winthrop was recalling troops, he urged him to reconsider, warning that it would give the Pequots more time to gain the allegiance of the Mohawks and "put many opportunities of occasionall revenge into their hand."[54]

The weeks after the Fort Mystic offensive gave Williams space to reflect on the nature of the war and evaluate his initial assumptions and goals. Throughout the remainder of his life, Williams would justify the Pequot War as a defensive war, but after the Mystic conflagration he became nervous that the leadership in the Bay colony saw this war as a religious war, a chance to stamp out all non-Christians. Some Puritans were creating pamphlets and sermons exalting a vengeful God who uprooted Satan's agents. John Underhill, for instance, defended the events at Mystic by referring to the story of David, which instructed that in the event that a people "sinne against God and man . . . the Scripture declareth women and children must perish with their parents."[55] Williams, on the other hand, increasingly invoked a God who wanted his followers to be guided more "by love and pitie then by futy, and wrath."[56] "Blessed be the holy name of the most High who breakes the Bow and cuts the spear," Williams wrote on July 10, 1637, characterizing God as an active agent of peace.[57] Though Williams's early letters were consistent with the writings of the Puritan elite in his detachment from Native American subjects, hostility toward the Pequots, and religious interpretations of the Pequots' military defeats, Williams ceased believing the Pequots were Satan's agents and instead viewed the war in civil terms. Rather than likening them to the devil, Williams wrote six weeks after the attack at Mystic that the Pequots' "treacheries exceede Machiavills."[58] Although the Pequots were "another miserable drove of Adams degenerate seede," they were, he contended, "our brethren by nature."[59] Williams himself was reevaluating his initial assumptions about Native American virtue. With surprise, he noted in the Narragansett leader Miantonomi "some sparkes of true Friendship," despite the fact that "there is no feare of God before their eye."[60] Williams was separating civil relationships from religious uniformity, and eventually he would suggest that peace was dependent on this separation.

Williams's developing devotion to peace is probably related to his growing distrust of existing churches, which culminated in his turn to Seekerism sometime between 1639 and 1643.[61] Seekers concluded that the line of apostolic succession had been broken and therefore valid churches did not exist on Earth and could not be convened until a second advent of Christ.[62] Instead of ensuring that churches were pure, as he did while in the Bay colony, Williams now shifted his goal to readying Earth for the coming apostles. As Williams explained in 1644, in the anonymously published pamphlet *Christening Make Not Christians*, apostles would not be sent to Earth until there was peace. As proof of this claim he referred to 2 Samuel 7, the story of David, who had to live in a tent until God permitted a peace that could sustain a standing house of God.[63]

Like those of most early modern ethnographers, Williams's cultural views were inseparable from his religious and civil views, and they developed in tandem.[64] He opened *The Bloudy Tenent* by promising to present "arguments from religion, reason, experience," and it was the experience of the Pequot War that allowed him to hone the peacemaking skills necessary to prepare the world for the Second Coming.[65] During July 1637, in "the midst of a multitude of barbarous distractions," Williams began to construct his first argument against religious persecution.[66] He had been carrying a letter from John Cotton for over a year. In dialogue with the Williams of 1635, Cotton's letter dealt exclusively with the topic of church purity and Williams's spiritual state. Cotton asserted that God was putting Williams in harm's way to fight against his "corrupt Doctrines." When the "sword of his mouth" did not convince Williams to change paths, God threatened Williams's life.[67] Cotton, in other words, was arguing that Williams was erring against his conscience, or willfully ignoring God's corrections.[68]

Christians called man's pipeline to God "conscience," and they struggled with the limits and accuracy of one's conscience.[69] Perpetrators of religious persecution were emboldened by their belief that they could "discern clearly the difference between such as are to be punished and persecuted, and such as are not," Williams explained in *The Bloudy Tenent*.[70] Williams had increasingly little faith in man's ability to discern another's spiritual state. As I will discuss more fully in the final section of this article, the basis of both Williams's criticism of the Pequot War and his criticism of using civil punishments for religious ends was his realization that humans lacked the ability to differentiate accurately between the godly and the ungodly.

His acknowledgment after the events at Mystic that colonists were carelessly killing all Native Americans heightened Williams's sensitivity to man's faulty judgment. During the Pequot War, Williams began to "feare that some innocent blood cryes at Qunnihticut."[71] He was suspicious of the "generall speech" circulating in New England that "all must be rooted" out for the sake of the Lord.[72] Williams believed that New Englanders were incapable of distinguishing loyal Indians from enemy Indians, and thus were killing friends whom they mistook as foes. He watched as Narragansett individuals who had fought alongside New England soldiers were hastily lumped with Indian enemies. This crisis of identification began at the attack on Fort Mystic, when the English mistakenly killed a substantial number of Narragansett Indians. Williams brushed the killings aside as an accident and asked that in future battles the New Englanders supply their Indian allies with "some yellow or red for their heads" to prevent confusion.[73] But these accidents continued to occur with great regularity, and Williams repeatedly complained that the Narragansetts and other allied Indians were being "much disregarded by many."[74] Further, loyalties and spiritual states were fluid, and the Pequots who were acting as enemies at one point might not be enemies later and thus should be spared execution. Whereas some Pequot individuals were "perswaded to fight," Williams explained, "the greater sort dissented." Williams criticized the Massachusetts Bay officials for failing to recognize that not all Pequot individuals were dangerous enemies. He became an advocate for those Pequot individuals who wanted peace, and he wrote to Massachusetts Bay in their behalf, asking for their lives to be spared.[75] In *The Bloudy Tenent*, Williams would similarly argue that God might plan to save an individual later in life, and thus man must not kill another man because of his current spiritual state or denominational membership.[76]

The summer of 1637 also marked a stylistic development: Williams's first use of transcription, or carrying verbatim messages between the Narragansetts and Massachusetts Bay officials. Miantonomi's brother Yotaash, who was transporting a letter to Winthrop, requested this method. Williams, uneasy with the prospect of Yotaash's words traveling unfiltered to Winthrop, insisted on interspersing Yotaash's request for Pequot captives with his own opinions on the matter: "Miantunnomu requests you to bestow a Pequt squaw upon him. I object, he had his share sent him. He answeres that Caunounicus receaved but a few women and keepes them: and yet he sayth his brother hath more right: for himselfe and his brothers men first laid hold upon that Company. I object, that all are disposed of. He answeres, if so, he desires to buy one or 2 of some English man."[77]

Initially a reluctant transcriber, Williams adopted the method in his subsequent letters and publications. He continued to record the dialogue between himself and the Native American speaker, sometimes transcribing the Algonquian words. Eventually, he expanded his participation from objections to questions, clarifications, and alternative explanations.[78] This role demanded that, instead of simply noting facts, he also included the logic behind the information. By so doing, he moved from being an outside observer to a participant-observer, engaging with, instead of just watching, Native Americans. Even as he objected to their claims, he began to recognize the coherence of the Native Americans' reasoning and the nature of their sense of justice.

Williams employed the transcription and dialogue method of mediation in *A Key* and *The Bloudy Tenent*. In *A Key*, an Englishman and a Narragansett engage in dialogue; in *The Bloudy Tenent*, Peace and Truth are interlocutors: peace is often charged with quoting the official positions of John Cotton or Massachusetts Bay, and Truth patiently offers counter positions. He allowed both sides to make their own judgments but also attempted to present them with a fuller picture of one another, and ultimately the interlocutors in both pieces find common ground. As Williams wrote to Winthrop, he believed that by recording the actual words of the Native Americans, he could better foster understanding. After transcribing a Narragansett leader's speech, Williams admitted he disagreed with the leader but explained, "I was willing to gratifie him in this because as I know your owne heart studies peace, and their soule good: So your Wisedome may make use of it unto others who happily take some more pleasure in Wars."[79] His determination that peace required dialogue prompted Williams to organize face-to-face meetings between New England Native Americans and English colonists who were at odds with each other.[80]

But Williams became increasingly convinced that dialogue between two peoples could not always dislodge deeply entrenched beliefs or stereotypes. He saw this clearly in his efforts to convert Native Americans to Christianity, a project he abandoned sometime after 1638.[81] He gave up on the goal of conversion because, he explained in 1644, "In matters of the Earth men will helpe to spell out each other, but in matters of Heaven (to which the soule is naturally so adverse) how far are the Eares of man hedged up from listening to all improper Language?"[82] In other words, Williams had found it possible for people to negotiate in most secular matters, but not in spiritual matters. In *A Key*, Williams revealed how tightly men held to their erroneous religious beliefs, even when confronted with the truth. For example, Englishmen who attempted to teach Native Americans the Genesis story of Creation would probably meet the following response: "Wee never heard of this before: and then will relate how they have it from their Fathers, that *Kautántowwit* made one man and woman of a stone, which disliking, he broke them in pieces, and made another man and woman of a Tree, which were the Fountaines of all mankind."[83] For Williams, this anecdote exemplified the resistance to change, particularly religious change, exhibited by all people. Williams proceeded to argue in *The Bloudy Tenent* that society could not be trusted with judging the veracity of religious beliefs, and thus all should be afforded the right to practice their religion as they saw fit. The epistemological basis of this argument, that man cannot fully recognize a new spiritual order, mirrors the conclusions he reached during the Pequot War and in *A Key*, that man could not easily read a new culture.[84]

If people could not easily understand a new culture, a mediator was needed to translate this culture into terms that were familiar and acceptable. Williams became this mediator. A year after the Mystic attack, Williams had completely replaced his earlier role of intelligence gatherer with a self-proclaimed duty to mediate disputes and dispel the rumors that ran rampant on the frontier.[85] While the Pequots no longer posed a threat to New England, the colonists continued to round up and enslave surviving Pequot individuals, sometimes treating them cruelly.[86] Even those Native American groups who had not been at war against the New England colonies were treated with immediate suspicion. Williams's goal, he wrote in August 1638, was to "negotiate their business, and save blood, whether the natives' or my countrymen's."[87] Judgment and justice were central to Williams's conception of peace after the Pequot War, and these two concepts would remain central to his argument for civil and religious peace in *The Bloudy Tenent*. He envisioned himself as "a patient and gentle hand to rectifie Misunderstanding of Each other and misprisions."[88] Williams acted as a judge by convincing the Massachusetts Bay authorities of the guilt of some Indians and the innocence of others in issues ranging from murder and theft to trespassing. His goal was to spare innocent Indians death, imprisonment, or economic dispossession. For instance, in the summer of 1638, Williams ascertained that a Pequot man named Pametesick had murdered three Englishmen who were traveling on the Connecticut River. He wrote to Winthrop, "I refer it humbly to your wisedome whether (although I desire not the destruction of the surviving Pequts but a safe dispersion of them yet) the actuall murtherers be not to be Surrendred up and this Pametesick (I am partly Confident this is he) at present apprehended."[89] He was insistent that only the guilty Pequot individual face sanction, not the entire Pequot people.

Significantly, at a time when many Puritan writers were claiming that Native Americans lacked morality, Williams had to rely on a shared sense of justice as he worked with Native Americans and New Englanders to locate, capture, and prosecute criminals on the frontier. Williams demonstrated that rather than being amoral rogues, the Native Americans professed "that what evil soever shall appeare to be done by any (Subject to them) against the Bodies or goods of the English, Satisfaction shall readily be made out of the Bodies or goods of the Delinquents."[90] Further, Williams insisted that Native American witnesses were as, if not more, reliable than English witnesses. For instance, when Massachusetts Bay officials accused Wattattaaguegin of unlawfully laying hunting traps that injured a number of horses in land newly acquired by Massachusetts Bay, Williams argued that the Natives had not been adequately informed of the new land boundaries and, further, that Wattattaaguegin saw two of the horses that the colonist claimed were maimed ride away from the traps unharmed. Williams insisted that Wattattaaguegin be allowed "to return to the Bay to enquire more perfectly the dammage." Although the Narragansetts, according to Williams, did not believe "that Wattattaaguegin broke any knowne covenant in laying his traps in that place, nor willingly wrought evil against the English," they promised that if found guilty by the English they would make any economic restitution required.[91] Williams's emerging conviction that Native Americans had a coherent and moral system of justice that was consistent with that of the English formed the basis of his arguments in *A Key* and *The Bloudy Tenent* that civil societies need not be founded on Christianity or religious uniformity.

Both Williams's New England and Narragansett contemporaries noted a transformation in him. The Narragansetts attested to Williams's competency in understanding their language, intentions, and desires; they were hesitant to attend councils with the English unless accompanied by Williams.[92] Williams's willingness to give credence to the Native Americans' views increasingly put him at odds with Massachusetts Bay elites. By the summer of 1640, he argued that the war against the Pequots had not been a holy war and criticized Europeans who used Christianity to justify murder. On catching wind "of another cause of Warr upon the Nayantaquits," Williams questioned "whether any other use of Warr and Arms be lawfull to the professours of the Lord Jesus but in Execution of Justice upon malefactors at home: or preserving of Life and the lives in defencive warr as was upon the Pequts etc.: Isay. 2. Mic. 4."[93] He recounted, with disgust, "How oft have I heard both the English and Dutch (not onely the most civill but the most debauched and profane) say, These *Heathen* Dogges, better kill a thousand of them then that we *Christians* should be indangered or troubled with them; Better they were all cut off, & then we shall be no more troubled with them: They have spilt our *Christian* bloud, the best way to make riddance of them, cut them all off, and so make way for Christians."[94] In 1654, he wrote a scathing account of the Puritan New Englanders' and Christian Indians' propensity to wage war on unconverted Native Americans. The Narragansetts, Williams claimed, were "daily visited with threatenings... that if they would not pray, they would be destroyed by war."[95] In response to these critiques, Puritan writers omitted Williams's name in all the contemporary accounts of the Pequot War, despite his indispensable contribution to the safety of the colonies.[96]

Williams protested against this marginalization. In the summer of 1638, presumably coming under suspicion for turning Indian, he wrote a letter to Winthrop asserting his English identity. He could not be considered an Indian, he argued, because he was not perfectly fluent in Algonquian: "Let me humbly beg belief, that for myself, I am not yet turned Indian, to believe all barbarians tell me.... I commonly guess shrewdly at what a native utters, and, to my remembrance, never wrote particular, but either I know the bottom of it, or else I am bold to give hint of my suspense."[97] Williams could have pointed to any number of traits while trying to set himself apart from the Native Americans. Europeans drew attention to the barbarity of Native American clothing, habitation, agricultural practices, marriage partners, and hairstyles.[98] Williams himself reported that William Baker, who was previously a Massachusetts Bay resident, had "turned Indian in nakedness and cutting of haire."[99] But Williams concentrated on one characteristic, language, and narrowly defined fluency as the ability to recognize every word, and identity as believing every word.[100]

Language and understanding were the cornerstones of mediation, and they became the focus of Williams's larger questions of religious identity. As his hopes for peace between the Native Americans and the New England settlers changed, so did his method of mediation, creating a dynamic in which understanding and peace were inextricably entwined; peace required the establishment of a shared language and the refusal to persecute those with a foreign tongue. During the war, Williams was an intelligence carrier, a transcriber, and, lastly, a cultural interpreter. Williams's mid-1637 through early 1638 letters that literally transcribed conversations he had had with the Narragansett leaders gave way to a more digested account of conversations. These post-1638 letters translated Native American demands and concerns, instead of just presenting intelligence information that would be useful to the New Englanders. Williams's role as cultural interpreter grew out of his realization that unfiltered words could easily be misconstrued if heard by a lazy or unsympathetic ear.[101] Therefore, he translated the logic of the Native Americans into cultural terms that the Puritans could understand and vice versa, ultimately constructing a cross-cultural code of morals and justice that he would present in *A Key* and refer to in *The Bloudy Tenent*.[102]

As religious sectarian violence started to brew in England, culminating in the English civil war, Williams offered the English the model for creating a peaceful civil government that he was devising in America. Williams's two manuals for peace, *A Key into the Language of America* and *The Bloudy Tenent of Persecution*, were founded on his determination that limited moral similarities could serve as the basis for peaceful civil relationships and ultimately aid in the progression of Christianity by creating a safe environment for the next apostles. Williams "drew the *Materialls*" for *A Key* "in a rude lumpe at sea" as he traveled back to London in 1643 to secure an official charter for Rhode Island.[103] While in London, he also published *The Bloudy Tenent of Persecution* in an effort to further the cause of religious tolerationist authors who were emerging in England in the 1640s.[104] In the seventeenth century, those who raised their voices in support of universal religious toleration were few, whereas "the voices in defense of religious intolerance were legion."[105] Situating himself within this budding debate about religious toleration, Williams began *The Bloudy Tenent* by reprinting parts of John Murton's anonymously published tract, *A Most Humble Supplication of the King's Majesty's Loyal Subjects* (1620). He followed Murton's tract with John Cotton's opposition to Murton's ideas of religious liberty and Cotton's "Model of Church and Civil Power," written to summarize the official position of Massachusetts Bay. Williams then rebutted Cotton's positions using biblical exegesis, historical examples, and arguments about human nature, thus reasserting Murton's key ideas: God is the only giver of truth, only spiritual weapons should be used against religious transgressions, men could be saved by God in their last hour and should be spared until then, civil government extends only to the goods and not the souls of men, and religious uniformity was not necessary for the existence of a peaceful polity. Although he did not mention previous writers on toleration, Williams supported many of the arguments made by writers in the sixteenth and early seventeenth centuries, such as Menno Simons, Sebastian Castellio, Jacob Acontius, John Smyth, Leonard Busher, and Thomas Helwys.

Like many Puritan writers, Williams cited only the Bible, making it hard to ascertain his wider intellectual influences.[106] But the similarity of his published writings on toleration and his observations and arguments that unfolded in his Pequot War letters suggests that Williams, who was an ocean away from the post-1640 emerging dialogue, arrived at these convictions and devised solutions by looking through the lens of the Pequot War. The Thirty Years' War was, for Williams, a distant atrocity; but he could begin understanding and preventing the "bloody, irreligious, and inhuman oppressions and destructions under the mask or veil of the name of Christ, &c" by analyzing the dynamics of the Pequot War.[107] This starting point is reflected in the fact that Williams roots many of his specific arguments for toleration in the dangers posed by foreign judgment.

The remaining portion of this article uncovers the arguments of *A Key* and *The Bloudy Tenent* that stemmed from Williams's Pequot War experiences. It argues that as a mediator Williams saw firsthand that humans were limited in their ability to grasp truths beyond what they already believed: the Native Americans did not accept Christianity, and the English did not accept that non-Christians could be trustworthy neighbors. But he also saw that when people concentrated on their similarities, they were able to discuss, and ultimately tolerate, their differences. The similarity common to all peoples was their desire to form moral societies and to act justly, regardless of religion. To obtain peace, he constructed a model that combined this hopefulness and this realization of human limitations. In *A Key*, Williams argued that Native Americans shared the same moral commitments as Europeans, despite the fact that the articulation of these moral commitments appeared foreign. In *The Bloudy Tenent*, he argued that peaceful societies should be based on these universal moral commitments, and therefore enforced religious uniformity was unnecessary, as well as harmful to individuals. These were both lessons he learned as a mediator during and after the Pequot War.

***

The Pequot War was still fresh in Williams's mind in 1643 when he constructed *A Key*. As he wrote about Narragansett culture in that work, he walked a fine line between presenting an unmediated Native voice and translating this voice into English.[108] Incorporating modes of mediation he devised during and after the Pequot War, Williams began each of his 32 chapters of *A Key* with the transcription method, which he called an "implicit dialogue" and which recorded Narragansett phrases across from their English translations (Figure 1). Many scholars argue that by placing a column of Algonquian words across from their English equivalents, and separating the words with a solid line, Williams perpetuated the distance the English saw between themselves and the Native Americans.[109] David Murray points out, "If we try to read across the page from Narragansett to English, we are bounced back off the Indian word increasingly quickly, so that we end up reading vertically down the English side, rather than operating in any linguistic middle ground."[110] Instead of being a failure of mediation, however, Williams deliberately used the "implicit dialogue" sections to acknowledge the gap that existed between the English and the Native Americans. He proceeded to mediate these cultural differences in each chapter's other sections.[111] Below the "implicit dialogues" Williams bridged the cultural chasms with explanatory notes and the identification of shared emotions and motives.

As you can see from the following illustration, Williams broke the solid line and spanned the two columns with a translation of Native American actions into English terms, enacting the role of cultural mediator that he perfected in his later Pequot War letters, in which he interspersed transcriptions of dialogue with explications.

His attention to war methods was particularly important, for, as Andrea Robertson Cremer has argued, New Englanders staked their claim to superiority on the argument that they embodied a more legitimate version of wartime manhood than Native American combatants. They described Native American warfare methods as chaotic and complained that in battle their Mohegan and Narragansett allies cowardly fell to the rear of the line or retreated.[112] Williams directly countered this argument by highlighting parallels in Native American and European warfare. He likened the startling war cries of the Native Americans to drums and trumpets, rendering the initially alien sounds familiar to the English. Elsewhere in the chapter he stressed that the Native Americans and the English began wars for similar reasons: anger, retribution, pride, and passion. They differed not in impulse but in actions: the Native Americans used words, sounds, and gestures to carry out

Figure 1

Page 175 from Roger Williams, *A Key into the Language of America* (London, 1643). Courtesy of the Clements Library, University of Michigan.

Of their Warre, &c.	175
Cummusquáunamuck	He is angry with you.
Matwaûog.	Souldiers.
Matwaûonck.	A Battle.
Cummusqnaúnamish	I am angry with you.
Cummusquawname?	Are you angry with me?
Miskisaûwaw.	A quarrelsome fellow.
Tawhitch niskqúekean?	Why are you so fierce?
Ntatakcómmuck qun ewò.	He strucke mee.
Nummokókunitch Ncheckéqunnitch.	I am robbed.
Mecaútea.	A fighter.
Mecâuntitea.	Let us fight.
Mecaúnteafs.	Fight with him.
Wepè cummécautch.	You are a quarreller.
Jûhettitea.	Let us fight.
Jûhetteke.	Fight, Which is the word of incouragement which they use when they animate each other in warre; for they use their tongues in stead of drummes and trumpets.

a war, whereas the English ultimately used weapons and violence. Williams explained that Native Americans "fight with leaping and dancing, that seldome an Arrow hits, and when a man is wounded . . . they soone retire and save the wounded."[113] Unlike other Puritan writers who deemed the English mode of war superior, Williams contended that because Native American wars stood on words and postures of power, they were executed, if at all, with more restraint: "Their Warres are farre lesse bloudy, and devouring then the cruell Warres of *Europe*,"[114] He continued to underline the peacefulness of Native Americans in *The Bloody Tenent* when he wrote that "the very Americans and wildest pagans keep the peace of their towns or cities, though neither in one nor the other can any man prove a true church of God in those places."[115]

His realization that non-Christian Native American communities maintained peace when Christian communities could not led Williams to unravel Christianity from a functioning civil government, a necessary step in his path toward arguing for the viability of societies that permitted liberty of conscience. Williams, like most Englishmen, believed that "a civil government is an ordinance of God, to conserve the civil peace of people so far as concerns their bodies and goods."[116] But unlike Williams, most Englishmen and New Englanders believed that, as Cotton wrote, "Civil peace cannot stand entire, where religion is corrupted," and thus orderly societies could not exist independently of Christianity.[117] As the historian Christopher Hill explains, "The function of a state church was not merely to guide men to heaven; it was also to keep them in subordination here on earth. Different societies, different churches: but to want no state church at all seemed to traditionalists a denial of all good order."[118] Secular and ecclesiastical authorities were responsible for protecting civil society from individuals who strayed from religious orthodoxy, for they could either spark divine retribution against the entire polity or engage in harmful immoral acts.[119] Thus, support for religious toleration was associated with a wide variety of social and political transgressions such as communism, sodomy, sedition, and murder.[120]

Williams vehemently disagreed with the supposition that civil peace depended on religious uniformity. He responded to the claim that "Civil peace cannot stand entire, where religion is corrupted" by retorting that the civil governments of the "wildest Indians in America" were "as lawful and true as any governments in the world," for they most effectively kept the peace by establishing "a uniformity of civil obedience" that protected the bodies and goods of individuals.[121] In *The Bloudy Tenent*, Williams was insistent that although "a civil government is an ordinance of God, to conserve the civil peace," the form of this government stemmed from man, and that "a people," including Native Americans, could "erect and establish what form of government seems to them most meet for their civil condition."[122] One could use the civil dictates of Old Testament when establishing a code of law, Williams argued, "yet who can question the lawfulness of other forms of government, laws, and punishments which differ, since civil constitutions are men's ordinances (or creation, 2 Pet. ii. 13)?"[123]

Williams laid the groundwork for the argument that non-Christian peoples could establish effective civil governments in *A Key*. He underlined his conclusion that Native Americans' moral values and sense of justice were commensurate with those of the English, a point he continually made in his post–Pequot War mediations. In fact, England's Christian communities fell far short of enacting many of these shared values, as Williams forcefully argued in his closing remarks about Narragansett government (Figure 2). Williams was not the first thinker to argue that nature, and not just the Bible, could lead people to moral actions. But for Calvin and other Christians of the Reformed tradition, who espoused a belief in natural law, sin could obscure one's ability to correctly identify and institute this universal law.[124] For Williams, moral rules were universally visible, even to pagans, despite the fact that their manifestations varied cross-culturally.[125] Take, for example, his general observation about marriage: "God hath planted in the Hearts of the Wildest of the sonnes of Men, an High and Honourable esteeme of the Mariage bed, insomuch that they universally submit unto it, and hold the Violation of that Bed, Abominable, and accordingly reape the Fruit thereof in the abundant increase of posterity."[126] God equipped every person with the knowledge of how to form the building blocks of societies. Though there were different ways of enacting the specificities of these unions (Native women, for example, performed different tasks from those undertaken by European women), respect for a social institution that ensured this sacred bond was universal.

This point must have seemed as obvious to Williams, who had spent close to a decade witnessing non-Christian Native Americans abide by a social system that was akin to that of the English, as it seemed ridiculous to his contemporaries. Williams pushed the point a step further, arguing that not only was religious uniformity unnecessary for civil uniformity but that state-enforced religious orthodoxy often unraveled civil peace and led to war, just as it did on the New England frontier. "[S]uppressing, preventing, and extinguishing such doctrines or practices by weapons of wrath and blood, whips, stocks,

Figure 2

Page 137 from Roger Williams, *A Key into the Language of America* (London, 1643). Courtesy of the Clements Library, University of Michigan.

Of their Government. 137

Observation generall, of their Government.

The wildeſt of the ſonnes of Men have ever found a necesſity, (for preſervation of themſelves, their Families and Properties) to caſt themſelves into ſome Mould or forme of Government.

More particular:

Adulteries, Murthers, Robberies, Thefts,
1 *Wild* Indians *puniſh theſe!*
And hold the Scales of Iuſtice ſo,
That no man farthing leeſe.

When Indians *heare the horrid filths,*
2 *Of* Iriſh, Engliſh *Men,*
The horrid Oaths and Murthers late,
Thus ſay theſe Indians *then.*

We weare no Cloaths, have many Gods,
And yet our ſinnes are leſſe:
You are Barbarians, Pagans wild,
Your Land's the Wilderneſſe.

L   CHAP. XIII.

imprisonment, banishment, death, & such," caused chaos, as such "alarum" hurled towns into "an uproar."[127] In contrast, the most peaceful societies permitted a range of religious beliefs and practices. "The permission of other consciences and worships than a state professeth, only can, according to God, procure a firm and lasting peace," Williams explained in his introduction to *The Bloudy Tenent*.[128] He used the example of the Native Americans to argue that peace sprung from the toleration of religious plurality. He depicted the Narragansetts as tolerant of all religions: "They have a modest Religious perswasion not to disturb any man, either themselves *English*, *Dutch*, or any in their Conscience, and worship, and therefore say: Aquiewopwauwash., Aquiewopwauwock., Peace, hold your peace."[129]

Williams's conviction that governments that permitted religious variability gave rise to peaceful societies was only one strand of his defense of freedom of conscience. His second argument, which grew out of the Pequot War, was based on his belief that individuals lacked the ability to accurately judge ideas that were foreign to them. Because of this fallibility of judgment, civil authorities should not be given the power to judge, and then punish, someone on the basis of his religious beliefs. This position stood contrary to the majority stance in England and Massachusetts Bay, where civil authorities were invested with enough disciplinary power to ensure the purity of the godly communities that were emerging with more regularity during the seventeenth century.[130] Civil authorities were charged with punishing blatant transgressions against fundamental religious doctrines, so as to protect an individual from doing irreparable harm to his soul.[131] Therefore, liberty was conceived of as the power to do what one ought and not what one willed.[132] But Williams questioned how one would be able to determine which actions were blatant transgressions. Because of his experience in New England, where he saw Massachusetts Bay officials erroneously punish non-Christian Native Americans who he knew were innocent and trustworthy, Williams was adamant that individuals were not capable of making spiritual distinctions, and thus all religious beliefs and practices should be protected in the civil sphere and corrected nonviolently in the church.

Unlike many other tolerationist arguments, which were based largely on historical precedent, much of Williams's argument was grounded in a determination about human nature: that individuals, including himself, were unable to accept and accurately judge one who was different from himself.[133] This was due to the fact that the judgments one made were always self-validating. He asked his readers early in *The Bloudy Tenent*, "If Paul, if Jesus Christ, were present here at London, and the question were proposed, what religion would they approve of—the papists, prelatists, Presbyterians, Independents, &c., would each say, Of mine, Of mine?"[134] Millions, he contended, were persuaded that their own conscience was truth, and the conscience of another was false.[135] Therefore, people simply could not be trusted as judges of each other's internal spirituality. Williams and Cotton spent a lifetime disagreeing with each other, but they agreed on most biblical dictates. What they did not agree on was one person's ability to determine if these dictates were being upheld.[136] As

Michael Kaufmann concludes after analyzing the Williams–Cotton debate, Williams's "lack of trust in interpretation" led him to argue "that ministers have no grounds upon which to base judgments about the state of an individual's soul." Williams simply did not have confidence that one's heart, language, and behavior would always be in alignment, and thus would be discernable to others.[137]

For Williams, who was eagerly awaiting the Second Coming, which would usher in a new religious order, this inability to recognize the validity of something foreign was particularly dangerous. Since "every conscience in the world is fearful, at least shy of the priests and ministers of other gods and worships, and of holding spiritual fellowship in any of their services," Williams feared that when God did send new messengers, the public would not recognize them.[138] Here he stood in unison with other tolerationist writers who feared that Jesus' messengers might be persecuted. Using the parable of the wheat and the tares, these writers claimed that because good and evil were intertwined, it was impossible for men to differentiate the saved from the damned.[139] For this reason, apostles would not be sent to Earth, Williams claimed, until there was peace and religious toleration.[140]

In developing his argument, Williams parted ways with some of the positions espoused by his contemporaries. Tolerationist writers often spoke in terms of light and darkness, claiming that the light of true religion would peacefully dispel the darkness of evil.[141] Williams rarely made such a claim about the clarity of truth. For him, "Precious pearls and jewels, and far more precious truth, are found in muddy shells and places. The rich mines of golden truth lie hid under barren hills, and in obscure holes and corners."[142] Those who were "deluded and captivated . . . against some fundamentals" were acting "not against the light, but according to the light or eye of a deceived conscience," Williams wrote, arguing against the supposition that truth dispelled all false beliefs.[143] Much like Montaigne, who also immersed himself in examples of cultural fixity, Williams concluded that belief systems were too deeply rooted to allow for the easy separation of truth from falsity.[144] How else could one explain the Massachusetts Bay officials' inability to see that although their customs were unfamiliar, neighboring Native Americans respected property rights, had a concept of just war, and abided by a system of morality? How else could one explain the Native Americans' resistance to Christianity? Watching the repeated foibles on the New England frontier, performed with an abundance of confidence, turned Williams, in many ways, into a skeptic.

There is a sense that what started as a rhetorical strategy of defending the rationality of the Native Americans after the Pequot War and in *A Key* spread far beyond that project. Now, everywhere he looked, he recognized that there was an underlying system of belief that was inaccessible to a casual, outside observer, but which, when seriously evaluated, must be classified as rational and moral. Williams went much further than many of his fellow tolerationists: he granted conscience to *every* individual. Within the first two pages of *The Bloudy Tenent* he claimed that Papists, pagans, Jews, and Turks acted according to conscience. Cotton stated that if an individual persisted in acting erroneously after several admonitions, he was no longer acting out of conscience but against his conscience; Williams denied this distinction, claiming that all individuals "are persuaded in their own belief and conscience, be their conscience paganish, Turkish, or anti-Christian."[145]

Although some historians have placed Williams in the very small group of individuals who argued unequivocally for universal religious toleration, there is evidence that he, like many tolerationist writers, saw toleration as a temporary policy that should be adopted before religious unity could be established.[146] Williams believed that only the apostles could forge this unity. Fearing that people were incapable of peacefully establishing religious unity, he lamented that only after the Second Coming, when all the irreligious people had been consumed by fire, would religious liberty be granted to everyone who was still on Earth.[147] As he had learned from his experience mediating between Native Americans and English colonists, unfiltered heterogeneity led to misunderstanding and intolerance; a bedrock of homogeneous values was a necessary precondition of acceptance. The fellowship of the godly who survived the fire would be homogeneous, Williams insisted, not consisting "of any more sorts or natures of ground [hearts of men] properly but one."[148] They would be uniform not only in heart but in action, for the new apostles would institute a uniformity of God's ordinances and an understanding of his Word. Until the time of uniformity, the most people could achieve was a dedication to peace that would provide a safe sanctuary for God's next messengers. Peace required people to establish agreement on civil principles, for people's religious state was too uneven to provide a basis for communication and peace.

In summary, after the Pequot War, Williams concentrated all his energy on revealing the injustices that ensued when an outsider who had only a superficial, and thus flawed, understanding of another group's motivations judged that group's spiritual or civil state. Following this train of logic, Williams concluded that a person could fairly judge, and be fairly judged by, only the group of which he was a part.[149] This group could be expansive; Williams presented a model in *A Key* and *The Bloudy Tenent* in which the English and the Native Americans were part of one group identified by a common moral system. But the criteria for judgment must either originate from or be adopted by the group itself.[150] Until the Second Coming, religious beliefs and practices would be disparate; thus, until that time a solid ground needed to be established through civil morality that Williams felt was universally understood and desired. Williams believed that an accepted moral system would lead, quite naturally, to secular concord if the leader united his people and acted according to their wishes. Once a person gave his consent to be ruled by a particular government, he also consented to be judged by this government in civil matters, for he was now being judged by a system to which he acceded. Only the church he consented to join could judge his spiritual beliefs and religious practices.

***

This article has suggested a reexamination of Roger Williams that looks throughout his life for transformative experiences. Much fine work has excavated the Calvinist and Baptist dimensions of Williams's thought. But it is time to consider how his experience after he arrived in Massachusetts Bay refined and altered his religious and social ideas. This article has explained the changes that occurred in Williams's ideas about religious uniformity between his first years in Massachusetts Bay in the mid-1630s, in which he was focused on church purity, and his publication of *The Bloudy Tenent* in 1644, in which he focused on civil peace, as a product of his extensive experience in various roles among the New England Native Americans during and after the Pequot War. As this article has shown, Williams personally evolved from viewing Native Americans as foreigners who were controlled by the devil to seeing them as friends who upheld the moral tenets that he was deeply committed to. He made this transition, but the majority of other colonists did not, and Williams watched with horror as they invoked Christianity to justify executions, enslavements, and other retributions, long past the point at which the Native Americans stopped posing a threat to New England security. Witnessing this process of repeated injustices made Williams skeptical of people's ability to accurately judge the virtues of, and dangers posed by, foreigners. This fear of people's capacity to judge others became a cornerstone of Williams's argument for religious toleration in *The Bloudy Tenent of Persecution*, where he argued that civil magistrates could not be trusted to evaluate the spiritual state of everyone in their jurisdiction, for nations would be, until the Second Coming, composed of people of various religious persuasions.

Williams's work as a mediator also taught him a strategy by which to establish peace among peoples who, at first glance, appeared to have different morals and customs. Williams experimented with a number of mediation methods before realizing that the transcription of Native American statements, combined with his own translation of these statements into English cultural terms, was most effective in negotiating peace between the English and Native Americans. In practicing this method, Williams began to see clearly that most of the Native American values had English equivalents. Williams explored both this methodology and this universal morality in *A Key into the Language of America*. Developing a reverence for Native American government convinced Williams that just and peaceful civil societies were not dependent on Christianity, a stance that stood counter to the majority opinion in New England and England that the only valid governments were those anchored to a Christian church. This argument provided Williams with a second major cornerstone of *The Bloudy Tenent of Persecution*: liberty of conscience would facilitate, not deter, the mission of a civil government, which was to establish peace and protect individuals. An obedience to civil morality and justice, which was universal among all people, could provide the uniformity necessary for a coherent form of government.

Although Williams's *Bloudy Tenent* did not found the call for liberty of conscience, its particular, and largely original, justifications strongly influenced the discourse of the English civil war.[151] In a discussion on the development of liberty of conscience, Nigel Smith writes, "A more durable and far-reaching method was developed by Roger Williams, whose *The Bloudy Tenent of Persecution* (1644) is one of the greatest and most original statements for religious toleration."[152] His argument caused such a stir in England that the House of Commons ordered the public hangman to throw *The Bloudy Tenent* to the pyre on August 9, 1644.[153] Religious radicals, including many individuals who later became part of the Leveller movement, found its message profound. More than 40 of the pamphlets recorded in the Thomason collection in 1644 and 1645 quote directly from *The Bloudy Tenent* and from two smaller, complementary works by Williams.[154] Suffice to say, arguments about religious toleration that took place in England owed much to the cultural encounters in America.

Notes

1. Jill Lepore, *The Name of War: King Philip's War and the Origins of American Identity* (New York: Alfred A. Knopf, 1998).

2. Andrea Robertson Cremer, "Possession: Indian Bodies, Cultural Control, and Colonialism in the Pequot War," *Early American Studies* 6, no. 2 (2008): 295–345; Michael L. Fickes, "'They Could Not Endure That Yoke': The Captivity of Pequot Women and Children," *New England Quarterly* (hereafter *NEQ*) 73, no. 1 (2000): 58–81; Ronald Dale Karr, "'Why Should You Be So Furious?': The Violence of the Pequot War," *Journal of American History* 85, no. 3 (1998): 876–909; Andrew Lipman, "'A meanes to knitt them togeather': The Exchange of Body Parts in the Pequot War," *William and Mary Quarterly* (hereafter *WMQ*) 65, no. 1 (2008): 3–28.

3. Cremer, "Possession," 300; Michael Freeman, "Puritans and Pequots: The Question of Genocide," *NEQ* 68, no. 2 (1995): 278–93; Steven T. Katz, "The Pequot War Reconsidered," *NEQ* 64, no. 2 (1991): 217–20. Ronald Karr only gingerly calls the attack of Fort Mystic genocide. He does claim that inflicting as much pain as possible against all members of society was premeditated. Karr, "'Why Should You Be So Furious?'" 902–3, 906, 908.

4. Alfred A. Cave, "Who Killed John Stone? A Note on the Origins of the Pequot War," *WMQ* 49, no. 3 (1992): 519–21; Cave, *The Pequot War* (Amherst: University of Massachusetts Press, 1996), 168–74; Karr, "Why Should You Be So Furious?" 877–78, 909; Katz, "The Pequot War Reconsidered," 221; Timothy L. Wood, "Worlds Apart: Puritan Perceptions of the Native Americans during the Pequot War," *Rhode Island History* 56, no. 3 (1998): 63–64, 71, 73.

5. Cave, *The Pequot War*, 168–78; Cremer, "Possession," 301–3.

6. Because his Puritan contemporaries wrote him out of the Pequot War, few scholars give him more than a brief mention. Francis Jennings notes that Williams was a dissenting voice; Francis Jennings, *The Invasion of America: Indians, Colonialism, and the Cant of Conquest* (Chapel Hill: University of North Carolina Press, 1975), 181. More recently, scholars have turned to Williams's letters to reconstruct the war. See Cremer, "Possession"; Lipman, "'A meanes to knitt them together.'"

7. For the emerging historiographical debate about the relationship between religious tolerance and cultural pluralism, see Marcy Norton, "Pluralism and Tolerance," *WMQ* 66, no. 2 (2009): 415–17; Stuart B. Schwartz, "Tolerance in Unexpected Places," *WMQ* 66, no. 2 (2009): 421–26. Historians of religious toleration are also beginning to examine the ways in which living in religiously pluralistic societies led individuals to come to conclusions about the meaning of toleration that were different from those held by intellectuals and political and ecclesiastical leaders; see Benjamin J. Kaplan, *Divided by Faith: Religious Conflict and the Practice of Toleration in Early Modern Europe* (Cambridge: Cambridge University Press, 2007); John Coffey, *Persecution and Toleration in Protestant England, 1558–1689* (London: Longman, 2000), 13, 116, 119, 123.

8. For a time line of Williams's publishing activities while in London, see Jonathan Beecher Field, "A Key for the Gate: Roger Williams, Parliament, and Providence," *NEQ* 80, no. 3 (2007): 357–58.

9. In his superb book on Williams's millenarian theology, W. Clark Gilpin concludes after a short discussion of *A Key* that both works were based on the same theological assertion that no existing political state was covenanted with God, and thus pagan and Christian governments were equally valid; W. Clark Gilpin, *The Millenarian Piety of Roger Williams* (Chicago: University of Chicago Press, 1979), 124. Also interested in the millenarian dimensions of Williams's theology, the literary critic David Read argues that Williams constructed *A Key* in anticipation of Christ's Second Coming, a topic that dominates *The Bloudy Tenent*. In the American wilderness represented in *A Key*, Williams could clearly see a divine plan and tentatively predict the process of conversion that would occur when Christ returned; David Read, *New World, Known World: Shaping Knowledge in Early Anglo-American Writing* (Columbia: University of Missouri Press, 2005), 95–130. Christopher Felker, a scholar of law and literature, suggests that Williams used *A Key* to explore the malleability of discourse that he first encountered in England when working as a court recorder for Sir Edward Coke. Felker proposes that this malleability gave way to the ideas of toleration in *The Bloudy Tenent*; Christopher Felker, "Roger Williams's Uses of Legal Discourse: Testing Authority in Early New England," *NEQ* 63, no. 4 (1990): 624–48.

10. Scott L. Pratt, *Native Pragmatism: Rethinking the Roots of American Philosophy* (Bloomington: Indiana University Press, 2002), 78–106; Patricia

E. Rubertone, *Grave Undertakings: An Archaeology of Roger Williams and the Narragansett Indians* (Washington, DC: Smithsonian Institution Press, 2001), 4–5; Martha Nussbaum, *Liberty of Conscience: In Defense of America's Tradition of Religious Equality* (New York: Basic Books, 2008), 47.

11. John Coffey, "Puritanism and Liberty Revisited: The Case for Toleration in the English Revolution," *Historical Journal* 41, no. 4 (1998): 962–63.

12. Williams, "To Lady Joan Barrington, ca. April 1629," in *Correspondence of Roger Williams*, ed. Glenn LaFantasie (hereafter cited as *CRW*) (Providence: Rhode Island Historical Society, 1988), 1:2.

13. Williams, "To John Winthrop, October 24, 1636?" *CRW* 1:66. Winthrop was discussing Williams's practices that caused his expulsion in 1635. William Bradford claimed that suddenly in 1633 Williams fell into some strange opinions and practices; Bradford, *Of Plymouth Plantation, 1620–1647* (New York: Modern Library, 1981), 286.

14. L. Raymond Camp, *Roger Williams, God's Apostle of Advocacy: Biography and Rhetoric* (Lewiston, N.Y.: Edwin Mellen Press, 1989), 105–6; Nicholas Tyacke, "Puritanism, Arminianism and Counter Revolution," in *The Origins of the English Civil War*, ed. Conrad Russell (London: Macmillan, 1973), 120; John A. Moore, "Roger Williams," *Baptist Quarterly* 13 (1950): 245.

15. Williams refers to the "new-England call" in "To Lady Joan Barrington, ca. April 1629," *CRW* 1:2. In a later letter, to Sir Edward Coke's daughter, he reveals why he left England; "To Mrs. Anne Sadleir, ca. April 1652," *CRW* 1:358. Williams took illness very seriously as a message from God that he had gone astray; see Williams, "To Lady Joan Barrington, ca. April 1629," *CRW* 1:5; James Ernst, *Roger Williams: New England Firebrand* (New York: Macmillan, 1932), 49.

16. Janice Knight, *Orthodoxies in Massachusetts: Rereading American Puritanism* (Cambridge: Harvard University Press, 1994), 11; Philip F. Gura, *A Glimpse of Sion's Glory: Puritan Radicalism in New England, 1620–1660* (Middletown: Wesleyan University Press, 1984), 8.

17. Bradford, *Of Plymouth Plantation*, 286.

18. John Winthrop, *Winthrop's Journal, "History of New England," 1630–1649*, ed. James Kendall Hosmer (New York: Charles Scribner's Sons, 1908), 61–62; Williams, "To John Cotton, Jr., March 25, 1671," *CRW* 2:630.

19. Immediately after his expulsion, Williams told John Cotton that it was the lack of visible saints within the New England churches and their insistence on remaining connected with the Church of England that made him break with the churches; John Cotton, summarizing Williams's argument in "To Roger Williams, ca. early 1636," *CRW* 1:35–44. For the veil controversy, see Gilpin, *Millenarian Piety*, 38–39.

20. David D. Hall, *The Faithful Shepherd: A History of the New England Ministry in the Seventeenth Century* (Chapel Hill: University of North Carolina Press, 1972), 6–7; Williston Walker, *The Creeds and Platforms of Congregationalism* (Philadelphia: Pilgrim Press, 1969), 103–4; John Robinson, *The Works of John Robinson*, ed. Robert Ashton (London: John Snow, 1851), 257; Edmund Sears Morgan, *Roger Williams: The Church and the State* (New York: Harcourt, Brace and World, 1967), 18–22; Gilpin, *Millenarian Piety*, 30–35.

21. "The Church at Salem to the Elders of the Church at Boston, after July 22, 1635," *CRW* 1:24. He was also critical of any actions taken by church elders or ministers that resembled a presbytery: Williams, "To Governor John Winthrop, between July and December 1632," *CRW* 1:8.

22. Williams, "To John Cotton, Jr., March 25, 1671," *CRW* 2:630.

23. John Cotton summarizing Williams's views in "To Roger Williams, ca. early 1636," *CRW* 1:39.

24. Winthrop, *Winthrop's Journal*, 61–62; Williams, "To John Cotton, Jr., March 25, 1671," *CRW* 2:630.

25. Winthrop, *Winthrop's Journal*, 116–17. Most scholars agree that in his 1633 treatise against the royal charter Williams was motivated against the concept of a Christian king rather than by a desire to defend the Native Americans. Field, "A Key for the Gate," 355; LaFantasie, "Road to Banishment," *CRW* 1:15; Gilpin, *Millenarian Piety*, 41.

26. Winthrop, *Winthrop's Journal*, 61–62.

27. Timothy L. Hall, *Separating Church and State: Roger Williams and Religious Liberty* (Urbana: University of Illinois Press, 1998), 31.

28. Winthrop, *Winthrop's Journal*, 149.

29. LaFantasie, "Road to Banishment," *CRW* 1:18.

30. Though Williams's letter does not survive, we do have Cotton's response, which addresses Williams's letter point by point, in *CRW* 1:33–44.

31. John Marshall, *John Locke, Toleration and Early Enlightenment Culture: Religious Intolerance and Arguments for Religious Toleration in Early Modern and "Early Enlightenment" Europe* (Cambridge: Cambridge University Press, 2006), 315; Coffey, "Puritanism and Liberty Revisited," 975.

32. Nussbaum, *Liberty of Conscience*, 41–42. Coffey claims that in *The Bloudy Tenent* Williams argues that Christendom is harmful to churches; Coffey, "Puritanism and Liberty Revisited," 975. My own reading of *The Bloudy Tenent* finds that while Williams does criticize the impure churches in existence, he does not do so to argue that freedom of conscience would lead to church purity but rather to claim that it is impossible to uphold the fundamentals of doctrine because the church is so corrupted; thus, if a civil government were to punish this fundamental it would have to punish every Christian (including Cotton); Roger Williams, *The Bloudy Tenent of Persecution for Cause of Conscience Discussed*, ed. Edward Bean Underhill (London: The Hanserd Knollys Society, 1848), 40–45. Williams also discusses church purity in his exegesis of the wheat and the tares parable, where he argues that the Bible dictates that the church, but not civil society, uphold certain religious dictates; ibid., 70–89.

33. Morgan, *Roger Williams*, 90.

34. Williams, "To Mrs. Anne Sadleir, ca. April 1652," *CRW* 1:358.

35. Ernst, *Roger Williams*, 5; Ola Elizabeth Winslow, *Master Roger Williams: A Biography* (New York: Macmillan, 1957), 9; Rubertone, *Grave Undertakings*, 7, 89–92.

36. Williams, "To an Assembly of Commissioners, November 17, 1677?" *CRW* 2:750.

37. Camp, *Roger Williams*, 18–19.

38. Williams, "To Thomas Thorowgood, December 20, 1635," *CRW* 1:30. He eventually abandoned the belief that the Native Americans sprang from one of the lost Hebrew tribes.

39. Some scholars, I believe mistakenly, talk about Williams as if he stepped off the boat with a respect for Native Americans and "always treated them as human beings, not as beasts or devils"; Nussbaum, *Liberty of Conscience*, 43. See also James Calvin Davis, *The Moral Theology of Roger Williams: Christian Conviction and Public Ethics*, Columbia Series in Reformed Theology (Louisville: Westminster John Knox Press, 2004), 7, 50–51.

40. Williams, "To an Assembly of Commissioners, November 17, 1677?" *CRW* 2:750. He included the phrase "Nippúckis: *Smoke Troubleth Me*" in *A Key into the Language of America* (1643; repr., Bedford, MA: Applewood Books, 1997), 32.

41. Williams, *A Key*, 14, 19, 29–30, 83.

42. Williams, "To the General Court of Massachusetts Bay, May 7, 1668," *CRW* 2:577.

43. Williams, "To Deputy Governor John Winthrop, before August 25, 1636," *CRW* 1:53.

44. The narrative of the events leading up to the Pequot War has been carefully laid out by Cave, *The Pequot War*, 59–76, 87–100, 104–10; Lipman, "'A meanes to knitt them together,'" 15–16.

45. Williams, "To Major John Mason and Governor Thomas Prence, June 22, 1670," *CRW* 2:611.

46. Williams, "To Deputy Governor John Winthrop, before August 25, 1636," *CRW* 1:53.

47. Cave, *The Pequot War*, 106.

48. Williams, "To Deputy John Winthrop, before August 25, 1636," *CRW* 1:54–55.

49. Timothy Wood interprets this letter similarly in "Worlds Apart," 70–71.

50. Felker, "Roger Williams's Uses of Legal Discourse," 632–33.

51. Williams, "To Governor Henry Vane or Deputy Governor John Winthrop, May 13, 1637," *CRW* 1:78.

52. Williams, "To Governor Henry Vane and Deputy Governor John Winthrop, May 1, 1637," *CRW* 1:73; John Underhill, *Newes from America; or, A new and experimentall discoverie of New England containing, a true relation of their war-like proceedings these two yeares last past, with a figure of the Indian fort, or palizado* (London, 1638).

53. Williams, "To John Winthrop, June 2, 1637," *CRW* 1:83.

54. Williams, "To Governor John Winthrop, June 30, 1637," *CRW* 1:88.

55. Underhill, *Newes from America*, 35–36.

56. Williams, "To Governor John Winthrop, July 10, 1637," *CRW* 1:98.

57. Ibid., 95.

58. Ibid., 94.

59. Williams, "To Governor John Winthrop, June 30, 1637," *CRW* 1:88.

60. Williams, "To John Winthrop, July 15, 1637," *CRW* 1:101.

61. Williams would not have known that a group of people who shared his beliefs were called Seekers until he returned to England in 1643; J. F. McGregor, "Seekers and Ranters," in *Radical Religion in the English Revolution*, eds. J. F. McGregor and B. Reay (Oxford: Oxford University Press, 1984), 122–23. There has been some resistance to the argument that Williams was a Seeker, see Morgan, *Roger Williams*, 152n56. A letter John Eliot wrote to John Cotton reveals that Williams was reading and disseminating Seeker writings; "John Eliot to John Cotton, June 6, 1651," in *The Correspondence of John Cotton*, ed. Sargent Bush Jr. (Chapel Hill: University of North Carolina Press, 2001), 447. A letter that Williams wrote to Winthrop in October 1636 provides strong proof that Williams had by that time shifted his focus from establishing a pure church to sowing the seed for the Second Coming; "To John Winthrop, October 24, 1636?" *CRW* 1:65–69.

62. Jesper Rosenmeier, "The Teacher and the Witness: John Cotton and Roger Williams," *WMQ* 25, no. 3 (1968): 417; Davis, *The Moral Theology of Roger Williams*, 41; Hall, *Separating Church and State*, 25–27.

63. Williams, *Christening Make Not Christians* (London, 1644), 19.

64. Margaret T. Hodgen, *Early Anthropology in the Sixteenth and Seventeenth Centuries* (Philadelphia: University of Pennsylvania Press, 1964); Anthony Pagden, *The Fall of Natural Man: The American Indian and the Origins of Comparative Ethnology* (Cambridge: Cambridge University Press, 1982); Gordon M. Sayre, *Les sauvages américains: Representations of Native Americans in French and English Colonial Literature* (Chapel Hill: University of North Carolina Press, 1997), 1–48.

65. Williams, *The Bloudy Tenent*, 4. James Calvin Davis also argues that "Williams's theological orientation permitted him to appeal to a number of sources for moral insight, including practical reason and the precedents of human experience"; Davis, *The Moral Theology of Roger Williams*, 21; see also 64–69.

66. Williams, "To Governor John Winthrop, July 21, 1637," *CRW* 1:106. The writings that Williams mentions in this letter have not been recovered, but his description reveals that he was still focused on the dangers of separatists listening to English preachers. Yet a new strand of his thought was emerging that focused on liberty of conscience and the separation of church and state. When Williams published his response to Cotton's letter in London, he similarly said: "This Letter I acknowledge to have received from Mr. Cotton (whom for his personall excellencies I truly honour and love.) Yet at such a time of my distressed wanders amongst the Barbarians, that being destitute of food, of cloths, of time I reserved it (though barely, amidst so many barbarous distractions) and afterwards prepared an Answer to be returned." Roger Williams, *Mr. Cottons Letter Lately Printed, Examined and Answered* (London, 1644), n.p. (first page).

67. John Cotton, "To Roger Williams, ca. early 1636" *CRW* 1:34.

68. This letter has not survived, but Cotton's letter and a different response by Williams were published in England in 1644, and dialogues between them served as the basis of *The Bloudy Tenent of Persecution*.

69. Conrad Wright, "John Cotton Washed and Made White," in *Continuity and Discontinuity in Church History: Essays Presented to George Huntson Williams*, eds. F. F. Church and T. George (Leiden: Brill Academic Press, 1979), 342.

70. Williams, *The Bloudy Tenent*, 157.

71. Williams, "To John Winthrop, July 15, 1637," *CRW* 1:102. For Williams's insistence that the Pequots be dispersed instead of murdered, see "To Governor John Winthrop, June 7, 1638," *CRW* 1:161. For Williams's horror at reports of Indian executions, see "To John Winthrop, after September 21, 1638," *CRW* 1:184.

72. Williams, "To John Winthrop, July 15, 1637," *CRW* 1:102.

73. Williams, "To John Winthrop, June 2, 1637," *CRW* 1:84.

74. Williams, "To Governor John Winthrop, August 20, 1637," *CRW* 1:114.

75. See Williams, "To Governor Winthrop, July 2, 1637," *CRW* 1:96–97; see also Williams, "To John Winthrop, August 1639," *CRW* 1:200.

76. Williams, *The Bloudy Tenent*, 11–12, 178.

77. Williams, "To John Winthrop, ca. August 12, 1637," *CRW* 1:110.

78. Williams, "To Governor John Winthrop, August 20, 1637," *CRW* 1:112–14; "To Governor John Winthrop, ca. September 9, 1637," *CRW* 1:118–19.
79. Williams, "To Governor John Winthrop, ca. September 9, 1637," *CRW* 1:119.
80. Williams, "To John Winthrop, January 10, 1637/8," *CRW* 1:140; "To Governor John Winthrop, February 28, 1637/8," *CRW* 1:145–46.
81. Williams, "To Governor John Winthrop, February 28, 1637/8," *CRW* 1:146.
82. Williams, *Christening Make Not Christians*, 18–19.
83. Williams, *A Key*, 134–35.
84. David Read has also noted Williams's particularly acute sensitivity to man's capacity for misjudgment in *A Key* and *The Bloudy Tenent*; see Read, *New World, Known World*, 100–101, 116, 118–19.
85. The most striking and potentially disastrous rumor that Williams had to dispel was that the Narragansett leader Miantonomi intended to kill Thomas Stantons. If the English had acted on this rumor, the results would have been calamitous: Williams, "To John Winthrop, January 10, 1637/8," *CRW* 1:140. Complicated tribal identities led to rumors implicating one group of Indians in a wrongdoing when another group was to blame; see "To Governor John Winthrop, June 7, 1638," *CRW* 1:161. Williams rectified disputes that did not stem directly from the Pequot War but that he feared could cause more bloodshed if left unresolved. For example, in the summer of 1639, Williams resolved a dispute regarding hunting lands; "To Governor John Winthrop, May 2, 1639," *CRW* 1:194–95.
86. Fickes, "'They Could Not Endure That Yoke,'" 59–62, 71–72; Cremer, "Possession," 301–4, 334–37.
87. Williams, "To John Winthrop, ca. August 1, 1638," *CRW* 1:171. See also "To Governor John Winthrop, June 7, 1638," *CRW* 1:162; "To Governor John Winthrop, August 14, 1638," *CRW* 1:176–77.
88. Williams, "To John Winthrop, ca. October 1638," *CRW* 1:192.
89. Williams, "To Governor John Winthrop, June 7, 1638," *CRW* 1:161. For other examples of Williams reporting on the guilt of particular Indians, see "To Governor John Winthrop, September 10, 1638," *CRW* 1:179–80; "To John Winthrop, after September 21, 1638," *CRW* 1:183–84; "To John Winthrop, ca. October 1638," *CRW* 1:189–90.
90. Williams, "To John Winthrop, ca. October 1638," *CRW* 1:192.
91. Williams, "To Governor John Winthrop, May 2, 1639," *CRW* 1:195.
92. Williams, "To Governor John Winthrop, February 28, 1637/8," *CRW* 1:145.
93. Williams, "To John Winthrop, July 21, 1640," *CRW* 1:203.
94. Williams, *Christening Make Not Christians*, 1–2; emphases in original.
95. "Letter of Roger Williams, President of Providence Colony, to the General Court of Massachusetts, 5, 8, 1654," *Records of Rhode Island and Providence Plantations in New England*, vol. 1, ed. John Russell Bartlett (Providence: Rhode Island Historical Society, 1856), 292–93.
96. Cave, *The Pequot War*, 126. This process of suspicion and exclusion based on a Puritan individual's defense of Native American groups occurred during King Philip's War as well. See J. Patrick Cesarini, "'What Has Become of Your Praying to God?' Daniel Gookin's Troubled History of King Philip's War," *Early American Literature* 44, no. 3 (2009): 500, 502.
97. Williams, "To Governor John Winthrop, ca. June 14, 1638," *CRW* 1:163. See also Ivy Schweitzer, *The Work of Self-Representation: Lyric Poetry in Colonial New England* (Chapel Hill: University of North Carolina Press, 1991), 188.
98. James Axtell, *The Invasion Within: The Contest of Cultures in Colonial North America* (New York: Oxford University Press, 1985), 131–328; James H. Merrell, "'The Customes of Our Countrey': Indians and Colonists in Early America," in *Strangers within the Realm: Cultural Margins of the First British Empire*, eds. Bernard Bailyn and Philip D. Morgan (Chapel Hill, NC: University of North Carolina Press, 1991), 117–56; Dane Anthony Morrison, *A Praying People: Massachusett Acculturation and the Failure of the Puritan Mission, 1600–1690* (New York: Peter Lang Press, 1995); Karen Ordahl Kupperman, *Indians and English: Facing Off in Early America* (Ithaca, NY: Cornell University Press, 2000), 41–76, 142–73.
99. Williams, "To John Winthrop, January 10, 1637/8," *CRW* 1:140. See also "To Governor John Winthrop, ca. October 26, 1637," *CRW* 1:126; Rubertone, *Grave Undertakings*, 94–95.

100. Williams undoubtedly saw language and cultural identity as interrelated. But we should not overlook the fact that it was not until the eighteenth century that Europeans believed that language was a societal invention. Before that point, most European linguists believed that all languages were divine, originating from Eden and diversified after the fall of Babel. One of the largest concerns was that after Babel language had lost its power to communicate. Throughout the seventeenth century, philosophers and other scholars began a search for this universal language that resembled that used before Babel. There was an effort among many New World missionaries, including Williams, to explain Native languages using grammar models derived from Greek, Latin, and Hebrew. See Edward G. Gray, *New World Babel: Languages and Nations in Early America* (Princeton: Princeton University Press, 1999); Lieve Jooken, "Descriptions of American Indian Word Forms in Colonial Missionary Grammars," in *The Language Encounter in the Americas, 1492–1800: A Collection of Essays*, eds. Edward Gray and Norman Fiering (New York: Berghahn Books, 2000), 293–309; David S. Katz, *Philo-Semitism and the Readmission of the Jews to England, 1603–1655* (Oxford: Oxford University Press, 1982); Rudiger Schreyer, "'Savage' Languages in Eighteenth-Century Theoretical History of Language," in *The Language Encounter in the Americas*, eds. Gray and Fiering, 310–26.

101. Williams, "To John Winthrop, January 10, 1637/8," *CRW* 1:140; "To Governor John Winthrop, February 28, 1637/8," *CRW* 1:145–46.

102. Williams occasionally continued to include direct dialogue in later letters as well. See, for example, "To Governor John Winthrop, May 9, 1639," *CRW* 1:196–98.

103. Williams, *A Key*, A2.

104. Williams, *The Bloudy Tenent*, 130. For the early tolerationist context, and Williams's place in it, see Marshall, *John Locke, Toleration and Early Enlightenment Culture*, 312–34.

105. Marshall, *John Locke, Toleration and Early Enlightenment Culture*, 6; see also 312–13; Andrew R. Murphy, "Complicating the Standard Narrative," *WMQ* 66 (2009): 432; Alexandra Walshram, *Charitable Hatred: Tolerance and Intolerance in England, 1500–1700* (Manchester: Manchester University Press, 2006), 234–35.

106. The one exception is his inclusion of a quote by Francis Bacon; *The Bloudy Tenent*, 6.

107. Ibid., 8.

108. Though the goal of this article is to locate the place of the Pequot War in Williams's developing discourse about toleration, I encourage readers who are interested in the accuracy of Williams's claims about Narragansett culture and history to see Rubertone, *Grave Undertakings*, 96–114.

109. Camp, *Roger Williams*, 228.

110. David Murray, *Indian Giving: Economies of Power in Indian-White Exchanges* (Amherst: University of Massachusetts Press, 2000), 98. See also Field, "A Key for the Gate," 369.

111. Even in his later letters, Williams was careful to keep his observations separate from those of his Native informants: "I shall humbly and faythfully submit to Consideracion: I, from them, 2, from my selfe." Williams, "To John Winthrop, ca. October 1638," *CRW* 1:192.

112. Cremer, "Possession," 327–31.

113. Williams, *A Key*, 189.

114. Ibid., 188–89.

115. Williams, *The Bloudy Tenent*, 46.

116. Ibid., 214.

117. Cotton, "A Model of Church and Civil Power," quoted ibid., 213; William Haller, *Tracts on Liberty in the Puritan Revolution, 1638–1647* (New York: Columbia University Press, 1934), 4; Schwartz, "Tolerance in Unexpected Places," 421.

118. Christopher Hill, *The World Turned Upside Down: Radical Ideas during the English Revolution* (New York: Penguin, 1972), 98.

119. Walshram, *Charitable Hatred*, 1–2, 4–5, 39–40, 46–49, 235–36; Coffey, *Persecution and Toleration in Protestant England*, 33–34, 38–41; Avihu Zakai, "Religious Toleration and Its Enemies: The Independent Divines and the Issue of Toleration during the English Civil War," *Albion* 21, no. 1 (1989): 1–33. See also Avihu Zakai, "Orthodoxy in England and New England: Puritans and the Issue of Religious Toleration, 1640–1650," *Proceedings of the American Philosophical Society* 135, no. 3 (1991): 401–41.

120. Marshall, *John Locke, Toleration and Early Enlightenment Culture*, 7, 281–311, 325, 332.

121. Williams, *The Bloudy Tenent*, 213, 215; Williams, *A Key*, 7.

122. Williams, *The Bloudy Tenent*, 214.
123. Ibid., 313.
124. Davis, *Moral Theology of Roger Williams*, 61.
125. Morgan, *Roger Williams*, 128; Hall, *Separating Church and State*, 82, 110.
126. Williams, *A Key*, 151.
127. Williams, *The Bloudy Tenent*, 53.
128. Ibid., Bl.
129. Williams, *A Key*, 129. Scott Pratt's recent work, mentioned at the beginning of this article as the first analysis of Native American influence on *The Bloudy Tenent*, focuses on explaining how Williams adopted his theory of accepting potentially dangerous outsiders from Native American treatment of cannibals; Pratt, *Native Pragmatism*, 78–106.
130. William Lamont, "Pamphleteering, the Protestant Consensus and the English Revolution," in *Freedom and the English Revolution*, eds. R. C. Richardson and G. M. Ridden (Manchester: Manchester University Press, 1986), 77.
131. John Cotton, "The Answer of Mr. John Cotton," in Williams, *The Bloudy Tenent*, 20, 24; Walshram, *Charitable Hatred*, 40–46, 228–29.
132. Blair Worden, "Toleration and the Cromwellian Protectorate," in *Persecution and Toleration: Papers Read at the Twenty-second Summer Meeting and the Twenty-third Winter Meeting of the Ecclesiastical History Society*, ed. W. J. Sheils (Padstow: Blackwell, 1984), 200–201, 209, 216.
133. Williams, *The Bloudy Tenent*, 175.
134. Ibid., 7.
135. Ibid., 53–54, 128, 234–35, 241, 248–50, 295–96, 301–302. On this point, Williams was similar to Sebastian Castellio (1515–1563), who argued that "heretic" was a term commonly used by religious groups to refer to those who did not agree with them. While Castellio argued, therefore, for the right of Christians to practice their religion as they saw fit, he did believe that the civil magistrate should punish atheists and that those who denied the creation of the world, resurrection, and the immortality of the soul could be punished with fines and banishment; Marshall, *John Locke, Toleration and Early Enlightenment Culture*, 320–23; Perez Zagorin, *How the Idea of Religious Toleration Came to the West* (Princeton, NJ: Princeton University Press, 2003), 112–14.
136. See, for example, Williams, *The Bloudy Tenent*, 44–45, 113–14, 143–44, 168. Alexandra Walshram has identified a handful of others who defended toleration using the uncertainty of knowledge; Walshram, *Charitable Hatred*, 244. For the scholarly debate about the role of skepticism in English toleration, see Coffey, *Persecution and Toleration in Protestant England*, 64–68.
137. Michael Kaufmann, *Institutional Individualism: Conversion, Exile, and Nostalgia in Puritan New England* (Hanover, NH: Wesleyan University Press, 1998), 59; see also 56. See Zagorin, *How the Idea of Religious Toleration Came to the West*, 205.
138. Williams, *The Bloudy Tenent*, 250; see also 152, 179, 284, 319–20. Unlike Cotton, who argued that religious time was cyclical and could be predicted and understood by looking at the Bible, Williams, like many other tolerationist writers, employed a historiographic-theological method of typology that distinguished between, rather than noted the similarity of, the Old and New Testaments. One who believed in the continuity between the two Testaments was inclined to believe that God's dictates were static. Williams, on the other hand, believed that God's message was active, not frozen. Just as the coming of Christ invalidated the laws of Moses, the next apostles would bring a new order. Sacvan Bercovitch, "Typology in Puritan New England: The Williams-Cotton Controversy Reassessed," *American Quarterly* 19, no. 2 (1967): 166–91; Richard Reinitz, "The Separatist Background of Roger Williams' Argument for Religious Toleration," in *Typology in Early American Literature*, ed. Sacvan Bercovitch (Amherst: University of Massachusetts Press, 1972), 107–38; Davis, *The Moral Theology of Roger Williams*, 31, 43; Zagorin, *How the Idea of Religious Toleration Came to the West*, 201–203; Rosenmeier, "The Teacher and the Witness."
139. Leonard Busher, *Religions Peace; or, A reconciliation, between princes & peoples, & nations* (London, 1614), ii, 31, 32, 36. See also Walshram, *Charitable Hatred*, 239. For an excellent analysis of how Williams uses the wheat and the tares parable, see James P. Byrd, *The Challenges of Roger Williams: Religious Liberty, Violent Persecution, and the Bible* (Macon, GA: Mercer University Press, 2002), 87–127.
140. Williams, *Christening Make Not Christians*, 19.
141. Busher, *Religions Peace*, 23; Thomas Helwys, *A Short Declaration of the Mystery of Iniquity (1611/1612)*, ed. Richard Groves (Macon, GA: Mercer University Press, 1998), 10–11, 14, 76.

142. Williams, *The Bloudy Tenent*, 150.
143. Ibid., 235.
144. Michel de Montaigne, *The Essays of Michael, Lord of Montaigne*, trans. John Florio, 3 vols. (London: J. M. Dent, 1927), 1:105–22, 145, 219.
145. Williams, *The Bloudy Tenent*, 170–71. For Cotton's stance, see ibid., 20.
146. Lamont, "Pamphleteering," 81–82.
147. Williams, *The Bloudy Tenent*, 83–84; see also Coffey, "Puritanism and Liberty Revisited," 980–81. Although some theorists during this time argued that at the Second Coming the reprobate would be removed from Earth, others claimed that there would be a universal peace that included all. Williams sided with the former, see Katherine Firth, *The Apocalpytic Tradition in Reformation Britain, 1530–1645* (Oxford: Oxford University Press, 1979), 211. Martha Nussbaum disagrees that Williams, in Andrew Delbanco's words, was "longing for the purifying inferno," claiming that in his writing he encouraged dialogue between all viewpoints; Nussbaum, *Liberty of Conscience*, 42. Though I agree with Nussbaum that Williams gave equal voice to differing arguments in this world, he still had his eye on a future world of uniformity.
148. Williams, *The Bloudy Tenent*, 76.
149. Williams insists that a person can judge only the religious group that he is, according to his conscience, a part of; see ibid., 170–71, 175, 183, 197, 215.
150. Williams was insistent that conversion must be voluntary and often takes place after the converter has exited; *A Key*, 136–38; *The Bloudy Tenent*, 152, 185, 187, 220, 222–23, 237–38; John Peacock, "Regions of the Soul: Ethnography as Narrative," *European Contributions to American Studies* 33 (1996): 192.
151. See Haller, *Tracts on Liberty in the Puritan Revolution*, 61.
152. Nigel Smith, *Literature and Revolution in England, 1640–1660* (New Haven, CT: Yale University Press, 1994), 121. On Williams's originality, see also Zagorin, *How the Idea of Religious Toleration Came to the West*, 200.
153. James Ernst, "Roger Williams and the English Revolution," *Rhode Island Historical Society Collections* 14, no. 1 (1931): 12.
154. Ibid., 20.

JESSICA R. STERN is an associate professor of History at California State University, Fullerton. Dr. Stern has a special interest in anthropology. Her research focuses on the interactions of American Indigenous communities and Euro-Americans. She is currently working on a biography of Roger Williams.

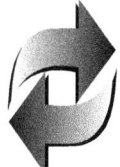

EXPLORING THE ISSUE

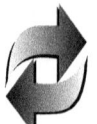

Did the Core Values in Colonial Ideology Lead to Conflict with Native Americans and U.S. Imperialism?

Critical Thinking and Reflection

1. In what ways did the abstract nature of liberal imperialism divest the United States of responsibility in its relationship with Indigenous Americans?
2. How and why was morality/religion used as a weapon against Indigenous Americans in colonial times?
3. Reflect on Roger Williams' assertion that humans were "limited in their ability to grasp truths beyond what they already believed: The Native Americans did not accept Christianity, and the English did not accept the non-Christians could be trustworthy neighbors." Do you agree or disagree? Why or why not?
4. Reflect on Roger Williams' belief that religious uniformity was unnecessary for civil uniformity and that state-enforced religious orthodoxy often unraveled civil peace and led to war. Do you agree or disagree? Why or why not?
5. How are moral codes developed and enacted?

Is There Common Ground?

Drawing on opposite ends of colonial chronology, both Stern (early–mid 17th century) and Konkle (18th–19th centuries) highlight the shifting relationship between Indigenous Americans and the colonies (and later the United States) and the material realities that underscored the changes in perception and engagement. Stern, in her discussion of Roger Williams, highlights his notion of moral codes and tolerance as a means toward peaceful and civil interactions between groups of differing beliefs. His thinking in this matter was a direct correlation to how he viewed colonial interactions with Indigenous Peoples after the attack on the Pequots at Mystic. Konkle states that while U.S. imperialism inexplicitly manifested in colonial relationships with Indigenous Americans, it did constitute a "way of life" that belies is depoliticized nature of never been expressly named as a course of action by the United States.

In both articles, a focus on expansion meant that colonists were often in close contact with Indigenous Peoples. For Stern, the focus is on Williams, who tried to find a workable peace after conflict. Whereas, Konkle outlines how the United States systematically changed its views on Indigenous land ownership made manifest in changes to the law. Perhaps common people represented Sterns view and were generally peaceful, but that propaganda developed their imperialist ideologies, as Konkle seems to suggest. Were and are Americans fearful of other cultures or do they find reasons to fulfill their divine imperial right or are both true? These authors help reveal the nature of colonial ideology through their historical analysis.

Additional Resources

Denevan, William M. "The Pristine Myth: The Landscape of the Americas in 1492." *Annals of the Association of American Geographers*, 82.3 (1992): 369–385.

Denevan, William M. "The "Pristine Myth" Revisited." *Geographical Review*, 101.4 (2011): 576–591.

Freeman, Michael. "Puritans and Pequots: The Question of Genocide." *The New England Quarterly*, 68.2 (1995): 278–293.

Harvey, Sean P. "Must Not Their Languages Be Savage and Barbarous Like Them? Philology, Indian Removal, and Race Science." *Journal of the early Republic*, 30.4 (2010): 505–532.

Jennings, Francis. *The Invasion of America: Indians, Colonialism, and the Cant of Conquest*. University of North Carolina Press, 1975.

Katz, Steven T. "Pequots and the Question of Genocide: A Reply to Michael Freeman." *The New England Quarterly*, 68.4 (1995): 641–649.

Lepore, Jill. *The Name of War: King Philip's War and the Origins of American Identity*. Vintage, 2009.

Sayre, Gordon M. *Les sauvages américains: Representations of Native Americans in French and English Colonial Literature*. University of North Carolina Press, 2000.

Silliman, Stephen W. "Change and Continuity, Practice and Memory: Native American Persistence in Colonial New England." *American Antiquity*, 74.2 (2009): 211–230.

Slotkin, Richard, and James K. Folsom, eds. *So Dreadfull a Judgment: Puritan Responses to King Philip's War, 1676–1677*. Wesleyan University Press, 1978.

Stevens, Laura M. *The Poor Indians: British Missionaries, Native Americans, and Colonial Sensibility*. University of Pennsylvania Press, 2004.

Wallace, Anthony FC. *Jefferson and the Indians: The Tragic Fate of the First Americans*. Harvard University Press, 2009.

Internet References...

First Encounters: Native Americans and Christians. The Pluralism Project—Harvard University

http://pluralism.org/encounter/historical-perspectives/first-encounters-native-americans-and-christians/

Gordon-Reed, Annette. "What if Reconstruction Hadn't Failed? *The Atlantic*. October 26, 2015

https://www.theatlantic.com/politics/archive/2015/10/what-if-reconstruction-hadnt-failed/412219/

Lynch, Jack. "A Principal Source of Dishonor": Indian Policies in Early America. Colonial Williamsburg

http://www.history.org/foundation/journal/spring09/policies.cfm

National Park Service. Captain John Smith Chesapeake

https://www.nps.gov/cajo/index.htm

Smithsonian.com. January 29, 2016

https://www.smithsonianmag.com/smart-news/colonial-america-depended-enslavement-indigenous-people-180957900/

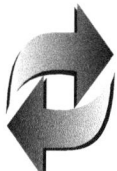

Selected, Edited, and with Issue Framing Material by:
Kevin R. Magill and Tony L. Talbert, *Baylor University*

ISSUE

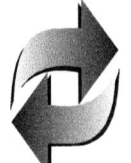

Was the Pequot War Largely a Product of Native American Aggression?

YES: Steven T. Katz, from "The Pequot War Reconsidered," *The New England Quarterly* (1991)

NO: Alfred A. Cave, from "The Pequot War and the Mythology of the Frontier," University of Massachusetts Press (1996)

Learning Outcomes

After reading this issue, you will be able to:

- Understand some of the differences between the traditional and revisionist interpretations of the causes of the Pequot War.
- Summarize several key events leading up to the Pequot War.
- Evaluate the role played by religion in the conflicts between Native Americans and British American colonists.
- Identify the competing perspectives of Native Americans and colonists with regard to the causes of the Pequot War.
- Explain the concept of a "clash of cultures" as it pertains to the interactions of Native Americans and colonists in New England and throughout the British North American colonies.

ISSUE SUMMARY

YES: Steven Katz believes the Pequots conducted a series of aggressive raids, ambushes, and murders in the 1630. He suggests the Pequot Indians attempted to destroy the European Colonies after the two sides failed in their negotiations. Katz further believes that the colonists conducted a defensive war in support of their New England settlements, which was justified in protecting themselves from Pequot aggression.

NO: Alfred A. Cave believes the Pequot War started because Puritanical leaders were able to convince settlers that the Indigenous Americans were Satanic. This European colonial perception led them to clash with the Pequots believing they needed to eliminate Indigenous autonomy, intimidate their population and controlling the land and recourses.

Relations between Native Americans and Europeans were marred by the difficulties that arose from people of very different cultures encountering each other for the first time. These encounters led to inaccurate perceptions, misunderstandings, and failed expectations. While at first the American Indians deified the explorers, experience soon taught them to do otherwise. European opinion ran the gamut from admiration to contempt; for example, some European poets and painters who expressed admiration for the Noble Savage while other Europeans accepted as a rationalization for genocide the sentiment that "the only good savage is a dead one."

Spanish, French, Dutch, and English treatment of Native Americans differed and was based to a considerable extent on each nation's hopes about the New World and how it could be subordinated to the Old. The Spanish exploited the Indians most directly, taking their gold and silver, transforming their government, religion, and society, and even occasionally enslaving them. The French were less of a menace than the others because there were fewer of them and because many French immigrants were itinerant trappers and priests rather than settlers. The Dutch presence in North America was relatively short-lived. In the long run, the emigration from the British Isles was the most threatening of all. Entire families came from England, and they were determined to establish a permanent home in the wilderness.

The juxtaposition of Native American and English from the Atlantic to the Appalachians resulted sometimes in coexistence, other times in enmity. William Bradford's account of the Pilgrims' arrival at Cape Cod describes the insecurity the new migrants felt as they disembarked on American soil. "[T]hey had now no friends to welcome them nor inns to entertain or refresh their weather beaten bodies; no houses or much less towns to repair to, to seek for succor. . . . Besides, what could they see but a hideous and deserted wilderness, full of wild beasts and wild men. . . . If they looked behind them there was the mighty ocean which they had passed and was now a main bar and gulf to separate them from all the civil parts of the world." Historical hindsight, however, suggests that if anyone should have expressed fears about the unfolding encounter in the Western Hemisphere, it should have been the Native Americans because their numbers declined by as much as 95 percent in the first century following Columbus's arrival. Although some of this decline can be attributed to violent encounters with Europeans, there seems to have been a more hostile (and far less visible) force at work. As historian William McNeill has suggested, the main weapon that overwhelmed indigenous peoples in the Americas was the Europeans' breath which transmitted disease germs for which most American Indians had no immunities.

Upon arrival, English settlers depended on the Indians' generosity in sharing the techniques of wilderness survival. Puritan clergymen tried to save their neighbors' souls, going so far as to translate the Bible into dialects, but they were not as successful at conversion as the French Jesuits and Spanish Franciscans. Attempts at coexistence did not smooth over the tension between the English and the Indians. They did not see eye to eye, for example, about the uses of the environment. Indian agriculture, in the eyes of English settlers, was neither intense nor efficient. Native Americans observed that white settlers consumed larger amounts of food per person and cultivated not only for themselves but also for towns and villages that bought the surplus. Subsistence farming collided with the market economy.

Large-scale violence erupted in Virginia in the 1620s, the 1640s, and the 1670s. In the latter decade, frontiersmen in the Virginia piedmont led by Nathaniel Bacon attacked tribes living in the Appalachian foothills. In New England, from the 1630s through the 1670s, Pequots, Wampanoags, Narragansetts, Mohegans, Podunks, and Nipmunks united to stop the encroachments into their woodlands and hunting grounds. King Philip's War lasted from June 1675 to September 1676, with isolated raids stretching on until 1678. Casualties rose into the hundreds, and Anglo-Indian relations deteriorated.

In the next century Spain, France, and England disputed each other's North American claims, and Native Americans joined sides, usually as the allies of France against England. These great wars of the eighteenth century ended in 1763 with England's victory, but disputes over territorial expansion continued. Colonial officials objected to the Proclamation of 1763 by which King George III's imperial government forbade his subjects from settling west of the Appalachian watershed. The area from those mountains to the Mississippi River, acquired from France at the recently negotiated Peace of Paris, was designated as an Indian reservation. From 1763 to 1783, as Anglo-colonial relations moved from disagreement to combat to independence, the London government consistently sided with the Native Americans.

The full range of experiences of Europeans encountering Native Americans in the New World does not lend itself to easy, unalterable conclusions regarding the nature of those contacts. The consequences of these interactions depended upon when and where they took place and which particular groups were involved, and there was rarely any constant or consistent pattern of behavior. One tribe might experience cordial relations with European colonists at one point in time but not another. A particular tribe would get along well with the French but not the English or Dutch; in another generation, the same tribe might enter into an alliance with its former enemies. A case in point is the history of Indian–white relations in early Virginia. The colonists participating in the Jamestown expedition, for example, were attacked by a group of Indians almost as soon as they set foot on American soil. A few months later, however, Powhatan, the dominant chief in the region, provided essential food supplies to the Jamestown residents who were suffering from disease and hunger. By the latter part of 1608, however, the colonists, under the leadership of John Smith, had begun to take an antagonistic stance toward Powhatan and his people. Smith attempted to extort food supplies from the Indians by threatening to burn their villages and canoes. These hostilities continued long after

Smith's departure from Virginia and did not end until the 1640s, when colonial leaders signed a formal treaty with the Powhatan Confederacy.

Similar experiences occurred in New England where colonists and Native Americans maintained reasonably cordial relations in the early years of settlement. Tensions over land usage, trade, and acts of violence, however, soon produced warfare in southern New England in the 1630s. Following the murder of several Englishmen, Puritan officials demanded that the Pequots, who were held responsible for the deaths despite evidence that members of other tribes in the region were culpable, turn over the guilty parties for prosecution by colonial courts. The Pequot sachem Sassacus refused but did provide restitution in the form of wampum, believing this to be a satisfactory response. Subsequently, in 1637, New England officials sent armed colonists to exact revenge on the Pequots at Fort Mystic, where raids resulted in the deaths of all but a few of the Indian inhabitants, and the village was put to the torch. Plymouth Colony governor William Bradford described the scene in his autobiography: "It was a fearful sight to see them [mainly Pequot women and children] thus frying in the fire and the streams of blood quenching the same, and horrible was the stink and scent thereof; but the victory seemed a sweet sacrifice, and they gave the praise thereof to God, who had wrought so wonderfully for them, thus to enclose their enemies in their hands and give them so speedy a victory over so proud and insulting an enemy."

Responsibility for the outbreak of the Pequot War (1636–1638) has become the topic of considerable debate among scholars of colonial America and specialists in Native American history. While most of the nineteenth-century treatments of this conflict are marred by racist characterizations of Native Americans generally, in the twentieth century, historians have traditionally recognized that New England Puritans certainly were guilty of the slaughter of their Pequot adversaries. At the same time, however, many like Alden Vaughan in *New England Frontier: Puritans and Indians, 1620–1675* (Little, Brown, 1965) have argued that the Pequots represented a threat to New England security and that Puritans acted in self-defense to resist Pequot aggression. Revisionists have been far more critical of the Puritans. Most notable in this regard is Francis Jennings, whose book *The Invasion of America: Indians, Colonialism, and the Cant of Conquest* (University of North Carolina Press, 1975) refocused the argument on Puritan greed, prejudice, and bigotry. For Jennings, the Pequots were trapped in the middle of an ongoing competition among colonial residents in Massachusetts Bay Colony, Plymouth, and Connecticut over land and control of trade in the region. Neal Salisbury avoids Jennings' polemical style and concludes in *Manitou and Providence: Indians, Europeans, and the Making of New England, 1500–1643* (Oxford University Press, 1982) that the conflict with the Pequots succeeded in bringing the New England Puritan community together to refocus on its divine mission of dispatching the indigenous peoples from their midst. In her book *Settling with the Indians: The Meeting of English and Indian Cultures in America, 1580–1640* (Rowman & Littlefield, 1980), Karen Ordahl Kupperman insists that the Pequot War was prompted by English efforts to exercise undisputed power in New England.

In the following essays, the reader will find two very different interpretations of the causes of the Pequot War. In the first selection, Steven T. Katz challenges revisionists who view the conflict as an act of racist genocide on the part of New England Puritans. According to Katz, Massachusetts Bay Colony leaders attempted unsuccessfully to negotiate with the Pequots in an effort to bring the murderers of John Stone, John Oldham, and other colonists to justice. English colonists, Katz argues, had every reason to fear for their safety and lives as the Pequots attempted to destroy English settlement throughout New England. The Puritans fought a defensive war that included the decision to burn the Pequot village at Fort Mystic and had no intention of carrying out a full-scale war against these Native American adversaries.

Alfred Cave views the Puritans as the aggressors in this conflict as they attempted to make the New England frontier safe for their followers. Cave disputes the argument that the Pequots were a threat to Puritan security except insofar as they attempted to control European trade and maintain a network of allied tribes throughout New England. Characterizing the Pequots (and all Native Americans for that matter) as savages, instruments of Satan, and enemies of Christianity, the Puritans overreacted to rumors promulgated by the Mohegan sachem Uncas that the Pequots were preparing to assault the expanding Puritan settlements. The attack at Fort Mystic resulted and ultimately destroyed Pequot hegemony in the region.

YES

Steven T. Katz

The Pequot War Reconsidered

It is well known that in the 1970s and 1980s traditional scholarly analyses and judgments of the motives and events surrounding the Pequot War of 1637 came to be revised. In place of the view that the English were simply protecting themselves by preemptively attacking the Pequots, the revisionists argued that the Europeans used earlier, limited threats against them as cause to bring mass destruction on the Pequots. That assault is then taken to be a harbinger, a symbol of a larger, premeditated exterminatory intent that characterized the invasion of the New World. While there is surely room for a more penetrating critical reconstruction of the meaning of America's conquest and settlement than has yet appeared, one must be cautious in allowing legitimate moral outrage at the treatment of the Indians to substitute for a careful sorting of the evidence about the Pequot War. If we examine the facts closely and try to analyze them within their particular historical context, our judgments of the wrongs done the Native Americans will be more nuanced, balanced, and discriminating than radicalizing polemics allow and thus ultimately will better serve our efforts to understand the processes and consequences of colonization.

I

My first cautionary comment regarding the war is that it should not be viewed in strictly racial or ethnic terms of Red vs. White I do not dispute that the colonists viewed the Indians through racial stereotypes, or that those stereotypes affected their behavior, but the particular circumstances of the Pequot War certainly seem to argue against the charge that It was a universal offensive against "Indianness" per se. The most telling of these circumstances is the presence of rival Indian groups on the side of the colonists. The crucial role of the Narragansetts, first in rejecting Pequot overtures to join a pan-Indian front against the English and then, in October 1636, in allying with the English against the Pequot, is but the earliest and most prominent case of European-Indian collaboration in the conflict. Following this alliance, the Mohegans, the Massachusetts and River Tribes, and later the Mohawks all sided with the British. Although the reasons for these alliances have been disputed for three centuries, seventeenth-century evidence—for example, the "Remonstrance of New Netherland," John Winthrop's *History of New England*, and John De Forest's *History of the Indians*—is clear that at least intermittent hostility between the Pequots and the Narragansetts and their tributaries preceded the war.

Once we are able to hold our charges of racism in reserve, we can attend to the specifics of the war. Our distance from the events obviously blurs our vision. Many facts about the war have been contested, including the particular causes for the outbreak of hostilities; however, there can be no doubt that both sides had cause to feel aggrieved. From the perspective of most Indians, exceptions notwithstanding, the very presence of the European was an act of aggression. Filling in the outlines of this generalized aggression was an already considerable and well-documented body of particular crimes committed by unscrupulous individuals like John Oldham, whose murder in 1636 set in motion the events that led to the war. Oldham was not, moreover, the only Englishman the Pequots or their tributaries had murdered. In 1634 they had killed two English captains, including the notorious and disreputable John Stone, who had kidnapped and held several Indians for ransom, and in the next two years they had killed at least six more colonists. Alternatively, the English leadership was disturbed that the Pequots had taken no action against the guilty among them and disheartened that the Pequots had abrogated the terms of the treaty they had signed. Fears increased when Jonathan Brewster, a Plymouth trader, passed word that Uncas, sachem of the Mohegans, had reported that

> the Pequents have some mistrust, that the English will shortly come against them (which I take is by indiscreet speeches of some of your people here to the Natives) and therefore out of desperate

madnesse doe threaten shortly to sett upon both Indians [Mohegans] and English, joyntly.

Uncas may well have fabricated the rumor, but the colonists were certainly in a frame of mind to take it seriously. Their numbers were small, and news of the Virginia uprising of 1622, with its 350 casualties, had still not faded from memory. What the Puritans sought was a stratagem that would put an end to unpredictable, deadly annoyances as well as forestall any larger, more significant Indian military action like that suggested by Uncas's report. However one estimates the "good faith" or lack thereof of the Massachusetts leadership, efforts were made to negotiate, but these efforts failed, or at least were perceived to have failed. The colonists then chose as their best course of action a retaliatory raid, intended both to punish and to warn, on the Indians of Block Island, who were specifically charged with Oldham's murder. The Pequots were involved, according to William Hubbard, because the murderers had "fled presently to the Pequods, by whom they were sheltered, and so became also guilty themselves of his blood."

Ninety Englishmen participated in the raid commanded by John Endecott. John Winthrop noted that Endecott was ordered

> to put to death the men of Block Island, but to spare the women and children, and to bring them away, and to take possession of the Island; and from thence to go to the Pequods to demand the murderers of Capt. Stone and other English, and one thousand fathom of wampom for damages, etc., and some of their children as hostages.

None of the mainland Pequot at Pequot Harbor were to be harmed if they capitulated to his demands. In the event, the raid on Block Island turned into an extensive assault, and the Indian settlement there was looted and burned. However, although property was destroyed and several Indians were wounded, "the Naymen killed not a man, save that one Kichomiquim, an Indian Sachem of the Bay, killed a Pequot." The fact that only one Indian was killed seems to confirm John Winthrop's belief that the colonists "went not to make war upon [the Pequots] but to do justice." Not all colonists defined "justice" as Winthrop did, however, for the Endecott raid on the Harbor Indians was condemned by the colonial leaders of Plymouth, Connecticut, and Fort Saybrook.

In response to Endecott's assaults, the Pequots plagued the settlers with a series of raids, ambushes, and annoyances. On 23 April, Wethersfield, Connecticut, was attacked. Nine were killed, including a woman and child, and two additional young women were captured. A number of other raids claimed the lives of thirty Europeans, or five percent of all the settlers in Connecticut. In addition to these offensive actions, the Pequot set about developing alliances, particularly with the Narragansett, to galvanize support for a war to destroy European settlement in their territory, if not in New England entirely. Many colonists who learned of the plan for a broad effort against them, which was frustrated only at the last minute through the intervention of Roger Williams, rightly felt, given their demographic vulnerability, that their very survival was threatened. Even Francis Jennings, the most severe critic of Puritan behavior, acknowledges that "Had these [Pequot] proposals [for alliance with the Narragansetts] been accepted by the Narragansetts, there would have without a doubt arisen a genuine Indian menace. . . . Whether the colonies could long have maintained themselves under such conditions is open to serious question."

The Pequot War was the organized reaction of the colonists of Connecticut and Massachusetts to these intimidating events. In choosing to make war, they were choosing to put an end to threats to their existence as individuals and as a community. They did not decide to fight out of some a priori lust for Indian blood based on some metaphysical doctrine of Indian inferiority, however much they may have held that view, or some desire for further, even complete, control over Indian territory, much as they coveted such land. They fought, initially, a defensive war. They may well have provoked events, as even Winthrop tacitly acknowledged, by their over-reactive raid on Block Island, but, in the early stages of the conflict, they did not intend to enter into a full-scale war with the Pequot until the Pequot raised the stakes with their response to the events at Block Island and Pequot Harbor. Of course the Indians cannot be blamed for so replying, for they too saw themselves as acting legitimately in self-defense, both narrowly and more generally in defense of traditional Indian rights to their own native lands. In effect, both sides acted to defend what they perceived as rightly theirs. In this context, if either side can be said to have harbored larger geo-political ambitions, it was the Pequot, though defeat would certainly bury those desires.

The major action of the war was an attack by 70 Connecticut and 90 Massachusetts colonists along with 60 Mohegans, plus some scattered Narragansett and Eastern Niantics, against the Pequot Fort at Mystic, which held an Indian population of between 400 and 700, including women and children. The colonists and their Indian allies surprised the Pequots and burned their fort to the ground. During the battle two English soldiers were killed and about 20 were wounded, while almost half the Indians allied with them were killed or wounded; almost all the Pequots were killed.

Richard Drinnon, in his *Facing West: The Metaphysics of Indian Hating and Empire Building* (1980), has argued that the unusual violence of the operation signals the colonists' "genocidal intentions." In evaluating the behavior of the English in this particular instance, however, it should be recognized that the tactics employed were neither so unconventional nor so novel that they can be taken to mark a turning point in Puritan-Indian relations, nor were they so distinctive as to indicate a transformation in Puritan awareness of the otherness of their adversaries. Given the relative strength of the enemy, the inexperience of the colonial forces, and the crucial fact that Sassacus, chief of the Pequot, and his warriors were camped only five miles from Mystic Fort and were sure to arrive soon, as in fact they did, one need not resort to dramatic theories of genocidal intentionality to explain the actions of the English. The simple, irrefutable fact is that had the battle been prolonged, Sassacus would have had time to reach Mystic and deflect the English attack.

II

Although he does not use the term *genocide* per se, it is clear from the rhetorical thrust of his argument and his use of phrases like "deliberate massacre" that Francis Jennings is an insistent advocate of the genocidal thesis. Given the force of his prose, the popularity of his work, and its long-standing influence, it is useful to deconstruct Jennings's argument to evaluate the legitimacy of the heinous charge leveled against the English colonists.

Jennings attributes to Capt. John Mason, the expedition's leader, an overt, *ab initio* desire to massacre the Indians. "Mason proposed," he writes,

> to avoid attacking Pequot warriors, which would have overtaxed his unseasoned, unreliable troops. Battle, as such, was not his purpose. Battle is only one of the ways to destroy an enemy's will to fight. Massacre can accomplish the same end with less risk, and Mason had determined that massacre would be his objective.

Ignoring all other reports of Mason's intentions and actions, Jennings bases his conclusions on Mason's own terse account of the event. Jennings cites Mason's reasons for his strategy, with special reference to his concluding "'and also some other [reasons],'" which he says "'I shall forebear to trouble you with.'" Even Jennings labels this comment cryptic, but he still does not forebear using it as unambiguous evidence of a hidden, premeditated plan to massacre all the Indians at Fort Mystic.

Jennings also refers to Mason's discussion with his colleagues Lt. Lion Gardiner and Capt. John Underhill as well as with the expedition's Chaplain Stone. He takes Mason's request that the chaplain "'commend our Condition to the Lord, that night, to direct how in what manner we should demean our selves'" to be a covert reference to the existence of a plan to massacre the Indians the next day. But on the eve of such a battle, especially given Puritan sensibilities, such a request is neither surprising nor, given the text before us, indicative of any special intent; to read it as an implicit confession of genocidal desire, Jennings has to overinterpret the brief original source dramatically.

Jennings charges that "all the secondary accounts of the Pequot conquest squeamishly evade confessing the deliberateness of Mason's strategy, and some falsify to conceal it." What Jennings adduces as confirmation of both the premeditated plot to massacre and the later conscious suppression of that fact emerges in the course of a curious argument, which I quote in full.

> Mason's own narrative is the best authority on this point. The Massachusetts Puritans' William Hubbard brazened out his own misquotation by telling his readers to "take it as it was delivered in writing by that valiant, faithful, and prudent Commander Capt. Mason." With this emphatic claim to authority he quoted Mason as saying, "We had resolved a while not to have burned it [the village], but being we could not come at them, I resolved to set it on fire." Despite Hubbard's assurance, these were not Mason's words. His manuscript said bluntly, "we had formerly concluded to destroy them by the Sword and save the Plunder."

Jennings's conclusion does not follow logically from the texts he cites nor from his juxtaposition of them. They neither suggest premeditation to massacre nor falsification of the record; instead, Hubbard's paraphrase of Mason's words accords perfectly with his stated intent to plunder the settlement. Jennings himself recognizes that such economic motives were central to the Block Island raid, as well as other actions by the English. Burning Fort Mystic would, of course, severely limit its economic potential; the sword was a less efficient tool of human destruction but would preserve goods of value to the English. In fact, Mason's vow to "destroy" the Pequots "by the Sword" is a phrase not at all unusual to the language of military conflict and in that context such comments almost always signal not the annihilation of the enemy but the disruption of its capacity to fight. This understanding of Mason's comment is supported by the Puritans' further prosecution of the war.

Jennings continues to press home his point in his increasingly confused and confusing reconstruction of events. I quote:

> The rest of Mason's manuscript revealed what sort of inhabitants had been occupying the Mystic River village and proved conclusively that mere victory over them was not enough to satisfy Mason's purpose. After telling how the attack was launched at dawn of May 26, and how entrance to the village was forced, the account continued thus:

> At length William Heydon espying the Breach in the Wigwam, supposing some English might be there, entred; but in his Entrance fell over a dead Indian; but speedily recovering himself, the Indians some fled, others crept under their Beds: the Captain [Mason] going out of the Wigwam saw many Indians in the Lane or Street; he making towards them, they fled, were pursued to the End of the Lane, where they were met by Edward Pattison, Thomas Barber, with some others; where seven of them were Slain, as they said. The Captain facing about, Marched a slow Pace up the Lane he came down, perceiving himself very much out of Breath; and coming to the other End near the Place where he first entred, saw two Soldiers standing close to the Pallizado with their Swords pointed to the Ground: The Captain told them that We should never kill them after that manner: The Captain also said, WE MUST BURN THEM: and immediately stepping into the Wigwam where he had been before, brought out a Fire Brand, and putting it into the Matts with which they were covered, set the Wigwams on Fire.

From this sparse, unsophisticated description, Jennings concludes that "It is terribly clear . . . that the village, stockaded though it was, had few warriors at home when the attack took place." Mason himself, however, asserts that just the day before the English attack, 150 braves had reinforced the Indian garrison holding the fort, but Jennings cavalierly dismisses this claim in a marvelous display of selective reading. The reasons he musters for denying Mason's express testimony on such a vital matter are offered both in Jennings's text and in a dizzying footnote. The burden of the main argument is that insofar as Mason's account portrays Indians fleeing and creeping under their beds for protection, those so described could only have been "women, children, and feeble old men," who had no other recourse but to resort to such cowardly stratagems. Surely 150 warriors—and the Pequots had already well demonstrated "their willingness to fight to the death"—would not have "suddenly and uncharacteristically turned craven." At the end of this convoluted denial of part—and only part, indeed the most straightforward and factual part—of Mason's account is Jennings's assumption that Mason marched on Fort Mystic because he had received advance intelligence from Narragansett allies that "there were no 'reinforcements.'" Destroying the "wretches" would be easily accomplished.

But the original narratives of the battle suggest a very different reading. Mason indicates that he found his first plan unworkable, that only after the attack had begun did he realize how costly it might prove for the English; only then, in self-protection, did he make the decision to burn rather than to plunder the settlement. This analysis of events is confirmed by Underhill's record of the battle, which also has the virtue of emphasizing the bravery of the Indians involved. "Most courageously," he writes, "these Pequots behaved themselves." Only when the battle grew too intense did the British, out of necessity, torch the fort. Even then, Underhill states, "many courageous fellows were unwilling to come out and fought most desperately through the palisadoes . . . and so perished valiantly. Mercy did they deserve for their valor, could we have had opportunity to bestow it." Jennings does not cite Underhill's crucial and disarming testimony; instead, he engages in some more verbal sleight of hand, carefully choosing the texts he wishes to manipulate.

[H]e replays his charge against Mason. Leaving out only the citations, I quote in full:

> . . . Underhill and Hubbard omitted the reinforcements assertion. Winthrop assigned as Pequot casualties "two chief sachems, and one hundred and fifty fighting men, and about one hundred and fifty old men, women, and children." . . . Mason's and Winthrop's "reinforcements" thus became Winthrop's total of warrior casualties. Even if this is true, it means that Mason planned the attack before those warriors arrived, but the likelihood of its truth is remote. No matter how these wriggly texts are viewed, they testify to Mason's deliberate purpose of massacring noncombatants. He had advance information of the Pequot dispositions.

First, it should be recognized that because Underhill and Hubbard do not mention the 150 Indian reinforcements, Jennings uses their silence as confirmation of the dishonesty of Mason's account. But arguments from silence "say" very little, and extreme caution should be exercised in employing them, especially in the face of explicit testimony to the contrary. Jennings next uses Winthrop's narrative, which supports Mason's claim about reinforcements, to diminish that claim by impugning Winthrop's veracity. But such doublethink will not do, for if Winthrop is unreliable, the truth of his account "remote," he cannot serve to discredit Mason; if he is reliable, his depiction of events cannot be taken lightly. Then, out of this morass of conflicting facts and conclusions, Jennings draws the non sequitur that Mason was intent on massacring noncombatant Pequots; in fact, all contemporary accounts simply state that noncombatants were massacred, not that there was any premeditated plan to do so. It appears that Jennings would have us believe that his highly ambiguous, contradictory reconstruction of the facts proposed 340 years after the event and premised on a dubious dialectical analysis of silence, a great deal of hermeneutical confusion, and a series of non sequiturs is to be given precedence over the description of circumstances provided by several contemporary and first-person accounts in our possession. Assuredly, the Connecticut militiamen acted reprehensibly and with unnecessary severity against noncombatants that spring day in 1637, but they did not do so for the reasons, nor in the manner, advanced in Jennings's moving, but untrue, retelling of the tale.

III

Following the destruction of Mystic Fort, the colonists and their Indian allies pursued the surviving Pequots. In the first major encounter of this subsequent stage in the conflict, approximately 200 Indians were captured, of whom 22 or 24 were adult males; these braves were executed. The remaining women and children, almost 80 percent of the total captured, were parceled up about evenly, as was common Indian practice, among the victorious Indian allies and the colonists of Massachusetts Bay. A second and larger engagement took place on 14 July near modern Southport, Connecticut, where Sassacus and the majority of the remaining Pequots, numbering several hundred, were surrounded. In the ensuing battle, women, children, and old men, again a majority of the Pequots present, were allowed to seek sanctuary while about 80 warriors fought to their death. In the final phase of the war, various Indian tribes in the area, vying for English friendship and seeking to settle old tribal debts, hunted down and murdered Pequot braves while dispersing their womenfolk and children. Sassacus was killed, and in early August the Mohawks sent his head to the British in Hartford.

Alden Vaughan describes the aftermath of these events:

> Toward the end of 1637 the few remaining sachems begged for an end to the war, promising vassalage in return for their lives. A peace convention was arranged for the following September. With the Treaty of Hartford, signed on September 21, 1638, the Pequots ceased to exist as an independent polity.

The treaty arrangement as well as the previous pattern of killing all adult males suggests that the anti-Pequot forces, both Indian and European, were determined to eliminate the Pequot threat once and for all. The 180 Pequots captured in the assault on Sassacus were parceled out among the victors: 80 to the Narragansett, 80 to the Mohegans, and 20 to the Eastern Niantics. The survivors were now no longer to be known as Pequots or to reside in their tribal lands, and the Pequot River was renamed the Thames and the Pequot village, New London. These treaty stipulations, which required the extinction of Pequot identity and the assignment of Pequot survivors to other tribes, and some to slavery, suggest an overt, unambiguous form of *cultural* genocide, here employed in the name of military security, However, the dispersement of the remaining communal members—the elderly, the women, and the children, almost certainly a majority of the tribe as a whole—directly contradicts the imputation of any intent to commit *physical* genocide, as some revisionists insist.

A more constrained reading of events would not deny that the Puritans, as their post-war writings reflect, were conscious that they had acted with great, perhaps even excessive, destructive force. Almost certainly composed as responses to English and Indian critics, these after-the-fact appraisals should not, however, be misconstrued as evidence of either genocidal intent prior to the event or even of genocidal behavior during and after the war. Rather, given the Puritan mentality, saturated as it was with concerns to detect God's providential design in temporal matters, these post-hoc accountings, even were we to call them rationalizations, were attempts to satisfy the Puritans' own internal axiological demand that their taking of lives on such a large scale, and in such a bloody way, was justified. Puritans had to know, and they wanted their critics to know, that what they had done was sanctioned by heaven. This concern for ethical legitimation should not be mistaken as evidence that the Puritans, however aware they were *after the event* of the contentious nature of the massacre they had wrought, looked upon this happening as signaling some fundamental re-orientation in their relationship either to their New World surroundings in general or with their New England Indian neighbors in particular. Neither Edward Johnson's approval of the Puritan preachers' exhortation to "execute vengeance upon the heathen," nor William Bradford's description of the burning of the inhabitants at Fort Mystic as a "sweet sacrifice" to the Lord, nor Underhill's appeal to scriptural precedent that in conquering a grossly evil people, such as the Pequot, "women and children must perish with their parents" are proof to the contrary. Indeed, they are exactly the sort of theological pronouncements one would expect within the Puritan conceptual environment, fed as it was by recycled scriptural paradigms.

In general, the English did not relish their victory in an unseemly way. John Mason, for example, "refused to publish his accounts of his exploits, deeming them too immodest and likely to detract from the glory ascribed to God in those events." Captain Underhill, by contrast, did publish his version of the tale, but as Richard Slotkin has written, "Captain Underhill was a man clearly out of step with the Massachusetts way and one proscribed and exiled by the Puritan community." Underhill's "enthusiasms," in fact, were repeatedly met with censure rather than emulation. Mason, by contrast, the modest, self-effacing, God-extolling leader, was considered a worthy model in early American literature.

IV

When the actions of the Puritans are placed in their appropriate context, when they are deconstructed as part and parcel of the historical reality of the seventeenth century, the accusations of genocide leveled against them are recognized to be exaggerations. However excessive the force wielded by the colonists, they had already seen—and would continue to see—their own die at the hands of the Indians. The Virginia Indian uprisings of 1622 have already been mentioned. In April 1644, a second uprising took the lives of approximately 500 whites, and in 1675, 300 more colonists were killed. The bloody events of King Philip's War (1675–76) would certainly have intensified the fears that had long plagued those living at the edge of the frontier. Much Indian violence was, of course, a response to English greed, but for those charged with protecting the members of expanding English communities, the violence had to be stopped at all costs. In the New World—an environment so uncertain, so hostile—the colonists' need to limit threats to their survival was intense. Their responses could be excessive, but their fears were not unfounded.

From our point of view, it is easy to sympathize with the Pequots and to condemn the colonists' actions, but the scope of our condemnation must be measured against the facts. After the Treaty of Hartford was signed, Pequots were not physically harmed. Indeed, in 1640 the Connecticut leadership "declared their dislike of such as would have the Indians rooted out," that is, murdered. Before the Pequots capitulated, many of their tribe had died, but the number killed probably totaled less than half the entire tribe. Sherburne Cook's estimate is even lower: "If the initial population [of Pequots] was 3,000 and 750 were killed, the battle loss was twenty-five percent of the tribe."

While many Pequots were absorbed by other tribes—it is estimated that Uncas's Mohegan tribe, for example, received hundreds—evidence clearly indicates that soon after the conclusion of the war, the Pequot began to regroup as a tribe. By 1650 four special towns were created to accommodate them, each ruled by a Pequot governor, and in 1667 Connecticut established permanent reservations for the tribe, which by 1675 numbered approximately 1,500–2,000 members. That year, no more than two generations after the Pequot War had ended, the Pequots allied with the colonists to fight King Philip's War. As recently as the 1960s, Pequots were still listed as a separate group residing in Connecticut. Such factors suggest that while the British could certainly have been less thorough, less severe, less deadly in prosecuting their campaign against the Pequots, the campaign they actually did carry out, for all its vehemence, was not, either in intent or execution, genocidal.

This revision of the revisionists is not meant to deny the larger truth that the conquest of the New World entailed the greatest demographic tragedy in history. The wrongs done to the Native Americans, the suffering they experienced, the manifest evil involved in the colonial enterprise is in no way to be deflected or minimized. However, this sorry tale of despoliation and depopulation needs to be chronicled aright, with an appropriate sense of the actuality of seventeenth-century colonial existence. False, if morally impassioned, judgments cannot substitute for carefully nuanced and discriminating appraisals. Thus, while it is appropriate to censure the excesses, the unnecessary carnage, of the Pequot War, to interpret these events through the radicalizing polemic of accusations of genocide is to rewrite history to satisfy our own moral outrage.

STEVEN T. KATZ earned his PhD at Cambridge University in 1972. He is the director of the Elie Wiesel Center for Judaic Studies at Boston University, where he holds the Alvin J. and Shirley Slater Chair in Jewish and Holocaust Studies. Katz is the author of *The Holocaust in Historical Context* (Oxford University Press, 1994) among numerous other books on Jewish history.

Alfred A. Cave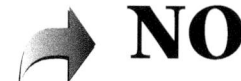

The Pequot War and the Mythology of the Frontier

Although the Pequot War was a small-scale conflict of short duration, it cast a long shadow. The images of brutal and untrustworthy savages plotting the extermination of those who would do the work of God in the wilderness, developed to explain and justify the killing of Pequots, became a vital part of the mythology of the American frontier. Celebration of victory over Indians as the triumph of light over darkness, civilization over savagery, for many generations our central historical myth, finds its earliest full expression in the contemporary chronicles and histories of this little war. The myth from its inception was grounded in a distorted conception of Indian character and behavior. The Pequot War was not waged in response to tangible acts of aggression. It cannot be understood as a rational response to a real threat to English security. It was, however, the expression of an assumption central to Puritan Indian policy. Puritan magistrates were persuaded that from time to time violent reprisals against recalcitrant savages would be necessary to make the frontier safe for the people of God. The campaign against the Pequots was driven by the same assumption that had impelled Plymouth to massacre Indians suspected of plotting against them at Wessagusett in 1623. The incineration of Pequots at Fort Mystic served the same symbolic purpose as the impalement of Wituwamet's head on Plymouth's blockhouse. Both were intended to intimidate potential enemies and to remind the Saints that they lived in daily peril of massacre at the hands of Satan's minions.

Two letters written by clergymen to civil authorities in 1637 tell us much about the Puritan mind-set. Both warn of the dangers of hesitation or leniency in dealing with the Pequots. The Reverend Thomas Hooker, responding to the attack on Wethersfield, predicted that any delay in undertaking a punitive war against them would lead other Indians to conclude that Englishmen were cowards. If that happened, Hooker predicted, all of the tribes would "turne enemyse against us." In a similar vein, the Reverend John Higginson, writing from Fort Saybrook, declared that "the eyes of all the Indians of the country are upon the English. If some serious and very speedie course not be taken to tame the pride and take down the insolency of these now insulting Pequots . . . we are like to have all the Indians in the country about our ears." The assumption, voiced here by Hooker and Higginson, that all Indians are natural enemies of Christians and that the English frontier in Connecticut can therefore be made secure only through the employment of extreme measures against the Pequots, was obviously shared by the English commanders whose cruelty to noncombatants and prisoners of war shocked their Indian allies.

In their reflections on the Pequot War, Puritan apologists argued that English troops were instruments of divine judgment. Early Puritan historians portrayed the war as a key episode in the unfolding of God's plan for New England. Captain John Mason, who believed that the English had been saved from a general Indian uprising only by divine intervention, ended his "Brief History of the Pequot War" with praise of the Almighty: "Let the whole Earth be filled with his Glory! Thus the lord was pleased to smite our Enemies in the hinder Parts, and give us their land for an Inheritance." Mason's colleague, Captain John Underhill, concurred. Through God's providence, "a few feeble instruments, soldiers not accustomed to war," defeated a barbarous and insolent nation," putting to the sword "fifteen hundred souls." Underhill rejoiced that through God's will "their country is fully subdued and fallen into the hands of the English," and he called on his readers to "magnify his honor for his great goodness." A dissenting note was struck by Lieutenant Lion Gardener who, in a work written in 1660, wondered why the Bay Colony leaders made war against the Pequots to avenge the worthless old reprobate Stone, while the Narragansetts, whom he presumed guilty of the murder of the worthy Captain Oldham, went scot-free. But Gardener, no less a Puritan than his colleagues, warned against trusting Indians

Cave, Alfred A. "The Pequot War and the Mythology of the Frontier." Reprinted from *The Pequot War*, pages 168–178. Copyright ©1996 by the University of Massachusetts Press. Used with permission.

and complained about lax military preparedness. After describing Indian tortures, he predicted that hundreds of Englishmen would die in agony and dishonor, "if God should deliver us into their hands, as justly he may for our sins."

No other Puritan writer expressed any misgivings about whether the English had attacked the right adversary in 1637. The Massachusetts Bay Colony historian Edward Johnson, writing of the English massacre of Pequots at Fort Mystic, declared that "by this means the Lord strook a trembling terror into all the Indians round about, even to this very day." Through righteous violence, Johnson believed, God had pacified the forces of Satan in the wilderness. That theme dominated Puritan thinking about Indian wars. The commissioners of the United Colonies of New England in 1646 called for the writing of histories that would record how God "hath cast the dread of his people (weak in themselves) upon the Indians." Increase Mather, in his *Brief History of the War with the Indians in New England* (1676), wrote that the defeat of the Pequots in 1637 "must be ascribed to the wonderful Providence of God, who did (as with Jacob of old, and after that with the children of Israel) lay the fear of the English and the dread of them upon all the Indians. The terror of god was upon them round about." Incorporating that notion into his grand history of New England, Cotton Mather later declared that, through God's providence, the Puritans were enabled to achieve not only "the utter subduing" of the Pequots but "the affrighting of all the other Natives" as well, and thereby secured several decades of peace.

As the evidence reviewed in this study demonstrates, Puritan preoccupation with the idea that Indians were part of a satanic conspiracy against God's true church in the wilderness led them to interpret Pequot recalcitrance as evidence of malevolent intent. But it does not follow that we can therefore explain the Pequot War solely and simply as the result of an unfortunate misunderstanding about certain specific occurrences, for the conflict was more fundamentally the outgrowth of a profound incompatibility of cultures. Puritan ideology precluded long-term coexistence with a "savage" people unwilling to acknowledge Christian hegemony. Clarification of Pequot intentions in the short run would not necessarily have changed the long-term outcome. A reading of their commentaries on Indian affairs suggests that our assumptions about the desirability of peaceful coexistence were not necessarily shared by the founders of Puritan New England or by their immediate successors. Although they feared Indian war and prayed that they be spared its horrors, they also suspected that it was both necessary and inevitable. Apologists for the Fort Mystic massacre did not invent the image of the Indian as a savage killer to excuse the Pequot War, nor did Pequot actions inspire a new view of Indian character. There is ample evidence, as we noted in the first chapter of this study, that from the founding of the first English settlements in North America onward, Englishmen in general and Puritans in particular saw in Native American culture only the "degeneracy" of those who follow the Devil rather than God; they accordingly were predisposed to regard Indians as untrustworthy and treacherous and were thus prone to overreact to rumors of impending Indian attacks.

Their acceptance of customary English anti-Indian prejudice in itself does not fully explain Puritan behavior. We must also examine Puritan ideas about the role of Indians in God's providential plan for New England. Here we encounter concepts quite alien to modern sensibilities, embedded in explanations so far removed from our sense of historical processes that it is tempting to dismiss them as irrelevant. But let us look more closely, for we must try to understand the seventeenth century on its own terms. Fundamental to the Puritan understanding of the dynamics of New England history was the assumption that only through God's special protection of his people could Christians survive in a wilderness realm dominated by Satan and inhabited by satanic savages. God intervened early to soften the hearts of the godless heathens who lurked in New England's forests and wastelands. Ultimately, he controlled their behavior. It therefore followed that troubled Indian relations might well be a frightening sign that God's protection had been, or was about to be, withheld for some reason. Throughout the seventeenth century, rumors of impending Indian attack occasioned deep soul-searching and calls for reformation in Puritan New England.

The Pequot War inspired the earliest expressions of the idea that Indian wars were providentially ordained events intended to test and chastise God's people. John Higginson suggested that the Lord had set "the Indians upon his servants, to make them cleave more closely together, to prevent contentions of brethern." Edward Johnson hinted that God had unleashed the Pequots in order to punish the Puritans for their lack of proper severity in dealing with Anne Hutchinson and the antinomians. Those suggestions foreshadowed the portrayals of the role of divine providence in Indian warfare that would dominate the literature inspired by King Philip's War half a century later. Historians of that conflict spoke of God's need to test his Saints in the fire of battle, punish his people for straying from the true way, and give them also opportunity to serve as the vehicles of God's wrath in exterminating heathen who refused to embrace the Gospel. Those themes were exploited most thoroughly by Puritan divines who, in later years, warned of the fearful consequences of declension. Thus, Increase Mather in a sermon preached in 1676 declared King Philip's War God's "heavy judgment," a punishment of the "sin of man's unfaithfulness. . . . Alas that New England should be brought so low in so short a time (for she is come down wonderfully) and that by such vile enemies by the Heathen, yea by the worst of the Heathen." Cotton Mather, in his 1689 election sermon, declared that the "molestations" the English in New England had suffered at the hands of the Indians had come about because God was angry that his people had "indianized"; in other words, they had allowed themselves to succumb to what Mather regarded as Indian vices: idleness, self-indulgence, and dishonesty. The belief that God used Indians as a rod with which to discipline his people became an enduring and vital aspect of the Puritan sense of the past. In his election sermon of 1730, the Reverend Thomas Prince, reviewing more than a century of New England history, exclaimed, "how often has he made the eastern Indians the rod of his anger and the staff of indignation with us! He has sent them against us and given them the charge to take the spoil and tread us down as the mire of the street. They came with open mouth upon us; they thrust thro' everyone they found abroad; they ensnared and slew our mighty men who went forth for our defense; they spoil'd our fields and pastures; they burnt up our houses; they destroy'd our towns and garrisons; they murdered our wives; they carried our young men and virgins into captivity; they had no pity on the fruit of the womb; their eyes spared not our children, they dashed them in pieces." Prince reminded the citizenry that they had survived only because the Lord, although rightly provoked, finally took pity on his own true people and turned against the savages. "He rebuk'd them and set them one against another . . . as wax melteth before the fire, so they perished at the presence of God." But his favor and protection were not to be taken for granted.

God's wrath, in Puritan formulations of the providential view of New England's history, was not reserved for errant Saints. Historians of King Philip's War assured their readers that, although the war was in part intended to punish the English in New England for straying from the true way, the Lord's anger against the Indians was far greater. For our purposes, perhaps the most revealing statement in the later Indian war literature was a declaration from the Bay Colony's superintendent of Indian affairs that God had ordained the war against King Philip in order to punish the Indians who had refused to embrace Puritan Christianity. This was not an entirely new theme. Although lack of receptivity to the Christian Gospel was not stated explicitly as a reason for killing Pequots by any of the chroniclers of that early war, the preacher's charge to the Connecticut militia to "execute vengeance against the heathen" rested upon the assumption that the English were indeed called upon by the Almighty to visit his wrath upon a very sinful people. Puritan literary celebrations of the Fort Mystic massacre, which strike us as rather grotesque, are grounded in the belief that the burning of Pequots was a righteous act of divine retribution.

Assessments of the causes and consequences of the Pequot War must take into account Puritan ideas about God's attitude toward the unregenerate. The Pequots were not the last indigenous group in New England to suffer what the Puritans believed to be divinely mandated punishment. The Narragansetts and the Wampanoags, friends of the English in 1636–37, both discovered, before the seventeenth century ended, that the Puritan conception of God's providential plan for New England ultimately left no room for vigorous assertions of Native American autonomy, for such assertions offended the Puritan sense of mission. Puritan toleration of Indian independence was never anything more than an expedient; as the population ratio between Englishmen and Native Americans in New England shifted in favor of the English, the Puritan authorities grew increasingly overbearing in their dealings with their Indian counterparts. Puritan Indian policy from its inception was driven by the conviction that, if the Puritans remained faithful to their covenant with the Almighty, they were destined to replace the Indians as lords of New England. Puritan ideology required that Indian control of land and resources be terminated, on the grounds that "savages" did not exploit natural bounty in the manner that God intended. The pressures created by the burgeoning of the English population in the latter half of the seventeenth century reinforced that ideological imperative. Economic changes, such as the declining importance of the fur trade and the expansion of English agriculture and industry, which reduced the need for Indian commerce, further jeopardized the status of Native American communities in a New England dominated by Euro-Americans. The Indian uprising led by Metacom (King Philip) in 1675 represented a desperate, belated, and ultimately futile effort to protect the last remnants of Indian sovereignty in southern New England.

Although Puritan apologists for the war against the Pequots provided one of the earliest English statements of the belief in Indian war as a divinely sanctioned means of extending the light of civilization and true religion into the wilderness, their version of the frontier drama contained some elements that later generations would find strange and uncongenial. Over the years, the myth of heroic struggle against savagery underwent some important changes in emphasis as secular doctrines of scientific progress and historical evolution, along with a new sense of "manifest destiny," largely but not entirely replaced Puritan notions of divine providence. The idea that Indians might be used by the Almighty to punish the sins of Christians fell from favor. Puritan misgivings about the wilderness as a place of spiritual peril gave way to a more optimistic and uncritical celebration of the frontier as the birthplace of uniquely American virtues. Indian rejection of progress replaced their disinterest in the Gospel or their presumed alliance with Satan as the reason most often advanced to explain their imminent extinction. But in one important particular, the central theme remained the same. On a succession of frontiers, as Winthrop Jordon reminds us, "conquering the Indian symbolized and personified the conquest of American difficulties, the surmounting of the wilderness. To push back the Indian was to prove the worth of one's own mission, to make straight in the desert a highway for civilization."

Once the eastern Indians were no longer a threat, some nineteenth-century writers transformed the Native American into a victim rather than a villain. In their pages, the American "savage" emerged as an innocent and hapless primitive doomed by the imperatives of historical progress, an object of pity for whom the sentimental might shed a tear. Historians, novelists, and dramatists now sometimes castigated Puritans and other pioneers for their mistreatment of such a simple and defenseless people. It goes without saying that such sympathy for the Indian as a "much injured race" is not to be found in seventeenth-century Puritan commentaries on Indian wars. But we must not assume that its appearance in later historical writing necessarily meant abandonment of the idea that the conquest and dispossession of Indians were historical imperatives. Until quite recently, the attitude of paternalistic benevolence cultivated by architects of Indian policy as well as by their critics was generally qualified by a condition: The Indian must now cease to be an Indian, must embrace the values, culture, and religion of his dispossessors, if he is to be deemed worthy of survival. Here we are once again face to face with the premise that drove Puritan Indian policy: denial of the validity and viability of Native American life. Whether the Indian was to be displaced by the workings of divine providence or by the inexorable march of progress, the outcome was much the same. Moreover, it did not matter whether Indians were portrayed as noble or degraded; white Americans over the years generally thought of them as a backward people without history and without a future.

While the frontier struggle for control of land continued, misgivings about mistreatment of Native Americans had only a very limited impact upon events. As Michael Paul Rogin notes, "not the Indians alive . . . but their destruction, symbolized the American experience." Violence against Indians cannot be explained fully as the outgrowth of the white man's acquisitive instincts. There were other motives at work. Rogin argues that Native American societies in their communal aspects "posed a severe threat," as they inspired "forbidden nostalgia for the nurturing, blissful and primitively violent connection to nature that white Americans had to leave behind." Hence, "the only safe Indians were dead, sanitized, or completely dependent upon white benevolence." Indians were "at once symbols of a lost childhood bliss, and, as bad children repositories of murderous negative projections." Those Indians who physically survived plague, war, and dispossession were therefore not only relegated to reservations, where they lived in abject poverty, but subjected to an onslaught on their cultural integrity through measures such as the so-called Religious Crimes Acts, which outlawed the sun dance and other expressions of Native American spirituality.

Intolerance of Indian cultures reflected the persistence of essential elements of the Puritan vision of the struggle between heathen savagery and Christian civilization. Puritan ideology as it pertained to encounters with Indians contained three premises which later provided vital elements in the mythology of the American frontier. One was the image, not original with the Puritans but embellished by them, of the Indian as the Other, primitive, dark, and sinister. Another was the portrayal, first developed in the Pequot War narratives, of the Indian fighter as the agent of God and of progress, redeeming the land through righteous violence. And finally, it is to the apologists for the Pequot War that we owe the justification of the expropriation of Indian resources and the extinction of Indian sovereignty as security measures necessitated by their presumed savagery.

Few historians today confuse these elements of our founding myth with historical fact. The "triumphalist" tone that once characterized the narration of Euro-American victories over presumably savage foes is now muted, or silenced, as scholars struggle to come to terms with the ambiguities as well as the cruelties and injustice now perceived in the encounters of indigenous peoples and European invaders. What place should the Pequots occupy in the new history of intercultural conflict? Despite the ample evidence of arrogance, ignorance, and brutality in the English treatment of Sassacus and his people, it will not do to cast them in the role of passive victims. They were not guilty of the enormities, real or anticipated, with which they are charged in the traditional, pro-Puritan literature. They were not a threat to the survival of the Puritan colonies. But in their efforts to establish and maintain a far-flung tributary network and to control European trade, the Pequots provoked powerful Indian opposition. Their murder of Indian rivals en route to trade at the House of Good Hope in 1632, the exile of the Mohegan sachems shortly thereafter and the occupation of their hunting preserves, along with the subsequent treatment of Mohegans living in Pequot villages after the final defection of Uncas, all give evidence of a ruthless determination to maintain power that suggests that Sassacus would be seriously miscast were we now to describe him simply as an inoffensive noble savage wronged by the white man. He was inept; he lost, but he was hardly a hapless innocent. Neither were the Mohegan, River Indian, and Narragansett sachems who engineered his downfall.

In seeking to use the English as pawns in their power struggles, the sachems made a serious miscalculation. The consequences of alliance with the Puritan colonies were not immediately apparent. The sachems no doubt believed that they could maintain control. The English, as we have seen, were susceptible to manipulation by those who knew how to play on their expectations and anxieties. It was a game that Uncas easily mastered, that Sassacus never learned how to play, and that Miantonomi ultimately lost. But the final outcome was loss of Algonquian autonomy. A revisionist history of the Pequot War written from the Native American point of view—and this present study does not pretend to accomplish that—might well deemphasize decisions made at Boston, Plymouth, Saybrook, and Hartford and focus instead on the miscalculations and blunders in Pequot, Mohegan, and Narragansett councils that paved the way for the early establishment of English hegemony in southern New England. Unfortunately, given the limitations in the source materials, such a reconstruction would be highly conjectural. But we do know enough about Native American politics in southern New England in the early seventeenth century to realize that viewing the conflict from an Algonquian perspective would immediately expose the absurdity of the English belief that they were engaged in some sort of holy war against murderous heathens determined to exterminate Christians. Although the Puritans believed that their actions were driven by their own security needs, and by divine providence, the conflicts that culminated in the Pequot War originally were the outgrowth of the ambitions of rival sachems, not of an anti-English conspiracy. Believing themselves endangered, the Puritan colonies, to the later sorrow of many of their Indian allies, transformed the quarrel with the Pequots into a successful campaign to establish English dominance.

In their justification of the war against the Pequots, Puritan mythmakers invoked old images of treacherous savages and told tales of diabolical plots. It is now clear that their portrayals of the Pequots bear little resemblance to reality. The Puritans transformed their adversary into a symbol of savagery. Rumors of Pequot conspiracy, although flimsy in substance and of dubious origin, reinforced expectations about savage behavior and justified preemptive slaughter and dispossession. Not only did the Pequot War engender its own myths in reinforcement and embellishment of Puritan ideology; it was the fulfillment of a prewar mythology that foretold conflicts in the wilderness between the people of God and the hosts of Satan. The fact that the triumph of Christians in such conflicts would open the way to English control of land and trade, and to the receipt of tribute, provided powerful material incentives to maintain intact ideas about savagery that justified the domination of indigenous peoples. Puritan apologists for their assault on the Pequots made a significant contribution to the development of an ideological rationale for Christian imperialism. The images they framed of their adversary have been remarkably persistent but now should be recognized as the products of wartime propaganda.

The Pequot War in reality was the messy outgrowth of petty squabbles over trade, tribute, and land among Pequots, Mohegans, River Indians, Niantics, Narragansetts, Dutch traders, and English Puritans. The Puritan imagination endowed this little war with a metahistorical significance it hardly deserved. But the inner logic of Puritan belief required creation of a mythical conflict, a cosmic struggle of good and evil in the wilderness, and out of that need the Pequot War epic was born.

ALFRED A. CAVE is Professor Emeritus of History at the University of Toledo. Previously, he held academic positions at the City College of New York, the University of Utah, and the University of Florida. Among his many publications in the fields of Native American and Jacksonian era history, he is the author of *Prophets of the Great Spirit: Native American Revitalization Movements in Eastern North America* (University of Nebraska Press, 2006) and *Lethal Encounters: Englishmen and Indians in Colonial Virginia* (University of Nebraska Press, 2013).

EXPLORING THE ISSUE

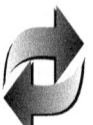

Was the Pequot War Largely a Product of Native American Aggression?

Critical Thinking and Reflection

1. Evaluate Steven Katz's perception of historical revisionism with regard to the Pequot War.
2. How does Alfred Cave support his argument that previous interpretations of the Pequot War were a product of Puritan mythmaking?
3. Compare and contrast the conclusions reached by Katz and Cave regarding the causes of the Pequot War.
4. What role did religion play in the outbreak of the Pequot War?
5. Based on your reading of these two essays, to what extent was the Pequot War inevitable?

Is There Common Ground?

The complexities associated with the relations between Native Americans and colonists from Europe are evident from the foregoing essays. Together they suggest the difficulty associated with efforts to generalize about the clash of cultures that occurred on New World shores.

By the end of the colonial period in British North America, the Native American populations in the original 13 colonies had been significantly reduced in terms of numbers and power. Was this reality an inevitable consequence of intercultural hostilities, or are their other viable explanations for Indian decline? Undoubtedly, many European colonists harbored attitudes that allowed them to rationalize aggressive action toward the indigenous peoples they encountered in America. As was the case with their European counterparts, Indians, too, saw themselves and their culture as superior to the new arrivals from across the Atlantic. Both sides viewed the other as uncivilized savages. These general attitudes, however, did not prevent cordial relations and other forms of beneficial alliances from developing. Trade alliances did not end conflict, but they did reinforce recognition of the mutual benefit derived from such connections.

As Gary Nash has observed, American culture derived much of its uniqueness from the interaction of Indian and European, as well as African, traditional folkways. The physical presence of each of these groups played a fundamental role in the emerging political, economic, and social development of early America. The day-to-day lives of the residents of the New World were dramatically affected by the presence of these various human populations and not solely in negative ways.

Additional Resources

James Axtell, *The Invasion Within: The Contest of Cultures in Colonial North America* (Oxford University Press, 1985)

Karen Ordahl Kupperman, *Indians and English: Facing Off in Early America* (Cornell University Press, 2000)

Jill Lepore, *The Name of War: King Philip's War and the Origins of American Identity* (Alfred A. Knopf, 1998)

Daniel R. Mandell, *King Philip's War: Colonial Expansion, Native Resistance, and the End of Indian Hegemony* (Johns Hopkins University Press, 2010)

Gary Nash, *Red, White, and Black: The Peoples of Early America*, 3rd ed. (Prentice-Hall, 1982)

Internet References . . .

Colonial Settlement, 1600s-1763: Virginia's Early Relations with Native Americans

http://www.loc.gov/teachers/classroommaterials/presentationsandactivities/presentations/timeline/colonial/indians/

Document Showcase: American Indians in Colonial New York

http://nysa32.nysed.gov/education/showcase/201111nativeamerican/index.shtml

Native American Archaeology

http://www.portal.state.pa.us/portal/server.pt/community/native_american_archaeology/3316

Native American Legends: Colonial Era Indian Wars, Battles & Massacres

http://www.legendsofamerica.com/na-colonialindianwars.html

Virginia's Indians, Past and Present

http://virginiaindians.pwnet.org/

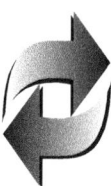

ISSUE

Selected, Edited, and with Issue Framing Material by:
Kevin R. Magill and Tony L. Talbert, *Baylor University*

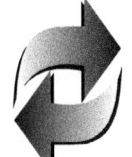

Was the Colonial Period a "Golden Age" for Women in America?

YES: **Gloria L. Main**, "Gender, Work, and Wages in Colonial New England," *William and Mary Quarterly* (1994)

NO: **Cornelia Hughes Dayton**, from "Women Before the Bar," University of North Carolina Press (1995)

Learning Outcomes

After reading this issue, you will be able to:

- Discuss the type of work women in colonial New England did for pay compared to men.
- Appreciate how women's opportunities to earn wages for their work changed over time in the colonial period.
- Understand the intersection of legal culture and gender relations in colonial New England.
- Discuss the ways in which women possessed a voice in colonial American courts.
- Realize how women's legal status declined in colonial Connecticut from the seventeenth to the eighteenth century.

ISSUE SUMMARY

YES: Gloria Main highlights that more New England women entered the paid work force, received higher wages, and saw increased recognition for their labors following the Seven Years War. She believes because women were more highly valued for their labor and that labor was relatively scarce in the early colonial period, that they received higher wages and economic autonomy.

NO: Cornelia Hughes Dayton challenges the "golden age" thesis, arguing that women were being used for their labor and that improvements in their condition benefited the patriarchy. She argues that increased access to county courts for women in seventeenth-century was negated as new rules and practices were implemented in the eighteenth century. The changes strengthen patriarchal authority and reversed many of the gains that had been made.

For generations students in American history classes have read of the founding of the colonies in British North America, their political and economic development, and the colonists' struggles for independence, without ever being confronted by a female protagonist in this magnificent historical drama. The terms "sons of liberty" and "founding fathers" reflect the end result of a long tradition of gender-specific myopia. In fact, only in the last generation have discussions of the role of women in the development of American society made their appearance in standard textbooks. Consequently, it is useful to explore the status of women in colonial America.

The topic is quite complex. The status of colonial women was determined by cultural attitudes that were exported to the New World from Europe, by the specific conditions confronting successive waves of settlers—male and female—in terms of labor requirements, and by changes produced by colonial maturation over time. It would be impossible to pinpoint a single, static condition in which all colonial women existed.

What was the status of women in the British North American colonies? To what degree did the legal status of women differ from their de facto status? For much of the past century, scholarship has produced the notion that colonial women enjoyed a more privileged status than either their European contemporaries or their nineteenth-century descendants. Support for the "golden age" theory can be found in Elizabeth Anthony Dexter, *Colonial Women of Affairs*, 2nd ed. (Houghton Mifflin, 1931); Mary Ritter Beard, *Woman as Force in History* (Macmillan, 1946); Eleanor Flexner, *Century of Struggle* (Belknap Press, 1959); and Richard B. Morris, *Studies in the History of American Law*, 2nd ed. (Octagon Books, 1964). This interpretation was reinforced in the 1970s in John Demos, *A Little Commonwealth: Family Life in Plymouth Colony* (Oxford University Press, 1970); Roger Thompson, *Women in Stuart England and America: A Comparative Study* (Routledge and Kegan, 1974); and Page Smith, *Daughters of the Promised Land: Women in American History* (Little, Brown, 1977). For example, Demos contends that despite the fact that Plymouth Colony was based on a patriarchal model in which women were expected to subordinate themselves to men, women still shared certain responsibilities with their husbands in some business activities and in matters relating to their children. N. E. H. Hull's *Female Felons: Women and Serious Crime in Colonial Massachusetts* (University of Illinois Press, 1987) concludes that men and women received equal justice in the colonial period.

Women were crucial to the economic success of the colonial experiments and performed numerous functions in various occupations and professions. They not only performed all the household duties but also assisted the menfolk with agricultural duties outside the home when the necessity arose. In colonial America and during the American Revolution, they practiced law, pounded iron as blacksmiths, trapped for furs and tanned leather, made guns, built ships, and edited and printed newspapers. In their path-breaking article "The Planter's Wife: The Experience of White Women in Seventeenth-Century Maryland," *William and Mary Quarterly* (October 1977), Lois Green Carr and Lorena S. Walsh assessed this issue against the backdrop of four factors in colonial Maryland: the predominance of an immigrant population; the early death of male inhabitants; the late marriages of women due to their indentured servitude; and the sexual imbalance in which men greatly outnumbered women. As a result of these conditions, according to Carr and Walsh, Maryland women experienced fewer restraints on their social conduct and enjoyed more power than did their English counterparts. Most who survived became planters' wives, enjoyed considerable freedom in choosing their husbands, and benefited from a substantial right to inherit property.

At the same time, colonial society viewed women as subordinate beings. They were closed off from any formal public power in the colonies even when they performed essential economic functions within the community. Society as a whole viewed them as "weaker vessels," physically, intellectually, and morally. Nor was it a coincidence that most suspected witches were female. Many of those accused of witchcraft in late-seventeenth-century New England were older women who had inherited land that traditionally would have gone to males. Such patterns of inheritance disrupted the normative male-dominated social order. Witchcraft hysteria in colonial America, then, was a by-product of economic pressures and gender exploitation. These views are developed particularly well in Lyle Koehler, *A Search for Power: The "Weaker Sex" in Seventeenth Century New England* (University of Illinois Press, 1980), and Carol F. Karlsen, *The Devil in the Shape of a Woman: Witchcraft in Colonial New England* (Random House, 1987).

As several of the titles cited above suggest, many of the scholarly monographs on the lives of colonial women focus on New England. These include Edmund S. Morgan, *The Puritan Family: Religion and Domestic Relations in Seventeenth-Century New England* (Boston Public Library, 1944) and Laurel Thatcher Ulrich, *Good Wives: Image and Reality in the Lives of Women in Northern New England, 1650–1750* (Knopf, 1980). For another Chesapeake colony, women in colonial Virginia are treated in Darrett B. Rutman and Anita H. Rutman, *A Place in Time: Middlesex County, Virginia, 1650–1750* (W. W. Norton, 1984) and Kathleen M. Brown, *Good Wives, Nasty Wenches, and Anxious Patriarchs: Gender, Race, and Power in Colonial Virginia* (University of North Carolina Press, 1996).

Women in the age of the American Revolution are the focus of Carol Ruth Berkin, *Within the Conjurer's Circle: Women in Colonial America* (General Learning Press, 1974); Linda Grant DePauw and Conover Hunt, *"Remember the Ladies": Women in America, 1750–1815* (Viking Press, 1976); Mary Beth Norton, *Liberty's Daughters: The Revolutionary Experience of American Women, 1750–1800* (Little, Brown 1980); Linda Kerber, *Women of the Republic: Intellect and Ideology in Revolutionary America* (North Carolina, 1980); Charles W. Akers, *Abigail Adams: An American Woman* (Little, Brown, 1980), and Joy Day Buel and Richard Buel, Jr., *The Way of Duty: A Woman and Her Family in Revolutionary America* (W. W. Norton, 1984). For the conclusion that the American Revolution failed to advance women's status, see Joan Hoff Wilson's "The Illusion of Change: Women and the American Revolution" in Alfred F. Young, ed., *The American Revolution: Explorations in the History of American Radicalism* (Northern Illinois University Press, 1976).

The following selections explore the status of women in the colonial period. Gloria Main focuses on women's economic status by comparing types of work, pay scales, and trends in wages in the seventeenth and eighteenth centuries and discovers that the division of labor between men and women was less clearly defined than traditionally assumed. Because they were relatively scarce, she concludes, women were valued for their labor and, as time passed, New England women developed a significant degree of economic autonomy.

Cornelia Hughes Dayton examines women's legal status in colonial Connecticut through a study of county court cases treating the subjects of debt, divorce, illicit consensual sex, rape, and slander in which women were involved. She finds that although the seventeenth-century Puritan sense of justice created opportunities for women to be heard in court in ways that had not been available within English legal tradition, these opportunities had begun to fade by the early eighteenth century, and women's presence in court declined dramatically as legal public space was transformed from an inclusive forum to an institution primarily serving the interests of commercially active men.

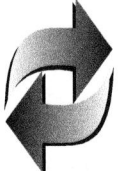

YES

Gloria L. Main

Gender, Work, and Wages in Colonial New England

...Historians of colonial women ... tend to ignore economic issues when debating trends in women's status and condition. Most believe that white women were more highly regarded in the colonies than at home, because of the higher value of their labor and their relative scarcity, at least in the seventeenth century in regions such as the Chesapeake. Others posit that economic opportunities for women narrowed as colonial society developed beyond primitive conditions in which women shouldered burdens customarily borne by men. Data presented below lend support to the first proposition but dispute the second.

This article examines the types of work women in early New England did compared to men, weighs relative pay scales, and explores trends in the wages of both sexes. Evidence comes from two types of sources: wage ceilings discussed or imposed by governments in 1670 and 1777 and pay rates found in account books, diaries, and probate records. These sources also supply the basis for estimating women's rates of participation in the paid labor force and for tabulating the types of work women performed for pay. All of this material can be conveniently summarized by dividing the colonial period into four phases: initial growth (1620–1674), crisis and recovery (1675–1714), stability (1715–1754), and expansion (1755–1774). The sequence, however, defies simple linear interpretations of progression, either from good conditions to bad, declension, or from bad conditions to good, progress. Both the status of women and the region's economy experienced cycles of good and bad times, but the closing decades of the period saw real improvement for both. Perhaps the most important lesson of this investigation is that even relatively modest economic changes can, by their cumulative actions, significantly alter family relations and living standards....

Settlers in a new land must find ways to acquire the goods they want and cannot make for themselves. For New Englanders, this proved a major challenge. Probably the most notable characteristic of the economy that is evident in probate inventories was the economy's dependence on England for manufactures of all sorts, including textiles. In the first generation after settlement, few women could have engaged in spinning, weaving, or dyeing simply because unprocessed textile fibers were in short supply. "Farmers deem it better for their profit to put away [sell] their cattel and corn for cloathing, then to set upon making of cloth." Flax production was labor intensive, and sheep did not thrive under pioneering conditions: wolves found them easy prey, and the woodland underbrush tore away their wool. By the 1670s these conditions had changed. An aggressive bounty system and the spread of settlements into the interior gradually exterminated the wolves and cleared enough pastureland so that sheep became a more familiar sight on mainland farms. Spinning wheels, mentioned in Plymouth Colony inventories as early as 1644, gradually became common, and most mid-century householders' inventories in Plymouth and neighboring colonies listed wool and flax, and some mention sheep, cotton, and even homemade cloth. Still, textile production must have continued to fall short of potential demand, because few people chose to invest their time in weaving. Of roughly 1,500 inventories dating from before 1675, only thirty, all for men, list looms. Similarly, when Carl Bridenbaugh recorded the occupations of men in the early volumes of Rhode Island land evidences, he identified only one weaver and one cloth worker out of forty-two artisans before 1670.

Nor did many early households possess the tools for such women's tasks as brewing, baking, or dairying. Only a few women appear anywhere in John Pynchon's Connecticut Valley accounts. Of the four women he mentioned in the 1640s, one received pay for chickens and eggs, one for weeding, one for making hay, and the fourth for domestic service. There is no mention of brewing, baking, or butter making, although in 1648 Pynchon paid Henry Burt for making malt, probably from the barley mowed by Richard Excell that year, and Pynchon paid another man for milking his cows in 1666–1667. The first reference to spinning appears in 1663, to knitting in 1668, and to sewing in 1669.

Most of New England's people were farmers. Women who were not tied down by young children probably spent their time outdoors working in gardens or with their men in the fields. Although English women did not customarily do heavy field work, they did garden with hoes, and in the colonies the hoe played a major role wherever families could use existing Indian fields. In early Saybrook Alice Apsley marketed medicinal herbs and onions from her garden. Goody Macksfield supplied a Boston shopkeeper with apples, squashes, beans, cucumbers, carrots, and cabbages, as well as honey, butter, cheese, and eggs. C. Dallett Hemphill examined the work activities of Salem women recorded in testimony before the Essex County court between 1636 and 1683 and found them engaged in men's work or working with men: servant Ann Knight winnowed corn, another woman carried grain to the mill, and others milked cows and branded steers in the company of men; a witness in one case remembered seeing the wife of Joseph Dalaber working alongside her husband planting and covering corn.

. . . [T]he ratio of women's pay to men's pay was at its highest point in this early period when the division of labor between men and women was less clearly defined than in contemporary England or as it later came to be in New England. Women could hoe in already-cleared Indian fields, and meadows and salt marshes supplied their small herds of animals with forage. When these sites filled up and the numbers of livestock expanded, newcomers had to break new ground and create meadows planted with English grasses. Inventories record the gradual advent of a more English farming style using heavy plows drawn by teams of oxen, while tax lists and town genealogies trace the growing supply of sturdy young sons. Similarly, the appearance of spinning wheels, firkins, brewing vats, and dye pots attests to the kinds of activities that came to employ women. The division of labor between the sexes widened and, as it did so, separated them physically.

The use of ox teams, restricted to older men, effectively segregated family members into field and home workers. Men and older boys also did the sowing and harrowing at the beginning of the farm year and the reaping and mowing at harvest. In early spring they planted and pruned orchards and carted and spread dung. In June they washed and sheared sheep. In fall they pressed cider and slaughtered hogs. In the slack seasons men cut and dragged timber, built and maintained fences, cleared underbrush, ditched bogs, and dug out stones. In most of these activities, handling draft animals was essential and was work for males only. The men used oxen to remove stumps and boulders, drag timber, cart dung, and haul hay and horses to drive cider presses. Only men and older boys paddled canoes, steered scows, piloted "gundalows" (gondolas), or rowed boats.

Women participated in none of these activities except at harvest time, when their help was welcomed. Even then, they did not mow grass or grain, because most did not have the height or upper body strength to handle scythes. Diaries after 1750 show them helping with the reaping, probably binding sheaves and sickling wheat and rye. Young Jabez Fitch of Norwich, Connecticut, reported enthusiastically in his diary on July 24, 1759, "there was a great Reeping[;] we Liv'd very well[;] we had Women anough & Some more." A story related in a town history about one woman's feat is no doubt apocryphal but interesting for its celebration of women's physical achievements in a less genteel age: a Mrs. Brown of Chester, New Hampshire, around the year 1800 or earlier, with others had sowed rye for its seed. At harvest time she prepared breakfast, nursed her child, walked five or six miles to the field, reaped her rye (finishing before any of the men), and walked back home.

Men's diaries also describe both sexes and all ages gathering corn by day and husking together at night, making the work an occasion for a frolic. Both sexes and all ages went berrying and nutting together. Young people often turned such occasions to their own devices, especially when gathering strawberries on long June evenings. The excitement these occasions could create is recorded in the diary of a Harvard undergraduate, who, with other young men, succeeded in transforming a quilting party into a late night gala.

Many farm tasks fell more or less exclusively to the female members of the household. Girls and women tended the fowl and small animals. They milked the cows at dawn and dusk, separated the cream, churned the butter, and made the cheese. They planted and hoed kitchen gardens in plots men had prepared by plowing and harrowing. Women boiled the offal for such by-products as sausage casings, head cheese, calf's foot jelly, and rennet after men killed, cleaned, and butchered animals. Gender-based assignment of many farm chores centered on objective differences in body height and strength rather than on what was deemed culturally appropriate to one sex or the other. Females carried out some of the same tasks as younger boys—they helped hay, hoe, weed, harvest crops, and husk corn.

Yet gender ordered male and female spheres in ways that went beyond obvious physical distinctions. For instance, men and older boys not only cut timber but operated sawmills, erected buildings, dug wells and cellars, laid stone, pointed chimneys, and shaved shingles and staves. Men tanned and curried hides, made saddles or gloves, and bound shoes. Older boys got the bark for tanning, shaved it, ground it, and laid the leather away.... [S]killed craftsmen in these trades earned substantially more than farm laborers. Females never participated in these activities. Nor did girls drive cattle or carry grain on horseback to the mill, as boys did. Women did not thresh grain, even though boys of thirteen or fourteen did so. Although men and boys traveled abroad freely in their duties, women's work more often kept them inside or near their own home or those of kinsmen or employers. In and around the home they earned income from tasks that males assiduously avoided: cleaning, cooking, sewing, spinning, washing clothes, nursing, and caring for children.

Thus, people allocated work among themselves based on physical capacity but also on gender. The advent of English-style agriculture, involving large draft animals and deep plowing, helped fix many boundaries between the sexes. The case of John Graves II of East Guilford is illustrative. Five daughters and four sons survived infancy; all of them appear in his accounts at one time or another credited for a day's or a week's work. Of the eighty-nine work occasions he recorded between 1703 and 1726 (the year he died), he identified daughters on twenty-one occasions and sons on sixty-eight. Thus, sons appeared more than three times as often. Graves hired occasional male help in addition to his sons and kept a young servant named Thome for two years when his younger boys were too small to hoe, make fences, or mow hay. Meanwhile, his girls did chores—but never farm work—for his neighbors. They sewed, spun, nursed, and kept house.

An account book of great interest because of the economic activities of women that it records is that of merchant Elisha Williams of Wethersfield, Connecticut, a commercial farm town situated on the Connecticut River just south of Hartford. Williams's ledger begins in 1738, and its pages are filled with references to women credited for onions. A bunch of roped onions weighed about three or four pounds, and Williams bought them for 5d. per bunch in 1738. Women earned a penny per bunch for tying them in the early 1740s. They generally took their pay in the form of store merchandise, mostly luxury imports such as sugar, chocolate, pepper, rum, cotton lace, and silk romall, a silken handkerchief used as a head covering. Other goods paid for by women's onions included medicine, a pair of spectacles, and a copy of Homer's *Iliad*.

So far, the evidence from account books and diaries has helped locate the boundaries demarcating women's work from men's work. Those boundaries, however, were permeable. Men could and did cross into women's domain when the size of the market justified a larger scale of operations than the home could provide. For example, baking and brewing were normally women's work, but men in port towns also made their living by these activities. Men in New England did not lose self-respect if they milked cows, but they did not normally make cheese or churn cream into butter.

If, however, the family began to specialize in dairying for sale, the men might take part. Matthew Patten of New Hampshire mentioned husbands as well as wives buying and selling butter. Thus, when nominally feminine tasks became important to household income, men undertook a share of the responsibility, even if only to keep track of the profits. Male account keepers commonly listed payments due from boarders and lodgers but never credited the work by their wives that made the hospitality possible. On the other hand, some male-dominated occupations were always open to women. Retail trade was perhaps the most common, although before 1740 such opportunities arose in only a few commercial areas. Most women in retailing were widows who had taken over a deceased husband's shop, although one Mary Johnson of Boston, who was not identified as a widow, owned shop goods worth over two hundred pounds, according to the 1669 inventory of her estate. Helen Hobart ran a shop in Hingham in 1682 with her husband's approval. By the late colonial period, such opportunities had spread deeper into the interior. In Worcester County in 1760, for instance, twelve out of 267 licensed dispensers of spirituous liquors (4.5 percent) were women.

Though women had always acted as midwives, nursed the sick, and disbursed homemade remedies, a few also "doctored." The administrator of the estate of David Clark of Wrentham listed payment to Mary Johnson, "Doctoress" for "Physick and Tendance." William Corbin, minister of the Anglican church in Boston, willed his medical books to Jane Allen of Newbury, spinster and daughter of the Honorable Samuel Allen, Esquire. In 1758 the Reverend Ebenezer Parkman went to see the widow Ruhamah Newton, who had broken her leg in a fall. Friends had called a Mrs. Parker to set the leg, and the time it took her to get her apparatus in order and carry out the operation delayed the diarist's return home "till night."

Women taught school, as did men. Generally speaking, women taught young pupils of both sexes to read and spell, and men instructed more advanced classes in writing and arithmetic. Seventeenth-century records occasionally identify "school dames" who took students for fees, but they do not seem to have been common outside the largest settlements.

In the eighteenth century, women usually taught the younger children and girls during the summer, often for only half the wages of the young male college graduates who took the older children the rest of the year. The town of Amesbury, Massachusetts, voted in 1707 that the selectmen "hire four or five school Dames for the town to teach children to read" and allowed five pounds to two men "to keep a school to teach young parsons to write and sifer two months this year." Most towns seem to have found the two-tier system a cheap and efficient way to comply with the provincial school laws. The town meeting of Hingham instructed its selectmen to "hire a schoolmaster as cheap as they can get one, provided they shall hire a single man and not a man that have a family."

There was also a two-tier system in making apparel. Men normally tailored coats and breeches, and women sewed shirts and gowns; however, women in the eighteenth century also engaged in tailoring to a limited extent. In 1708, the estate of Simon Gross, deceased mariner of Hingham, paid for forty weeks of training as a tailor for his daughter Allis. John Ballantine, minister at Westfield, Massachusetts, mentioned two occasions in 1768 when Ruth Weller came for a week to make garments; in 1773 he noted that "Sally Noble, Tailer" was working at his house.

Gender distinctions were very clear in the processing of textiles. Females did not comb worsted or hackle flax, which was men's work, although women, along with boys, pulled flax, carded wool, and picked seeds out of cotton. Girls and women spun, dyed, and knitted yarn, but few engaged in weaving, traditionally a male occupation in England. Women did take up the craft in the eighteenth century, doing simple weaves while men concentrated on more complex patterns.

Few inventoried estates mention looms in the seventeenth century, and only 6 percent in Essex County, Massachusetts, list them around 1700. By 1774, the proportion of inventories with looms in Alice Hanson Jones's New England sample ranged from a low of 17 percent in Essex County to a high of 37.5 percent in Plymouth County. The spread of looms did not mean that the region's textile industry was in the throes of protoindustrialization. Rather, households in less commercial areas were producing more cloth for home use in order to spend their cash and vendible products on new consumer goods like tea and sugar. The newer weavers included women who took up weaving as a nearly full-time activity in the years before marriage or during widowhood. Growing numbers of married women also wove part time to conserve or expand family income.

Weaving may be the only occupation in the colonial period for which there is sufficient documentation to compare men's and women's pay for the same type of work. Women weavers appear in account books as early as 1704 in Norwich, Connecticut, and in 1728, when Mary Stodder purchased a loom from John Marsh of Litchfield. Altogether, eighteen women weavers appear in the diaries, probate records, and account books consulted for this study, of whom just four are identified as "widow." Of those for whom pay rates are available, comparisons with contemporary male weavers show that the sexes earned similar rates per yard for common kinds of cloth. We can conclude that, in this instance, women did earn equal pay for equal work. However, only two women weavers in the sample, Mary Parker and Hannah Smith of Hingham, received credit for weaving more than the common fabrics— "plain," drugget, shirting, linen, tow, and "blanketing." Men produced a much wider variety, including relatively fancy weaves. Judging from these examples, an expanding demand for domestic cloth created opportunities for women to do simple weaving. They could do so without driving down piece rates, which rose by a third between the 1750s and the 1770s; from 4.1d. to 5.4d. and then to 5.5d. in the early 1770s. Although the sources do not reveal great numbers of women working at looms, women's growing presence in the late colonial period signals a trend that accelerated during the Revolution.

The history of weaving and tailoring in New England illustrates the flexibility inherent in the region's gender-based work roles. The further removed the activity was from hard-core masculine tasks associated with oxen, plows, and heavy equipment, the more likely that respectable women did it. The history of work and gender in New England during the colonial years divides readily into four periods of unequal duration. In the earliest period, before the 1670s, the economy simplified compared to England's economy, and the variety of occupations open to either sex contracted sharply. Women spent more time outdoors and working alongside men. The second period came with the proliferation of activities by which men habitually and strictly segregated themselves from women, and women undertook domestic manufacturing tasks with which historians have so often associated them: brewing beer, baking bread, churning butter, making cheese, spinning yarn, and knitting stockings and mittens. Not every housewife practiced all these arts, and specialization encouraged exchange between them.

The third period, beginning about 1715, constituted the farm maintenance stage in older settlements during which demand for unskilled labor declined relative to skilled labor. Increasing population densities created exchange opportunities that encouraged both men and women to specialize and invest more time in nonfarm occupations. This stage might have continued indefinitely, with population growth putting continuous downward pressure on wages, but outside forces intervened, creating the fourth and final phase of New England's colonial development. Beginning in 1739, wars and their aftermaths administered a succession of shocks to the system, creating sudden demands for men and provisions and putting large amounts of money into circulation. The conclusion to the Seven Years' War opened up northern New England and Nova Scotia to British settlement, and the treaty that ended the War for Independence swung open the gates to Iroquoia in New York, as did the Battle of Fallen Timbers (1794) for the Ohio Valley. Much of the labor supply that might have depressed wage rates emigrated instead; in New England, it was not replaced by immigrants.

Despite New England's limited resources and the absence of technological change, demand generated by war and export markets drove the region's economy at a faster rate than its population grew. Evidence for economic expansion appears in both account books and probate inventories. First, stores with new consumer wares appeared. Storekeepers began moving into the rural interior during the 1740s, and their numbers grew dramatically in the ensuing decades. Proportionately, there were nearly as many retailers in Massachusetts in 1771 as there were in the United States in 1929. Many hopeful young businessmen were assisted by merchants in port cities who had advanced their wares on credit to the neophytes.

The lure was the money jingling in farmers' pockets from increasing prices for their products, beginning with the preparations against Louisbourg in 1744–1745. Prices for livestock began to soar faster than inflation, offering strong inducements to farmers to expand their herds. The sterling equivalent of Connecticut inventory values of oxen, for instance, jumped 19 percent in the 1740s, continued to rise in the 1750s, and by the early 1760s reached 80 percent above levels of the 1730s. During the height of the Seven Years' War, Connecticut prices for cows and barreled pork climbed 50 percent, while prices for sheep doubled. After dropping modestly in the late 1760s, prices for oxen and cows rose sharply in the early 1770s, attaining levels not seen since the 1640s. Livestock values in Massachusetts did not keep up with this torrid pace, but the cost of oxen ballooned by more than 70 percent in 1758–1763 and grew again in the early 1770s. Connecticut wheat prices ascended a bit more demurely: 43 percent in the 1750s and 48 percent in 1772–1774. Farmers in newer settlements sent off, besides barreled meat and draft animals, loads of lumber products, such as staves and shingles, potash, tar, turpentine, and maple syrup. New Englanders also shipped thousands of pounds of well-preserved butter and cheese every year.

For men with resources, the rational reaction to such prices would have been to devote more of their own and their sons' time to farming and less time to crafts such as weaving. To raise and feed more livestock, farmers had to create more pasture and mowing lands, plant more timothy and clover, maintain longer fence lines, and store many more tons of hay in their newly erected barns. Winter chores expanded, cutting the time available for craft activities.

When farmers endeavored to raise more livestock and the grass to feed them, and when farm wives found themselves milking more cows, churning more butter, and making more cheese, men and women were putting pressure on a labor force that in the short run could expand only by crossing the gender division of labor. Every attempt by the colonial governments during the Seven Years' War to recruit soldiers for the summer campaigns further reduced the available pool of young men, and farmers found themselves engaged in a bidding war that raised wages and bounties. According to Fred Anderson, men in military service during these years could earn far more than a fully employed farm laborer. With an eight-month enlistment, plus bounty, minimum income for soldiers in Massachusetts rose from £10.1 sterling in 1755 to £13.9 in 1757, and bounced between a high of £21.75 and a low of £15.75 thereafter. When bounties for *re*enlistment are figured in, estimated maximum incomes reached £32.3 in 1760 and £29.2 in 1762. Anywhere from one-fourth to one-third of men aged sixteen to twenty-nine served with Massachusetts forces at some point during the war.

The rise in wages beginning in the 1740s at first touched only men but in the long term affected everyone by loosening the bonds between parents and their grown children as daughters found work outside the home and sons joined the military or emigrated. The account books show that men abruptly began employing greater numbers of women in the final two decades of the colonial period. Women had already begun moving into tailoring and weaving, but the labor shortages of the Seven Years' War boosted demand for their services, and the migration out of southern New England in the 1760s apparently worked to cushion the postwar depression in farm wages and prices.

Rising wages and expanding employment meant higher incomes for those who did not emigrate. The probate inventories of the late colonial period show that most New England families were prospering. The estimated sterling value per capita of consumer goods in 1774 was

10 percent higher than in the middle colonies, for instance, and an index of amenities in probate inventories from rural New England registered substantial gains in the decades before 1774, catching up and then keeping pace with Chesapeake households that had long been engaged in a commercial economy.

The New England economy took time to recover from the crises of war and destruction in 1675–1694; it grew only slowly for a long period before heating up during the Seven Years' War. That war accelerated economic change, bringing more women into the paid labor force and expanding the penetration of the market into the rural interior. The growing proportion of young women working outside the home in the final decades of the colonial period accompanied a rise in their wages, which no doubt helped attract them. When combined with evidence that increasing numbers of country girls were attending school and learning how to write, the growing ability of women to earn money and conduct business at the local store can be viewed as a positive good, giving them greater control over their own lives. Furthermore, the addition of tea, sugar, and spices to their diets, painted earthenware to their tables, featherbeds to sleep on, and greater privacy, all surely added pleasures to generally hard lives. Although marriage still meant coverture, more women chose to remain single and access to divorce became easier. There is also a demographic indicator that women's lot was improving: life expectancy of married women rose. Mean age at death increased from sixty-two to sixty-six for women marrying between 1760 and 1774 and to sixty-eight for those marrying between 1775 and 1800. On balance, these changes appear beneficial. Women would not gain politically or legally from American Independence, and equality was never even a prospect, but in the decades before 1776 they had won a little liberty, and comfort is no mean thing.

GLORIA L. MAIN is professor of history at the University of Colorado, Boulder. She is also the author of *Tobacco Colony: Life in Early Maryland, 1650–1720* (Princeton University Press, 1983) and *Peoples of a Spacious Land: Families and Cultures in Colonial New England* (Harvard University Press, 2001).

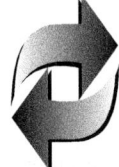

Cornelia Hughes Dayton

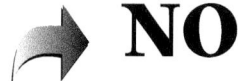

Women Before the Bar

More than half a century separated the first and last courtroom appearances of Rebecca Baldwin of Milford, Connecticut. In 1719, when she was seventeen, Rebecca came before the bar in the New Haven courthouse to confess to the crime of fornication; her father, a prosperous wheelwright, paid her fine of forty-three shillings. The man whom Rebecca named as the father of her infant was a newly married local physician, from whom the court extracted a pledge of child support. Despite the embarrassment of bearing a child out of wedlock, Rebecca avoided forfeiting the respectable status of the family she was born into. At age 24, she married her first cousin Phineas Baldwin; they soon became full church members and had three children, all of whom survived to marry well. In her thirties Rebecca inherited two small tracts of land and one hundred pounds from her father and in her sixties a generous testamentary property settlement when her husband died. In 1775 and 1778—well before her death at age 89—Rebecca again crossed the threshold of the courthouse, now as a widow and the sole surviving executor of her husband's estate.

Rebecca Baldwin's adult life was thus bracketed by two quintessential encounters with the law among those experienced by the hundreds of New England women in each county jurisdiction who found their way into court. Although many women never made the trip to the courthouse, the presence of women in court was not unusual. In the early part of the colonial period, spectators on court days would have found it routine that one-third of those waiting to plead or to give testimony were women. Taking shame upon oneself for the illicit act of fornication, as young Rebecca Baldwin did, and suing to collect a debt, as Rebecca did as a widow, were the most common guises in which Connecticut women appeared before the judges of the county courts, the forums to which the bulk of civil and criminal cases were funneled. In addition, scores of women came into county court to sue over slanderous words or inheritance disputes. In Connecticut, the Superior Court, which rode circuit holding sessions in each county seat, heard a smattering of felony and capital cases inherently involving women—rape, adultery, infanticide—amid a much larger stream of divorce petitions, most of which were brought by deserted wives.

This study takes as its central subjects the many women who entered early Connecticut courtrooms: women suing and being sued over debt and slander, women petitioning for divorce, women prosecuted for sexual transgressions, women advancing rape charges. To ask what the everyday practice of the law courts meant for women is to ask how both women *and* men used available legal procedures to advance their own interests and in what ways they were treated by magistrates and the panoply of community members who, as grand jurors, jurors, and witnesses, made the legal system function. Drawing on colonywide criminal cases and the extensive court records of one jurisdiction, New Haven, in its incarnation as a separate colony until 1665 and afterward as a Connecticut county, this work traces how the gendered patterns of civil, criminal, and divorce litigation changed over 150 years.

Although it follows a design uniquely its own, this investigation builds on three types of scholarly works: analyses of litigation patterns in a single jurisdiction over time, in-depth community studies of towns and their inhabitants, and inquiries into specific aspects of women's relationship to the law. When I began this project, excellent work was emerging on women's legal position as it was defined by colonial statutes, early modern English treatises, and late-eighteenth-century appellate case law, but gender as an important analytical category was missing from new studies on the actual workings of early American courts. Setting out to remedy the deficit, I chose to eschew sampling, a traditional social science technique that can yield a useful portrait of a legal system but that fails to capture all the courtroom encounters that individuals like Rebecca Baldwin might have had over their lifetime. In order to paint an accurate and telling portrait of the early

From WOMEN BEFORE THE BAR: GENDER, LAW, AND SOCIETY IN CONNECTICUT, 1639–1789 by Cornelia Hughes Dayton. Published for the Omohundro Institute of Early American History and Culture. Copyright © 1995 by the University of North Carolina Press. Used by permission of the publisher. www.uncpress.unc.edu

American courts, treatment of subordinate groups such as women, African-Americans, and Indians, the best strategy, I believe, is a systematic profiling of everything occurring in court in a given jurisdiction.

The extensive, nearly complete records surviving for colonial Connecticut and New Haven make this study possible. For the seventeenth and eighteenth centuries, court records provide an extraordinary window in to behaviors, self-fashionings, and idiomatic uses of language that would otherwise go unrecorded. In a period when few adults left letters or diaries, women and men speak through court records more openly than through almost any other set of documents. Slander writs quote speech fragments verbatim, depositions offer a person's deliberate construction of events, and local magistrates' records transcribe criminals' examinations in a question-and-answer format. Thus we can hear women talking and being talked to, we can see the extent to which they were recognized or ignored in the courtroom, in a more tangible way than is possible for other public settings, such as the tavern, the street, and the meetinghouse.

Besides their usefulness in capturing random, individual voices and in documenting the literal and symbolic work of an important public institution, court records disclose the agency of laypersons. In the seventeenth and eighteenth centuries the legal system could function only with the cooperation of ordinary men and women. New Englanders with legal standing could choose, after all, whether to submit their disputes to the magistrates and courts or resort instead to other forms of mediation, such as the parish or neighborhood arbitration. Indeed, because civil litigation occupied the bulk of the courts' business, local inhabitants by their decisions on whom to sue and how to plead gave shape to the rhythms of court sessions and breathed life into, spelled atrophy for, or prompted modification of legal forms and actions. Similarly, in the realm of criminal justice, without the modern-day apparatus of police, prosecutors, and investigators, the colonial court's effectiveness in keeping the peace depended on the public's willingness to bring complaints and testimony to it.

As members of the lay population, women could contribute to the dynamics of legal business as litigants, witnesses, and criminal defendants. Indeed, they did so with unparalleled frequency in the earliest decades of settlement, when simplified legal rules and a ban on lawyers gave all residents direct access to the legal system. But women stood outside the loose group of brokers who coalesced in the early eighteenth century, a group I call the legal fraternity. Wider than the clusters of judges, justices of the peace, and professional attorneys serving each county, the legal fraternity should be seen as encompassing the many propertied heads of household who rotated on and off duty as trial jurors and grand jurors. Since the men chosen as jurors were typically in their thirties or forties with average landholdings and dense kinship networks in Connecticut, the system ensured that legal decisions were influenced by men of middling ranks, not just the wealthiest, most prominent figures in the county or those few trained in the law. Thus, after 1700, women's cases were filtered through several layers of men dispensing legal advice and decrees. For New Haven women encountering the law in the eighteenth century, this arrangement represented a different sort of paternalism from that exemplified by the unmediated power of seventeenth-century magistrates. As in affairs of church governance, women operated informally, behind the scenes, to shape legal outcomes, but with the expansion of the legal fraternity through the century their activities became more and more invisible to the public record.

Alongside any brief for the value of early modern court records must come recognition of their recalcitrance. Writs in certain civil actions, notably debt, assault, and trespass, usually fail to record the actual nature of the underlying transaction or conflict. Moreover, no matter how voluminous the depositions surviving in a particular case, as historians we can capture only a small fraction of the information that came before the bench and jury. There were no stenographers in colonial Connecticut courtrooms to transcribe oral testimony, lawyers' arguments, and defendants' exact words. The gestures of the various participants, the gasps and sighs and catcalls of the audience, and in general the dramaturgy of early New England courtrooms—these are almost always lost to us. Much of what the judges said from the bench went unrecorded, including instructions to juries in criminal trials. The practice of issuing judicial opinions to explain rulings and verdicts began, spottily, only in the 1780s. Few eighteenth-century Connecticut judges and lawyers wrote diaries or left papers containing legal briefs and correspondence. Lay men and women, introspective over spiritual matters but not yet inspired to self-revelatory consciousness by Romanticism or modernist impulses, would never have conceived the value of recording in detail what motivated them to attend court, what they observed in the courtroom, or why they might have altered their testimony from one hearing to the next.

Thus our interpretations of what happened in court are inevitably dependent on records full of omissions and silences and on testimonies refracted through faulty memories and calculation. Supplemental information from nonlegal sources can shed light on such issues as who was in court by age or social status and what sorts of disputes failed to come before the bar, but it rarely supplies direct evidence on the attitudes and motivations of courtroom actors. Court records, of course, can be a springboard to investigations of all sorts of topics—from witchcraft beliefs and courtship rituals to credit networks. Yet principally the record books and file papers speak to what issues came before the courts and how laypeople and officials negotiated the terrain marked as law. Thus, the present study keeps a steady focus on the courtroom itself. In its pursuit of the story of New Englanders' use of and reception by the courts over time, it is institutional history. In its close attention to the gender, age, and social standing of litigants, it relies heavily on social history methods. Above all, it is meant to contribute to our understanding of change in early American legal culture and in gender relations and gender ideology.

. . . Five topical categories—debt, divorce, illicit consensual sex, rape, and slander—were chosen because of the sheer quantity of cases or the utility of the legal record for illuminating important aspects of women's relationship to the courts over time. For example, women were party to more than a thousand debt suits in New Haven County alone in the seventeenth and eighteenth centuries, A comparison of women's and men's litigated debt significantly expands our grasp of an understudied aspect of colonial development—the gendered dimensions of commercialization and rural economic growth. In contrast, cases involving rape were few, yet file papers permit us to reconstruct women's and men's conflicting stories and to compare community responses to charges against acquaintances and outsiders, whites and blacks. Considering major aspects of civil, criminal, and divorce law together highlights important currents of legal and social change that can remain obscured when legal actions are studied in isolation.

I make no claim, however, that the study covers every aspect of women's experience before the courts in early New England. Readers will not find extended discussions of several issues. Witchcraft is omitted because the number of cases in New Haven was small and because two fine, in-depth studies of early New England witch-hunting exist that cover Connecticut, including one that makes gender central to its analysis. Furthermore, singular criminal cases in which women played a central role, like a rare 1740s Connecticut abortion prosecution of a doctor and his alleged accomplices, did not fit easily into a study that was geared to examine change in legal actions over time. Finally, legal scholars may argue for the importance of studying women's roles in land and inheritance disputes, but I found it difficult to tease conclusions about gender out of the records for trespass, ejectment, trover, or inheritance suits, since most involved joint heirs—siblings suing together. To my mind, the differential pattern of men's and women's participation in debt litigation was the most important area of private law to address: debt, after all, was the major engine of change in the colonial legal system.

[T]he courtrooms of the seventeenth-century New Haven and Connecticut colonies had a very different character from those of the late eighteenth century. I argue that the most critical period of change for women's relation to the public space of the courtroom came in the decades surrounding the end of the seventeenth century. By then a collective commitment to upholding a God-fearing society through the courts had been abandoned, and Puritan resistance to the technicalities of English common law practice had faded. From the 1690s to the 1720s rules were implemented that shifted New Haven courtrooms from the utopian reform platform of the Puritan founders to a selective embrace of English formalism. Toward the end of that transition, an enormous expansion in indebtedness reshaped civil litigation. As a result of these transformations in law and society, by the end of the colonial period women's presence in court declined dramatically.

In essence, women's courtroom participation throws into sharp relief the realignment of court and community. The seventeenth-century courts had been occupied by the sorts of community activities to which women were integral: maintaining harmonious neighborly relations, ensuring equitable local trading, and monitoring sexual and moral conduct. After the turn of the century, the courts increasingly became adjuncts and facilitators of vast credit networks that provided farmers and tradesmen with the capital to expand their farms and enterprises. The constituency served by the courts narrowed to propertied men active in the expanding economy; at the same time the volume of court business was growing exponentially. Women's economic and social activities did not change markedly at the beginning of the eighteenth century, but in a schematic sense what was happening in court reveals a new set of divergences in men's and women's spheres taking hold gradually throughout the century. These divergences—in women's and men's relations to commercialization, to the public theater of the courtroom, and to religious attitudes toward sin and human culpability—were silent foreshadowings of the more explicit nineteenth-century ideology that reserved the public realms of commerce, law, and politics to men and gave white women moral dominion over privatized families.

If New Haven's evolving courtroom scenes illumine the restructuring of public and private space, putting law at the center of the story of gender and social change in early New England also enables us to perceive important shifts in a system of power relations that is often viewed as static: patriarchy, or the legal and cultural rules by which men held authority over women in the household and polity. It is my contention that the seventeenth-century Puritan courtroom occupies an anomalous position in the long histories of Anglo-American law and of patriarchy. The New England Puritans struck out on idiosyncratic legal paths, the twisted strands of which included some policies harshly intolerant of unsubmissive women and others remarkably unforgiving of men's ungodly behavior.

On the one hand, the familiar characterization of Puritan justice as repressive of women is borne out in many respects. Puritan legal regimes across New England unquestioningly cast women as witches and condoned a prosecutorial double standard for accused men and women such that twenty-eight women and only seven men were hanged for the crime of witchcraft. In the 1630s and 1640s, New England's leaders used showcase trials against Anne Hutchinson and other female dissenters to silence women as political beings and religious leaders. Finally, the Puritan compulsion to punish a wide range of moral lapses with whippings meant that women were frequently haled before the bar to confess their sins publicly and to submit to the lash.

On the other hand, Puritan jurisprudence, by encouraging lay pleading and by insisting on godly rules, created unusual opportunities for women's voices to be heard in court. The prohibition against lawyers, the simplification of procedural rules, and the magistrates' confidence that God would help them discern the truth behind a dispute or criminal charge meant that women's testimony was invited and encouraged in ways that clashed with English legal traditions. Not only was women's access to courts eased, but the Puritans' emphasis on each individual's obedience to God's strictures led them to insist on punishing men's abuse of authority and sinful behavior. In cases of sexual assault, wife-abuse, and premarital sex, seventeenth-century magistrates gave credence to women's charges and meted out swift, severe sentences to men. Indeed, New Haven Colony came close to establishing a single standard for men and women in the areas of sexual and moral conduct. In sum, policies that were intended to create the most God-fearing society possible operated to reduce the near-absolute power that English men by law wielded over their wives, to undercut men's sense of sexual entitlement to women's bodies, and to relieve women in some situations from their extreme dependency on men. Thus, when Puritanism ceased to be the organizing force in New England society and courtrooms, there were losses for women as well as gains.

Along with new work on the Chesapeake, this study urges that we examine the early and middle decades of the eighteenth century as a period that saw the return to a more traditional type of patriarchy in Britain's New World colonies. Quite different material and ideological conditions explain why some traditional supports of patriarchy were loosened in seventeenth-century colonies as distinct as Virginia and Connecticut and why women in various regions encountered a tightening of patriarchal authority in the eighteenth century. I attempt to account only for women's experience in New Haven as suggestive of the cultural shifts characterizing colonies that began as intensely Puritan settlements. Here, judges, lawmakers, and other men of influence and wealth launched no coordinated, self-conscious campaign to roll back the slight openings and advances women had enjoyed under seventeenth-century legal approaches. Rather, their implicit endorsement of rules and practices that would reinforce male authority was integrally bound up in their promulgation of two pervasive cultural trends: anglicization and embourgeoisement.

Anglicization, the importation of English ways by colonists newly and self-consciously eager to bind themselves to the cultural sophistication of the empire's urban centers, has gained much attention in recent years. In the realm of law, the process can be discerned in early-eighteenth-century New England not only in the licensing of professional attorneys but also in the stricter attention paid to common law procedures and rules of evidence. These shifts internal to the legal system raised barriers to women's easy use of the courts and introduced skeptical attitudes toward the reliability of women's charges of male abuse. Beyond the law, newspapers and almanacs show that by midcentury New England culture also became more English (and more European) in its new toleration of misogynist, antimatrimonial, and bawdy themes. Having been invoked by historians to illuminate such diverse areas as professionalization, political culture, consumer tastes, and national integration, anglicization needs also to be recognized as the bearer of ideas about woman's nature that had been largely suppressed in seventeenth-century New England.

Although there has been much hesitation over applying the language of class to early America before wage dependency was extensive, a social stratum and a set of practices later identified as middle-class were emerging in the eighteenth century. The various processes that one scholar calls the "refinement of America" reflect not just the formation of a distinct American gentry but also the fact that many colonials were taking on genteel habits that the post-Independence, republican context would remake into bourgeois habits. The signs of interest in acquiring the badges of cultivation appeared as early as the 1690s. Expanded trade and sources of credit, denser kinship networks, and ideological shifts released New Englanders from insular preoccupations with family and community survival. Wealthy and ambitious families became caught up in elaborating their material world by adding rooms to their dwelling houses, dividing household space into public and private areas, and acquiring luxury goods. Along with those trends came a new ethic of privacy among the emergent bourgeoisie. The social, religious, and political values of the men who breathed life into the legal system no longer called upon them to insist that their dependents or peers submit moral transgressions—slander, premarital sex, drunkenness—to the regulation of the community embodied in the county court. In the area of regulating premarital sexual relations, for example, Connecticut officials moved toward a narrowly selective approach targeting poor, marginal women and sheltering the middling classes from public scrutiny, humiliation, and penalty. These changes in the types of transgressors and transgressions subject to legal action point to a general reformulation of status and identity, a reformulation that authorized propertied male family heads to distance themselves from . . . some of the key communal values espoused by Puritan founders. What was at work was a simultaneous intensification of class definitions and a "restructuring of morality as a category of private or individual rather than communal life."

Studying gendered patterns of litigation and criminal prosecution over 150 years of New Haven's and Connecticut's shared early history allows us to glimpse not only forces that dramatically changed the face of court business but also divergences in women's and men's lives that led to a redefinition of the public space of the courtroom as a male arena. Crucial to this process were both material conditions, as in women's increasingly attenuated link to their menfolks' economic dealings, and cultural fashions, notably perceptions of appropriate behavior for respectable women. Moreover, that women's voices were largely emptied out of the theater of the courtroom by the era of the new Republic was not a maneuver engineered by elites. Laypersons, through their strategies in civil suits, their pleas in criminal cases, and the wording of their writs and petitions, were critical participants in the renegotiations played out in the courts over how reputation was measured, how culpability for sexual transgressions was calculated, how male power within marriage would be buttressed, and how much women could manage property and have access to credit networks.

Men's and women's actions together, then, over the eighteenth century reshaped the county court from an inclusive forum representative of community to a rationalized institution serving the interests of commercially active men. The refashioning of the court into a public space designed solely to shape and nurture the civic identity of bourgeois men powerfully illustrates that fraternity in its deliberately gendered sense would determine access to the new nation's political and public spheres. The refusal of the statesmen, jurists, and political pamphleteers of the Revolutionary and nation-building era to see women as anything but dependent, apolitical beings emerges clearly in their writings. It is through the narrative trail left in court records predating the Constitution that we can discern that writing women out of the original American political contract had a structural history and experiential base many decades in the making.

CORNELIA HUGHES DAYTON, a specialist in early British North American, legal, and women's history, currently serves as associate professor of history at the University of Connecticut. She earned her PhD at Princeton University in 1986 and taught at the University of California–Irvine from 1988 to 1997.

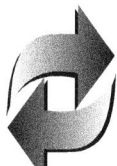

EXPLORING THE ISSUE

Was the Colonial Period a "Golden Age" for Women in America?

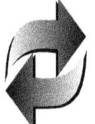

Critical Thinking and Reflection

1. How did the economic status of New England women change over the course of the seventeenth and eighteenth centuries?
2. How did the jobs assigned to New England women differ from those deemed appropriate for men?
3. What are the basic assertions that support the "golden age" thesis as presented by Main?
4. According to Hughes, how did the legal status of New England women change over the course of the seventeenth and eighteenth centuries?
5. What factors contributed to the transformation of the county courts in Connecticut from a gender-inclusive venue to an arena primarily serving the interests of men?

Is There Common Ground?

Both of these essays address the "golden age" thesis that became a significant focus of historical debate in the 1970s and 1980s at a time when the women's liberation movement was at high tide. Both authors ground their research in New England and trace change in women's status from the seventeenth to the eighteenth centuries, although Gloria Main finds improving economic opportunities for women as time passes, while Cornelia Hughes Dayton identifies a clear decline in women's legal status by the early eighteenth century. Both authors also appear to be evaluating the status of white women. What might happen to the conclusions of each had they also factored in the status of nonwhite women in the colonies, or if data from Virginia, Maryland, Pennsylvania, or some other British North American colony had been added to their analyses?

The British North American colonies were clearly a part of a larger, Western European patriarchal structure, so similarities in the status of women undoubtedly existed. Some interesting comparisons could be made between colonial families and modern families. The status of women in the two eras is markedly different, especially in the political realm, but what about average family size and the age of women at first marriage? How were women treated outside of the traditional domestic sphere? This question is central to Hughes's study. To what degree have these spheres changed over time since the colonial period? One obvious difference is the extent to which women have become the focus of historical research.

Mary Beth Norton explores the changes in the status of colonial women more fully in "The Evolution of White Women's Experience in Early America," *American Historical Review*, vol. 89 (June 1984), pp. 593–619. Here she surveys the basic elements of the "golden age" theory and perceptively pronounces the thesis to be "simplistic and unsophisticated" because it concentrates primarily upon the economic function of women in colonial society. Hughes's essay, therefore, represents a corrective to traditional analysis by focusing upon women's roles in the courts.

Additional Resources

Carol Berkin, *First Generations: Women in Colonial America* (Hill & Wang, 1997)

Nancy F. Cott, "Divorce and the Changing Status of Women in Eighteenth-Century Massachusetts," *William and Mary Quarterly*, 3rd series, vol. 33, pp. 586–614 (October 1976)

Mary Beth Norton, *Founding Mothers & Fathers: Gendered Power and the Forming of American Society* (Alfred A. Knopf, 1996)

Elizabeth Reis, *Damned Women: Sinners and Witches in Puritan New England* (Cornell University Press, 1999)

Marylynn Salmon, *Women and the Law of Property in Early America* (University of North Carolina Press, 1986)

Internet References . . .

A Colonial Lady's Clothing: A Glossary of Terms

www.history.org/history/clothing/women/wglossary.cfm

American Women's History: A Research Guide: The Colonial Period

capone.mtsu.edu/kmidlet/history/women/wh-colonial.html

Women of the American Revolution

www.americanrevolution.org/women/women.html

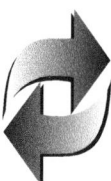

ISSUE

Selected, Edited, and with Issue Framing Material by:
Kevin R. Magill and Tony L. Talbert, *Baylor University*

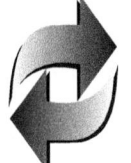

Was Encephalitis Responsible for the Salem Witchcraft Hysteria?

YES: **Laurie Winn Carlson**, from "A Fever in Salem: A New Interpretation of the New England Witch Trials," Ivan R. Dee (1999)

NO: **Lyle Koehler**, from "The Salem Village Cataclysm: Origins and Impact of a Witch Hunt, 1689–92," University of Illinois Press (1980)

Learning Outcomes

After reading this issue, you will be able to:

- Present the sociological and biological factors that affect historical agency.
- Critically analyze several of the multiple theses that contextualize the Salem Witch Trials.
- Develop the foundational knowledge to conduct further historical inquiry into the Salem Witch Trials and the social order of the time period.
- Consider the relationship between the trials and contemporary interpretations.

ISSUE SUMMARY

YES: Laurie Winn Carlson suggests that witchcraft hysteria occurred because of the Colonist's physical and neurological responses to an unrecognized outbreak of encephalitis. She suggests the outbreak affected physical and neurological behaviors causing people to act hysterically.

NO: Lyle Koehler points out that most of the Witchcraft accusers were women and likely seeking to overcome their own feelings of personal powerlessness by speaking out in a patriarchal and oppressive world. These women relished the sense of power they received from the community's attention to their allegations that were designed to conquer the supernatural forces around them.

The Salem witch trials have a mythological place in the U.S. cultural and historical imagination. Though witchcraft is no longer seen as a threat to social organization, it is still present in media, literature, and holiday celebrations, and is an undeniable part of our social consciousness. Salem was a confluence of extremes, politics, and fear, which led to isolationism, persecutions, religious ideology, vendetta accusations, and legal failures. The Salem affair also represents one of the most infamous instances of mass hysteria in American history. Because of its strange and macabre nature, the trials have been well explored in many fields including history, literature, economics, and political science. In addition to academic explorations, media portrayals have shaped the mythologies framing how we understand these interesting historical events. Certain historians fear the fervor caused by the gregarious and over the top media portrayals of Salem has led to egregious misrepresentations of the event and inappropriately elevated its importance. Other historians have conversely argued that the trials have significantly influenced U.S. History in the areas of justice (innocent until proven guilty) and are historical markers that represent a transition from the extreme theocratic organization of the

English North American colonies. In any case, much historical debate and conversation have occurred related to this interesting time in Colonial history.

In past times, witchcraft was understood as a legitimate concern in many European societies. The ideology and inter-relational sociological effects of this tradition became dogma in some of the largely Christian European societies during the 16th and 17th centuries. Many have argued this was the legacy of the Inquisition, which saw officials encouraging local citizens to rid themselves of the manifestations of paganism. Many historians suggest the culture of the European hysteria traversed the Atlantic and was a foundational part of Colonial consciousness. Puritans believed one's heavenly destiny was preordained and that life was about struggling and looking for signs from God of what the afterlife might be. The psychological impact of this worldview was no doubt a challenging burden. In addition to these cultural ideological similarities, European societies and Salem also shared other similar social conditions and environmental realities.

The witch trials themselves were a series of prosecutorial events that occurred across Europe during the 16th to 18th centuries and in North America between 1650 and 1700. Over 100 witchcraft trials happened in the British North American colonies between 1600 and 1700. Of those trials, 40 percent of the accused were executed. Despite being held in several towns, the Salem witch trials have a particularly notorious place within historical discussions, having resulted in the executions of 20 people, 19 of which were by hanging. Fourteen of the twenty executed persons were women. Originally, the accused were the poor and outcast (not uncommon because of the Protestant belief that God blessed the chosen-on earth), but when accusations shifted to the affluent, the trials came to an end.

Much discussion has occurred on who or what is to blame for the trials. Historians have identified several patterns that can help us understand causes of the witchcraft hysteria. Some historians point to the fact that the trials occurred during a time of great political turmoil, economic strife, and or social strain, perhaps requiring scapegoats for Colonial failures. The political reality of this time is one of chaotic transformation in a sea of ideological conservatism, puritanical fear, and significant stress. In Salem, these factors were most certainly present, as in other parts of witch-fearing Europe and the colonies. Supporting research has also suggested that the Massachusetts Bay Colony was politically at odds with the English authorities, which created increased economic tensions and stress on the people. Salem was also divided by internal disputes between villages and villagers. Conflicts and struggles for regional power existed between politicians, those with farming versus commercial interests, and between the church factions. Many of these quarrels were about social relations of production and included property and land right claims. In the east, the fishermen were wealthier, less susceptible to raids, less isolated, and less superstitious which is notable because the accusations came from the west. Disputes and accusations were also grounded in privilege and concerns over who were to be the social and moral leaders of the community. The conflicts naturally led to intersectional power struggles between and among ministers, leaders, fishermen, and farmers. Often these quarrels emerged from desires of the more religious of the refugees who settled New England and the Provence of Massachusetts Bay, perhaps to maintain a theocratic society based on a purely biblical devotion. It is perhaps likely that the ideological dogma was used as a political tool to further political interests. This may have occurred by carefully developing myths about witches and divergent thinkers and their families. Local churches had a documented history of disseminating satanic and abnormal stories. Similarly, artifacts like paintings and relics were developed and circulated. These representations depicted Christian women succumbing to temptations by the devil and paying the price for their failing. One such story gained significant notoriety when four of six children of a particular woman died with no medical explanation. Therefore, the story created whispers of satanic temptation when many of the symptoms presented mirrored what churchgoers had historically and mythologically understood to be manifestations of demonic possession. Her temptation became a sermon championing a particular type of Christian adherence to Protestantism. Some historians claim that what befell this woman and her family was due to biological factors such as disease and crop contamination. Subsequently, some authors argue that diseases presenting like encephalitis were associated with the Devil and witchcraft.

Others have suggested that the secret of the Hysteria lays in the stories of the accusers. These girls acted as if possessed—but were their behaviors the result of disease, drug-like effects from infected crops, or notoriety. Perhaps, their accusations were designed to eliminate political rivals, gain fame, or take agency in a society that marginalized women. Regardless, the accusers were seen as local celebrities of their time and their stories spread across Massachusetts Bay Colony. These experiences would have been in stark contrast to the normal lives of women in this time and place.

Looking at much of the historical scholarship, puritanical ideology is a common way to describe the community's conflicts. Charles Upham and Marion Starkey, for example, suggest this time period would have been a natural reaction of Puritans in this an age of superstition. Therefore, they have argued that religious control and social organization are most to blame for the witchcraft hysteria. Still others suggest that some of the accusers purposefully represented themselves as possessed to express resistance to puritanical oppression. Different historians of this time period argue that it was several of these truly complex sociological relationships that were to blame. Newer research points to environmental and economic issues such as drought, which caused food storages and economic hardship. Emily Oster's *Witchcraft, Weather and Economic Growth in Renaissance Europe*, for example, offers a compelling historical picture of the conditions under which witchcraft hysteria occurred in Europe between 1520 and 1770. Oster analyzes the extreme weather patterns that caused poor economic conditions in the regions in which the witchcraft hysteria occurred. These conditions also existed in Salem in 1692. She also offers many historical examples of capital punishment that have been used to scapegoat certain persons during challenging economic times like these. Her analysis of American lynching is a troubling yet compelling historical parallel. We can likely make a case that the "Red Scare" and anti-Muslim sentiment were, and are, similar phenomena.

Paul Boyer and Stephen Nissenbaum also believe that the Salem witchcraft hysteria of 1692 was a result of the economic and social tensions, suggesting that the beginnings of commercial capitalism, religious conflicts between ministers and their congregations, and the loss of family lands in the emerging society led to extreme civil unrest between Salem Town and Salem Village. The authors note, "The alleged witches and those who accused them resided on opposite sides of the village." Benjamin Ray similarly highlights the factionalism in Salem. He argues that geographical factors played a part in cultivating the community's tribal nature. Carol F. Karlsen argues that gender issues were partly to blame for the trials. She suggests women at the time were understood as the embodiment of evil in the Puritanical and European ideologies. She acknowledges that New Englanders did not make an explicit connection between women and witchcraft, but she suggests that many of attitudes and depictions of women as witches created a strong correlation between the activities of women and witchcraft in the minds of Salem residents. She therefore suggests these perceptions became a self-fulfilling prophecy in Salem. Mary Beth Norton believes external threats were also to blame for much of the hysteria. Concerns regarding the "Godless" Native Americans, the vicious French, or the external "other" intensified the angst and religious fervor in Salem. She argues the borderlands' threats were seen as an extension of the social unrest many believed to be caused by witches and was used as a way to explain the many of the problems that existed within Massachusetts Bay Colony. It was convenient for many residents to believe God was punishing them.

The following articles provided in this chapter offer other insights into this strange and heated time. In *A Search for Power: The 'Weaker Sex' in Seventeenth Century New England*, Lyle Koehler notes that ¾ of those accused of witchcraft in the colonies were females and that of the 56 men accused half of them were related to these women. Those men who were executed were seen as culpable for their relatives becoming "witches" or to their non-confessions. Many young puritan girls of the place and time wished to understand themselves and increase their autonomy and agency. In a changing world, these women were being tethered to the supremely rigid social and moral ideology of restrictive society that was losing power and status. Koehler asserts that those accused of witchcraft were largely the victims of a society looking to restore self-worth, social recognition, and status in a changing society. The accusers, he claims, were happy to be a part of something that made them feel like they had a sense of agency in a changing world. Koehler also suggests that women had historically been linked to witchcraft and when some women looked for their own sense of agency outside Puritanism, for which they were scapegoated for many social issues. He believed that these episodes were a way for those in power to blame the families of these women who had rejected the social rules of the community or for those jealous and without means to target those women who had inherited wealth from their husbands that had died in ways that were unexplainable at the time. Laurie Winn Carlson takes a significantly different perspective in her analysis of the witchcraft hysteria. She believes Koehler and many other historians fail to account for the clear biological symptoms exhibited by many of the Salem residents. She suggests that the symptoms commonly associated with demonic possession very likely resembled those described during the encephalitis pandemic that significantly affected the United States in the early 20th century. Carlson believes that encephalitis is a more reasonable explanation then what has been presented for many of the unanswered questions that historians have about the hysterical events that occurred in Salem.

Regardless of what or who is to blame for the hysteria, we are the historical benefactors of this hysterical and antiquated ideology. We still live in a society that still has different rules for men and women. We still punish people for differences. We still punish those who do are not successful in the capitalist society. We still elect leaders who scapegoat those who are different. We still downgrade certain religions and religious interpretations. We still marginalize those who look to cultivate their agency. We still mis-educate people with myths and stories developed for particular purposes. We still reject scientific interpretation to suit our political agenda. We still are puritanical in the ways we consider identity. We still impose our beliefs on others. Therefore, we claim the ideologies present in Salem may be alive and well within the liminal fabric of our so-called postmodern, postfeminist, post-racial, postcapitalist, society. Perhaps, we are not as far removed from this hysteria than we might like to believe.

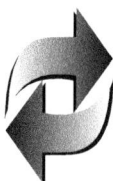

YES ✐

Laurie Winn Carlson

A Fever in Salem: A New Interpretation of the New England Witch Trials

During the latter part of the seventeenth century, residents of a northeastern Massachusetts colony experienced a succession of witchcraft accusations resulting in hearings, trials, imprisonments, and executions. Between 1689 and 1700 the citizens complained of symptoms that included fits (convulsions), spectral visions (hallucinations), mental "distraction" (psychosis), "pinching, pin pricking and bites" on their skin (clonus), lethargy, and even death. They "barked like dogs," were unable to walk, and had their arms and legs "nearly twisted out of joint."

In late winter and early spring of 1692, residents of Salem Village, Massachusetts, a thinly settled town of six hundred, began to suffer from a strange physical and mental malady. Fits, hallucinations, temporary paralysis, and "distracted" rampages were suddenly occurring sporadically in the community. The livestock, too, seemed to suffer from the unexplainable illness. The randomness of the victims and the unusual symptoms that were seldom exactly the same, led the residents to suspect an otherworldly menace. With the limited scientific and medical knowledge of the time, physicians who were consulted could only offer witchcraft as an explanation.

These New Englanders were Puritans, people who had come to North America to establish a utopian vision of community based upon religious ideals. But, as the historian Daniel Boorstin points out, their religious beliefs were countered by their reliance on English common law. The Puritans did not create a society out of their religious dogma, but maintained the rule of law brought from their homeland. They were pragmatic, attempting to adapt practices brought from England rather than reinventing their own as it suited them. When problems arose that were within the realm of the legal system, the community acted appropriately, seeking redress for wrongs within the courts.

Thus when purported witchcraft appeared, church leaders, physicians, and a panicked citizenry turned the problem over to the civil authorities. Witchcraft was a capital crime in all the colonies, and whoever was to blame for it had to be ferreted out and made to stop. Because no one could halt the outbreak of illness, for ten months the community wrestled with sickness, sin, and the criminal act of witchcraft. By September 1692, nineteen convicted witches had been hanged and more than a hundred people sat in prison awaiting sentencing when the trials at last faded. The next year all were released and the court closed. The craze ended as abruptly as it began.

Or did it? There had been similar sporadic physical complaints blamed *on* witchcraft going back several decades in New England, to the 1640s when the first executions for the crime of witchcraft were ordered in the colonies. Evidence indicates that people (and domestic animals) had suffered similar physical symptoms and ailments in Europe in still earlier years. After the witch trials ended in Salem, there continued to be complaints of the "Salem symptoms" in Connecticut and New Hampshire, as well as in Boston, into the early eighteenth century. But there were no more hangings. The epidemic and witchcraft had parted ways.

By examining the primary records left by those who suffered from the unexplainable and supposedly diabolical ailments in 1692, we get a clear picture of exactly what they were experiencing. *The Salem Witchcraft Papers*, a three-volume set compiled from the original documents and preserved as typescripts by the Works Progress Administration in the 1930s, has been edited for today's reader by Paul Boyer and Stephen Nissenbaum. It is invaluable for reading the complete and detailed problems people were dealing with. Like sitting in the physician's office with them, we read where the pain started, how it disappeared or progressed, how long they endured it.

A similar epidemic with nearly exact symptoms swept the world from 1916 to 1930. This world-wide pandemic, sleeping sickness, or encephalitis lethargica, eventually claimed more than five million victims. Its cause has never been fully identified. There is no cure. Victims

---

Carlson, Laurie Winn, *A Fever in Salem: A New Interpretation of the New England Witch Trials*, pp. xiii–xvi, 114–125, 142–146. Copyright ©1999 by Rowman & Littlefield Publishers. Used with permission.

of the twentieth-century epidemic continue under hospitalization to the present day. An excellent source for better understanding encephalitis lethargica is Oliver Sacks's book *Awakenings,* which is now in its sixth edition and has become a cult classic. A movie of the same title, based on the book, presents a very credible look at the physical behaviors patients exhibited during the epidemic. While encephalitis lethargica, in the epidemic form in which it appeared in the early twentieth century, is not active today, outbreaks of insect-borne encephalitis do appear infrequently throughout the country; recent outbreaks of mosquito-borne encephalitis have nearly brought Walt Disney World in Florida to a halt, have caused entire towns to abandon evening football games, and have made horse owners anxious throughout the San Joaquin Valley in California.

Using the legal documents from the Salem witch trials of 1692, as well as contemporary accounts of earlier incidents in the surrounding area, we can identify the "afflictions" that the colonists experienced and that led to the accusations of witchcraft. By comparing the symptoms reported by seventeenth-century colonists with those of patients affected by the encephalitis lethargica epidemic of the early twentieth century, a pattern of symptoms emerges. This pattern supports the hypothesis that the witch-hunts of New England were a response to unexplained physical and neurological behaviors resulting from an epidemic of encephalitis. This was some form of the same encephalitis epidemic that became pandemic in the 1920s. In fact, it is difficult to find anything in the record at Salem that *doesn't* support the idea that the symptoms were caused by that very disease. . . .

What Happened at Salem?

. . . Historical explanations of witchcraft dwell on what Thomas Szasz calls the "scapegoat theory of witchcraft," which explores who was accused and why in the context of larger societal issues. Inevitably they fail to examine the accusers or the "afflicted," who themselves were often tried for witchcraft.

Sociologists have pointed to community-based socioeconomic problems as the causative agent in the events at Salem. They propose that there were really two Salems: Salem Town (a prosperous sector on the well-developed east side of town) and Salem Village (a less-developed, very swampy and rocky area on the west side). Likening Salem Village to a troubled backwater, the accusations and afflictions emanated from the west side, where the residents directed their animosity toward their wealthier, more powerful eastern counterparts by accusing individuals on the east side of witchcraft. Examining the struggles, failures, broken dreams, and lost hopes of the Salem Village residents, sociologists began to view the village as "an inner city on a hill." Social conflict, in this case between prosperous merchants and struggling subsistence farmers, was examined. In the case of the Salem witch hunts, the theory may better explain who was accused and convicted of witchcraft than why individuals were afflicted. Division along class and religious lines has been well documented in determining criminal accusations.

Other investigators have blamed the situation on village factionalism, claiming that Salem Village was rife with suspicious, disgruntled, jealous settlers whose frustrations had festered for years before exploding in the court record with witchcraft accusations and trials. But that does not explain why twenty-two *other* towns in New England were eventually connected to the proceedings in some way; villagers throughout Maine, New Hampshire, Connecticut, Massachusetts, and Rhode Island were brought into the trial records. Victims, accused witches, and witnesses came from other locales as far away as the Maine frontier. Other locations, such as Connecticut, conducted witch trials that preceded or coincided with those at Salem. Choosing to view the problems as power struggles or personality differences within a small village strikes one as too parochial. Many of the possessed claimants barely knew the people they named as their tormenters, in fact several had never even met the persons they accused of fostering their problems—hardly enough tension to support the idea that the entire uproar was based on long-standing animosities. Socioeconomic divisions did engender problems in the region, and while they ultimately may be used to explain who was accused and why, they do not explain the many physical symptoms or who experienced them.

Carol Karlsen has viewed what happened at Salem in her book *The Devil in the Shape of a Woman,* which relates the events to women's oppressed status within Puritan society. She considers New Englanders' "possession" to have been a cultural performance—a ritual—performed by girls, interpreted by ministers, and observed by an audience as a dramatic event. Karlsen claims the possessed individuals exhibited learned behavior patterns and that words and actions varied only slightly among them. The affected women experienced an inner conflict which was explained by ministers as a struggle between good and evil: God versus Satan. The outcome revolved around whether or not the young women would later lead virtuous lives or fall into sin. Karlsen suggests that a woman's possession was the result of her indecision or ambivalence about choosing the sort of woman she wanted to be. She views the possession as a "collective phenomenon" among women in Connecticut between 1662 and 1663, and in Massachusetts from 1692 to 1693. It was a "ritual expression of Puritan belief and New England's gender arrangements," and a challenge to society. It was ultimately a simple power struggle between women and their oppressors.

As to the physical symptoms: the fits, trances, and paralyzed limbs, among others, Karlsen attributes them to the afflicted girls' actual fear of witches as well as the idea that once they fell into an afflicted state they were free to express unacceptable feelings without reprisal. The swollen throats, extended tongues, and eyes frozen in peripheral stares were manifestations of the inner rage they felt toward society; they were so upset they literally *couldn't* speak. Their paralysis was based on anger over having to work; their inability to walk meant they could not perform their expected labor—in other words, a passive-aggressive response to a situation that incensed them. Karlsen views witchcraft possession in New England as a rebellion against gender and class powers: a psychopathology rooted in female anger.

Misogyny may well explain who was accused of witchcraft, but it lacks an explanation for the wide-ranging symptoms, the ages of the afflicted, and the patterns of symptoms that occurred across time and distance in seventeenth-century New England. Scholars who take this route, however, conveniently ignore the fact that men too were accused, tried, and hanged for witchcraft, both in the colonies and in Europe. In fact, Robin Briggs states that though "every serious historical account recognizes that large numbers of men were accused and executed on similar charges, this fact has never really penetrated to become part of the general knowledge on the subject." His research shows that a misogynistic view of witch-hunts lacks complete credibility.

Many researchers have proposed that mass hysteria affected the young women of Salem. The term *hysteria*, essentially a female complaint, has recently been dropped from use by the psychiatric profession in favor of "conversion symptom," which describes the manner in which neurotic patients suffer emotional stress brought on by an unconscious source. This stress or tension can undergo "conversion" and reveal itself in a variety of physical ailments. Conversion, a very pliable disorder, can be explained by almost any societal pressure in any particular culture. It is a psychological catchall for unexplained neurological or emotional problems. But its victims are always the same, according to analysts: unstable females.

Jean-Martin Charcot, a French physician, worked extensively with epileptic and hysteric female patients at the Salpêtrière Hospital in Paris between 1862 and 1870. He laid the groundwork for hysteria theory, calling it hystero-epilepsy. He accused his patients of being deceitful, clever actresses who delighted in fooling the male physician. Charcot's medical students claimed to be able to transfer diseases from hysterics with the use of magnets, something they called the "metal cure." Eventually his professional standing as a neurologist diminished and faded, and he turned to faith healing. Sigmund Freud, one of his students, began his work under Charcot's direction.

A more modern version of the hysteria complex is called Mass Psychogenic Illness, or MPI, which is defined as the contagious spread of behavior within a group of individuals where one person serves as the catalyst or "starter" and the others imitate the behavior. Used to describe situations where mass illness breaks out in the school or workplace, it is usually connected to a toxic agent—real or imagined—in a less than satisfactory institutional or factory setting. MPI is the sufferer's response to overwhelming life and work stress. It relies on the individual's identification with the index case (the first one to get sick, in effect the "leader") and willingness to succumb to the same illness. A classical outbreak of MPI involves a group of segregated young females in a noisy, crowded, high-intensity setting. It is most common in Southeast Asian factories crowded with young female workers; adults are not usually affected. Symptoms appear, spread, and subside rapidly (usually over one day). Physical manifestations usually include fainting, malaise, convulsions with hyperventilation, and excitement. Transmission is by sight or sound brought about by a triggering factor which affects members of the group, who share some degree of unconscious fantasies. A phenomenon more related to the industrial world of the nineteenth and twentieth centuries than to pastoral village life in colonial New England, MPI does not address the question of why men and young children, who would not have identified emotionally and psychologically with a group of young girls, suffered. The New England colonists scarcely fit the pattern for this illness theory that demands large groups of people of similar age, sex, and personality assembled in one confined location.

Salem's witches cannot, of course, escape Freudian critique. Beyond the hysteria hypothesis, John Demos, in *Entertaining Satan*, looked at the evidence from the perspective of modern psychoanalysis. He pointed out that witchcraft explained and excused people's mistakes or incompetence—a failure or mistake blamed on witches allowed a cathartic cleansing of personal responsibility. Witches served a purpose; deviant people served as models to the rest of society to exemplify socially unacceptable behavior. But Demos's explanation that witch-hunts were an integral part of social experience, something that bound the community together—sort of a public works project—does not address the physical symptoms of the sufferers.

For the most part, examinations of the afflicted individuals at Salem have focused on the young women, essentially placing the blame on them instead of exploring an organic cause for their behaviors. Freudian explanations for the goings-on have attributed the activities of the possessed girls to a quest for attention. Their physical manifestations of illness have been explained as being conversion symptoms due to intrapsychic conflict. Their physical expression of psychological conflict is a compromise between unacceptable impulses and the mind's attempt to ignore them. Demos uses the example of Elizabeth Knapp, whose fits became increasingly severe while strangers gathered to view her behavior. Instead of considering that she was beset by an uncontrollable series of convulsions which were likely worsened by the excited witnesses who refused to leave her alone, he attributes her worsening condition to her exhibitionist tendencies, motivated by strong dependency needs. Elizabeth's writhing on the floor in a fetal position is seen as an oral dependency left over from childhood, causing her regression to infancy.

But "inner conflict" simply does not explain the events at Salem. Neither does the idea that the young afflicted girls were motivated by an erotic attraction to church ministers who were called in to determine whether Satan was involved. The girls' repressed adolescent sexual wishes (one girl was only eleven years old) and their seeking a replacement for absent father figures scarcely explains the toll the disease was taking on victims of both sexes and all ages. No Freudian stone has been left unturned by scholars; even the "genetic reconstruction" of Elizabeth Knapp's past points out that her childhood was filled with unmet needs, her mother's frustration because of an inability to bear additional children, and her father's reputation as a suspected adulterer. "Narcissistic depletion," "psychological transference," "a tendency to fragment which was temporarily neutralized"—the psycho-lingo just about stumbles over itself in attempts to explain the afflicted girls at Salem. But unanswered questions remain: Why the sharp pains in extremities? The hallucinations? The hyperactivity? The periods of calm between sessions of convulsions? Why did other residents swear in court that they had seen marks appear on the arms of the afflicted?

The opinion that the victims were creating their own fits as challenges to authority and quests for fame has shaped most interpretations of what happened in 1692. But would the colonists have strived for public notice and attention? If the afflicted individuals were behaving unusually to garner public notice, why? Did women and men of that era really crave public attention, or would it have put them in awkward, critical, and socially unacceptable situations? How socially redeeming would writhing on the ground "like a hog" and emitting strange noises, "barking like a dog," or "bleating like a calf" be for a destitute young servant girl who hoped to marry above her station? It is difficult to accept that these spectacles, which horrified viewers as well as the participants themselves, were actually a positive experience for the young women. That sort of suspicious activity usually met with social stigma, shunning, or, at the least, brutal whipping from father or master.

Puberty, a time of inner turmoil, is thought to have contributed to the victims acting out through fits, convulsions, and erratic behavior. The victims' inability to eat is explained away as a disorder related to the youthful struggle for individuality: anorexia nervosa. What about the young men who reported symptoms? Freudian interpretation attributes their behavior to rebellion against controlling fathers. How have psycho-social interpretations explained the reason witch trials ended after 1692 in Salem? As communities grew into larger urban units, people no longer knew their neighbors, grudges receded in importance as a factor in social control, and witches were no longer valuable to society. John Demos observes that witchcraft never appeared in cities, and that it lasted longest in villages far removed from urban influence. That linkage between witchcraft outbreaks and agricultural villages is important when establishing a connection with outbreaks of encephalitis lethargica, which appeared largely in small towns and rural areas in the early twentieth century. Rather than accepting the idea that witchcraft receded because it was no longer useful in a community context, one must examine why epidemics occurred in waves and how particular diseases affected isolated population groups.

The situation in seventeenth-century New England fails psycho-social explanation because too many questions remain unanswered. Not only can we not make a strong case that infantilism, sexual repression, and a struggle for individuality caused the turmoil in Salem, but a psycho-social explanation does not answer why the symptoms, which were so *obviously physical,* appeared with such force and then, in the autumn of 1692, largely disappeared from Salem.

Because the complexity of psychological and social factors connected with interpreting witchcraft is so absorbing, the existence of a physical pathology behind the events at Salem has long been overlooked. Linnda Caporeal, a graduate student in psychology, proposed that ergot, a fungus that appears on rye crops, caused the hallucinogenic poisoning in Salem. Her article appeared in 1976 in *Science* while Americans were trying to understand the LSD drug phenomenon. Hers is one of the few attempts made to link the puzzling occurrences at Salem with biological evidence.

Ergot was identified by a French scientist in 1676, in an explanation of the relation between ergotized rye and bread poisoning. It is a fungus that contains several potent pharmacologic agents, the ergot alkaloids. One of these alkaloids is lysergic acid amide, which has ten percent of the activity of LSD (lysergic acid diethylamide). This sort of substance causes convulsions or gangrenous deterioration of the extremities. Caporeal proposed that an ergot infestation in the Salem area might explain the convulsions attributed to witchcraft. If grain crops had been infected with ergot fungus during the 1692 rainy season and later stored away, the fungus might have grown in the storage area and spread to the entire crop. When it was distributed randomly among friends and villagers, they would have become affected by the poisoned grain.

Caporeal's innovative thinking was challenged by psychologists Nicholas Spanos and Jack Gottlieb, who were quick to point out that her theory did not explain why, if food poisoning were to blame, families who ate from the same source of grain were not affected. And infants were afflicted who may not have been eating bread grains. Historically, epidemics of ergotism have appeared in areas where there was a severe vitamin A deficiency in the diet. Salem residents had plenty of milk and seafood available; they certainly did not suffer from vitamin A deficiency. Ergotism also involves extensive vomiting and diarrhea, symptoms not found in the Salem cases. A hearty appetite, almost ravenous, follows ergotism; in New England the afflicted wasted away from either an inability to eat or a lack of interest in it. The sudden onset of the Salem symptoms in late winter and early spring would be hard to trace to months of eating contaminated grain. Ergot was never seriously considered as the cause of problems at Salem, even by the colonists themselves who knew what ergotism was (it had been identified sixteen years earlier) and were trying desperately to discover the source of their problems.

An explanation that satisfies many of the unanswered questions about the events at Salem is that the symptoms reported by the afflicted New Englanders and their families in the seventeenth century were the result of an unrecognized epidemic of encephalitis. Comparisons may be made between the afflictions reported at Salem (as well as the rest of seventeenth-century New England) and the encephalitis lethargica pandemic of the early twentieth century. This partial list, created from the literature, reveals how similar the two epidemics were, in spite of the variation in medical terms of the day:

1692 SALEM	1916–1930s ENCEPHALITIS EPIDEMIC
fits	convulsions
spectral visions	hallucinations
mental "distraction"	psychoses
pinching, pricking	myoclonus of small muscle bundles on skin surface
"bites"	erythmata on skin surface, capillary hemorrhaging
eyes twisted	oculogyric crises: gaze fixed upward, downward, or to the side
inability to walk	paresis: partial paralysis
neck twisted	torticollis: spasm of neck muscles forces head to one side, spasms affect trunk and neck
repeating nonsense words	palilalia: repetition of one's own words

In both times, most of the afflicted were young women or children; the children were hit hardest, several dying in their cradles from violent fits. The afflictions appeared in late winter and early spring and receded with the heat of summer.... Von Economo noted that most encephalitis lethargica epidemics had historically shown the greatest number of acute cases occurring in the first quarter of the year, from midwinter to the beginning of spring. The "pricking and pinching" repeated so often in the court records at Salem can be explained by the way patients' skin surfaces exhibited twitches—quick, short, fluttering sequences of contractions of muscle bundles. Cold temperatures cause them to increase in number and spread over the body. Twitches were seldom absent in cases of hyperkinetic encephalitis lethargica during the 1920s epidemic. The skin surface also exhibited a peculiar disturbance in which red areas appeared due to dilation and congestion of the capillaries. Red marks that bleed through the skin's surface would explain the many references in court documents to suspected bites made by witches.

Examining the colonists' complaints in the trial papers uncovers many other symptom similarities: inability to walk, terrifying hallucinations, sore throat, or choking—the list goes on and on....

Ultimately the witch-hunts—or at least the complaints of afflictions—ended in Salem in the autumn of 1692, and there were no more complaints the following year. An arboviral encephalitis epidemic would have receded in the fall, when the air and water grew too cold for mosquitoes' survival. By the time spring arrived, the situation had altered, and the epidemic appeared to fade. Encephalitis epidemics, like many other contagious epidemics, often recede for years—sometimes decades—between recrudescence periods. Either the agents mutate and disappear to return years later, or they run out of susceptible hosts—the only ones left are those who have an immunity to the infection.

Ticks too might have been to blame. Just as in the spread of tick-borne encephalitis throughout the northern region of Russia, ticks played a part in spreading the disease across the virgin forests of temperate North America. Peasants who worked in the forest as woodcutters were affected in Russia during the epidemic of the 1950s; in Salem, in the seventeenth century, residents also worked as woodcutters and loggers. The Putnam family, in particular, were engaged in logging and woodcutting (and in fact were involved in arguments over whether they were taking logs from property they did not own). If the Putnams brought ticks bearing disease into their homes on their bodies or clothing, other members might have been affected. Reverend Parris's household could have been infected from the large amount of firewood he negotiated to supply his family, as part of his salary. Because they were his strongest supporters, the Putnams would likely have been the ones to cut and deliver the wood to his doorstep. Firewood, in the form of large logs used in colonial fireplaces, might have harbored wood ticks that had gone into winter hibernation but came out of the bark when logs were stored beside the hearth in a warm New England house. Infestations of ticks and body lice were common in colonial homes where laundry could not be done during the winter (nowhere to dry the wet clothing) and baths were rarely taken.

Another disease that results in encephalitis is endemic to the New England area even today. *Lyme disease* is a contemporary problem in New England, and there is little reason to think that it would have been absent from the area in colonial times. It is an infectious disease caused by bacteria spread by deer ticks. Both people and animals can be infected with Lyme disease. It is a serious but not fatal disease today. Found throughout the United States, it is most common along the East Coast, the Great Lakes, and the Pacific Northwest. In Massachusetts, deer ticks are most often found along the coast and are common in the Connecticut River Valley. The disease most likely spreads between late May and early autumn, when ticks are active. So tiny that the larvae are no bigger than a pencil point, the ticks live for two years, during which they can infect wild and domestic animals as well as people.

Symptoms of Lyme disease include a rash where the tick was attached—which may appear anywhere between three days and a month after the innocuous bite. Sometimes the rash looks like a small red doughnut. Other signs include itching, hives, swollen eyelids, and flulike symptoms such as fever, headache, stiff neck, sore muscles, fatigue, sore throat, and swollen glands. The symptoms go away after a few weeks, but without medical treatment nearly half the infected people will experience the rash again in other places on their bodies. In the later stages, three major areas—the joints, the nervous system, and the heart—may be affected even months after the tick bite. People with Lyme disease can develop late-stage symptoms even if they have never had the rash. About 10 to 20 percent of the people who do not get treatment develop nervous system problems: severe headache, stiff neck, facial paralysis, or cranial nerve palsies, and weakness and/or pain in their hands, arms, feet, or legs. Symptoms may last for weeks, often shifting from mild to severe and back again.

These symptoms are found in the present form of Lyme disease; the disease could likely have mutated over the centuries, because hallucinations and paranoia, along with lethargy, are not found in today's tick-borne version of Lyme disease. Questions and problems arise when connecting Lyme disease to the situations in 1692 or 1920, but it is another factor to consider. Could ticks have been common in Salem? The colonists did not bathe regularly, and they lived close by their domestic animals. Ticks could have wintered inside the home, carried in on firewood. They would have found ample hiding places in the seams of the heavy woolen clothing commonly worn by the colonists.

What about 1920? A common nuisance of that era was the "bedbug," chinch bug, or *Cimex lectularius*. Jar lids filled with arsenic were placed under bedsteads to keep the critters from climbing into bed and feeding on people's blood. Head lice have been common throughout the ages; today's rampant epidemics in schools are nothing to ignore, though scientists reassure us that neither bedbugs nor head lice carry any type of disease. Perhaps they did at one time. Many avenues must be explored, much research must be done. Perhaps we will never know what caused encephalitis lethargica. . . .

LAURIE WINN CARLSON is an assistant professor of history at Western Oregon University. She is the author of several scholarly historical studies, including *Cattle: An Informal Social History* (Ivan R. Dee, 2002); *Seduced by the West: Jefferson's America and the Lure of Land Beyond the Mississippi* (Ivan R. Dee, 2003); and *William J. Spillman and the Birth of Agricultural Economics* (University of Missouri Press, 2005).

Lyle Koehler

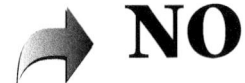

The Salem Village Cataclysm: Origins and Impact of a Witch Hunt, 1689–92

An Epidemic of Witchcraft

The Salem Village witch mania began easily enough, when several young girls experimented with fortune-telling and read occult works. In late January 1692, these girls began creeping under chairs and into holes, uttering "foolish, ridiculous speeches," assuming odd postures and, on occasion, writhing in agony. Their antics soon became full-fledged hysterical fits. Their tongues extended out to "a fearful length," like those of hanged persons; their necks cracked; blood "gushed plentifully out of their Mouths." A local physician named William Griggs, unable to explain the girls' behavior in medical terms, warned that it must be due to an "Evil hand." The fits quickly spread to other youngsters ranging in age from 12 to 19, as well as to married women like Ann Pope, Sarah Bibber, and Ann Putnam, and "an Ancient Woman, named Goodall."

The afflicted girls initially charged Sarah Good, Sarah Osborne, and the minister's Indian slave Tituba with practicing *maleficium* upon them. Local magistrates served warrants on these designated witches, who faced a courtroom examination on March 1. Twenty days later, Deodat Lawson, an ex-Salem Village pastor visiting from Boston, delivered a rousing anti-witchcraft sermon after observing the convulsive fits of Mary Walcott and Abigail Williams. A week later, Samuel Parris called his congregation to search out the many devils in the church. Parris was an old-line Puritan—a man anxious about his declining ministerial power, intensely suspicious of his neighbors, obsessed with thoughts of his own filthiness, and fearing the subversion of the Biblical Commonwealth.

The half dozen afflicted girls had accused only three witches in February and four in March, but after the ministers' warnings, no fewer than 15 girls and women of Salem Village accused witches—at least 25 additional during April, and 51 in May. "Witch" Martha Corey warned the authorities in March, "We must not believe all these distracted children say," but prosecutions continued. More persons from areas outside Salem Village were added to the list of accused witches—15 from Topsfield, most of whom had previously quarreled with the Putnam family over land boundaries, 12 others from Gloucester; 13 from the port of Salem; and 55 from Andover, a locale torn by land stress. Twenty-eight different persons, including four Andover women, fell subject to hysterical attacks in five outlying towns. Altogether, these ostensibly bewitched persons denounced almost all of the 56 men and 148 women accused of practicing witchcraft in 1692–1693. Not only were ¾ of the accused persons females, but of the 56 men half were singled out only after a close female relative or a wife had been accused—a sort of guilt by association. The reverse pattern holds true for only one, or possibly three, of the remaining male witches. Thus the traditional notion of the witch as a specifically female type held true for most Essex County accusations—even during times of severe stress, when virtually anyone might suffice as a scapegoat.

The Accusers

For many people who were already struggling against spiritual, political, and economic deprivation, and against the force of late seventeenth century changes, making a witchcraft accusation expressed their anxiety while it reasserted a sense of their own potency. Sociologist Dodd Bogart's conclusion that demon or witch charges are attempts to restore "self-worth, social recognition, social acceptance, social status, and other related social rewards" is pertinent to the Salem Village situation. Accusations allowed the angry, the helpless, and sometimes the sensitive to fight the imagined malign powers that frustrated them by scapegoating suitable incarnations of evil. By testifying against a witch, they not only exposed but also conquered their own feelings of powerlessness in a changing world. By blaming witches, men and women attempted to reestablish some feeling of order, of control, when confronted by the discomforting effects of threats both external (e.g., Indians, political anarchy, urban materialism)

Koehler, Lyle. "The Salem Village Cataclysm: Origins and Impact of a Witch Hunt, 1689–92," from *A SEARCH FOR POWER: The 'Weaker Sex' in Seventeenth Century New England*, pages 108–129. Copyright ©1980 by Lyle Koehler. Used with permission of University of Illinois Press.

and internal (e.g., the inability to achieve assurance of justification before God, or to understand, if assured, why God had chosen to "providentially" destroy a given animal or person).

The 63 men and 21 women who testified as corroborating witnesses against accused witches had much in common with the six males and 37 females whose hysterical fits initiated proceedings. In specifically sex-role-defined ways, members of each sex responded to an apparent condition of helplessness. Men primarily appeared before the magistrates and, in typically straightforward fashion, gave accounts of the witches' *maleficium;* women usually made their accusations more circuitously, behind the cover of a fit. Men revealed their feelings of fear and impotence by describing how witches had pressed them into rigid immobility; bewitched women demonstrated dramatically, before the very eyes of the justices, how that—and far worse—could happen.

Women, particularly those adolescents who experienced fits, used the witchcraft accusation as a viable form of self-expression in 1692–1693. Burdened by the restrictive contingencies of the ideal feminine role, with its dictum (reinforced in church and school) that good girls must control their longings for material joy and submit to stronger adult authority figures, many young females probably felt a great deal of frustration as they searched for gaiety, attention, accomplishment, and individual autonomy. This was especially true considering the recent fits of the Goodwin children in Boston (1688), the occupational assertiveness of female innkeepers and school dames, and the patent examples of so many women who violated Puritan laws—all of which had an impact upon the consciousnesses of developing adolescents.

After studying spirit possession and shamanism in primitive societies, I. M. Lewis concluded that accusatory fits are "thinly disguised protest movements directed against the dominant sex. They thus play a significant part in the sex-war in traditional societies and cultures where women lack more obvious and direct means of forwarding their aims. To a considerable extent, they protect women from the exactions of men and offer an effective vehicle for manipulating husbands and male relatives." Lewis's conclusion is equally applicable to Salem Village. There, in the paranoid atmosphere of 1692, girls used the fit—although not necessarily consciously—as a vehicle to invert the traditional social status hierarchy. Similarly, adult women, those perpetual children, expressed, through the fit, a need for excitement and dominion. For females, such assertion entailed, symbolically and on occasion literally, the elimination of the immediate oppressing force—the adult, the husband, or, in Mercy Short's case, the Indians.

The bewitched parties, through their accusations, did help to eliminate authority figures—if not actual parents or husbands, whose destruction would be *too* discomforting or would deprive them of necessary support, then surely "representative" substitutions. A female figure suggestive of parental authority by her mature years, or one closely associated with a male of high position, was frequently chosen as a safer but still satisfactory surrogate. Later, as the afflicted girls achieved more self-confidence, they actually attacked men, including at least two ministers.

All of the afflicted women, most particularly the Salem Village girls, exercised fantastic power. The public watched spellbound while the girls contorted their bodies into unbelievable shapes. Magistrates hung on their every word, believing them even when the girls were caught in outright lies. At least one justice changed his opinion of a prominent friend after that man came under accusation. Accused witches hardly knew what to say, save to maintain their innocence, when confronted by the awesome spectacle of girls throwing themselves about the courtroom, pulling four-inch-long pins and broken knife blades out of their own flesh. Some accused witches even became confused as to their own complicity in such goings on. Anyone who criticized the court proceedings or the afflicted quickly fell under accusation as another witch, including even defecting members of the girls' own group.

As early as March 20, the afflicted proved they could also, on occasion, assume a more self-consciously assertive stance. When Deodat Lawson prepared to give a Sabbath lecture, eleven-year-old Abigail Williams shouted out, "Now stand up, and Name your Text." In the beginning of his sermon, Goodwife Ann Pope told him, "Now there is enough of that," and after it was finished, Williams asserted, "It is a long Text." Twelve-year-old Anne Putnam shouted out that an invisible yellow bird, a witch's familiar, sat on Lawson's hat as it hung on a pin. In the afternoon sermon, Williams again spoke up: "I know no Doctrine you had," she informed the minister, "If you did name one, I have forgot it." Such outspokenness dumbfounded the congregation. Here, three females had violated the biblical injunction against women speaking in church; furthermore, a little girl had criticized the minister. Obviously, witches were to blame!

Not only had such females assumed the power to speak in church and to designate men and women as witches, they also claimed the ability to vanquish supernatural creatures. They asserted that they could see and talk to the Devil, yet emerge unscathed from those encounters. Tituba, powerless both as servant and as woman, told imaginative tales of her own fearless contact with frightening spectral creatures—hairy upright men and great black dogs. Another "very sober and pious woman," uncowed by a malign specter's appearance, disputed with it about a scriptural text.

The choice of victims, many of them eccentrics, suggests that the bewitched females were most discomforted by those women who had acted upon their own inner needs to ignore or defy the ideal feminine sex role, i.e., those women who best illustrated the projected desires of the afflicted. Unable to be similarly assertive, the accusers turned instead to equally unfeminine, but disguised and purely destructive, aggression in punishing those nontraditional women. The psychoanalyst Merell Middlemore appears correct when he writes that the Salem Village girls could not "consolidate a female identification"—but only if his remark is qualified to read Puritan, or perhaps seventeenth-century, female identification.

Scapegoating witches did not always work for the individual accuser, as the shocking inhumanity of sending people to the gallows sometimes became too much for the afflicted girls to handle. Some initial accusers ceased to have fits or to denounce witches long before the frenzy abated. Mary Warren, after actively accusing a number of witches, suddenly began to charge that the "afflicted children did but dissemble." Immediately she was cried out upon as a witch, but in prison she continued to speak out against the proceedings, asserting several times that the magistrates "might as well examine Keysar's daughter that had been distracted many years." She explained, "when I was afflicted, I thought I saw the apparitions of 100 persons," but then added that her head had been "distempered." In court, however, the other girls, Ann Pope, and John Indian attributed their violent fits to her, and under stringent cross-examination, Mary Warren fell once again into fits. Imprisoned for a month, she finally retracted her criticism, admitted her own witchcraft, and once more began accusing others. Similarly, when Deliverance Hobbs wavered from her accusatory affliction, the bewitched girls denounced her. She, like Mary Warren, denied signing the Devil's book, but then, under the magistrates' relentless questioning, also admitted her witchcraft. Another of the girls, Sarah Churchill, fell under suspicion of practicing witchcraft, probably for the same reason. After her examination, she cried and appeared "much troubled in spirit." She explained to Sarah Ingersoll that she had confessed her *maleficium* only "because they threatened her and told her they would put her into the dungeon."

The line between witch and bewitched was dangerously thin, both on the psychological level and in terms of the social distribution of Power which an accuser manipulated. Once a woman began having fits in which she declared herself afflicted by agents of Satan, she could afford no second thoughts, however sane and humane. Once she had "sold her soul"—that is, disavowed responsibility for her own deepest impulses—she could not recover it without sharing the fate of her accused victims, without becoming as powerless as they in the grip of the larger Puritan community.

The Accused: Nontraditional Women

While many witches served as scapegoat-victims of various men's land greed, others more clearly fitted the image of social deviants. Women who did not toe the ideal feminine line offered the afflicted females a superb opportunity to work out their own projected aggressions and needs for dominion—those unacceptable urges which the afflicted found desirable yet incompatible with their Puritan training. In what was probably an overstatement, Thomas Maule estimated that ▨ of the accused were either guilty of rebellion against their parents (who included, in Puritan terms, husbands and magistrates) or of adultery. One, Sarah Osborne, had lived in a common law relationship with her "wild" Irish servant; another, Martha Corey, had given birth to a mulatto child. "Witch" Susannah Roots had earned a reputation as a "bad woman" who entertained company late at night.

Those women who had openly flouted the ideal role in the changing world of the late century received quick convictions. One of the first three persons accused, Sarah Good, was such a woman. Born into a wealthy family, she had been cheated out of her inheritance after her father's suicide in 1672. She married twice, both times to men who became debt ridden. By 1689, her second husband, William Good, had lost all of his land and 17 head of cattle to his creditors. Too poor to own a house, he lived with Sarah and their infant daughter in neighbors' houses, barns, and sometimes open ditches. Turbulent and vitriolic, Sarah Good often scolded and "fell to muttering" when people extended charity to her. When one neighbor refused her lodging, she was not above setting his cattle loose. In court, she answered the magistrates "in a very wicked spiteful manner, reflecting and retorting against the authorities with base and abusive words." After the minister Nicholas Noyes urged her of confess, since "she knew she was a witch," Sarah pulled no punches in lashing out, "you are a liar; I am no more a Witch than you are a Wizard; and if you take away my Life, God will give you Blood to drink." She died on July 19, protesting to the end.

Bridget Bishop, the first "witch" hanged, would not be dominated by her three husbands. She operated an unlicensed tavern where visitors congregated late at night to play the illegal game of shuffleboard, and she dressed provocatively—some of her contemporaries might say whorishly—in a red paragon bodice. Once she had driven an accusatory stranger off her porch with a spade. Like so many other alleged witches, she protested her innocence, asserting, "I know not what a witch is."

Martha Carrier, accused of no less than 13 witchly murders at Andover, had actively disputed with neighbors over land, physically shaken up one twelve-year-old girl in church, and threatened a male opponent by saying that "She would hold his Nose close to the Grindstone as ever it was held since his Name was Abbot." Her interrogator asked at the witch trials, "What black man did you see?" She retorted, "I saw no black man but your own presence." She charged the magistrates with not listening to what she said while they "shamefully" paid attention to every little utterance of the bewitched girls. Cotton Mather, detesting her outspokenness termed her "this rampant hag."

Many other witches revealed their deviance both in and out of court. Abigail Hobbs expressed no fear of lying out in the woods at night, explaining that "she was not afraid of anything." Disobedient to her parents, she had once sprinkled water in her mother's face, saying she "baptized her in the name of the Father, Son, and Holy Ghost." Susannah Martin of Amesbury, long accounted a witch, spoke harshly to neighbors, accused the girls of "dealing in the Black Art," and pointed out (to the magistrates' chagrin) that the Old Testament described Satan's appearance in the shape of an innocent, one "glorified Saint." Mary Parker had once shocked her associates by coming to the tavern after her husband and there "railing" at him. Ann Pudeator possessed a long-standing reputation as "an ill-carriaged woman," while Mary Obinson several times abused Thomas Hill, calling him "cuckold & old foole." Mammy Read had the gall to tell Mistress Symmes, after an argument, that she wished her antagonist "might never piss, nor shit, if she did not go [i.e., leave]." Read, Pudeator, Martin, Carrier, and Bishop all swung from the gallows, but Hobbs received a reprieve after her conviction. No further record exists of Obinson's case. Whether any of these women actually practiced witchcraft cannot now be deemed, but it is unlikely. The fact that women in 1692 had more freedom than ever before—a reality produced in part by the lack of witchcraft prosecutions after 1665—would presumably have decreased the need for "rebels" against the feminine ideal to assume the totally malign inversion of the proper role. The clarity and force of the earlier typologies of Witch and Whore, as well as Virgin and Wife, had considerably weakened by the 1690s, only to dramatically resurface in 1692.

Despite their realizations that they faced a death sentence, most of the accused women refused to insure their own releases by concocting confessions. Instead, they "would neither in time of Examination, nor Trial, Confess anything of what was laid to their Charge; some would not admit of any Minister to Pray with them, others refused to pray for themselves." Nineteen women died protesting their innocence, including five in prison. One of the hanged "witches," Mary Easty, knowing that she could not save her own life, wished to save those "that are going the same way with myself." She urged the Salem Court to examine carefully all confessing witches who accused others, for, she explained, they "have belyed themselves and others."

Those women who walked bravely to the gallows may have summoned strength from their religious faith, or from recognition of the integrity of their own personhood. Other women signed petitions supporting accused witches, even though such petitioners should have been aware that the afflicted girls quickly accused their critics. Two Putnam opponents, Israel and Elizabeth Porter, headed a petition signed by 16 other women and 21 men on behalf of Rebecca Nurse. Another 13 men and seven of their wives requested leniency for the Proctors.

During the trials, from time to time, an occasional unaccused woman went so far as to attack the character of one or more of the afflicted. For example, Lydia Porter charged Goody Bibber with mischief-making and lying. Mary Phips, the wife of the governor, expressed her own disagreement by pardoning one convicted witch in the governor's absence, although she had no legal power to do so. Lady Phips, Lydia Porter, and the almost 100 female petitioners, as well as many of the "witches," were acting assertively in varying degrees, reflecting and contributing to the style of the nontraditional woman.

An End to Witchcraft

As witchcraft accusations increased in number, protests also mounted, from men as well as from women. Husbands spoke up in defense of their wives. Ex-deputy Robert Pike told Justice Corwin that "diabolical visions, apparitions, or representations" were "more commonly false and delusive then real," also pointing out that the afflicted women raised the dead, like the Witch of Endor in biblical times. A Salem Quaker named Thomas Maule anonymously blasted the Puritans for murdering one another under the Devil's influence, and as early as June the Anabaptist William. Milbourne protested to the General Court against the use of "bare specter testimony" to convict "persons of good fame and of unspotted reputations." A Boston merchant by the name of Thomas Brattle, in an October letter, penned a scathing criticism of the Salem proceedings. At about the same time Samuel Willard published a disapproving analysis of the arguments used against witches, in *Some Miscellany Observations on our Present Debates Respecting Witchcraft, In a Dialogue between S[alem] and B[oston]*. Cotton Mather had begun to doubt the reality of specter evidence, while other *ministers*, including Joshua Moody, John Hale, John Wise, Francis Dane, James Allen, and John Baily, raised objections to the proceedings. Willard and Moody took occasion to preach the text, "they that are persecuted in one city, let them flee to another," and then counselled four "witches" to escape from prison.

The afflicted girls ultimately insured that the witchcraft proceedings would halt—by accusing the most prestigious members of Puritan society. The girls had first charged contentious, penniless Sarah Good, disreputable Sarah Osborne, and the exotic Barbadian Indian slave Tituba. Sensing their own power in the court's re*sponse*, they subsequently broadened their attack by clamoring not only against low-status eccentrics but also against virtuous women like Rebecca Nurse, and even against men. On May 31, attorney Thomas Newton would assert that they "spare no person of what quality so ever." By November, the bewitched had charged the wives of critics Moody, Hale, and Dane, as well as several members of Boston's ruling elite. However, the authorities were reluctant to prosecute. Margaret Thatcher, the widow of Boston's wealthiest merchant and mother-in-law of Judge Jonathan Corwin, who presided at witchcraft trials, escaped apprehension, even though she was much complained about by the afflicted. So did Mary Phips, Samuel Willard, and Mistress Moody. The magistrates did issue a warrant for the arrest of a prominent merchant named Hezekiah Usher, but he received lodging in a private house and then was permitted to leave the colony.

Bostonians had less respect for the orders of the Salem Court than did the citizenry of any other area; their constables ignored warrants. Accused witches broke out of prison altogether too easily, suggesting complicity on the part of the jailor. In fact, the keeper had no apparent hesitancy about releasing one "witch" upon receipt of Lady Phips's pardon. Other Bostonians hid "witches" who had escaped from prison or fled apprehension.

The Salem Village girls who accused proper Bostonians quite possibly exploited the resentment of many rural Salem Villagers for those alien yet very powerful urbanites who often valued capital over land, commerce over husbandry, ornamentation over simplicity, and new ideas over old. The Putnams, in particular, facing diminishing land resources and declining status, had a good deal to resent; they listened with open ears while the girls accused nine prominent Bostonians and denounced Nathaniel Saltonstall, the Haverhill Councilor who had resigned his seat on the witch court. Those with Boston connections also faced prosecution. In Andover, for example, three prominent Bradstreets—a family with close marital and political ties to Boston's ruling elite—fled prosecution. Before the witchcraft frenzy had abated, even the secretary of Connecticut had been denounced.

Perhaps, nothing better illustrates many people's dislike for the merchant class than the destruction wrought against the property of the wealthy French Huguenot, Philip English. (There was undoubtedly some anti-French feeling involved in English's case as well.) After English and his "aristocratic" wife, Mary, escaped from Salem prison, an irate group of citizens sacked their "great house" at Salem, destroying or carrying away various old family portraits and furniture and robbing storehouses of goods valued at £2,683. When English later returned, he found a single servant's bed, the only furniture remaining in the house.

The colony's economic and political leaders objected to the accusations levied against so many of their friends and wives. Quite probably their objections were crucial in bringing the frenzy to a halt. Robert Calef credited one prominent Bostonian with stopping proceedings at Andover by threatening to sue his accusers there in a £1,000 defamation action. Governor William Phips initially left all witchcraft affairs to the Court of Oyer and Terminer, but after returning to Boston from an expedition against the Maine Indians, he found "many persons in a strange ferment of dissatisfaction." Soon the royal governor forbade the issuance of any new literature on the subject, asked the Crown for counsel, and dissolved the Court of Oyer and Terminer. In the winter of 1692–1693 Phips pardoned some convicted witches, caused some to be let out on bail, and "put the Judges upon considering a way to relieve others and prevent them from perishing in prison." The General Court on December 16, 1692, directed the newly created Superior Court to try the "witches" still in custody within Essex County. The Superior Court, meeting on January 3, 1692/3, acquitted 49 "witches" and convicted three. Deputy Governor Stoughton, the chief justice, ordered the execution of those three, as he had of other "witches," but Phips pardoned these and five other convicted persons. Stoughton, enraged, refused to sit on the bench of the next court at Charlestown. That body released all the accused persons tried before it.

Before the Superior Court met at Salem, the bewitched girls had ceased their afflictions. Perhaps, by then, they had realized that their reach exceeded their grasp. Perhaps, they felt guilty over precipitating the deaths of 25 persons. Perhaps, their power impulses had been satiated. (After all, for some time people as far away as Boston, Andover, and Gloucester had sought their advice in pointing out witches.) Perhaps, they were drained by the physical and emotional strain which attended fits. Perhaps, they felt purged, for a time, of their own unfeminine longings. For whatever reasons, they *had* had their day; now it seemed only appropriate that they return to their status as unobtrusive members of the Puritan community.

Only in eastern Massachusetts, with its intense and numerous frustrations, could a sustained witch hunt be mounted. There the reality of the nontraditional woman loomed larger, helping to precipitate fits in powerless adolescents and religious Puritan wives, as well as aggravating the already established tendency to view unfeminine behavior as witchlike. Those independent-spirited women who faced prosecution as witches were the victims of other, more conservative women's unconscious search for power.

LYLE KOEHLER (1944–2015) was a Professor of History, an archeologist, and an accomplished writer. His most famous book was "*A Search for Power: The 'Weaker Sex' in Seventeeth Century New England*" (University of Illinois Press, 1980), which earned him finalist honors for the 1981 Pulitzer Prize in history.

EXPLORING THE ISSUE

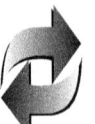

Was Encephalitis Responsible for the Salem Witchcraft Hysteria?

Critical Thinking and Reflection

1. What is the specific evidence Laurie Winn Carlson gives to support her interpretation of the events in Salem in 1692? Do you believe her argument?
2. What evidence does Koehler provide for suggesting witchcraft being related to women's search for power? Do you believe his argument?
3. How did the relationship between the residents of Salem Town and Salem Village affect the witchcraft hysteria?
4. Does the complex system of ideological and material conditions stand out as being particularly important in allowing the Salem witchcraft hysteria to occur or can we blame disease, socioeconomic tensions, a history of sexism, or other factors as being particularly integral to unraveling this history?
5. What does Koehler suggest about the way women were understood in seventeenth century New England?

Is There Common Ground?

The Salem hysteria, trials, and executions were not historically unique when we consider the factors that existed. We may never be able to distill the precise reasons that witchcraft hysteria occurred in Salem; however, both authors offer compelling evidence that provide a more complete picture of this interesting historical period. There is no doubt that examining the micro and macroelements of the period will provide a slightly different picture informing the ways we understand this issue. On one hand, there is little doubt that the broader political, economic, and social transformations occurring during this time generated increased hysteria. Study of the sociology of the time also helps us understand this period. Examination of accusers and accused reveals a distinct split between where acquisitions originated, the ways people conceived of puritanical religious beliefs, and the sociopolitical contexts in which these people lived. Women were likely targeted based on gender, economic jealousy, and historical mythology. Many other factors may have been relevant in a town interested in restoring self-worth, social recognition, and status in a changing society. For some living as part of a puritanical public, these issues were undoubtedly related to the eternal struggle between God and the Devil. We can also likely assume that ambitious leaders would use the social changes as a way to further certain religious and political agendas. From a micro perspective, compelling evidence suggests that the symptom described as demonic closely resembled encephalitis and no known cure existed. We know that weather had caused fungus to develop in rye crops, which affected the health and economic wellbeing of the colony. The warm and humid summer preceding the Salem trials leading to the outbreak of this fungus likely presents similar symptoms to encephalitis and what was understood at the time to be "demonic possession." Or were the accusers interested in fame and personal agency in a culture when women had little.

There are several facts that support the arguments of both authors. What is interesting is that similar events happened across Western Europe and in other parts of the American Colonies. Witchcraft could account for the outbreaks, the weather, and the economic conditions, which could all be considered punishments from God. Similarly, raids, economic instability, jealousy, and disease could have been explained through the religious dogma of the time to explain how a society had lost its way. Interestingly, we can also see that these factors affected the economic wellbeing of those in the colony. Accusations largely came from an area with more religious and dogmatic poor farmers. What is more, 14 of the victims had large fortunes and land that they inherited from relatives that likely died from disease. When combining the encephalitis outbreak, socioeconomic tensions, and religious fervor, we can see how military, economic, biological, and political elements intersecting with religious, historical, and social ones (i.e., gender) might have created mass hysteria. These and even more complex historical arguments paint an interesting picture of why the trials occurred.

Therefore, there is not only common ground for this question, but each side may help reveal the nuanced historical portrait of this interesting time in American history. The question may not be is encephalitis to blame for witchcraft hysteria, but rather, what were the complex intersectional events that led to the conditions that allowed the Salem hysteria to occur? This question has been and continues to be explored by interested students, teachers, and researchers.

Additional Resources

Boyer, P. S., & Nissenbaum, S. (Eds.). (1993). *Salem-Village Witchcraft: A Documentary Record of Local Conflict in Colonial New England*. UPNE.

Breslaw, E. G. (1995). *Tituba, Reluctant Witch of Salem: Devilish Indians and Puritan Fantasies*. NYU Press.

Gragg, L. D. (1992). *The Salem Witch Crisis*. Praeger Publishers.

Hill, F. (2000). *The Salem Witch Trials Reader*. Perseus Books Group.

Hoffer, P. C. (1996). *The Devil's Disciples: Makers of the Salem Witchcraft Trials*. Johns Hopkins University Press.

Internet References . . .

Famous American Trials: Salem Witchcraft Trials, 1692

http://famous-trials.com/salem

Salem Witch Trials Documentary Archive and Transcription Project

salem.lib.virginia.edu/home.html

Salem Witch Trials: Can You Survive Salem's Witchcraft Hysteria?

https://www.nationalgeographic.org/interactive/salem-interactive/

The 1692 Salem Witch Trials: The Salem Witch Museum

https://salemwitchmuseum.com/

The Library of Congress

https://www.loc.gov/item/today-in-history/march-01

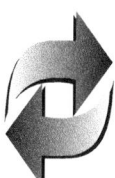

ISSUE

Selected, Edited, and with Issue Framing Material by:
Kevin R. Magill and Tony L. Talbert, Baylor University

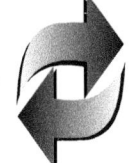

Should the Great Awakening Be Understood Primarily through Religious Evangelicalism?

YES: Thomas S. Kidd, from "The Great Awakening: The Roots of Evangelical Christianity in Colonial America," Yale University Press (2007)

NO: David A. Varel, from "The Historiography of the Second Great Awakening and the Problem of Historical Causation, 1945–2005," *Madison Historical Review* (2011)

Learning Outcomes

After reading this issue, you will be able to:

- Describe the cause and effect relationships of the role of religion in Great Britain's North American Colonies.
- Discuss the competing ideological ideas as promoted by prominent Christian leaders such as George Whitfield, Jonathan Edwards, Benjamin Coleman, Jonathan Barber, Timothy Cutler, et al., in the British colonies of North America.
- Compare and contrast the antecedents, characteristics, and impact of the first and second Protestant Christian Great Awakening movements on the political landscape of the British North American Colonies.
- Explain the relationship between the Protestant Christian Great Awakening movements and the rise of democratic social and political activism in the British North American colonies of the mid- to late 18th century.
- Develop a conceptual connection between the multiple theological and philosophical movements that influenced the intersections of religious and political life in mid- to late 18th century British North American colonies.

ISSUE SUMMARY

YES: Thomas S. Kidd believes that a Great Awakening occurred because influential preachers engineered divinely inspired revivals in the mid-eighteenth century causing an evangelical movement that spread across the colonies, changing the nature of Christianity.

NO: David A. Varel tracks the historiography of the Second Great Awakening and suggests that historian need to consider more that evangelicalism. He believes that factors such as social control, democratization, and denominational concentration present a problem in determining historical causation. He therefore suggests that the Second Great Awakening should be understood through the many intersectional aspects that helped create this evangelical movement. He additionally notes, though it was a national phenomenon, the Second Great Awakening greatly varied in its local and regional manifestations and should not be understood solely through its most famous preachers.

"Thus religion lay as it were dying, and ready to expire its last breath of life in this part of the visible church: and it was in the spring of 1740, when the God of salvation was pleased to visit us with the blessed effusions of his Holy Spirit in an eminent manner" (Tracy, 1845).

Joseph Tracy's words have become the fundamental characterization that have defined our general understanding of the origins and causes of the First Great Awakening (FGA) and Second Great Awakening (SGA) movements in the 18th and 19th centuries' British North American colonies. For generations, public school and university textbooks have offered a relatively consistent version of the FGA and SGA as being solely rooted in religious revivalism. However, there have been and continue to be rival historical interpretations of these initial North American *Awakenings Movements* that are not simply revisionist conspiracy but indeed reasoned conjecture offering evidence that challenges the notion that the FGA and SGA in the colonial and frontier eras of America are to be understood primary through religious evangelicalism.

It is essential that we first provide the outline of what is commonly understood as the FGA and SGA in North America. The FGA is most often placed within the time frame of 1735–1743 C.E. Although, as will be noted in the selected reading, Thomas Kidd challenges this conventional segmentation of the FGA and offers a convincing argument for the notion of a *long Great Awakening* that begins in the 1670s and closes at the end of the American Revolution in 1783. The SGA's timeframe is relatively uncontested by historians being placed within a date range of approximately 1795 C.E. as to near the 1850s C.E.

The FGA and SGA shared common characteristics with their geographical boundaries, unique American social, economic, and political contexts, and certainly the significant impact on religious and moral teachings through the rise of new Christian Protestant sects. The theological and ideological impact of the FGA and SGA is evidenced in the historical records and cultures of the people groups throughout the New England colonies, the North East territories, including Canadian Nova Scotia, New Brunswick, and Prince Edward Island, and the so-called American "backcountry" encompassing a wide swath of the Blue Ridge range, Shenandoah Valley, the Virginia's and Kentucky counties, and the Ohio Valley. Although we can develop a cursory understanding of the FGA and SGA through the common characteristic manifest in their origins and outcomes, it is only when we take a closer look at the distinctive variations of each *Awakening* as evidenced through the voices of the persons who came to be most closely identified with them.

Against the backdrop of colonial British America with rival sentiments of loyalty to the crown versus liberty through revolution, the FGA's most prominent voices must certainly be identified with the writings and teaching of Jonathan Edwards and George Whitefield. Both Edwards' and Whitefiled's influence in the origins and impact of the FGS's theological and ideological significance cannot be understated. Edwards' theology, rooted in Calvinism and nurtured in Puritan/Congregationalist spirituality, is considered by many historians to be America's greatest theologian. Edwards' influence in the hearts and minds of the people who would eventually form a new nation extends beyond treatises of *an angry God*. His blending of rhetoric of sensation and intellectual vivid imagery resulted in a powerful elixir that inspired and instigated both religious and sociopolitical activism. George Whitefield's dynamic oratory and sonorous voice attracted crowds of tens of thousands of adherents, agnostics, and acolytes in gatherings across the British colonies of New England, the Southern regions, and so-called "backcountry" of 18th century North America. Already well known in England holding equal stature with John Wesley, Whitefield's persona, passion, and prolific public preaching regimen (i.e., reported to have held 18,000 preaching engagements before 10 million listeners) elevated him to the status of a public celebrity allowing him interact with other famous cultural contemporaries as well as offer spiritual counsel and friendship to such luminaries as Dr. Benjamin Franklin.

The emergence of the SGA in the late 18th century's newly birthed United States is best represented by the voices of Nathaniel Taylor and Charles Grandison Finney. Taylor and Finney, less Calvinistic than their predecessors Edwards and Whitefield, were nonetheless just as theologically and ideologically aligned with vast swaths of the U.S. population as Edwards and Whitefield during their most active years. Taylor and Finney captured the zeitgeist of the age through the integration of religious, social, political, and economic issues that seemed most pressing to a newly formed nation and her people who had just won a victory through stalemate against the world power Great Britain (Howe, 2007). The momentum of Christian Evangelical Revivalism would continue under the tutelage of Nathaniel Taylor and Charles G. Finney as both men took up the mantel of cause célèbre as they preached a *freewill* theology (though contrasting on specific points of the Divine and human will) that complimented the *freewill* ideology that spurned the new American nation's people to a promise of manifest destiny and self-determination on such issues as acquisition of native people's lands, abolition of slavery, women's rights, universal suffrage, temperance, prison reform, and so on. Though less popular among Southern slaveholders, Taylor's and Finney's brand of revivalism and revolution gained influenced their current and future generations throughout the former New England colonies (now states), southern Appalachian regions, the old and new backcountry areas, and beyond. Evidence by the rise of new Christian sects (e.g., Methodists, Baptists, Mormons, Seventh Day Adventists, et al.), the SGA, like the FGA, blurred the lines of religion, society, politics, and economics.

Given the traditional historical record's emphasis on religion, spirituality, and morality as the fundamental characteristics of the FGA and SGA, one would consider the matter settled on whether the *Great Awakening movements should be understood primarily through religious evangelicalism*. However, it is precisely the notion of *traditional historical record* vs. *revisionist historical record* that frames this inquiry as evidenced by the writings of Thomas S. Kidd and David A. Varel. Both Kidd and Varel represent two rival, though collegial, camps of historians who have sustained this debate on the fundamental characteristics and historical causation of the FGA and SGA. Perhaps, it is precisely the nuanced nature of the overlap of Kidd's and Veral's analyses of the phenomenon of the Christian Evangelical FGA and SGA movements in North America that offers the reader an intriguing glimpse into the conjecture of historical causation whether founded primarily in theological antecedents (Kidd) or a multiplicity of ideological antecedents (Veral) or dare one venture to hypothesize a different conclusion.

In the following selections, Thomas S. Kidd asserts that notion of segmented FGA and SGA movements in the British North American Colonies with a multiplicity of foundational antecedents obscures the reality of a *long series of Awakening Movements* that were continuously sustained through religious fervor and spiritual manifestations inspired by the ideological momentum of Christian Evangelicals. According to Kidd, the FGA and SGA's historical causation can be traced to the influence of Christian Evangelical leaders and their adherents successful engineering of what some might attribute to divinely inspired revivals that paved the way for the intersection of well-established Christian Evangelical and fledgling Patriot-Democracy movements that simultaneously spread across the colonies, changing the nature and trajectory of Christianity's influence in North America and around the globe.

David A. Varel offers a historiographical explanation for the antecedents of the 18th century's North American Christian Evangelical Great Awakening movements. Varel suggests that four competing historical interpretations of the origins of the American Great Awakening movements is the evidence of the multifaceted historical causation of the so-called *Awakenings* in the British colonies of North America. Varel contends that religion alone cannot be ascribed to the rise of the SGA. Instead, democratization and denominational concentration present a problem in determining historical causation. He therefore suggests that the SGA should be understood through the many intersectional aspects that helped create this evangelical movement. He additionally notes, though it was a national phenomenon, the SGA greatly varied in its local and regional manifestations and should not be understood solely through its most famous preachers. Moreover, while he acknowledges the significant corollary of religion as an influence on the social, political, and economic impact of the Great Awakening Movements, it would be an oversimplification of the complexity of the rise of revolutionary Democracy movements to over emphasize the role of Christian Evangelicalism given the dominant revolutionary and reform ideologies that were present in colonial and new nation building America.

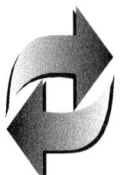

YES

Thomas S. Kidd

The Great Awakening: The Roots of Evangelical Christianity in Colonial America

... Until 1982, historians took the Great Awakening as a given, but then historian Jon Butler argued that it was only an "interpretative fiction" invented by nineteenth-century Christian historians. Although Butler's argument was overextended, it helpfully provoked a revaluation of what we actually mean by "the Great Awakening." He contended that the event really amounted to just "a short-lived Calvinist revival in New England during the early 1740s." No doubt the eighteenth-century awakenings were centered in New England, but over time they came to influence parts of all the colonies, and more important, they helped birth an enormously important religious movement, evangelicalism, which shows no sign of disappearing today.

Butler also asserted that the "revivals had modest effects on colonial religion" and that they were "never radical." But if the revivals helped create evangelicalism, then not only did the awakenings make a profound change in colonial religion, but they began a major alteration of global Christian history. Moreover, ... the revivals featured all manner of radical spiritual manifestations, unnerving antirevivalists and moderate evangelicals alike. Butler's critique does show, however, that it is not enough to evaluate evangelicalism as a homogenous whole. It had radical implications, but those implications were hotly contested by moderates, and its social potential often came to naught for women, African Americans, and Native Americans. Some evangelicals also began a great assault on the churchly establishments of colonial America, and the revolutionary move for disestablishment on the federal and state levels can largely be attributed to evangelical and deist cooperation in favor of the separation of church and state.

Butler finally claimed that, contrary to the suggestions of previous scholars, "the link between the revivals and the American Revolution is virtually nonexistent." ...

I am in substantial agreement with Butler on this point. Moreover, evangelicals' responses to the Revolution covered the whole range of opinions from enthusiastic Patriotism to staunch Loyalism. But we should also note that evangelical rhetoric and ideology helped to inspire and justify the Patriot cause for both evangelical and nonevangelical leaders. Evangelicalism did not start the Revolution, but the Patriot side certainly benefited from the support of many evangelicals.

... I contend that there was, indeed, a powerful, unprecedented series of revivals from about 1740 to 1743 that touched many of the colonies and that contemporaries remembered for decades as a special visitation of the Holy Spirit. Calling this event "the" Great Awakening does present historical problems. Chief among them is that the standard framework of the "First" and "Second" Great Awakenings may obscure the fact that the evangelical movement continued to develop after 1743 and before 1800. There were important, widespread revivals that happened before the First, and between the First and Second, Great Awakenings. ... I examine, instead, what we might call the *long* First Great Awakening and the contest to define its boundaries. Although many revivals, including the major season from 1740 to 1743, happened during this period, revivals alone did not delineate the early evangelical movement. Instead, persistent desires for revival, widespread individual conversions, and the outpouring of the Holy Spirit distinguished the new evangelicals. The long First Great Awakening started before Jonathan Edwards's 1734–35 Northampton revival and lasted roughly through the end of the American Revolution, when disestablishment, theological change, and a new round of growth started the (even more imprecise) "Second" Great Awakening. The controversial emergence of the religion of the new birth demarcated the long First Great Awakening and the first generation of American evangelical Christianity.

. . . New Englanders began to hear about George Whitefield in 1739, and many hoped that he would soon visit them. Benjamin Colman of Boston's Brattle Street Church wrote to Whitefield in December 1739 after having received a letter from him. Whitefield estimated that he might come to New England by summer 1740. Colman was deeply impressed by what he had learned about Whitefield. He had read Whitefield's *Journals,* as well as some of his sermons. Colman wrote that he had never encountered anything comparable to Whitefield's ministry, although he had witnessed "uncommon Operations of the holy Spirit . . .; as in our Country of Hampshire of late; the Narrative of which by Mr. Edwards, I suppose you may have seen." If Whitefield would come to New England, he would find the churches' Calvinist doctrine to his liking, "how short soever we may come of your Fervours." Colman told him that the churches had been praying for him publicly, and that when he arrived he could use the commodious Brattle Street Church for meetings. In a letter to Gilbert Tennent, Whitefield wrote that he found Colman's published sermons "acute and pointed, but I think not searching enough by many degrees." If anything, Colman was too polite for Whitefield. Nevertheless, Whitefield wrote back to Colman and promised that when he came to New England "I shall endeavour to recommend an universal charity amongst all the true members of CHRIST's mystical body." Because of this universal spirit, he suggested that he might stay in the fields to preach, and out of the meetinghouses. He appreciated Colman's latitudinarianism, and they both hoped that the old division of Anglican versus dissenter would become irrelevant in light of the ministry of the new birth.

Jonathan Edwards also received word of Whitefield's revivals, and in November 1739 Whitefield wrote to him, desiring to visit Northampton to see for himself the fruit of the 1734–35 awakening. Edwards wrote back in February 1740, encouraging Whitefield to travel to Northampton but warning him not to expect much. Edwards was heartened by God's raising up Whitefield in the Church of England "to revive the mysterious, spiritual, despised, and exploded doctrines of the gospel." This might be a sign of the coming Kingdom of God, Edwards thought.

The Boston and Philadelphia newspapers began picking up stories about Whitefield's prodigious meetings in England in spring 1739, and Whitefield's fame began to spread into the hinterlands by early 1740. For instance, pastor Nicholas Gilman of Exeter, New Hampshire, on a visit to Boston, began reading Whitefield's *Journals* in mid-January 1740 and commented with admiration on Whitefield's "most Indefatigable labours to Advance the Kingdom of Christ." He borrowed more of Whitefield's sermons from Colman. In June, Gilman noted that "Mr. Whitefield [was] Now much the Subject of Conversations."

In July, Whitefield wrote to Colman to announce that he was coming soon, perhaps within a month, and to ask Colman to spread the word in friendly churches. This advance publicity worked wonderfully, and when Whitefield arrived in Newport. Rhode Island, on September 14, 1740, New England was abuzz with talk of his coming. In Newport, Whitefield was welcomed by Nathaniel Clap, a venerable Congregational minister, and the wandering Jonathan Barber of Oysterponds, Long Island. Whitefield had earlier written the disconsolate Barber, telling him that he did not presume to judge whatever dealings God had with him. As for his visionary experiences, "I rather rejoice in them, having myself been blessed with many experiences of the like nature." He told Barber to expect persecution when God dealt with him in extraordinary ways. These encouraging words led Barber to come to Newport to receive Whitefield. Upon meeting, they agreed that Barber would become part of Whitefield's entourage.

After some successes in preaching, particularly at Clap's meetinghouse, Whitefield traveled north to Boston, where he arrived on September 18. Boston was the largest town in the colonies but still only a small provincial capital with about 17,000 people. In 1740, it was in decline, and it would slowly lose population up through the American Revolution. War with Spain, and later with France, left many widows in Boston, and the city faced high taxes and inflation. The poor in Boston were many, and they responded exuberantly to Whitefield, as they would to the radical piety of James Davenport and others.

As usual, Whitefield met with Anglican authorities in Boston, most notably the Commissary Timothy Cutler, the former Congregationalist rector of Yale turned Anglican "apostate." Cutler was the most formidable proponent of Anglicanism in the colonies, and he and Whitefield did not see eye to eye about Whitefield's relationship with non-Anglicans. Cutler argued that dissenters had no legitimate ordination because they did not follow in the line of apostolic succession. Whitefield thought their ordinations were legitimate, primarily because they preached the new birth: "I saw regenerate souls among the Baptists, among the Presbyterians, among the Independents, and among the Church folks—all children of God, and yet all born again in a different way of worship," he told Cutler. Whitefield was able to leave Cutler on friendly terms, but he would receive a much warmer welcome among the Congregationalists, especially from Benjamin Colman. After visiting Cutler he preached at the Brattle Street Church to about four thousand.

Whitefield spoke from supporters' Boston pulpits as well as on Boston Common. On September 20, he preached at Joseph Sewall's Old South Church to about six thousand, and in the afternoon he addressed a crowd at the common that he estimated at eight thousand, although the papers guessed five thousand. The next day he attended Sunday morning services at the Brattle Street Church and spoke at Thomas Foxcroft's Old Brick Church in the afternoon. The crowd pressing to see him was so large that he went out to the common again and preached to an enormous assembly he totaled at fifteen thousand, close to the whole population of Boston (the newspapers guessed eight thousand). On Monday morning he sermonized at John Webb's New North Church to about six thousand. Then, in the afternoon, tragedy struck the tour. At Samuel Checklcy's New South Church, the sound of a breaking board in the gallery triggered a stampede among the overflow crowd. A number of people were severely trampled, and some jumped from the balcony. Five people died. Whitefield decided to go on with the message he planned to deliver, only moving out to the common. No doubt this suggested insensitivity in Whitefield's character, but the crowd wanted him to go on, and one could hardly imagine a better moment for people to contemplate their mortality.

Whitefield visited Harvard and was not impressed with the size of the school or its spirit. He noted that "bad books," such as those by John Tillotson and Samuel Clarke, defenders of natural religion, were popular there, not the Puritan classics. Whitefield would later regret his harsh assessment of Harvard and Yale and would become a great supporter of the colleges. Whitefield also toured neighboring towns, including Roxbury and Charlestown, in his circuit. On September 27, Whitefield preached to one of his greatest crowds yet, fifteen thousand, on the common. Many were deeply affected, and Whitefield himself wrote that he felt like shouting, "This is no other than the House of God and the Gate of Heaven." Boston Common had become a portal to divine glory.

Whitefield began taking collections for the Bethesda Orphanage, and the number of pounds given was truly remarkable: perhaps £3,000 in local currency. Boston outpaced collections even in London. On September 28 alone, he collected more than £1,000 in services at the Old South and Brattle Street churches. After speaking at Brattle Street in the afternoon, Whitefield held two private meetings that showed the breadth of his appeal. The first was with the governor, Jonathan Belcher, who was an evangelical supporter of Whitefield. The second was with "a great number of negroes," who requested a private session with him. He preached to them on the conversion of the Ethiopian in Acts 8.

Whitefield visited towns up the coast from Boston from September 29 to October 6, finding some successes but also a great deal of passivity. Maine and New Hampshire had a substantial revival tradition, having seen large numbers of conversions and admissions to full communion in the 1727–28 earthquake awakening, and to a lesser extent in 1735–36 as a devastating "throat distemper" (diphtheria) raged there. He preached as far north as York, Maine, at the church of the well-respected Samuel Moody. His northern tour gave Nicholas Gilman of Exeter, who had been reading Whitefield's *Journals* and sermons for almost a year, a chance to meet him. Gilman was perhaps not as adulatory in his initial response to Whitefield as one might expect, noting that "there are Various Conjectures about Mr. Whitefield," but expressing hope that he truly was "a Man of an Excellent Spirit." Whitefield's appearance precipitated a conversion crisis for Gilman, as well, and set him on the path to becoming one of the most radical of New England's evangelicals. Whitefield won some notable converts in Maine, especially John Rogers. The pastor at Kittery, Rogers had been in the ministry for thirty years when he heard Whitefield, but he had never experienced conversion. Whitefield's ministry convinced him of his need for the new birth, and afterwards he became one of Whitefield's foremost proponents in Maine. Rogers's son Daniel, a tutor at Harvard, would soon join Whitefield's entourage and seek his own assurance of salvation. The revivals in Maine and New Hampshire would not begin in force until late 1741, however.

Returning to Boston, Whitefield continued seeing large audiences, but he also gravitated toward Tennent's confrontational style as he spoke against unconverted ministers. "I am persuaded," he wrote in his journal, "[that] the generality of preachers talk of an unknown and unfelt Christ." He felt energized by confronting the unsaved clergy: "Unspeakable freedom God gave me while treating on this head." Although some of the ministers may have grown uneasy at such talk, Whitefield drew ever-larger crowds, until he finally announced a farewell sermon on October 12, which drew a crowd estimated at twenty thousand. If reasonably accurate, this was the largest crowd ever assembled in America up to that time.

From Boston, Whitefield traveled west through New England. Delivering on his promise, Whitefield went slightly out of his way to visit Northampton. It was a poignant occasion for Edwards, who had waited five long years for revival fire to reignite in Northampton. Edwards shed tears during Whitefield's preaching. Whitefield, too, was deeply affected by his visit and impressed with Edwards's wife and children, who seemed to him models of piety and propriety. Whitefield's preaching in Northampton reached a crescendo on the Sabbath, as "Mr. Edwards wept during the whole time of exercise" in the morning. "Mr. Whitefield's sermons were suitable to the circumstances of the town," Edwards wrote later to Thomas Prince, "containing just reproofs of our back-slidings." He reported to Whitefield that the revival bore lasting fruit, including the conversion of some of the Edwardses' children. Immediately after Whitefield's departure, however, Edwards did begin a sermon series on the parable of the sower (Matthew 13), including warnings that short-lived episodes of heated preaching and crying did not make for saving religion. He subtly warned that Whitefield's brand of revivalism was ripe for religious hypocrisy. Edwards would continue to support Whitefield, but he insisted that Northampton would experience revival on his terms.

Accompanied by Edwards, Whitefield made his way south to East Windsor, the home of Edwards's parents. Along the way Whitefield kept preaching on unconverted ministers, and at one point Edwards cautioned Whitefield about not judging other ministers too harshly or trying to ascertain whether they were converted. Edwards supported Whitefield overall, but he certainly had doubts about the emotionalism and rash judgments that seemed to characterize the itinerant's ministry. In East Windsor, Whitefield preached to Timothy Edwards's congregation and then visited the elderly pastor and his wife Esther Stoddard Edwards, sharing supper and staying the night in their home.

Out of Whitefield's journey through Connecticut came two remarkable testimonies of conversion. The first was from the East Windsor saddler Samuel Belcher. Though Belcher grew up in the family of Joseph Belcher, pastor at Dedham, Massachusetts, he became "Cold and Dull" in matters of salvation, and though he experienced some concerns for his soul before 1740, they had not lasted. Whitefield's arrival signaled the beginning of a six-month-long conversion crisis. When "mr Whitefield p[re]ached here, . . . I was Greatly effected with his preaching both here and att Hartford," Belcher wrote. Belcher grew cold again, but then in April he met a man in Lebanon, Connecticut, who told of the revival there, which deeply impressed him. Then pastors Eleazar Wheelock of Lebanon and Benjamin Pomeroy of Hebron preached at East Windsor, and Belcher fell under deeper convictions than ever before. He felt the terrors of sin and the threat of damnation, "but God was pleased to enable me to Cry mightily unto him in the bitterness of my Soul for mercy in and through Jesus Christ." While he was praying, "I felt my Load Go of and my mouth was Stopt and I Could not utter one word for Some time and I felt as if my heart was Changed." When Belcher could speak again, he began praising God and he knew he had been saved. For Belcher, Whitefield's exhortations began the conversion process, but Wheelock's and Pomeroy's preaching, and his own prayers, finished the ordeal.

Whitefield's appearance also represented a beginning point for the conversion of Nathan Cole, a farmer and carpenter from Kensington, Connecticut. Cole grew up as what he called an "Arminian," likely meaning that he casually assumed that good works would save him. He began to hear reports about Whitefield's tour, and he "longed to see and hear him, and wished he would come this way." News arrived in October that Whitefield had left Boston for Northampton. Then on October 23, a messenger arrived and told him that Whitefield was coming to nearby Middletown later that morning. Cole ran in from the field to tell his wife that they were leaving immediately, fearing they would not have time to get there. As they neared the road to Middletown, he wrote that

> I saw before me a Cloud or fogg rising; I first thought it came from the great River, but as I came nearer the Road, I heard a noise something like a low rumbling thunder and presently found it was the noise of Horses feet coming down the Road and this Cloud was a Cloud of dust. . . . I could see men and horses Sliping along in the Cloud like shadows . . . every horse seemed to go with all his might to carry his rider to hear news from heaven for the saving of Souls, it made me tremble to see the Sight, how the world was in a Struggle.

When they arrived at the Middletown meeting house, Cole guessed that perhaps three or four thousand had assembled there, the countryside having emptied of its residents. Then Whitefield came to the scaffold:

> He Looked almost angelical; a young, Slim, slender, youth before some thousands of people with a bold undaunted Countenance . . . he looked as if he was Cloathed with authority from the Great God. . . . And my hearing him preach, gave me a heart wound; By Gods blessing: my old Foundation was broken up, and I saw that my righteousness would not save me; then I was convinced of the doctrine of Election: and went right to quarrelling with God about it; because that all I could do would not save me; and he had decreed from Eternity who should be saved and who not.

Cole's "quarrelling" with God lasted almost two years. Like Jonathan Edwards, he wrestled with the doctrine of predestination, thinking it abhorrent, while at the same time wondering if he himself was damned. "Hell fire was most always in my mind; and I have hundreds of times put my fingers into my pipe when I have been smoking to feel how fire felt." In the midst of his fears of hell's torments, however, God gave him a vision:

> God appeared unto me and made me Skringe: before whose face the heavens and the earth fled away; and I was Shrinked into nothing; I knew not whether I was in the body or out, I seemed to hang in open Air before God, and he seemed to Speak to me in an angry and Sovereign way what won't you trust your Soul with God; My heart answered O yes, yes, yes. . . . Now while my Soul was viewing God, my fleshly part was working imaginations and saw many things which I will omitt to tell at this time. . . . When God appeared to me every thing vanished and was gone in the twinkling of an Eye, as quick as A flash of lightning; But when God disappeared or in some measure withdrew, every thing was in its place again and I was on my Bed. My heart was broken; my burden was fallen of[f] my mind; I was set free, my distress was gone.

Cole's long conversion culminated, as it did for many early evangelicals, with a vision of God.

In New Haven, Whitefield visited with Rector Thomas Clap, who would later become one of his most bitter opponents. For now, Whitefield received a universally polite, if not entirely zealous, reception at Yale, despite his speaking to the students about "the dreadful ill consequences of an unconverted ministry." Whitefield then continued toward New York, and when he reached the border, he evaluated New England as impressive because of its godly heritage, but he feared that "Many, nay most that preach . . . do not experimentally know Christ." He loved the excitement his visit generated, though, and he thought New England was pliable enough for true revival. Pastor William Gaylord of Wilton, Connecticut, brother-in-law of James Davenport, wrote that many thought Whitefield "has a Touch of Enthusiasm" but that overheatedness could be forgiven more easily than lukewarmness. He believed Whitefield's most profound effect might have been "stirring up" the ministers themselves, though he did have reservations about Whitefield's comments on unconverted ministers. Much of the power of Whitefield's tours lay in his ability to excite the local ministers to more fervent gospel preaching.

As Whitefield's band crossed into New York, the Harvard tutor Daniel Rogers came to the spiritual awakening he had sought during weeks of travel. After a meeting at King's Bridge (now a part of the Bronx), Rogers wrote,

"It pleased God of his free Sovereign Grace to come into my poor Soul with Power and so to fill me with Peace: yea with Such Joy in the Holy Ghost as I never Experienced before—I cd not forbear Smiling nay Laughing for Joy and Gladness of Heart." Rogers shared the news with an elated Whitefield, but soon after Satan was tormenting Rogers with "Abominable Horrible Shocking Tho'ts." Assurance was not always easily gained by the new evangelicals. . . .

Whitefield continued to preach with considerable success in New York City, then moved on to Staten Island where he rendezvoused with Gilbert Tennent and John Cross. Tennent told him of his recent itineration through south Jersey, Delaware, and northern Maryland, while Cross reported that he had recently "seen great and wonderful things in his congregations." They arrived at Cross's Basking Ridge congregation on November 5, where James Davenport had been preaching in the morning. At an affecting afternoon service, Daniel Rogers recalled that a nine- or ten-year-old boy began speaking loudly, at which time Whitefield called on the crowd "to hear this Lad preaching to them." This led to a "General motion" during which many cried out, some fainted, and some fell into fits. A young man near Rogers was so moved that he had to lean on Rogers during much of the sermon until he finally fell to his knees.

The large crowd then retired to Cross's barn for the evening lecture. Tennent preached first, followed by Whitefield. Whitefield estimated that he had spoken for six minutes when one man began to shout, "He is come, He is come!" (Rogers recalled the man as crying "I have found him!") Many others began crying out "for the like favour," and Whitefield stopped to pray over them, which only heightened their fervent emotions. Rogers struggled to adequately describe the meeting, but noted that many were "weeping, Sighing, Groaning, Sobbing, screaching, crying out." The ministers finally retired, but Rogers and Davenport returned at one o'clock in the morning to resume preaching. Many in the congregation stayed up all night in the barn, praying and worshipping. "Tis a night to be remembered," Rogers wrote.

The next morning many penitents approached the departing Whitefield, including a "poor negro woman," a slave, who asked to join his entourage. Her master actually agreed to this idea (it is unlikely that he had permanent emancipation in mind), but Whitefield told her to go home and "serve her present master." Whitefield and most white evangelicals were unprepared to let the social implications of his gospel run a course to abolitionism. . . .

. . . Whitefield's tour moved on to New Brunswick, where Whitefield began telling Gilbert Tennent and Daniel Rogers to go to New England to follow up on the work there. Tennent initially refused, but after encouragement from Whitefield and an apparent vote by the entourage, Tennent agreed. Whitefield headed south with Davenport while Rogers and Tennent began planning their new tours. In Philadelphia, Whitefield began preaching in the so-called New Building, a structure erected by supporters specifically for his visits. The one-hundred-by-seventy-foot building became Whitefield's usual pulpit in Philadelphia, and though the fervor of his earlier visit had abated, wondrous visitations continued. At one meeting, many reported experiencing the sensation of being pierced by "pointed arrows" as he preached, and a young woman fell down senseless during the meeting and had to be carried home. On another occasion Whitefield reported that he spontaneously spoke against "reasoning unbelievers," and he later found out that "a number of them were present" at his sermon. He attributed his well-timed admonition to the leading of the Holy Ghost.

Through November, Whitefield continued his tour of southern New Jersey, Pennsylvania, Delaware, and Maryland, making stops at friendly congregations in Whiteclay Creek, Fagg's Manor, Nottingham, and Bohemia Manor. Whitefield, as was often the case, fell terribly ill at Fagg's Manor, writing that "straining caused me to vomit much." But he continued preaching and praying, and "soon every person in the room seemed to be under great impressions, sighing and weeping." On December 1, Whitefield departed for South Carolina and Georgia, noting with satisfaction that he had preached perhaps one hundred seventy-five times since he arrived in Rhode Island two-and-a-half months earlier. The presence of God that attended his meetings convinced him that the British American provinces would remain his "chief scene for action." The fall 1740 tour had been a gigantic success for Whitefield. His method of theatrical field preaching rejuvenated New England's substantial revival tradition and captivated tens of thousands of listeners. His incautious remarks about unconverted ministers, however, and his friendship with such figures as Tennent, Davenport, and Cross laid the groundwork for great controversies concerning the awakenings in the years ahead.

DR. THOMAS S. KIDD is a Distinguished Professor of History at Baylor and an associate director of Baylor Institute for Studies of Religion, where he also codirects the Program on Historical Studies of Religion. His interests include eighteenth-century North America, particularly the history of evangelicalism. Some of his books include *Benjamin Franklin: The Religious Life of a Founding Father* (Yale University Press, 2017); *American Colonial History: Clashing Cultures and Faiths* (Yale University Press, 2016); *George Whitefield: America's Spiritual Founding Father* (Yale University Press, 2014); *Patrick Henry: First Among Patriots* (Basic Books, 2011); *God of Liberty: A Religious History of the American Revolution* (Basic Books, 2010); *American Christians and Islam: Evangelical Culture and Muslims from the Colonial Period to the Age of Terrorism* (Princeton University Press, 2008); *The Great Awakening: The Roots of Evangelical Christianity in Colonial America* (Yale University Press, 2007); *The Great Awakening: A Brief History with Documents* (Bedford Books, 2007); *The Protestant Interest: New England after Puritanism* (Yale University Press, 2004). He has written editorials for outlets including *USA Today* and *The Washington Post*, is a regular contributor for *WORLD* Magazine and Patheos.com, and been quoted in reports by CNN, NPR, and Scripps News. In 2010, he was named a Baylor University Outstanding Professor.

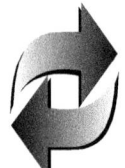

David A. Varel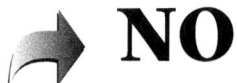

The Historiography of the Second Great Awakening and the Problem of Historical Causation, 1945–2005

Few historiographical debates have been as lively and enduring as those regarding the origins of the Second Great Awakening (SGA), which were the religious revivals that swept through the early American republic and forever transformed American culture. Prone to radical revision, this historiography suggests the difficulty in determining historical causation. This essay tracks that process of revision from 1945 to 2005, highlighting four central historiographic threads. The first thread, characterizing 1940s and 1950s scholarship, borrowed from Frederick Jackson Turner to interpret the SGA as a product of the unique features of the American frontier. The second thread, prominent in scholarship of the 1960s through the 1980s, understood the religious revivals as a means to assert social control amid disruptive social and economic changes. The third thread, reaching its height in the 1980s and 1990s, perceived the SGA as a democratic means to resist traditional sources of authority. Finally, the fourth thread, beginning in the 1990s, saw the SGA as a means of concentrating religious or social authority within expanding denominations.[1] Though these two most recent threads produced the most sophisticated and convincing interpretations of the SGA, future scholarship needs to aim at synthesis of these competing historiographies. Though it was a national phenomenon, the SGA varied extensively in its local and regional manifestations. A more nuanced interpretation of the SGA needs to consider the multiplicity of origins contributing to the revivals and how issues of social control, democratization, and denominational concentration interacted with and competed against one another in various contexts.

The first major historiographic thread to attempt a systematic explanation of the origins of the SGA drew directly from Frederick Jackson Turner's "Frontier Thesis." In 1893, Turner, an obscure historian at the University of Wisconsin, presented a paper to a group of historians at the Chicago World's Fair entitled "The Significance of the Frontier in American History." Here, he argued that Americans' unique experiences with the frontier shaped a distinctive American character and society. He described the frontier as a "free land" at the "meeting point between savagery and civilization," where Americans continually "return[ed] to primitive conditions" only to transform the wilderness into a civilized territory. "This perennial rebirth," he insisted, "furnish[ed] the forces dominating American character." Individualism and democracy were, for Turner, the two prominent features of American society. Away from the comforts and technologies of civilization, Turner described frontiersman as rugged individualists who survived through their own hard work and ingenuity. This frontier individualism produced "antisocial" behavior, but still "promoted democracy."[2]

This description of the frontier, though based more on myth than reality, dominated the historical discipline for half a century and formed the framework through which the first generation of historians explained the SGA. Since the SGA first began in the western territories of Kentucky and Tennessee, this first group of historians saw the unique conditions of the frontier as linked to the rise of evangelical religion. William Warren Sweet was one of the first historians to develop this interpretation with his *Revivalism in America* (1945) and later his *Religion in the Development of American Culture* (1952).[3] His interpretations dominated the historical landscape for the next twenty or thirty years, and even those scholars who disagreed continued to see the revivals as an expression of frontier democracy.

One of Sweet's students, Charles A. Johnson, provides a clear example of the Turner-thesis-driven historiography in his monograph entitled Frontier Camp Meeting (1955).[4] Focusing on the first revivals on the

Kentucky frontier at the beginning of the nineteenth century, Johnson attempted to explain why these revivals first occurred on the American frontier. His central argument was that the frontier was the birthplace of the SGA because of its unique historical conditions. Drawing directly from Turner, he described the frontier as individualistic, democratic, morally lax, and in need of an authority structure. These unique features, he contended, paved the way for and set the tone of the SGA.

Johnson first described the social need for religion on the frontier. He said that the frontier was a "moral desert," which "seemed to be coming apart at the seams." Away from the conventional forms of restraint from government, family, and church, men resorted to a pattern of "brawling, debauchery, and drunkenness." The disproportionate number of young men, the social isolation, and the focus on the bare necessities of life all contributed to this "uncivilized" society. Yet, Johnson insisted that these frontier settlements nevertheless "contained God-fearing men" who longed for social order as well as religious experience. When zealous missionaries and bold Methodist circuit riders made their way to the frontier, according to Johnson, they found a receptive audience.[5]

Though frontiersmen were ready to accept the social order, moral values, and religious experience that missionaries and circuit riders had to offer, Johnson argued that they were nevertheless active in shaping the character of their religious experiences. Johnson again drew directly from Turner in describing the frontiersmen as rugged individualists inclined toward egalitarianism and exhibiting a "bold nature in revolt of society's restraints" as a result of the "leveling influence of poverty." It is unsurprising, then, that the Methodist Episcopal Church, with its "democratic theology" stressing freedom of will and "instruction rather than castigation," resonated with the individualism and egalitarianism of the pioneers.[6] The diverse peoples on the frontier, moreover, coupled with their proximity toward nature and made the camp meeting, and its emotional fervor "ar[i]se logically out of the circumstances surrounding it."[7] Johnson, then, linked the origins of the SGA to the unique conditions historical conditions of the frontier and the pioneers who inhabited it.

Though this interpretation has some merits, such as its plausible linkage with aspects of life on the frontier and religious revival, the historical discipline later experienced a tectonic shift which raised serious questions regarding this Turner-thesis-driven historiography. In the 1960s, the United States and much of the rest of the world were shaken by an incredible surge of grassroots reform movements, such as the American civil rights movement. The incredible potency of the global student movements, women's movements, gay and lesbian movements, and civil rights movements cast doubt on the traditional approach to history, which emphasized elites and structural constraints as the principal determinants of continuity and change. Suddenly, historians perceived that ordinary people, from slaves to factory workers, had agency in daily life and could be the principal drivers of historical change. Previous interpretations soon demanded revision, and new areas of inquiry warranted exploration. For example, historians' neglect of the daily lives of African-Americans under slavery seemed appropriate when historians assumed that only elites made history and that slaves lacked any power. The civil rights movement, however, casts doubt on this assumption. Suddenly, a new wave of social histories reexamined the lives of slaves and demonstrated how they did, in fact, have some control over their daily lives and how they were key actors in winning their own freedom.

This huge shift in the historical discipline facilitated scholarship that delegitimized Turner's romanticized notion of the frontier and much of the historiography of the SGA—like Johnson's—which rested upon its foundations. To be sure, Turner in some ways preempted and anticipated the new scholarship foregrounding novel historical actors. His writing revised earlier interpretations stressing the centrality of eastern elites in determining American politics and culture, pointing instead to western frontiersmen as the pillars of American society. Still, Turner's romantic descriptions of the American West and its inhabitants remained problematic. A new generation of historians, labeled the "New Western Historians," soon reinterpreted Turner's conception of the frontier as a bastion of individualism and democracy.[8] These historians emphasized how family and community were actually at the center of not only success, but survival, on the frontier.[9] Additionally, the egalitarianism of frontier life appeared shallow amid the violent displacement and persecution of Native peoples. Whereas Turner described the West as "free land," subsequent historians revealed how the West was heavily populated with Indian tribes.[10] At the same time, while Turner conceived of westward expansion as unidirectional, New Western Historians described the complex and multiracial borderlands of the frontier to reveal the multidirectional character of the frontier. Therefore, while these points did not completely delegitimize Johnson's depiction of the frontier and, thus, his explanation for the SGA, they nevertheless cast serious doubt on the merits of this historiographic interpretation.

Another issue with the Turner-thesis-driven explanations of the SGA was their inability to explain how and why the revivals were a national phenomenon, affecting places very distant from the frontier, such as major cities like New York or Boston. The next major historiographic thread tackled this issue directly, as studies in the 1970s and 1980s often targeted regions in the Northeast. In line with the larger shift toward social history, this thread saw the religious revivals of the SGA as a means for marginalized, or self-perceived marginalized, people to assert social control. Again conceiving of the revivals as a product of earthly experiences rather than spiritual ones, this group of scholars explained religion's appeal through the disruptive nature of social and economic change. Most of these historians linked these changes to the Market Revolution, with its refashioning of the nature and organization of work, of social relations among classes and between the sexes, and of the political process.[11] These changes, according to this line of thinking, produced anxieties over marginalization which prompted people to reassert their authority through the apparatus of the church.

Paul E. Johnson's *A Shopkeeper's Millennium* is an important example of this historiography.[12] In this book, Johnson targeted Rochester, NY, from 1815–1837, insisting that it was a "center of both the religious and the social transformations" of this period.[13] For this reason, Rochester was not representative of most American towns and cities, but he maintained that it nevertheless embodied a dramatized example of the same processes occurring across the country. Discouraged by previous scholarship that provided only theoretical explanations for the causes of the SGA, Johnson sought to systematically test who "found comfort in revivals, and why."[14] To accomplish this, he used a quantitative approach that analyzed "family structure, kinship relations, political conflict, occupational and geographic mobility, [and] patterns of association."[15] Johnson scrutinized church records, city directories, tax lists, and newspapers in attempting this ambitious project. In this way, he sought to explain the origins of the SGA by examining the socioeconomic backgrounds of the people who participated in the revivals.

With this approach, Johnson argued that an emerging industrial bourgeoisie dominated the revivals in Rochester, finding in them a means to reassert their authority and resolve moral anxieties stemming from the Market Revolution. Johnson explained how the transformations of the Market Revolution spawned the development of two distinct cultures—working class and middle class. Suddenly, the middle class moved into separate neighborhoods and distanced themselves at work, since producing for the market demanded different functions, like supervising and advertising, than did traditional manufacturing and artisanship. This separation, according to Johnson, produced a loss of status for the masters and manufacturers, as well as a loss of control over the behaviors of the working class. Significantly, masters assumed a moral responsibility for what they saw as a decline in working-class behavior, and they "experienced disobedience and disorder as religious problems."[16] In Rochester, the elite's political efforts to resolve these issues failed miserably, as the middle class became hopelessly divided over how to enforce moral behavior—coercion or persuasion. Therefore, the resentment over loss of status, the moral responsibility for causing the disorder, and the inability of the government to resolve these conflicts paved the way for the religious revival of 1830–1831, when Charles Finney visited.

Johnson argued that Rochester's middle class saw in evangelicalism a means to resolve their personal tensions and to once again dominate society. Finney's evangelical message insisted that each individual had the ability to determine his/her own salvation, emphasized the social nature of conversion and prayer, and stressed immediate activism to inspire conversion. These features resolved the political issue over coercion versus persuasion, as Finney declared that "authoritarian controls were not necessary," and the middle class then united into "an active and united missionary army."[17] Individual responsibility for salvation, moreover, alleviated the bourgeoisie's responsibility for continued working-class debauchery, such as excessive drinking. Finally, the united activism that the movement created provided an effective avenue to convert many of the working-class to middle-class norms and values. This turn to evangelicalism was not, according to Johnson, a conscious effort to dominate society. Rather, it just so happened to provide resolutions to issues that plagued the middle class with the transformations attending the Market Revolution.

This interpretation of the SGA suffers from a number of problems, some of which other scholars within this historiographic thread addressed. Most notably, Johnson almost entirely excluded the role of women in the revivals. When he did mention them, he said simply that "the evangelicals assigned crucial religious duties to wives and mothers."[18] Here he assumed "evangelicals" as men who designated responsibilities to passive women, when, in reality, women exhibited leadership over the entire revival phenomenon and consistently made up the majority of the congregants. Mary P. Ryan's *Cradle of the Middle Class*, as but one example, revised this interpretation by placing women at the center of the religious revivals.[19] For Ryan, middle-class women were the central agents of the SGA, as the social changes stemming from the Market Revolution created a separate, domestic sphere for middle-class women in which they had less public authority. Providing public religious and moral leadership, then, provided middle-class women an avenue to reassert the authority they perceived they had lost in the transition from a home-based to a market-based economy.

Other scholars within this school of historiography revised Johnson's overly determinist interpretation. In *Religion and the Rise of the American City*, for instance, Carroll Smith-Rosenberg insisted that the guiding force for evangelical reform was more than simply a wanton attempt by the middle class to assert authority over lower classes. In examining city missions in New York City, she argued that "reformers desired both to save souls and to control social stress—but saw the two goals as essentially the same."[20] In other words, middle-class reformers genuinely wanted to save the souls of the unconverted at the same time that they wanted to retain secular authority. This interpretation departed from the conspiratorial nature of Johnson's argument and, therefore, provided a more sophisticated portrayal of the actions of middle-class evangelicals.

Still, the similarities far outweigh the differences within this historiographic thread. Randolph Roth's *The Democratic Dilemma* is a nice example of this. In his monograph, Roth similarly focused on one small area in the Northeast—the Connecticut River Valley of Vermont—and he claimed it was representative of the revivals of the SGA all across the country. He also perceived the revivals in Vermont as the product of a middle-class dilemma stemming from social changes in the antebellum era. Specifically, he argued that the middle class was anxious over "how to reconcile their commitment to competition, toleration, and popular sovereignty with their desire to defend an orderly and pious way of life."[21] For Roth, as for the other scholars in this historiographic thread, middle-class evangelicals resolved this dilemma by using the apparatus of the church to restrain democratic impulses and assert their own authority.

This social control thread suffered from a number of problems. The most damning of these was that the social control thesis was reductive of religious experience. While these scholars were right to examine the influence that changes in social status and power had on religious conversion, they were naïve to contend that phenomena as complex and contradictory as religious revivals can be explained primarily through these changes. Johnson's language, characteristic of some monographs of the 1970s and 1980s that first utilized quantitative analysis, did not help. For instance, he made the grandiose claim that he could "systematically trace the social origins of revival religion."[22] In the preface to the 25th anniversary edition of *A Shopkeeper's Millennium* in 2004, he toned down this language in his admission that he would "make only the most modest effort to explain religious conversion in terms of [work relationships, family forms, and residential patterns]."[23] Yet, even this scaling down did not sidestep the criticism that any interpretation of religious experience that attempts to explain it only through anxieties over social change ultimately is reductive of the great complexity that is religious experience.

The social control historiography was also limited in its wider explanatory power. Many scholars of this generation, including Paul Johnson and Mary Ryan, narrowed the scope of their research to one major community. This made sense given their approach to quantify history, as such quantification becomes untenable for much larger regions. These historians then justified their selection of certain communities by claiming that they were representative of larger processes. Yet it was precisely this claim of representativeness that was problematic. Johnson justified his selection of Rochester, for instance, by declaring that it was a dramatic microcosm of the same economic transformations that were occurring across the country during the Market Revolution. He then uses evidence from this one community to explain the national phenomenon of the SGA. But how, then, could he explain why the SGA swept rural communities as well, which were very distant from economic transformations affecting cities like Rochester? How could he explain the birth of the SGA on the frontier? How could he explain that the SGA was a national phenomenon that affected communities of very different social and economic compositions? And, finally, if religious revival was tied to anxieties over social and economic changes that people experienced throughout the world, how could he explain that the SGA was a distinctively American phenomenon?

The next major historiographic thread had answers to these questions. The neoprogressive scholarship on the American Revolution directly influenced this generation of scholars. Due to the turmoil of the 1960s and 1970s, historians began to pay more attention to the social context of the Revolution. This led some scholars, such as Gordon Wood, to examine how the radical ideas of freedom and equality espoused by the elite took root in the American populace.[24] The neoprogressives, on the other hand, foregrounded the class conflict in Revolutionary-era society, and they paid attention to the grassroots activism of ordinary people fighting for equality. In this line of thinking, the American Revolution was a social revolution that transformed—from the bottom-up—a society of deference to one insistent on equality. For the neoprogressives, then, the American Revolution galvanized strong democratic impulses as well as a powerful opposition to traditional sources of authority within American society.[25]

This new conception of Revolutionary-era America as democratic and antiauthoritarian drove a new set of interpretations of the SGA. Sudden historians paid attention to the mass appeal of the religious revivals as well as their central features, which often ran in the face of traditional liturgy and religious expression. Moreover, scholars began to reinterpret the democratic and egalitarian nature of much of the SGA, not as an expression of frontier democracy, but rather as a byproduct of the social revolution that swept the colonies during the Revolutionary war.

The most influential book of this historiographical thread was Nathan O. Hatch's *The Democratization of American Christianity* (1989).[26] Hatch adopted the neoprogressives' argument about the American Revolution, and he used it as a premise through which to understand the SGA. He proclaimed, "[t]he American Revolution is the most crucial event in American history" because it "dramatically expanded the circle of people who considered themselves capable of thinking for themselves." Moreover, he described how "[r]espect for authority, tradition, station, and education eroded," and "leaders could not survive" who refused to defer to the interests of the people. Hatch, therefore, saw the nature and extent of the SGA as an outgrowth of democratic populism, egalitarianism, and antiauthoritarianism stemming from the Revolution.[27]

Starting from this premise, Hatch organized his book around the theme of democratization. His central argument was that the "rise of evangelical Christianity in the early republic is . . . a story of the success of the common people in shaping the culture after their own priorities rather than the priorities outlined by gentleman." His focus, then, was on the SGA as a national phenomenon, rather than a regional or local one like Charles and Paul Johnson's books. He therefore emphasized the commonalities among religious revival across the country, which in his mind centered on the democratic impulse. In making his case, he examined five religious traditions or movements, including the Methodists, Baptists, Mormons, the black churches, and the Christian movement. He analyzed the written and verbal rhetoric as well as the nontraditional ecclesiastical methods of the leaders of these movements in order to demonstrate why these leaders were so popular. For instance, he pointed to the vernacular language of populist preachers like Elias Smith, Lorenzo Dow, and others who evinced a "coarse language, earthy humor, biting sarcasm, and commonsense reasoning" that appealed to the masses.[28] Hatch justified his focus on elites by arguing that the religious marketplace during this period was a largely open one where people flocked to the sects that matched their democratic impulses. Thus, the democratic dispositions of the masses were matched by an equally democratic competition among religious denominations for the patronage of the people.

Indeed, the numbers seemed to support Hatch's claim, as the period from 1780 to 1830 witnessed a vast growth in radical denominations. The Methodist membership, for instance, doubled to 500,000 between 1820 and 1830. The Baptist membership increased tenfold in the first three decades of following the Revolution. The Mormons, Disciples of Christ, and other radical new sects soon dotted the religious landscape as well.[29] The fact that these were the denominations and sects that thrived during the SGA certainly suggested that they offered something unique and important to people at the time.

But how could historians be so sure that it was the democratic and antiauthoritarian inclinations of these denominations that made them so successful? Hatch himself conceded that "[t]he rise of popular sovereignty . . . often has involved insurgent leaders glorifying the many as a way to legitimate their own authority."[30] One of the leaders of the Disciples of Christ, Alexander Campbell, for instance, spearheaded a decidedly undemocratic ecclesiastical structure despite his professed claims otherwise. Hatch addressed this by arguing that people's hopes for a democratic upsurge, unfortunately, often took form in highly undemocratic ways. But the extent of these undemocratic forms may be more significant than Hatch contended. Perhaps, Hatch borrowed too heavily from the neoprogressives in their insistence on the American Revolution as a social revolution, and this may have led him to overplay the centrality of the democratic impulse to the SGA.

Other historians who similarly interpreted revivalism as a democratic movement have focused on more specific regions. In *Religion in the Old South*, for instance, Donald Mathews explained revivalism in the South as an attempt by a "rising lower middle/middle-class" to "reject as authoritative . . . the lifestyle and values of traditional elites." For Mathews, evangelicalism was a "social process" through which middle-class Southerners, but also impoverished and oppressed groups of Southerners like slaves, resisted traditional authority and empowered themselves.[31] In *Religion in Antebellum Kentucky*, John Boles focused instead on the West. Harkening back to the frontier-thesis school of thought, Boles partly explained religious revival in Kentucky as a product of social and cultural conditions in the West. Specifically, he pointed to Kentuckians' desires for a sense of community in a mobile and rapidly changing society, and he suggested a perceived lack of religiosity and a "climate of expectation."[32] Even more, he stressed how revival religion was a "democratic faith that was profoundly comforting to most Kentuckians."[33] For poorer, subsistence-level Kentuckians, according to Boles, evangelical religion not only leveled the playing field in heaven but it also stressed the egalitarian nature of each individual in this world. In these ways, historians of this thread perceived revival religion as a democratic movement in its various regional manifestations.

Still other historians in line with this historical school stressed revivalism as a democratic process for particular groups. Jama Lamerow's *Religion and the Working Class in Antebellum America* is an important example of this historiography. In a direct refutation of interpretations like that in *A Shopkeeper's Millennium*, which perceived working-class religiosity as little more than a source of disunity or a result of coercion by the middle class, Lazerow argued that working-class people actively used religion as a tool to fight against their oppression. For Lazerow, the workers "internalized their own version of the religion being employed to control them and used it to impose their own form of control."[34] This is but one example of how other scholars within this historical school interpreted revivalism as primarily a democratic movement employed by people of all socioeconomic conditions—from middle-class artisans to factory workers to slaves.

The great achievement of this historiographic thread portraying the revivals as democratic expressions was its accounting for the SGA as a national movement during the early American republic. Since the American Revolution affected the entire nation, using democratic expression as an analytic framework helped explain why the SGA occurred throughout the entire country. Indeed, when different sections of the country had very different social and economic conditions, the Revolution was an event—a transformative event—that plausibly transformed the entire nation. Moreover, this explanation helped explain why the SGA was a distinctly American phenomenon. While other Western nations experienced similar social and economic transformations from a burgeoning capitalist order, the American Revolution was uniquely American. Finally, this thread also explained the clearly egalitarian and antiauthoritarian impulses that Americans of all backgrounds exhibited during this period. The scholars of this historiographic thread have offered the best explanations for these facts.

Despite these achievements, in their attempts to explain the SGA as a national movement, the historians of this school downplayed unfairly the importance of local and regional differences. After all, although the SGA was indeed a national phenomenon, it did not affect each region or local community equally. In fact, powerful local and regional variations of the SGA persisted. Though some of these scholars did focus on specific regions, the framework of democratization predominated their thinking. As a consequence, they portrayed narrowly all of the regional and local revivals as the product of only a national democratic impulse. Other factors certainly contributed to these revivals, and these factors undoubtedly varied within their disparate contexts. Furthermore, though Americans clearly evinced democratic impulses during the SGA, might not the elite have continued to direct the impulses of the masses?

The fourth and final major historiographic thread was more sensitive to regional differences and critical of the democratization thesis. Emerging in the 1990s largely as a reaction to the democratization thread, this group of historians saw the revivals as a means of concentrating social or religious authority within expanding denominations. This questioning of the democratic underpinnings of the movement naturally led many historians to focus on the South, where hierarchy and rank continued to permeate society.

One example of this thread, which remains prominent today, is Christine Heyrman's *Southern Cross* (1997).[35] Focusing on the South from 1780–1830, Heyrman attempted to explain the origins of the Bible Belt and its unlikely turn to evangelicalism during the SGA. She described how evangelicalism in the eighteenth century "aroused [southerners'] sharpest fears" because it "struck at those hierarchies that lent stability to their daily lives: the deference of youth to age; the submission of children to parents and women to men; the loyalties of individuals to family and kin above any other group; and the rule of reserve over emotion within each person."[36] In other words, the democratic nature of eighteenth-century evangelicalism that Hatch described struck fear into the hearts of southerners who saw this new radical religion as a threat to their social order. But, rather than infusing the South with egalitarianism, Heyrman showed how the radical nature of evangelicalism assured its marginalization in the eighteenth century. Heyrman, then, explained why evangelicalism took root in the nineteenth century when it was so marginal and threatening to "southern whites of all classes" only years before. She employed quantitative methods tracking membership within the various religious denominations, and she analyzed letters, sermons, speeches, pamphlets, and other materials to make sense of this transition.

Heyrman's main contention was that the evangelicalism that did prosper in the South represented a sharp break with the more democratic and egalitarian nature of the movement in the eighteenth century. She contended that southern evangelicalism "was being reinvented during the very decades that it took root in that region, transformed by the demands of laymen and women and the responses of clerical leaders."[37] Her interpretation thus turned the democratization theory on its head: instead of evangelicalism transforming southern society by making it more democratic, southern society transformed evangelicalism by making it more conducive to hierarchy and order. Although these two processes certainly played off one another, the evidence she presented explained convincingly just how far evangelicalism changed in its southern manifestation. For example, she detailed how southern evangelicals adopted a more conciliatory stance toward the gentry and even "muted evangelical testimony against slavery."[38] Yet more significantly, she showed how religious leaders went further by "altering, often drastically, many earlier evangelical teachings and practices concerning the proper roles of men and women, old and young, white and black, as well as their positions on the relationship between the church and the family."[39] In these ways, she demonstrated how the nature of evangelicalism in the South adapted to the southern environment.

Heyrman explained this adaptation as a result of the actions of evangelical leaders in the South. She argued that these leaders "realized that the future of their churches" depended on significant alteration of evangelical teachings and practices.[40] These leaders then made the conscious decision to compromise some religious principles in order to assure their churches' success. She identified these leaders as a "minority composed of clergy and laity who claimed that privilege by virtue of being white male heads of household." It was these men, she continued, "who decided that the ultimate success of evangelicalism in the South lay in appealing to those who . . . esteemed maturity more than youth, put family before religious fellowship, upheld the superiority of white over black and of men over women, and prized honor above all else."[41] A powerful and privileged few, then, according to Heyrman, spearheaded the revivals in the South along rather conservative and undemocratic lines.

This thread, though, has examined more than only the South, which clearly had a different culture. As a result of slavery and the South's very different historical evolution, the South continued to be dominated by hierarchy and rank in a way that the North did not. Other historians showed how these same impulses to institutionalize denominations operated in other regions of the U.S. Stephen Marini in *Radical Sects of Revolutionary New England*, for instance, argued that the institutionalization of radical denominations in New England explained religious growth in that region. Particularly, he explained how, in the 1780s, the Shakers, Universalists, and Freewill Baptists all labored to develop coherent structures that could consolidate the chaotic inclinations of revival. Indeed, without a coherent structure, leaders of these revivals understood that their success could only be as fleeting as the religious fervor itself. As a result of this urge to consolidate, religious groups managed to successfully meld their radical and disparate beliefs into a cohesive denomination with an authority structure and concrete theological principles. It was, for Marini, precisely their success in consolidating into distinct denominations that fueled the religious revivals of the SGA. Because these radical denominations responded to the new social, economic, and material conditions of rural New England in the late eighteenth century, and because they did so in an institutionalized way that allowed them to proselytize effectively, these radical denominations gave impetus and form to the SGA.[42]

Still other books within this historiographic thread emphasized the national character of this process of denominational institutionalization. For example, in *Awash in a Sea of Faith*, Jon Butler argued that "[d]enominational institutions became the engine of national spiritual development."[43] He contended that denominational authority expanded at the same time that the state's authority in religion declined during the Revolutionary era. Though he admitted that Americans contested this new form of authority amid the democratic environment of the Revolution, he argued that the ultimate cause of the SGA was precisely the expansion of this new form of authority. Specifically, he attributed the incredible growth of national church denominations to their own initiative and effort. He pointed to each denomination's appointment and regulation of itinerant ministers, publication of books and other print culture espousing its distinctiveness, and construction of sacred landscapes to argue that "congregations sprang up infrequently from lay initiative" and arose instead from "nurturing on the part of competing denominations."[44] In this fashion, Butler and other historians of this thread contested Hatch's democratization thesis and instead emphasized the importance of the consolidation and institutionalization of competing denominations.

This latest historiographic thread remains prominent today for its ability to complicate the democratization theory. Instead of the SGA being solely a national movement that represented the onward march of democratization, egalitarianism, and antiauthoritarianism, this thread explains the important regional variations of the SGA. Moreover, this thread provides a more sophisticated interpretation of the local contexts through which Americans not only accepted or rejected but also negotiated, contested, and compromised on religious ideas.

Most importantly, this thread complicates the argument that "the people" were the primary determinants of the nature and course of revival religion. The historians of this thread revealed how elites—even though they were elites of radical denominations—continued to direct and shape the latent religious fervor within the populace. For this reason, scholarship stressing the ways in which the SGA was a product of expanding denominations attempting to consolidate control has been important in furthering our understanding of the revivals.

Nevertheless, future scholars should aim more at synthesis of these competing historiographies. The democratization thesis continues to provide the best broad conceptual framework. As the SGA was a national phenomenon imbued with democratic impulses stemming from the American Revolution, certainly this theory wields much explanatory power over a movement that was national and democratic in significant ways. Indeed, even if denominations played a more prominent role in the process than democratization scholars maintained, it remained the common people who ultimately shaped the message of the elites and chose to accept or reject each denomination's theology and authority. Yet historians must now be sensitive to the important local and regional variations of the SGA, and they must realize that different forces interacted with one another to give rise to the movement in different places. The democratization thesis, for instance, simply did not operate in the same ways in the South as it did in the North. Moreover, in the city of Rochester where social and economic changes convulsed the town, it is likely true that social anxieties combined with but also played a more important role than democratic impulses in shaping the character and extent of the SGA. It is also plausible that similar anxieties infused the religious leadership of the various denominations and sects. An analysis that synthesizes anxieties over social control stemming from the Market Revolution and fears over religious control arising from denominational expansion is yet to be attempted. How might democratic impulses have informed and contested these competing anxieties over loss of control?

This advocacy of synthesis as a new direction for historical scholarship on the SGA stems from the realization that for too long these alternative interpretations have failed to benefit from one another's insights. Contrary to how many historians have approached the SGA, it is possible that the revivals evinced simultaneously authoritarian and antiauthoritarian impulses. Moreover, it is plausible that the frontier, the burgeoning urban environment, and the Deep South shared similar, yet distinct, contexts that facilitated revival. The task for the next generation of historians is to analyze the similarities within these contexts to further elucidate how the disparate impulses for social control, egalitarianism, religious control, and social order interacted to give shape and impetus to the SGA. Increasingly, historians will have to deal with the importance of theology and ideas in the revivals, as a new group of historians are reinterpreting American religious experience with theology at the center.[45] E. Brook Holifield's publication of *Theology in America* in 2005 embodies this nascent historiographic thread, which has the potential to move the field in new directions. Though ideas must be taken seriously, however, historians are right to continue to emphasize the social, economic, and political conditions in which people generated and adopted those ideas. By utilizing a comparative framework sensitive to regional and local variations, historians of the next generation should be able to provide a more sophisticated interpretation of the SGA that does justice to the complex and contradictory phenomena that are religious revivals.

Notes

1. A nascent thread stressing the centrality of theology and ideas to the origins of the SGA is perceptible in the work of Mark Knoll (*America's God: From Jonathan Edwards to Abraham Lincoln* (Oxford: Oxford University Press, 2002)) and E. Brooks Holifield (*Theology in America: Christian Thought from the Age of the Puritans to the Civil War* (New Haven: Yale University Press, 2005)). These works are a departure from the four main threads dominating the field, which have explained the revivals as a result of social and economic conditions. The chronology of this essay, then, correlates with the four major threads in this historiography and the state of field at a moment when a new thread may be emerging.

2. Frederick Jackson Turner, "The Significance of the Frontier in American History" (1893) in *The American Intellectual Tradition*, vol. II, eds. David A. Hollinger and Charles Capper (New York: Oxford University Press, 2006), 55–59.

3. William Warren Sweet, *Revivalism in America: Its Origin, Growth and Decline* (New York: Charles Scribner's Sons, 1945); William Warren Sweet, *Religion in the Development of American Culture, 1765–1840* (Gloucester, MA: P. Smith, 1963). See also, William Warren Sweet, *The Methodists, a Collection of Source Materials*, Volume 4 (New York: Cooper Square Publishers, 1964).

4. See also Walter B. Posey, *Frontier Mission: A History of Religion West of the Southern Appalachians to 1861* (Lexington: University of Kentucky Press, 1966). For books which revised the Turner-thesis-driven work but still operated within its framework, see Whitney R. Cross, *The Burned-Over District: The Social and Intellectual History of Enthusiastic Religion in Western New York, 1800–1850* (New York: Harper & Row, 1950); Charles I. Foster, *Errand of Mercy: The Evangelical United Front, 1790–1837* (Chapel Hill: University of North Carolina Press, 1960); and T. Scott Miyakawa, *Protestants and Pioneers: Individualism and Conformity of the American Frontier* (Chicago: University of Chicago Press, 1964).
5. Charles A. Johnson, *The Frontier Camp Meeting* (Dallas: Southern University Methodist Press, 1955), 8–13.
6. Charles A. Johnson, 13–18.
7. Charles A. Johnson, 38.
8. The best example of this scholarship is Patricia Nelson Limerick's *The Legacy of Conquest: The Unbroken Past of the American West* (New York: W.W. Norton and Company, 1987).
9. See John Mack Faragher, *Sugar Creek: Life on the Illinois Prairie* (New Haven: Yale University Press, 1986).
10. Turner, "Significance of the Frontier," 55.
11. For the classic statement on the Market Revolution, see Charles Sellers, *The Market Revolution: Jacksonian America, 1815–1846* (Oxford: Oxford University Press, 1994). For a recent book critiquing the idea of a "market revolution" during antebellum American, see Daniel Walker Howe, *What God Hath Wrought: The Transformation of America, 1815–1848* (Oxford: Oxford University Press, 2007).
12. See also Carroll Smith-Rosenberg, *Religion and the Rise of the City: The New York City Mission Movement, 1812–1870* (Ithaca, NY: Cornell University Press, 1971); and Randolph A. Roth, *The Democratic Dilemma: Religion, Reform, and the Social Order in the Connecticut River Valley of Vermont, 1791–1850* (Cambridge: Cambridge University Press, 1987).
13. Paul E. Johnson, *A Shopkeeper's Millennium: Society and Revivals in Rochester, New York, 1815–1837* (New York: Hill and Wang, 2004), xiv.
14. Paul E. Johnson, 10.
15. Paul E. Johnson, 13.
16. Paul E. Johnson, 140.
17. Ibid.
18. Paul E. Johnson, 108.
19. Mary P. Ryan, *Cradle of the Middle Class: The Family in Oneida County, New York, 1790–1865* (Cambridge: Cambridge University Press, 1981).
20. Carroll Smith-Rosenberg, *Religion and the Rise of the City*, 8.
21. Randolph A. Roth, *The Democratic Dilemma*, 6.
22. Roth, 13.
23. Roth, xix.
24. See Gordon Wood, *The Radicalism of the American Revolution* (New York: Vintage Books, 1991).
25. John E. Hollitz, "Evaluating One Historian's Argument: The 'Other Side' of the American Revolution," in *Thinking through the Past, Volume I: to 1877* (Boston: Houghton Mifflin Company, 2005), 57–59.
26. See also Donald G. Mathews, "The Second Great Awakening as an Organizing Process, 1780–1830: An Hypothesis," *American Quarterly* 21 (Spring 1969): 23–43; Donald G. Mathews, *Religion in the Old South* (Chicago: University of Chicago Press, 1977); John B. Boles, *Religion in Antebellum Kentucky* (Lexington: University of Kentucky Press, 1995); Paul K. Conkin, *Cane Ridge: America's Pentecost* (Madison: University of Wisconsin Press, 1990); and Jama Lazerow, *Religion and the Working Class in Antebellum America* (Washington: Smithsonian Institution Press, 1995).
27. Nathan O. Hatch, The Democratization of American Christianity (New Haven; Yale University Press, 1989), 3–7.
28. Hatch, 134–35.
29. Hatch, 3.
30. Hatch, 9.
31. Donald G. Mathews, *Religion in the Old South*, xv–xvii.
32. John B. Boles, *Religion in Antebellum Kentucky*, 21.
33. Boles, 32.
34. Jama Lazerow, *Religion and the Working Class in Antebellum America*, 6.
35. See also Stephen A. Marini, *Radical Sects of Revolutionary New England* (Cambridge, MA: Harvard University Press, 1982); John Butler, *Awash in a*

Sea of Faith (Cambridge, MA: Harvard University Press, 1990); Catherine A. Brekus, *Strangers and Pilgrims: Female Preaching in America, 1740–1845* (Chapel Hill: University of North Carolina Press, 1998); Ellen Eslinger, *Citizens of Zion: The Social Origins of Camp Meeting Revivalism* (Knoxville: The University of Tennessee Press, 1999); and Amy DeRogatis, *Moral Geography: Maps, Missionaries, and the American Frontier* (New York: Columbia University Press, 2003).

36. Christine Leigh Heyrman, *Southern Cross: The Beginnings of the Bible Belt* (New York: Alfred A. Knopf, Inc., 1997), 26.
37. Heyrman, 27.
38. Heyrman, 24.
39. Heyrman, 27.
40. Ibid.
41. Heyrman, 255–56.
42. Stephen A. Marini, *Radical Sects of Revolutionary New England*.
43. John Butler, *Awash in a Sea of Faith*, 274.
44. Butler, 274.
45. See Mark A. Noll, *America's God: From Jonathan Edwards to Abraham Lincoln* (Oxford: Oxford University Press, 2002); and E. Brooks Holifield, *Theology in America: Christian Thought from the Age of the Puritans to the Civil War* (New Haven: Yale University Press, 2005).

Bibliography

Boles, John B. *Religion in Antebellum Kentucky*. Lexington: University of Kentucky Press, 1995.

Brekus, Catherine A. *Strangers and Pilgrims: Female Preaching in America, 1740–1845*. Chapel Hill: University of North Carolina Press, 1998.

Butler, John. *Awash in a Sea of Faith*. Cambridge, MA: Harvard University Press, 1990.

Conkin, Paul K. *Cane Ridge: America's Pentecost*. Madison: University of Wisconsin Press, 1990.

Cross, Whitney R. *The Burned-Over District: The Social and Intellectual History of Enthusiastic Religion in Western New York, 1800–1850*. New York: Harper & Row, 1950.

DeRogatis, Amy. *Moral Geography: Maps, Missionaries, and the American Frontier*. New York: Columbia University Press, 2003.

Eslinger, Ellen. *Citizens of Zion: The Social Origins of Camp Meeting Revivalism*. Knoxville: The University of Tennessee Press, 1999.

Faragher, John Mack. Sugar Creek: *Life on the Illinois Prairie*. New Haven: Yale University Press, 1986.

Foster, Charles I. *Errand of Mercy: the Evangelical United Front, 1790–1837*. Chapel Hill: University of North Carolina Press, 1960.

Hatch, Nathan O. *The Democratization of American Christianity*. New Haven: Yale University Press, 1989.

Heyrman, Christine Leigh. *Southern Cross: The Beginnings of the Bible Belt*. New York: Alfred A. Knopf, Inc., 1997.

Holifield, E. Brooks. *Theology in America: Christian Thought from the Age of the Puritans to the Civil War*. New Haven: Yale University Press, 2005.

Hollitz, John E. "Evaluating One Historian's Argument: The 'Other Side' of the American Revolution." In *Thinking Through the Past, Volume I: to 1877*. Boston: Houghton Mifflin Company, 2005.

Howe, Daniel Walker. What God Hath Wrought: *The Transformation of America, 1815–1848*. Oxford: Oxford University Press, 2007.

Johnson, Charles A. *The Frontier Camp Meeting*. Dallas: Southern University Methodist Press, 1955.

Johnson, Paul E. *A Shopkeeper's Millennium: Society and Revivals in Rochester, New York, 1815–1837*. New York: Hill and Wang, 2004 (orig. 1978).

Lazerow, Jama. *Religion and the Working Class in Antebellum America*. Washington: Smithsonian Institution Press, 1995.

Limerick, Patricia Nelson. *The Legacy of Conquest: The Unbroken Past of the American West*. New York: W.W. Norton and Company, 1987.

Marini, Stephen A. *Radical Sects of Revolutionary New England*. Cambridge, MA: Harvard University Press, 1982.

Mathews, Donald G. "The Second Great Awakening as an Organizing Process, 1780–1830: An Hypothesis." *American Quarterly* 21 (Spring 1969): 23–43.

Mathews, Donald G. *Religion in the Old South*. Chicago: University of Chicago Press, 1977.

Miyakawa, T. Scott. *Protestants and Pioneers: Individualism and Conformity of the American Frontier*. Chicago: University of Chicago Press, 1964.

Noll, Mark A. *America's God: From Jonathan Edwards to Abraham Lincoln*. Oxford: Oxford University Press, 2002.

Posey, Walter B. *Frontier Mission: a History of Religion West of the Southern Appalachians to 1861*. Lexington: University of Kentucky Press, 1966.

Roth, Randolph A. *The Democratic Dilemma: Religion, Reform, and the Social Order in the Connecticut River Valley of Vermont, 1791–1850*. Cambridge: Cambridge University Press, 1987.

Ryan, Mary P. *Cradle of the Middle Class: The Family in Oneida County, New York, 1790–1865*. Cambridge: Cambridge University Press, 1981.

Sellers, Charles. *The Market Revolution: Jacksonian America, 1815–1846*. Oxford: Oxford University Press, 1994.

Smith-Rosenberg, Carroll. *Religion and the Rise of the City: the New York City Mission Movement, 1812–1870*. Ithaca: Cornell University Press, 1971.

Sweet, William Warren. *Revivalism in America: Its Origin, Growth and Decline*. New York: Charles Scribner's Sons, 1945.

Sweet, William Warren. *Religion in the Development of American Culture, 1765–1840*. Gloucester, MA: P. Smith, 1963.

Sweet, William Warren. *The Methodists, a Collection of Source Materials*, Volume 4. New York: Cooper Square Publishers, 1964.

Turner, Frederick Jackson. "The Significance of the Frontier in American History" (1893). *In the American Intellectual Tradition*, vol. II, edited by David A. Hollinger and Charles Capper, 54–62. New York: Oxford University Press, 2006.

Wood, Gordon. *The Radicalism of the American Revolution*. New York: Vintage Books, 1991.

DAVID A. VAREL is an intellectual historian of the modern United States who specializes in race, the history of social science, and the civil rights movement. Last year he served as a postdoctoral fellow in African American Studies at Case Western Reserve University. Varel's research explores the struggle against scientific racism, and he specializes in the generation of black scholars who transformed the academy in the second quarter of the twentieth century. His forthcoming book, *The Lost Black Scholar: Resurrecting Allison Davis in American Social Thought* (University of Chicago Press, spring 2018), is the first study of the pioneering anthropologist Allison Davis. Davis was the first African American appointed full time to a predominantly white university. Among other accomplishments, his research contributed to *Brown v. Board of Education*, the federal Head Start program, and the abolition of culturally biased intelligence tests. His marginalized career is a testament to the troubled politics of race in the academy. Varel's work has also appeared in the Journal of Negro Education and Knowledge Cultures, and it has been supported by fellowships from the New York Public Library, the University of Chicago Library, and the University of Colorado. He is currently working on a project on the black history movement.

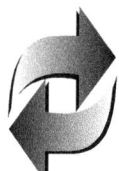

EXPLORING THE ISSUE

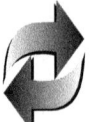

Should the Great Awakening Be Understood Primarily Through Religious Evangelicalism?

Critical Thinking and Reflection

1. In what ways did the First Great Awakening (FGA) and Second Great Awakening (SGA) influence religious, political, social, and economic beliefs and actions in the 18th century British American colonies and the 19th century newly founded nation of the United States?
2. Compare and contrast the main points of disagreement between Thomas S. Kidd and David A. Veral regarding the historic causation of the FGA and SGA movements in 18th and 19th century North America?
3. Compare and contrast the main points of agreement between Thomas S. Kidd and David A. Veral regarding the historic causation of the FGA and SGA movements in 18th and 19th century North America?
4. Have the ideological sentiments of revolution or the theological sensitivity of revivalism had a greater sustaining influence in the cultural, social, political, and economic institutions of the United States?
5. How might the notion of *freewill* as understood through the theological writings of Edwards, Whitefield, Taylor, and Finney influence the rise of liberty and equality sentiments during the 18th century colonial revolutionary and 19th century abolitionist and women's rights periods?
6. You are asked to take a stand on whether you believe the Great Awakening should be understood primarily through religious evangelicalism (Kidd) or a multiplicity of ideological Understood Primarily through Religious Evangelicalism? What would be your three to four main points of evidence to support your position?

Is There Common Ground?

Which came first? The religious fervor or the revolutionary spirit?

The rival interpretations of the historical causation of the North American FGA and SGA movements of the 18th and 19th centuries are unlikely to be settled any time soon. Upon first reading of Thomas S. Kidd's and David A. Veral's historical conjecture and interpretations, one might argue that Kidd's focus on what he redefines as the *long Great Awakening* (i.e., FGA) and Veral's emphasis of analyses on the Second Great Awakening (SGA) present an apples and oranges comparison. However, it is precisely Kidd's redefinition of the traditional historical timeline for the FGA (roughly 1670s C.E. to the close of the American Revolution in 1783) that raises the specter of an interdependent theological and ideological zeitgeist whose momentum blurs the lines of between the FGA and SGA movements. This is where Veral's contention of a *multiplicity of social, political, economic, and certainly religious* factors emerges to challenge Kidd's nod to religious evangelicalism antecedent causation argument.

Thomas S. Kidd certainly does not approach this matter of historical causation with a myopic worldview that offers a single-minded answer that the Great Awakenings movements are solely religious in origin and outcome. Quite frankly, Kidd's compelling argument is inclusive of some of Veral's multifaceted factors contention but is well-grounded in his evidentiary proof texts supporting the position that indeed the Great Awakening should be understood primarily through religious evangelicalism. Thomas S. Kidd has clearly established his reputation as a scholar of renown through meticulously researched and intricately constructed theses that support his arguments. Kidd's resonate and reasoned contention that the historical causation of the *long Great Awakening* can be traced to the influence of Christian Evangelical leaders and their adherents successful engineering of what some might attribute to divinely inspired revivals paved the way for the intersection of well-established Christian Evangelical and fledgling Patriot-Democracy movements that simultaneously spread across the colonies, changing the nature and trajectory of Christianity's influence in North America and around the globe. "He presents a compelling, clear narrative, oriented in the service of his interlocking rubrics of 'the Long Great Awakening,' the importance of the Holy Spirit, and the diversity among evangelical revivalists. In so doing, he reveals a single resonant tradition that does not oversimplify their difference but refuses to let them be unduly atomized by their diversity" (Kidd, 2010; Maskell, 2010).

Just as Kidd does not approach this topic of historical causation of the Great Awakenings movements as a one-note song, David A. Varel does not discount the importance of religious evangelicalism in the causation narrative of the 18th and 19th centuries Great Awakening movements of North America. However, Varel's fundamental premise does place religious evangelicalism's role in the Second Great Awakening as an integrated component of the growth of new sectarian and denominational groups' influence amidst an already robust democratization movement in pre and post 18th century revolutionary and 19th century reform inspired America. The Second Great Awakening, and presumably the near intersecting *long Great Awakening* movements (Kidd, 2008), should be considered as one of the diverse cultural, social, political, economic, and even geographic ingredients that contributed to the recipe of a democracy movement stew that had been simmering in multiple contexts over many years. Simply put, Veral contends that religion is a significant corollary to the equally important social, political, and economic antecedents to the Great Awakening Movements. To overemphasize the role of Christian Evangelicalism, given the dominant revolutionary and reform ideologies that were present in the colonial and nation building eras of America, would at best be an oversimplification of the causation of the Great Awakening movements and at worst a promotion of revivalism over the more significant rise of revolutionary Democracy movements that continues to have a global impact today.

References

Blosser, J.M. (2009). The great awakening: The roots of evangelical Christianity in Colonial America (review). *American Studies, 50*(1), 146–147. Mid-American Studies Association. Retrieved September 1, 2018, from Project MUSE database.

Gaustad, E.S. (1957). *The great awakening in New England.* New York, NY: Harper & Brothers.

Goen, C.G. (ed.) (1972). *Works of Jonathan Edwards: The great awakening.* New Haven, CT: Yale University Press.

Kidd, T.S. (2008). *The great awakening: A brief history with documents.* Boston, MA: Bedford/St. Martin's Press.

Kidd, T.S. (2010). The great awakening: The roots of evangelical Christianity in Colonial America. *The Journal of Religion, 90*(3), 414–415.

Lambert, F. (1994). *Pedlar in divinity: George Whitefield and the transatlantic revivals, 1737–1770.* Princeton, NJ: Princeton University Press.

Smith, J.E., Stout, H.S., & Minkema, K.P. (eds) (2003). *A Jonathan Edwards Reader.* New Haven, CT: Yale University Press.

Wood, G. (1991). *The Radicalism of the American Revolution.* New York: Vintage Books.

Additional Resources

Conforti, J. (1991). The invention of the great awakening, 1795–1842. *Early American Literature, 26*(2), 99–118. Retrieved from http://www.jstor.org/stable/25056853

Hatch, N.O. (1989) *The democratization of American Christianity.* New Haven, CT: Yale University Press.

Howe, D.W. (2007). *What Hath God Wrought: The transformation of America 1815–1848.* New York: Oxford University Press.

Johnson, P.E. (1978). *A shopkeeper's Millennium: Society and Revivals in Rochester, New York, 1815–1837.* New York: Hill and Wang.

Lambert, F. (1995). The first great awakening: Whose interpretive fiction? *The New England Quarterly, 68*(4), 650–659. doi:10.2307/365880

Stout, H.S. (1991). *The divine dramatist: George Whitefield and the rise of modern Evangelicalism.* Grand Rapids: Eerdmans Publishing.

Tracy, J. (1845). *The great awakening: A history of the revival of religion in the time of Edwards and Whitefield.* Boston: Tappan & Dennet.

Wood, G. (1991). *The Radicalism of the American Revolution.* New York: Vintage Books.

Internet References . . .

America's True History of Religious Tolerance

https://www.smithsonianmag.com/history/americas-true-history-of-religious-tolerance-61312684/

Divining America: Religion in American History

http://nationalhumanitiescenter.org/tserve/divam.htm

Edsitement: The First Great Awakening

https://edsitement.neh.gov/lesson-plan/first-great-awakening

Gilder Lehrman Institute: Religion in the Colonial World

https://www.gilderlehrman.org/site-search?keys=religion+colonial+world

History.Org: Religious Transformation and the Second Great Awakening

http://nationalhumanitiescenter.org/tserve/divam.htm

The Association of Religious Data Archives: The First and Second Grate Awakenings

http://www.thearda.com/Timeline/events/event_324.asp

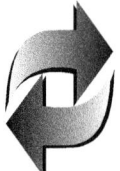

ISSUE

Selected, Edited, and with Issue Framing Material by:
Kevin R. Magill and Tony L. Talbert, *Baylor University*

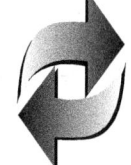

Was the American Revolution "Common Sense"?

YES: **Thomas Paine**, from *Common Sense, Jan. 1776, Introduction, Pt. III-IV*, Primary Source Collection, www.americainclass.org (1776)

NO: **Rev. Charles Inglis**, from *A Loyalist Rebuttal to Common Sense, 1776*, Primary Source Collection, www.americainclass.org (1776)

Learning Outcomes

After reading this issue, you will be able to:

- Identify the factors that influenced the primary arguments in the independence debate.
- Identify the factors that influenced the publication of each piece.
- Evaluate the rhetorical styles of political authors.
- Compare the logical and rhetorical devices from the articles to those used with regard to a contemporary issue.

ISSUE SUMMARY

YES: Thomas Paine's 1775 pamphlet titled *Common Sense* presents the author's case for independence from Britain. Written in common vernacular and widely read, *Common Sense* is considered to be the most influential text of the Revolutionary period. It remains the all-time best selling American title to this day. In this piece, Paine makes a fiery case for American independence by concentrating on moral and political arguments related to advocating for independence. His argument begins with general and theoretical reflections about government and religion. Paine then applies these intellectual traditions to the colonial situation.

NO: Charles Inglis's 1776 *The Deceiver Unmasked; Or, Loyalty and Interest United: In Answer to a Pamphlet Entitled Common Sense* is the author's rebuttal to Thomas Paine's *Common Sense*. Written to consolidate the support of American Loyalists, Inglis makes a case for American reconciliation with Britain. His response to *Common Sense* is a repudiation of Paine's revolutionary ideas and a call for an English cultural revival in her colonies. Inglis's argument suggests Paine is naive to think that a new government would be less tyrannical than England.

Issue Framing with Chris G. Lemley

In the American colonies of 1776, the time for the idea of independence had undoubtedly arrived. The viability of that idea, however, and the feasibility of its enactment were steeped in skepticism for a large swath of the masses that populated the cities, bergs, and homesteads of the fledgling colonies. Not until the publication of Thomas Paine's *Common Sense* did popular opinion irrevocably shift away from reconciliation or reform and set the colonies on a path to revolution. Even with the fiery rhetoric and revolutionary fervor, Paine's missive was opposed from within or outside of the movement.

Indeed, the success of Paine's argument swaying the American colonists toward the cause of independence is deemed so astonishing precisely because of the resistance to full-scale revolution in the months prior to the pamphlet's publication. Evidence of this opposition is found in the proliferation of rebuttals to *Common Sense*, foremost among them being Charles Inglis's *The Deceiver Unmasked; Or, Loyalty and Interest United: In Answer to a Pamphlet Entitled Common Sense*, which makes a case that rebellion would be lunacy in both ideological and practical terms. Inglis's earnest entreaty for the Englishmen of the colonies to repent and return to the good graces of the King as contrasted with the urgency of Paine's plea for freedom hint at the degree to which the matter remained unsettled in the months prior to the Declaration of Independence. A consideration of the events preceding and surrounding the publication of Paine and Inglis's works yields insight into the authors' respective motives.

Ironically for a man who would ultimately become renowned for his scathing criticism of monarchies and the oppression of their tax regimes, Thomas Paine would achieve his first measure of notoriety as an excise tax collector in the service of the English crown. Advocating for wage raises for his fellow taxmen in 1772, Paine honed his style of plain prose punctuated with biting satire. His eloquence would soon accord him a measure of notoriety within London's intellectual circles, among whom he would eventually make the acquaintance of a visitor from the American colonies, Dr. Benjamin Franklin. Inspired by the Enlightenment ideals he saw in practice in Franklin's Atlantic errands and eager to put his own skills to work in the service of such a worthy cause, Paine sailed for Philadelphia in 1774.

Almost immediately upon arriving in America, Paine found common cause with his Pennsylvania brethren. Struck by the egalitarianism and worldly optimism of the colony's Quaker meetings, invigorated by the revolutionary sentiments which were gaining traction in Philadelphia's tavern society, and incensed by the British repression he witnessed, Paine found a receptive audience for his increasingly radical writings in his adopted city. Impressed by Paine's eloquence in an antislavery pamphlet whose 1775 publication ultimately led to the establishment of the first abolitionist society in America, local physician and early member of the Sons of Liberty, Benjamin Rush sought out the budding writer. Rush would later recount soliciting Paine's assistance in crafting an argument "preparing our citizens for a perpetual separation of our country from Great Britain, by means of a work of such length as would obviate all the objections to it. He seized the idea with avidity and immediately began his famous pamphlet in favor of that measure."

In fact, Paine had been steadily crafting just such a document since his arrival in the colonies, but Rush's encouragement would throw the author into the project with renewed clarity and precision. Paring his argument with its most potent themes and writing in a style matching the simple vernacular of his adopted Pennsylvania home, Paine initially dubbed his argument "Plain Truth." Rush suggested the name be changed to "Common Sense." When Paine assented, the most influential document of the Revolutionary period was complete.

Like his future enemy in the battle for the fate of the American colonies, Charles Inglis's first stay in the Americas was in Pennsylvania, where the seminarian taught at an Anglican school in 1755. Following ordination in England, Inglis worked as a missionary to the Mohawk Native American tribe in Dover, DE, before pursuing and ultimately securing a position as an assistant at Trinity parish in New York in 1773. Inglis's strong loyalist inclinations were an ideal match for his congregation, which counted members of the colonial bureaucracy and upwardly mobile merchant class among its parishioners.

Convinced that the crown's leniency with regard to religious exercise, government, and trade had engendered many within the colonies with a rebellious spirit that must be Anglicized, Inglis's response to *Common Sense* is both a repudiation of Paine's ideas and a call for a revival of English culture in her colonies. Though Inglis's writings might appear self-serving, given his loyalist congregation and residence in New York City where British troops maintained firm control until the waning days of the war, the reverend's actions indicate that he had the courage of his convictions. When Inglis's writings drew the ire of American revolutionaries and the Sons of Liberty destroyed the press that published the *The Deceiver Unmasked*, Inglis personally financed a second imprint. He also drew the admiration of his fellow Anglican clergy for continuing the practice of offering prayers for the king, even as a company of armed patriots stormed the Trinity sanctuary, drums pounding and flutes tweeting.

At the time of the respective publications in 1776, the American colonists were faced with a vexing dilemma. Having enjoyed the relative freedom of a forgotten colony in their nescient stages, the American colonies were beginning to feel the weight of the multitudinous legislative remedies intended to assist the mother country in financing her wars of protection and conquest. The skirmishes at Lexington, Concord, and Bunker Hill were less than a year old and public opinion remained very much divided as to whether these constituted the beginning of a popular insurrection or were instead the work of trigger-happy firebrands. On the day that *Common Sense* hits the press, the Second Continental Congress sat in session and American troops stood frigid in the Quebec snow, waiting for orders to march. The times demanded a decision be made for independence or reconciliation. It was in this context that Thomas Paine and Charles Inglis offered their proposals. The question for the colonists was whether a war with Britain or an uncertain reunification made "common sense."

Common Sense would prove to be a runaway success, generating numerous follow-up editions and permanently shifting the public's disposition toward revolution. Paine's sequential logic and biting invective were seemingly written as an oration rather than as a reading and fomented ideas of liberty and insurrection across the colonies. Several prominent revolutionary figures, such as John Adams, feared that Paine's stirring call to arms might undermine the more deliberate and delicate work of the Continental Congress. In subsequent years, however, Adams along with Washington and other founding fathers noted the publication of Paine's work as the watershed that not only emboldened American ideas of independence but also cast a vision of what a new republic might mean.

Historian Robert Ferguson suggests that *Common Sense* was absorbed into the national memory and produced American culture like no other document before or since. Owen Aldredge argues that Paine's text was so effective because he was able to develop a style that spoke both to common Americans and could inform those intimately involved in Enlightenment era philosophical debates about morals, government, and the nature of democracy. We might also consider, what is the legacy of *Common Sense* in current media representations? The mixture of fact, opinion, and rhetoric is carefully cultivated to frame particular political perceptions within the media landscape. *Common Sense* may have created template for the foundation for modern propaganda and ways political information is prepared for public consumption. Given the masterful efforts of Paine to persuade just enough of his fellow countrymen to revolt, we ask the question was the American Revolution Common Sense? Or was the American Revolution the result of propaganda that was "equally inconsistent with learned and common sense"?

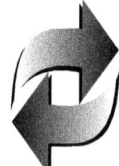

YES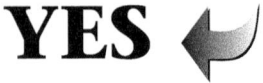

Thomas Paine

Common Sense

Jan. 1776, Introduction, Pt. III–IV, EXCERPTS

On January 10, 1776, while the Second Continental Congress was deliberating on the future of the "united colonies," a pamphlet was put on sale in Philadelphia. Simply titled *Common Sense*, it became a publishing phenomenon, a popular best seller that sold up to 150,000 copies in America and Europe. Written by an Englishman, Thomas Paine, who had arrived in America only 15 months earlier, it expressed America's pent-up rage against the mother country in fighting words, urging Americans to abandon the goal of reconciliation and fight for independence. While many of Paine's arguments were not new, his accessible prose and insistent incendiary style *were* revolutionary, spurring the spirit of INDEPENDENCE among the "common people," eliciting contempt from Loyalists, and disturbing Patriot leaders who feared the popular uproar would jeopardize the deliberative work of the Congress.

Introduction

PERHAPS, the sentiments contained in the following pages are not yet sufficiently fashionable to procure them general favor. A long habit of not thinking a thing wrong gives it a superficial appearance of being right, and raises at first a formidable outcry in defense of custom. But tumult soon subsides. Time makes more converts than reason.

As a long and violent abuse of power is generally the means of calling the right of it in question (and in matters too which might never have been thought of, had not the sufferers been aggravated into the inquiry), and as the King of England hath undertaken in his own Right to support the Parliament in what he calls Theirs, and as the good people of this country are grievously oppressed by the combination, they have an undoubted privilege to inquire into the pretensions of both, and equally to reject the usurpation of either....

The cause of America is in a great measure the cause of all mankind. Many circumstances hath and will arise which are not local, but universal, and through which the principles of all Lovers of Mankind are affected, and in the event of which their Affections are interested. The laying a Country desolate with Fire and Sword,[1] declaring War against the natural rights of all Mankind, and extirpating the Defenders thereof from the Face of the Earth, is the Concern of every Man to whom Nature hath given the Power of feeling, of which Class, regardless of Party Censure, is the

Thoughts of the Present State of American Affairs

In the following pages, I offer nothing more than simple facts, plain arguments, and common sense; and have no other preliminaries to settle with the reader than that he will divest himself of prejudice and prepossession, and suffer [permit] his reason and his feelings to determine for themselves; that he will put *on*, or rather that he will not put *off*, the true character of a man, and generously enlarge his views beyond the present day.

Volumes have been written on the subject of the struggle between England and America. Men of all ranks have embarked in the controversy, from different motives and with various designs; but all have been ineffectual, and the period of debate is closed. Arms, as the last resource, decide the contest; the appeal was the choice of the king, and the continent hath accepted the challenge.

It hath been reported of the late Mr. Pelham (who tho' an able minister was not without his faults)[2] that on his being attacked in the House of Commons on the score that his measures were only of a temporary kind, replied, "they will last my time." Should a thought so fatal and unmanly possess the colonies in the present contest, the

---

Paine, Thomas, "Common Sense, Jan. 1776, Introduction, Parts III–IV," http://americainclass.org/sources/makingrevolution/rebellion/text7/painecommonsense3and4.pdf. Copyright ©2010/2013 by National Humanities Center. Used with permission.

name of ancestors will be remembered by future generations with detestation.

The sun never shined on a cause of greater worth. 'Tis not the affair of a city, a country, a province, or a kingdom, but of a continent—of at least ⅛ part of the habitable globe. 'Tis not the concern of a day, a year, or an age; posterity are virtually involved in the contest and will be more or less affected, even to the end of time, by the proceedings now. Now is the seed time of continental union, faith, and honor. The least fracture now will be like a name engraved with the point of a pin on the tender rind of a young oak; the wound will enlarge with the tree, and posterity read it in full grown characters.

The sun never shined on a cause of greater worth. 'Tis not the affair of a city, a country, a province, or a kingdom, but of a continent—of at least one eighth part of the habitable globe.

By referring the matter from argument to arms, a new area for politics is struck; a new method of thinking hath arisen. All plans, proposals, &c. [etc.] prior to the April 19, that is, to the commencement of hostilities,[3] are like the almanacs of the last year which, though proper [accurate] then, are superseded and useless now. Whatever was advanced by the advocates on either side of the question then terminated in one and the same point, viz. [that is], a union with Great Britain. The only difference between the parties was the method of affecting it—the one proposing force, the other friendship; but it hath so far happened that the first hath failed and the second hath withdrawn her influence.

As much hath been said of the advantages of reconciliation, which like an agreeable dream hath passed away and left us as we were, it is but right that we should examine the contrary side of the argument and inquire into some of the many material injuries which these colonies sustain, and always will sustain, by being connected with and dependent on Great Britain. To examine that connection and dependence on the principles of nature and common sense, to see what we have to trust to, if separated, and what we are to expect if dependent.

I have heard it asserted by some that as America hath flourished under her former connection with Great Britain, that the same connection is necessary toward her future happiness, and will always have the same effect. Nothing can be more fallacious than this kind of argument. We may as well assert that because a child has thrived upon milk that it is never to have meat or that the first twenty years of our lives is to become a precedent for the next twenty. But even this is admitting more than is true, for I answer roundly that America would have flourished as much, and probably much more, had no European power had anything to do with her. The commerce by which she hath enriched herself are the necessaries of life, and will always have a market while eating is the custom of Europe.

But she has protected us, say some. That she hath engrossed us is true, and defended the continent at our expense as well as her own is admitted, and she would have defended Turkey from the same motive, viz., the sake of trade and dominion.

Alas, we have been long led away by ancient prejudices and made large sacrifices to superstition. We have boasted the protection of Great Britain without considering that her motive was *interest* not *attachment*, that she did not protect us from *our enemies* on *our account*, but from *her enemies* on *her own account*, from those who had no quarrel with us on any other account, and who will always be our enemies on the *same account*. Let Britain wave her pretensions to the continent, or the continent throw off the dependence, and we should be at peace with France and Spain were they at war with Britain. The miseries of Hanover last war[4] ought to warn us against connections [political alliances].

It hath lately been asserted in Parliament that the colonies have no relation to each other but through the parent country, *that is*, that Pennsylvania and the Jerseys, and so on for the rest, are sister colonies by the way of England. This is certainly a very roundabout way of proving relationship, but it is the nearest and only true way of proving enemyship, if I may so call it. France and Spain never were, nor perhaps ever will be our enemies as *Americans*, but as our being the *subjects of Great Britain*.

But Britain is the parent country, say some. . . Europe, and not England, is the parent country of America. This new world hath been the asylum for the persecuted lovers of civil and religious liberty from every part of Europe.

But Britain is the parent country, say some. Then the more shame upon her conduct. Even brutes do not devour their young nor savages make war upon their families,[5] wherefore the assertion, if true, turns to her reproach; but it happens not to be true, or only partly so, and the phrase *parent* or *mother country* hath been jesuitically adopted by the King and his parasites, with a low papistical design[6] of gaining an unfair bias on the credulous weakness of our minds. Europe, and not England, is the parent country of America. This new world hath been the asylum for the persecuted lovers of civil and religious liberty from *every part* of Europe. Hither have they fled, not from the tender embraces of the mother but from the cruelty of the monster; and it is so far true of England that the same tyranny which drove the first emigrants from home pursues their descendants still.

In this extensive quarter of the globe, we forget the narrow limits of three hundred and sixty miles (the extent of England) and carry our friendship on a larger scale. We claim brotherhood with every European Christian and triumph in the generosity of the sentiment. . . .

But admitting that we were all of English descent, what does it amount to? Nothing. Britain, being now an open enemy, extinguishes every other name and title: And to say that reconciliation is our duty is truly farcical. The first king of England of the present line (William, the Conqueror) was a Frenchman, and half the peers of England are descendants from the same country; wherefore by the same method of reasoning, England ought to be governed by France.

Much hath been said of the united strength of Britain and the colonies, that in conjunction they might bid defiance to the world. But this is mere presumption; the fate of war is uncertain. Neither do the expressions mean anything, for this continent would never suffer [permit] itself to be drained of inhabitants to support the British arms in either Asia, Africa, or Europe.

Besides, what have we to do with setting the world at defiance? Our plan is commerce, and that, well attended to, will secure us the peace and friendship of all Europe because it is the interest of all Europe to have America a *free port*. Her trade will always be a protection, and her barrenness of gold and silver secure her from invaders.

I challenge the warmest advocate for reconciliation to show a single advantage that this continent can reap by being connected with Great Britain. I repeat the challenge: not a single advantage is derived. Our corn will fetch its price in any market in Europe, and our imported goods must be paid for, buy them where we will.

But the injuries and disadvantages we sustain by that connection are without number, and our duty to mankind at large, as well as to ourselves, instructs us to renounce the alliance: because any submission to or dependence on Great Britain tends directly to involve this continent in European wars and quarrels and sets us at variance with nations who would otherwise seek our friendship and against whom we have neither anger nor complaint. As Europe is our market for trade, we ought to form no partial connection with any part of it. It is the true interest of America to steer clear of European contentions, which she never can do, while by her dependence on Britain she is made the makeweight in the scale of British politics.

Europe is too thickly planted with kingdoms to be long at peace, and whenever a war breaks out between England and any foreign power, the trade of America goes to ruin *because of her connection with Britain*. The next war may not turn out like the last, and should it not, the advocates for reconciliation now will be wishing for separation then, because neutrality in that case would be a safer convoy than a man of war [warship]. Everything that is right or natural pleads for separation. The blood of the slain, the weeping voice of nature cries, 'TIS TIME TO PART. Even the distance at which the Almighty hath placed England and America is a strong and natural proof that the authority of the one over the other was never the design of heaven. The time, likewise, at which the continent was discovered adds weight to the argument, and the manner in which it was peopled increases the force of it. The [Protestant] reformation was preceded by the discovery of America as if the Almighty graciously meant to open a sanctuary to the persecuted in future years, when home should afford neither friendship nor safety.

Everything that is right or natural pleads for separation. The blood of the slain, the weeping voice of nature cries, 'TIS TIME TO PART.

The authority of Great Britain over this continent is a form of government which sooner or later must have an end: and a serious mind can draw no true pleasure by looking forward, under the painful and positive conviction that what he calls "the present constitution" is merely temporary. As parents, we can have no joy knowing that *this government* is not sufficiently lasting to ensure anything which we may bequeath to posterity: and by a plain method of argument, as we are running the next generation into debt, we ought to do the work of it, otherwise we use them meanly and pitifully. In order to discover the line of our duty rightly, we should take our children in our hand and fix our station a few years farther into life; that eminence will present a prospect which a few present fears and prejudices conceal from our sight.

Though I would carefully avoid giving unnecessary offense, yet I am inclined to believe that all those who espouse the doctrine of reconciliation may be included within the following descriptions—interested men who are not to be trusted, weak men who *cannot* see, prejudiced men who *will not see*, and a certain set of moderate men who think better of the European world than it deserves, and this last class by an ill-judged deliberation will be the cause of more calamities to this continent than all the other three.

It is the good fortune of many to live distant from the scene of sorrow. The evil is not sufficiently brought to *their* doors to make *them* feel the precariousness with which all American property is possessed. But let our imaginations transport us for a few moments to Boston: that seat of wretchedness will teach us wisdom and instruct us forever to renounce a power in which we can have no trust. The inhabitants of that unfortunate city, who but a few months ago were in ease and affluence, have now no other alternative than to stay and starve or turn out to beg[7]—endangered by the fire of their friends if they continue within the city and plundered by the soldiery if they leave it. In their present condition, they are prisoners without the hope of redemption, and in a general attack for their relief they would be exposed to the fury of both armies.

Men of passive tempers look somewhat lightly over the offenses of Britain and, still hoping for the best, are apt to call out, *"Come, come, we shall be friends again for all this."* But examine the passions and feelings of mankind. Bring the doctrine of reconciliation to the touchstone of nature and then tell me whether you can hereafter love, honor, and faithfully serve the power that hath carried fire and sword into your land? If you cannot do all these, then are you only deceiving yourselves and by your delay bringing ruin upon posterity? Your future connection with Britain, whom you can neither love nor honor, will be forced and unnatural, and being formed only on the plan of present convenience, will in a little time fall into a relapse more wretched than the first. But if you say you can still pass the violations over, then I ask, Hath your house been burnt? Hath your property been destroyed before your face? Are your wife and children destitute of a bed to lie on or bread to live on? Have you lost a parent or a child by their hands and yourself the ruined and wretched survivor? If you have not, then are you not a judge of those who have. But if you have and can still shake hands with the murderers, then are you unworthy the name of husband, father, friend, or lover, and, whatever may be your rank or title in life, you have the heart of a coward and the spirit of a sycophant.

This is not inflaming or exaggerating matters, but trying them by those feelings and affections which nature justifies and without which we should be incapable of discharging the social duties of life or enjoying the felicities of it. I mean not to exhibit horror for the purpose of provoking revenge, but to awaken us from fatal and unmanly slumbers that we may pursue determinately some fixed object. It is not in the power of Britain or of Europe to conquer America, if she did not conquer herself by *delay* and *timidity*. The present winter is worth an age if rightly employed, but if lost or neglected the whole continent will partake of the misfortune; and there is no punishment which that man will not deserve, be he who or what or where he will, that may be the means of sacrificing a season so precious and useful.

It is repugnant to reason, to the universal order of things, to all examples from the former ages, and to suppose that this continent can longer remain subject to any external power. The most sanguine in Britain does not think so. The utmost stretch of human wisdom cannot at this time compass a plan short of separation, which can promise the continent even a year's security. Reconciliation is *now* a fallacious dream. Nature hath deserted the connection and art cannot supply her place. For, as Milton wisely expresses, "never can true reconcilement grow where wounds of deadly hate have pierced so deep."[8]

Every quiet method for peace hath been ineffectual. Our prayers have been rejected with disdain and only tended to convince us that nothing flatters vanity or confirms obstinacy in Kings more than repeated petitioning—and nothing hath contributed more than that very measure to make the Kings of Europe absolute: Witness Denmark and Sweden. Wherefore since nothing but blows will do, for God's sake let us come to a final separation, and not leave the next generation to be cutting throats under the violated unmeaning names of parent and child.

To say they will never attempt it again is idle and visionary. We thought so at the repeal of the Stamp Act. Yet a year or two undeceived us, as well may we suppose that nations, which have been once defeated, will never renew the quarrel.

Wherefore since nothing but blows will do, for God's sake let us come to a final separation, and not leave the next generation to be cutting throats under the violated unmeaning names of parent and child.

As to government matters, it is not in the powers of Britain to do this continent justice. The business of it will soon be too weighty and intricate to be managed with any tolerable degree of convenience by a power so distant from us and so very ignorant of us. For if they cannot conquer us, they cannot govern us. To be always running three or four thousand miles with a tale or a petition, waiting four or five months for an answer which, when obtained, requires five or six more to explain it in, will in a few years be looked upon as folly and childishness—there was a time when it was proper, and there is a proper time for it to cease.

Small islands not capable of protecting themselves are the proper objects for kingdoms to take under their care, but there is something very absurd in supposing a continent to be perpetually governed by an island. In no instance hath nature made the satellite larger than its primary planet, and as England and America, with respect to each Other, reverses the common order of nature, it is evident they belong to different systems—England to Europe, America to itself.

I am not induced by motives of pride, party, or resentment to espouse the doctrine of separation and independence. I am clearly, positively, and conscientiously persuaded that it is the true interest of this continent to be so; that everything short of *that* is mere patchwork, that it can afford no lasting felicity—that it is leaving the sword to our children and shrinking back at a time when, a little more, a little farther, would have rendered this continent the glory of the earth.

As Britain hath not manifested the least inclination toward a compromise, we may be assured that no terms can be obtained worthy the acceptance of the continent, or any ways equal to the expense of blood and treasure we have been already put to....

... No man was a warmer wisher for reconciliation than myself before the fatal April 19, 1775,[9] but the moment the event of that day was made known, I rejected the hardened sullen-tempered Pharaoh of England forever and disdain the wretch that, with the pretended title of FATHER OF HIS PEOPLE, can unfeelingly hear of their slaughter and composedly sleep with their blood upon his soul.

But admitting that matters were now made up,[10] what would be the event? I answer, the ruin of the continent. And that for several reasons:

First: The powers of governing still remaining in the hands of the King, he will have a negative[11] over the whole legislation of this continent. And as he hath shown himself such an inveterate enemy to liberty and discovered such a thirst for arbitrary power, is he or is he not a proper man to say to these colonies, "*You shall make no laws but what I please?*" And is there any inhabitant in America so ignorant as not to know that, according to what is called the *present constitution*,[12] that this continent can make no laws but what the King gives leave to, and is there any man so unwise as not to see that (considering what has happened) he will suffer [permit] no law to be made here but such as suit *his* purpose? We may be as effectually enslaved by the want [lack] of laws in America as by submitting to laws made for us in England. After matters are made up (as it is called), can there be any doubt but the whole power of the crown will be exerted to keep this continent as low and humble as possible? Instead of going forward, we shall go backward or be perpetually quarreling or ridiculously petitioning. We are already greater than the King wishes us to be and will he not hereafter endeavor to make us less? to bring the matter to one point. Is the power who is jealous of our prosperity, a proper power to govern us? Whoever says *No* to this question is an *independent*, for independence means no more than whether we shall make our own laws or whether the King, the greatest enemy this continent hath or can have, shall tell us, "*there shall be now laws but such as I like.*" . . .

America is only a secondary object in the system of British politics. England consults the good of *this* country no farther than it answers her *own* purpose. Wherefore her own interest leads her to suppress the growth of *ours* in every case which doth not promote her advantage or in the least interfere with it. A pretty state we should soon be in under such a secondhand government, considering what has happened! Men do not change from enemies to friends by the alteration of a name; and in order to show that reconciliation now is a dangerous doctrine, I affirm that *it would be policy in the King, at this time, to repeal the acts for the sake of reinstating himself in the government of the provinces* in order that HE MAY ACCOMPLISH BY CRAFT AND SUBTLETY, IN THE LONG RUN, WHAT HE CANNOT DO BY FORCE AND VIOLENCE IN THE SHORT ONE. Reconciliation and ruin are nearly related.

Second: That as even the best terms which we can expect to obtain can amount to no more than a temporary expedient, or a kind of government by guardianship which can last no longer than till the colonies come of age, so the general face and state of things in the interim will be unsettled and unpromising. Emigrants of property will not choose to come to a country whose form of government hangs but by a thread, and who is every day tottering on the brink of commotion and disturbance; and numbers of the present inhabitant would lay hold of the interval to dispose of their effects [property] and quit the continent.

Third: But the most powerful of all arguments is that nothing but independence, that is, a continental form of government, can keep the peace of the continent and preserve it inviolate from civil wars. I dread the event of a reconciliation with Britain now, as it is more than probable that it will be followed by a revolt somewhere or other, the consequences of which may be far more fatal than all the malice of Britain.

Thousands are already ruined by British barbarity (thousands more will probably suffer the same fate). Those men have other feelings than us who have nothing suffered. All they *now* possess is liberty, what they before enjoyed is sacrificed to its service, and having nothing more to lose, they disdain submission. Besides, the general temper of the colonies toward a British government will be like that of a youth who is nearly out of his time—they will care very little about her. And a government which cannot preserve the peace is no government at all, and in that case we pay our money for nothing, and pray what is it that Britain can do whose power will be wholly on paper should a civil tumult break out the very day after reconciliation? I have heard some men say, many of whom I believe spoke without thinking, that they dreaded independence, fearing that it would produce civil wars. It is but seldom that our first thoughts are truly correct, and that is the case here, for there are 10 times more to dread from a patched-up connection than from independence. I make the sufferers' case my own and I protest that, were I driven from house and home, my property destroyed, and my circumstances ruined, that as man, sensible of injuries, I could never relish the doctrine of reconciliation or consider myself bound thereby.

The colonies have manifested such a spirit of good order and obedience to continental government as is sufficient to make every reasonable person easy and happy on that head. No man can assign the least pretense for his fears on any other grounds that such as are truly childish and ridiculous, viz. [namely], that one colony will be striving for superiority over another. . . .

If there is any true cause of fear respecting independence, it is because no plan is yet laid down. Men do not see their way out. Wherefore, as an opening into that business I offer the following hints, at the same time modestly affirming that I have no other opinion of them myself than that they may be the means of giving rise to something better. Could the straggling thoughts of individuals be collected, they would frequently form materials for wise and able men to improve to useful matter.

If there is any true cause of fear respecting independence, it is because no plan is yet laid down. Men do not see their way out. Wherefore, as an opening into that business [of forming a new government] I offer the following hints. . . .

LET the assemblies be annual with a President only. The representation more equal. Their business wholly domestic and subject to the authority of a Continental Congress.

Let each colony be divided into six, eight, or ten convenient districts, each district to send a proper number of delegates to Congress, so that each colony send at least 30. The whole number in Congress will be at least 390. Each Congress to sit[13] and to choose a president by the following method. When the delegates are met, let a colony be taken from the whole 13 colonies by lot, after which let the whole congress choose (by ballot) a president from out of the delegates of that province. In the next Congress, let a colony be taken by lot from 12 only, omitting that colony from which the president was taken in the former congress, and so proceeding on till the whole 13 shall have had their proper rotation. And in order that nothing may pass into a law but what is satisfactorily just, not less than $3/5$ of the Congress to be called a majority—he that will promote discord under a government so equally formed as this would join Lucifer in his revolt.

But as there is a peculiar delicacy from whom, or in what manner, this business must first arise, and as it seems most agreeable and consistent that it should come from some intermediate body between the governed and the governors, that is, between the Congress and the people, let a CONTINENTAL CONFERENCE be held in the following manner and for the following purpose:

A committee of 26 members of Congress, viz., two for each colony. Two members for each House of Assembly or Provincial Convention and five representatives of the people at large to be chosen in the capital city or town of each province, for and in behalf of the whole province by as many qualified voters as shall think proper to attend from all parts of the province for that purpose; or, if more convenient, the representatives may be chosen in two or three of the most populous parts thereof. In this conference, thus assembled, will be united the two grand principles of business, *knowledge* and *power*. The members of Congress, Assemblies, or Conventions, by having had experience in national concerns, will be able and useful counselors, and the whole, being empowered by the people will have a truly legal authority.

The conferring members being met, let their business be to frame a CONTINENTAL CHARTER, or Charter of the United Colonies (answering to what is called the Magna Carta of England), fixing the number and manner of choosing members of Congress, members of Assembly, with their date of sitting, and drawing the line of business and jurisdiction between them (always remembering that our strength is continental not provincial)—securing freedom and property to all men and, above all things, the free exercise of religion according to the dictates of conscience, with such other matters as is necessary for a charter to contain. Immediately after which, the said conference to dissolve, and the bodies which shall be chosen conformable to the said charter to be the legislators and governors of this continent for the time being: Whose peace and happiness may God preserve, Amen.

Should any body of men be hereafter delegated for this or some similar purpose, I offer them the following extracts from that wise observer on governments *Dragonetti*. "The science," says he, "of the politician consists in fixing the true point of happiness and freedom. Those men would deserve the gratitude of ages who should discover a mode of government that contained the greatest sum of individual happiness with the least national expense." *Dragonetti on virtue and rewards*.[14]

But where, say some, is the King of America? I'll tell you, Friend: he reigns above and doth not make havoc of mankind like the Royal Brute of Britain. Yet that we may not appear to be defective even in earthly honors, let a day be solemnly set apart for proclaiming the charter. Let it be brought forth placed on the divine law, the word of God. Let a crown be placed thereon by which the world may know that, so far as we approve of monarchy, that in America THE LAW IS KING. For as in absolute governments the King is law, so in free countries the law *ought* to be king; and there ought to be no other. But lest any ill use should afterward arise, let the crown at the conclusion of the ceremony be demolished and scattered among the people whose right it is.

> *... in America THE LAW IS KING. For as in absolute governments the King is law, so in free countries the law ought to be king; and there ought to be no other.*

A government of our own is our natural right: and when a man seriously reflects on the precariousness of human affairs, he will become convinced that it is infinitely wiser and safer to form a constitution of our own in a cool deliberate manner, while we have it in our power, than to trust such an interesting event to time and chance. If we omit it now, some Massenello[15] may hereafter arise who, laying hold of popular disquietudes, may collect together the desperate and the discontented and, by assuming to themselves the powers of government, may sweep away the liberties of the continent like a deluge. Should the government of America return again into the hands of Britain, the tottering situation of things will be a temptation for some desperate adventurer to try his fortune, and in such a case what relief can Britain give? Ere [before] she could hear the news the fatal business might be done, and ourselves suffering like the wretched Britons under the oppression of the conqueror. Ye that oppose independence now, ye know not what ye do—ye are opening a door to eternal tyranny by keeping vacant the seat of government. There are thousands, and tens of thousands, who would think it glorious to expel from the continent that barbarous and hellish power which hath stirred up the Indians and Negroes to destroy us. The cruelty hath a double guilt—it is dealing brutally by us, and treacherously by them.

To talk of friendship with those in whom our reason forbids us to have faith, and our affections, wounded through 1,000 pores, instruct us to detest, is madness and folly. Every day wears out the little remains of kindred between us and them, and can there be any reason to hope that as the relationship expires the affection will increase, or that we shall agree better when we have ten times more and greater concerns to quarrel over than ever?

Ye that tell us of harmony and reconciliation, can ye restore to us the time that is past? Can ye give to prostitution its former innocence? Neither can ye reconcile Britain and America. The last cord now is broken; the people of England are presenting addresses against us. There are injuries which nature cannot forgive; she would cease to be natural if she did. As well can the lover forgive the ravisher of his mistress, as the continent forgive the murders of Britain. The Almighty hath implanted in us these inextinguishable feelings for good and wise purposes. They are the guardians of his image in our hearts. They distinguish us from the herd of common animals. The social compact would dissolve, and justice be extirpated the earth, or have only a casual existence were we callous to the touches of affection. The robber and the murderer would often escape unpunished, did not the injuries which our tempers sustain provoke us into justice.

> *O ye that love mankind! Ye that dare oppose not only the tyranny but the tyrant, stand forth!*

O ye that love mankind! Ye that dare oppose not only the tyranny but the tyrant, stand forth! Every spot of the old world is overrun with oppression. Freedom hath been hunted round the globe. Asia and Africa have long expelled her. Europe regards her like a stranger, and England hath given her warning to depart. O! receive the fugitive and prepare in time an asylum for mankind.

Of the Present Ability of America,
With Some Miscellaneous Reflections

I HAVE never met with a man, either in England or America, who hath not confessed his opinion that a separation between the countries would take place one time or other. And there is no instance in which we have shown less judgment than in endeavoring to describe what we call the ripeness or fitness of the continent for independence.

As all men allow the measure [admit the prospect] and vary only in their opinion of the time, let us, in order to remove mistakes, take a general survey of things and endeavor if possible to find out the *very* time. But we need not go far, the inquiry ceases at once, for the time hath found us. The general concurrence, the glorious union of all things prove the fact.

It is not in numbers but in unity that our great strength lies, yet our present numbers are sufficient to repel the force of all the world. The continent [i.e., the American colonies] hath at this time the largest body of armed and disciplined men of any power under Heaven and is just arrived at that pitch of strength in which no single colony is able to support itself, and the whole, who united can accomplish the matter, and either more or less than this might be fatal in its effects. Our land force is already sufficient, and as to naval affairs, we cannot be insensible that Britain would never suffer [allow] an American man of war [warship] to be built while the continent remained in her hands. Wherefore we should be no forwarder a hundred years hence in that branch than we are now; but the truth is we should be less so, because the timber of the country is every day diminishing, and that which will remain at last will be far off and difficult to procure.

Were the continent crowded with inhabitants, her sufferings under the present circumstances would be intolerable. The more seaport towns we had, the more should we have both to defend and to lose. Our present numbers are so happily proportioned to our wants that no man need be idle. The diminution of trade affords an army[16] and the necessities of an army create a new trade. Debts we have none, and whatever we may contract on this account will serve as a glorious memento of our virtue. Can we but leave posterity with a settled form of government, an independent constitution of its own; the purchase at any price will be cheap. But to expend millions for the sake of getting a few vile acts repealed and routing the present ministry [king's officials] only is unworthy the charge, and is using posterity with the utmost cruelty, because it is leaving them the great work to do and a debt upon their backs, from which they derive no advantage.[17] Such a thought is unworthy a man of honor, and is the true characteristic of a narrow heart and a peddling politician. . . .

> In editions of *Common Sense* after the first, Paine presents specific facts and figures to prove that the colonies can raise and support an adequate navy.

Youth is the seed time of good habits, as well in nations as in individuals. It might be difficult, if not impossible, to form the Continent into one government half a century hence. The vast variety of interests, occasioned by an increase of trade and population, would create confusion. Colony would be against colony. Each being able might scorn each other's assistance: and while the proud and foolish gloried in their little distinctions, the wise would lament that the union had not been formed before. Wherefore, the *present time* is the *true time* for establishing it. The intimacy which is contracted in infancy and the friendship which is formed in misfortune are, of all others, the most lasting and unalterable. Our present union is marked with both these characters—we are young and we have been distressed, but our concord hath withstood our troubles and fixes a memorable area for posterity to glory in.

The present time, likewise, is that peculiar time, which never happens to a nation but once, viz. [namely], the time of forming itself into a government. Most nations have let slip the opportunity, and by that means have been compelled to receive laws from their conquerors instead of making laws for themselves. First, they had a king, and then a form of government; whereas, the articles or charter of government should be formed first, and men delegated to execute them afterward; but from the errors of other nations, let us learn wisdom and lay hold of the present opportunity — *To begin government at the right end*. . . .

TO CONCLUDE: however strange it may appear to some, or however unwilling they may be to think so, matters not; but many strong and striking reasons may be

---

It is not in numbers but in unity that our great strength lies, yet our present numbers are sufficient to repel the force of all the world.

given to show that nothing can settle our affairs so expeditiously as an open and determined declaration for independence. Some of which are:

First: It is the custom of nations, when any two are at war, for some other powers not engaged in the quarrel to step in as mediators and bring about the preliminaries of a peace. But while America calls herself the Subject of Great Britain, no power, however well disposed she may be, can offer her mediation. Wherefore in our present state, we may quarrel on forever.

Second: It is unreasonable to suppose that France or Spain will give us any kind of assistance, if we mean only to make use of that assistance for the purpose of repairing the breach and strengthening the connection between Britain and America because those powers would be sufferers by the consequences.

Third: While we profess ourselves the subjects of Britain, we must, in the eye of foreign nations, be considered as rebels. The precedent is somewhat dangerous to *their peace* for men to be in arms under the name of subjects. We, on the spot, can solve the paradox: but to unite resistance and subjection requires an idea much too refined for common understanding.

Fourth: Were a manifesto to be published and dispatched to foreign courts, setting forth the miseries we have endured and the peaceable methods we have ineffectually used for redress; declaring at the same time that not being able any longer to live happily or safely under the cruel disposition of the British court, we had been driven to the necessity of breaking off all connection with her; at the same time assuring all such courts of our peaceable disposition toward them and of our desire of entering into trade with them—such a memorial would produce more good effects to this Continent than if a ship were freighted with petitions to Britain.

Under our present denomination of [status as] British subjects, we can neither be received nor heard abroad. The custom of all courts [European monarchs] is against us and will be so until, by an independence, we take rank with other nations.

. . . until an independence is declared, the continent will feel itself like a man who continues putting off some unpleasant business from day to day, yet knows it must be done, hates to set about it, wishes it over, and is continually haunted with the thoughts of its necessity.

These proceedings may at first appear strange and difficult; but, like all other steps which we have already passed over [discussed here], will in a little time become familiar and agreeable; and, until an independence is declared, the continent will feel itself like a man who continues putting off some unpleasant business from day to day, yet knows it must be done, hates to set about it, wishes it over, and is continually haunted with the thoughts of its necessity.

Notes

1. See footnote 5, p. 3.
2. HenryPelham (1696–1754), Prime Minister of Great Britain (1743–1754).
3. April 19, 1775: Battle of Lexington and Concord.
4. French and Indian War (1754–1763), fourth of the imperial wars fought in Europe and North America. George I, II, and III were monarchs of the House of Hanover.
5. "[Paine's] October 1775 essay, 'A Serious Thought,' fairly shouted at his readers to wake up to their peril. 'When I reflect on the horrid cruelties exercised by the British in the East-Indies,' he proclaimed, and 'read of the wretched natives being blown away, for no other crime than because, sickened with the miserable scene, they refused to fight—When I reflect on these and a thousand instances of similar barbarity, I firmly believe that the Almighty, in compassion to mankind, will curtail the power of Britain.' The atrocities in South Asia were the most recent and relevant clues as to British intentions. And they had gone *unpunished*, mocking the sovereignty of nature's God over the moral world. Paine's 'Serious Thought' went on to report that the British had also 'ravaged the hapless shores of Africa, robbing it of its unoffending inhabitants to cultivate her stolen dominions in the West.' Plunder and atrocity followed the British sword as night followed day." J. M. Opal, "*Common Sense* and Imperial Atrocity: How Thomas Paine Saw South Asia in North America," *Common-Place*, July 2009, www.common-place.org/vol-09/no-04/forum/opal.shtml.
6. *Jesuitically* and *papistical*: Paine is disparaging the place of the Roman Catholic Church in French governance.
7. Siege of Boston by American militiamen, encircling British troops in the city (April 19, 1775–March 17, 1776).

8. John Milton (British poet), *Paradise Lost*, ca. 1660–1670.
9. Massacre at Lexington (Paine footnote).
10. That is, but considering if matters were now reconciled with Britain.
11. *Negative*: in effect, executive veto power.
12. English constitution of 1688.
13. Blank space in original, perhaps intended for the length of each congressional session.
14. Giacinto Dragonetti, Italian statesman and political theorist, *Treatise of Virtues and Rewards*, 1765.
15. Thomas Amello, otherwise Massanello, a fisherman of Naples, who after spiriting up his countrymen in the public market place against the oppression of the Spaniards, to whom the place was then subject, prompted them to revolt and in the space of a day became king. [Paine footnote]
16. That is, the end of trade with Britain will release many working men to join the army.
17. That is, to spend millions only to reconcile with Britain (by gaining the repeal of some unjust laws and replacing the despised members of the king's cabinet), would be a terrible waste, and would leave to future generations the burden of final separation from Britain.

THOMAS PAINE was an American philosopher, political theorist, and revolutionist and is considered a Founding Father of the United States. He authored some of the most influential writings of the Enlightenment and Revolutionary eras in America and France including: *Common Sense, The American Crisis, Rights of Man, The Age of Reason,* and *Agrarian Justice. Common Sense* is considered vital to crystalizing the revolutionary ideas in such a way that allowed for its success.

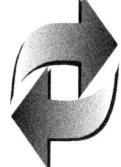

Rev. Charles Inglis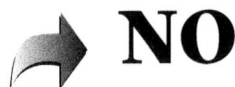

A Loyalist Rebuttal to Common Sense, 1776

The Deceiver Unmasked; Or, Loyalty and Interest United:
In Answer to a Pamphlet Entitled Common Sense
_____Preface; Answer to Section III _EXCERPTS

"a crack-brained zealot for democracy"

Horrified by Thomas Paine's pro-revolution *Common Sense*—widely read and reprinted after its initial appearance in January 1776—several Loyalists published immediate rebuttals. The most disturbing to the Patriots, perhaps, was that penned a month later by Rev. Charles Inglis, a British-born Anglican clergyman whose congregation at Trinity Church in New York City was largely Loyalist. Soon after *The Deceiver Unmasked* was advertised in a city newspaper, Sons of Liberty broke into the printer's office and destroyed all copies of the provocatively named pamphlet. Inglis published new copies and later in the year released his work under the title *The True Interest of America Impartially Stated*. Presented here are excerpts from his Preface and his rebuttal to Part III of *Common Sense* ("Thoughts on the Present State of American Affairs").

Preface

The following pages contain an answer to one of the most artful, insidious, and pernicious pamphlets I have ever met with. It is addressed to the passions of the populace at a time when their passions are much inflamed. At such junctures, cool reason and judgment are too apt to stop. The mind is easily imposed on, and the most violent measures will, *therefore*, be thought the most salutary [beneficial]. Positive assertions will pass for demonstration [proof] with many, rage for sincerity, and the most glaring absurdities and falsehoods will be swallowed.

The author of COMMON SENSE has availed himself of all those advantages. Under the mask of friendship to America, in the present calamitous situation of affairs, he gives vent to his own private resentment and ambition and recommends a scheme which must infallibly prove ruinous. He proposes that we should renounce our allegiance to our sovereign [king], break off all connection with Great Britain, and set up an independent empire of the republican kind. Sensible that such a proposal must, even at this time, be shocking to the ears of Americas, he insinuates that the novelty of his sentiments is the only obstacle to their success—that "perhaps they are not yet sufficiently fashionable to procure them general favor. . . ."

I find no *Common Sense* in this pamphlet, but much *uncommon* frenzy. It is an outrageous insult on the common sense of Americans, an insidious attempt to poison their minds and seduce them from their loyalty and truest interest. The principles of government laid down in it are not only false but such as scarcely ever entered the head of a crazy politician. Even Hobbes[1] would blush to own the author for a disciple. He unites the violence of a republican[2] with all the folly of a fanatic. . . . I think it a duty which I owe to God, to my King and country, to counteract in this manner the poison it contains . . . .

Answer to Section III

("Thoughts on the Present State of American Affairs")

In the section before me [III], this Gentleman unfolds his grand scheme of a revolt from the crown of England and setting up an independent republic in America. He leaves no method untried, which the most experienced practitioner in the art of deceiving could invent to persuade any people to a measure which was against their inclinations and interest, that was both disagreeable and destructive. He unsays in one place what he had said in another

Inglis, Rev. Charles, "A Loyalist Rebuttal to Common Sense, 1776," http://americainclass.org/sources/makingrevolution/rebellion/text7/inglisdeceiverunmasked.pdf, Copyright ©2010/2013 by National Humanities Center. Used with permission.

if it happens to serve the present purpose. He cants and whines; he tries wit, raillery, and declamation by turns. But his main attack is upon the passions of his readers, especially their pity and resentment—the latter of which is too apt to be predominant in mankind. As for himself, he seems to be everywhere transported with rage—a rage that knows no limits and hurries him along like an impetuous torrent. Everything that falls not in with his own scheme, or that he happens to dislike, is represented in the most aggravated light and with the most distorted features. Such a malignant spirit I have seldom met with in any composition. As often as I look into this section, I cannot forbear imaging to myself a guilty culprit, fresh reeking from the lashes of indignant justice, and raging against the hand that inflicted them. Yet I cannot persuade myself that such fire and fury are genuine marks of patriotism. On the contrary, they rather indicate that some mortifying disappointment is rankling at heart, that some tempting object of ambition is in view, or probably both. I always adopt the amiable Bishop Berkeley's maxim in such cases—"I see a man rage, rail and rave, I suspect his patriotism." . . .

> "I cannot persuade myself that such fire and fury are genuine marks of patriotism."

. . . My most ardent wish—next to future happiness—is to see tranquility restored to America—our liberties, property, and trade settled on a firm, generous, and constitutional plan, so that neither the former should be invaded nor the latter impoliticly or unjustly restrained; that in consequence of this a perfect reconciliation with Great Britain were effected, a union formed by which both countries, supporting and supported by each other, might rise to eminence and glory and be the admiration of mankind till time shall be no more. . . .

I think it no difficult matter to point out many advantages which will certainly attend our reconciliation and connection with Great Britain on a firm constitutional plan. I shall select a few of these; and that their importance may be more clearly discerned, I shall afterward point out some of the evils which inevitably must attend our separating from Britain and declaring for independency. On each article, I shall study brevity.

1. By a reconciliation with Britain, a period [end] would be put to the present calamitous war by which so many lives have been lost, and so many more must be lost if it continues. This alone is an advantage devoutly to he wished for. This author says—"The blood of the slain, the weeping voice of nature cries, 'Tis time to part." I think they cry just the reverse. The blood of the slain, the weeping voice of nature cries—It is time to be reconciled. It is time to lay aside those animosities which have pushed on Britons to shed the blood of Britons. It is high time that those who are connected by the endearing ties of religion, kindred and country should resume their former friendship and be united in the bond of mutual affection, as their interests are inseparably united.
2. By a Reconciliation with Great Britain, peace—that fairest offspring and gift of Heaven—will be restored. In one respect, peace is like health: we do not sufficiently know its value but by its absence. What uneasiness and anxiety, what evils has this short interruption of peace with the parent state brought on the whole British empire! Let every man only consult his feelings—I except my antagonist[3]—and it will require no great force of rhetoric to convince him that a removal of those evils and a restoration of peace would be a singular advantage and blessing.
3. Agriculture, commerce, and industry would resume their wonted vigor. At present, they languish and droop, both here and in Britain, and must continue to do so while this unhappy contest remains unsettled.
4. By a connection with Great Britain, our trade would still have the protection of the greatest naval power in the world. England has the advantage in this respect of every other state, whether of ancient or modern times. Her insular situation, her nurseries [training] for seamen, and the superiority of those seamen above others—these circumstances, to mention no other, combine to make her the first maritime power in the universe. Such exactly is the power whose protection we want for our commerce. To suppose, with our author, that we should have no war were we to revolt from England is too absurd to deserve a confutation. I could just as soon set about refuting the reveries of some brainsick enthusiast. Past experience shows that Britain is able to defend our commerce and our coasts, and we have no reason to doubt of her being able to do so for the future.
5. The protection of our trade, while connected with Britain, will not cost a 50th part of what it must cost were we ourselves to raise a naval force sufficient for the purpose.
6. While connected with Great Britain, we have a bounty on almost every article of exportation, and we may be better supplied with goods by her than we could elsewhere. What our author says is

true—"that our imported goods must be paid for, buy them where we will"—but we may buy them dearer [at more cost] and of worse quality in one place than another. The manufactures of Great Britain confessedly surpass any in the world—particularly those in every kind of metal which we want [lack] most, and no country can afford linens and woolens of equal quality cheaper.

7. When Reconciliation is effected and things return into the old channel, a few years of peace will restore everything to its pristine state. Emigrants will flow in as usual from the different parts of Europe. Population will advance with the same rapid progress as formerly, and our lands will rise in value.

These advantages are not imaginary but real. They are such as we have already experienced; and such as we may derive from a connection with Great Britain for ages to come. Each of these might easily be enlarged on and others added to them; but I only mean to suggest a few hints to the reader.

"Suppose we were to revolt from Great Britain, declare ourselves independent, and set up a Republic of our own—what would the consequences be? I stand aghast at the prospect—my blood runs chill when I think of the calamities, the complicated evils that must ensue, and may be clearly foreseen."

Let us now, if you please, take a view of the other side of the question. Suppose we were to revolt from Great Britain, declare ourselves independent, and set up a Republic of our own—what would the consequences be? I stand aghast at the prospect—my blood runs chill when I think of the calamities, the complicated evils that must ensue, and may be clearly foreseen. It is impossible for any man to foresee them all.

1. All our property throughout the continent would be unhinged. The greatest confusion and most violent convulsions would take place. It would not be here as it was in England at the Revolution in 1688. That revolution was not brought about by a defeasance[4] or disannulling the right of succession. James II, by abdicating the throne, left it vacant for the next in succession; accordingly his eldest daughter and her husband stepped in. Every other matter went on in the usual regular way, and the constitution,[5] instead of being dissolved, was strengthened. But in case of our revolt, the old constitution would be totally subverted. The common bond that tied us together, and by which our property was secured, would be snapped asunder. It is not to be doubted but our Congress would endeavor to apply some remedy for those evils; but with all deference to that respectable body, I do not apprehend that any remedy in their power would be adequate, at least for some time. I do not choose to be more explicit; but I am able to support my opinion.

2. What a horrid situation would thousands be reduced to who have taken the oath of allegiance to the King: yet contrary to their oath, as well as inclination, must be compelled to renounce that allegiance or abandon all their property in America! How many thousands more would be reduced to a similar situation; who, although they took not that oath, yet would think it inconsistent with their duty and a good conscience to renounce their sovereign. I dare say these will appear trifling difficulties to our author; but whatever he may think, there are thousands and thousands who would sooner lose all they had in the world, nay life itself, than thus wound their conscience.

3. By a declaration for independency, every avenue to an accommodation with Great Britain would be closed. The sword only could then decide the quarrel, and the sword would not be sheathed till one had conquered the other. The importance of these colonies to Britain need not be enlarged on; it is a thing so universally known. The greater their importance is to her, so much the more obstinate will her struggle be not to lose them. The independency of America would, in the end, deprive her of the West Indies, shake her empire to the foundation, and reduce her to a state of the most mortifying insignificance. Great Britain therefore must, for her own preservation, risk everything and exert her whole strength to prevent such an event from taking place. This being the case—

4. Devastation and ruin must mark the progress of this war along the sea coast of America. Hitherto, Britain has not exerted her power. Her number of troops and ships of war here at present is very little more than she judged expedient in time of peace—the former does not amount to 12,000 men—nor the latter to 40 ships, including frigates. Both she, and the colonies, hoped for and expected an accommodation. Neither of them has lost sight of that desirable object. The seas have been open to our ships, and although some skirmishes have unfortunately happened, yet a

ray of hope still cheered both sides that peace was not distant. But as soon as we declare for independency, every prospect of this kind must vanish. Ruthless war, with all its aggravated horrors, will ravage our once happy land our seacoasts and ports will be ruined, and our ships taken. Torrents of blood will be spilt, and thousands reduced to beggary and wretchedness.

This melancholy contest would last till one side conquered. Supposing Britain to be victorious, however high my opinion is of British generosity, I should be exceedingly sorry to receive terms from her in the haughty tone of a conqueror. Or supposing such a failure of her manufactures, commerce, and strength that victory should incline to the side of America; yet who can say in that case what extremities her sense of resentment and self-preservation will drive Great Britain to? For my part, I should not in the least be surprised if, on such a prospect as the independency of America, she would parcel out this continent to the different European powers. Canada might be restored to France, Florida to Spain, with additions to each. Other states also might come in for a portion. Let no man think this chimerical or improbable. The independency of America would be so fatal to Britain that she would leave nothing in her power undone to prevent it. I believe as firmly as I do my own existence that, if every other method failed, she would try some such expedient as this to disconcert our scheme of independency; and let any man figure to himself the situation of these British colonies if only Canada were restored to France!

5. But supposing once more that we were able to cut off every regiment that Britain can spare or hire, and to destroy every ship she can send—that we could beat off any other European power that would presume to intrude upon this continent: yet, a republican form of government would neither suit the genius of the people nor the extent of America.

In nothing is the wisdom of a legislator more conspicuous than in adapting his government to the genius, manners, disposition, and other circumstances of the people with whom he is concerned. If this important point is overlooked, confusion will ensue. His system will sink into neglect and ruin. Whatever check or barriers may be interposed, nature will always surmount them and finally prevail. It was chiefly by attention to this circumstance that Lycurgus and Solon[6] were so much celebrated and that their respective republics rose afterward to such eminence and acquired such stability.

The Americans are properly Britons. They have the manners, habits, and ideas of Britons, and have been accustomed to a similar form of government. But Britons never could bear the extremes either of monarchy or republicanism. Some of their kings have aimed at despotism but always failed. Repeated efforts have been made toward democracy, and they equally failed. Once indeed republicanism triumphed over the constitution; the despotism of one person[7] ensued: both were finally expelled. The inhabitants of Great Britain were quite anxious for the restoration of royalty in 1660, as they were for its expulsion in 1642 and for some succeeding years. If we may judge of future events by past transactions in similar circumstances, this would most probably be the case if America were a republican form of government adopted in our present ferment. After much blood was shed, those confusions would terminate in the despotism of some one successful adventurer; and should the Americans be so fortunate as to emancipate themselves from that thraldom, perhaps the whole would end in a limited monarchy after shedding as much more blood. Limited monarchy is the form of government which is most favorable to liberty—which is best adapted to the genius and temper of Britons; although here and there among us a crackbrained zealot for democracy or absolute monarchy may be sometimes found.

Besides the unsuitableness of the republican form to the genius of the people, America is too extensive for it. That form may do well enough for a single city, or small territory; but would be utterly improper for such a continent as this. America is too unwieldy for the feeble, dilatory administration of democracy. Rome had the most extensive dominions of any ancient republic. But it should be remembered that, very soon after the spirit of conquest carried the Romans beyond the limits that were proportioned to their constitution, they fell under a despotic yoke. A very few years had elapsed from the time of their conquering Greece and first entering Asia, till the battle of Pharsalia where Julius Caesar put an end to the liberties of his country....

"Limited monarchy is the form of government which is most favorable to liberty—which is best adapted to the genius and temper of Britons; although here and there among us a crack-brained zealot for democracy or absolute monarchy may be sometimes found."

6. In fine [summary]. Let us for a moment imagine that an American republic is formed, every obstacle having been surmounted, yet a very serious article still remains to be inquired into, viz. [namely], the expense necessary to support it. It behooves those who have any property to think of this part of the business. As for our author, it is more than probable he has nothing to lose and, like others in the same predicament, is willing to trust to the chapter of accidents and chances for something in the scramble. He cannot lose, but may possible gain. His own maxim is certainly true—"The more men have to lose, the less willing are they to venture," and vice versa, say I. . . .

For my part, I look upon this pamphlet to be the most injurious in every respect to America of any that has appeared since these troubles began. The Continental Congress, the several Provincial Congresses and Assemblies, have all unanimously and in the strongest terms disclaimed every idea of independency.

. . . They have repeatedly declared their abhorrence of such a step. They have as often declared their firm attachment to our sovereign and the parent state. They have declared that placing them in the same situation that they were at the close of the last war[8] was their only object; that when this was done, by repealing the obnoxious acts, our former harmony and friendship would be restored. I appeal to the reader whether all this has not been done from one end of the continent to the other. . . .

. . . The welfare of America is what I wish for above any earthly thing. I am fully, firmly, and conscientiously persuaded that in a reconciliation and union with Great Britain, on constitutional principles, the welfare of America is only to be found. I am fully, firmly, and conscientiously persuaded that our author's scheme of independence and republicanism is big with ruin—with inevitable ruin to America. Against this scheme, therefore, as an honest man, as a friend to human nature, I must and will bear testimony. . . .

The author of *Common Sense* is a violent stickler for democracy or republicanism only—every other species of government is reprobated [condemned] by him as tyrannical. I plead for that constitution which has been formed by the wisdom of ages—is the admiration of mankind—is best adapted to the genius of Britons, and is most friendly to liberty. . . .

America is far from being yet in a desperate situation. I am confident she may obtain honorable and advantageous terms from Great Britain. A few years of peace will soon retrieve all her losses. She will rapidly advance to a state of maturity whereby she may not only repay the parent state amply for all past benefits but also lay it under the greatest obligations. America, till very lately, has been the happiest country in the universe. Blest with all that Nature could bestow with the profusest bounty, she enjoyed, besides, more liberty, greater privileges than any other land. How painful is it to reflect on these things and to look forward to the gloomy prospects now before us! But it is not too late to hope that matters may mend. By prudent management, her former happiness may again return, and continue to increase for ages to come, in a union with the parent state.

However distant humanity may wish the period, yet, in the rotation of human affairs, a period may arrive, when (both countries being prepared for it) some terrible disaster, some dreadful convulsion in Great Britain, may transfer the seat of empire to this western hemisphere—where the British constitution, like the Phoenix from its parent's ashes, shall rise with youthful vigor and shine with redoubled splendor.

But if America should now mistake her real interest—if her sons, infatuated with romantic notions of conquest and empire ere things are ripe, should adopt this republican's scheme, they will infallibly destroy this smiling prospect. They will dismember this happy country—make it a scene of blood and slaughter, and entail wretchedness and misery on millions yet unborn.

I am fully, firmly, and conscientiously persuaded that our author's scheme of independence and republicanism is big with ruin—with inevitable ruin to America. Against this scheme, therefore, as an honest man, as a friend to human nature, I must and will bear testimony.

Notes

1. Thomas Hobbes (1588–1679), English political philosopher who argued for strong central government against which rebellion was justifiable only in response to grievous tyranny and abuse.
2. Republican, i.e., a proponent of a republic as a nation's form of government.
3. I.e., every man but Paine.
4. Defeasance: annulment, forfeiture.

5. English constitution of 1688.
6. In ancient Greece, the creators of the Spartan and Athenian legal systems.
7. Oliver Cromwell, who established a brief republic in England in the mid-1650s, after the execution of King Charles I, but exercised tyrannical authority.
8. French and Indian War (1754–1763).

REV. CHARLES INGLIS was the Bishop of Nova Scotia and the first consecrated Anglican Bishop in North America. He was a Loyalist who wrote a series of essays that he hoped would lead the American colonists to realize the folly of revolution. At Trinity Church in New York City, he prayed openly for King George III in front of parishioners like George Washington. Ingils developed an academy for the children of Anglican elite and backed unsuccessful Anglican missions intended to promote Loyalist support.

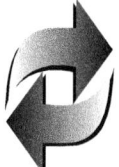

EXPLORING THE ISSUE

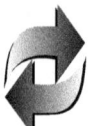

Was the American Revolution "Common Sense"?

Critical Thinking and Reflection

1. Which historical precedents does Inglis site as evidence of the inherent failures of republican democracy? Are these valid in your opinion?
2. What fears do the respective authors hope to allay or magnify?
3. Compare Paine and Inglis's rhetorical styles. Which seems more relatable and decorous?
4. Paine and Inglis seem to disagree as to whether Americans are still British. What evidence do they cite for these conclusions? Do you agree or disagree?
5. What role does the geography of Europe and America play in each author's argument?

Is There Common Ground?

Revolutionary era authors Thomas Paine and Charles Inglis could hardly be more dissimilar. Paine, an ardent revolutionary and radical with little respect for an empire that he regarded as tyrannical and oppressive was the very embodiment of the immoral, foolhardy mobs that Inglis and many others from across the colonial political spectrum feared. These ignorant masses had been so manipulated and enraged, Inglis reasoned, that they would be apt to thoughtlessly discard their privileges as British citizens in exchange for unprecedented economic and cultural isolation. Yet ultimately, it was Paine's prediction of a prosperous and vibrant independent republic that would materialize in the years following the respective publications.

On one matter, however, it seems that Paine and Inglis undoubtedly agreed. Having taken stock of their times, both concluded that a drastic measure was necessary. In Inglis's estimation, this grand action meant a total rejection of the independence movement in a bid to reenter the good graces of the English crown. That a Declaration of Independence was signed mere months after the publication of *Common Sense* demonstrates the strength and allure of Paine's preferred alternative.

Additional Resources

Foner, Eric (2004), *Tom Paine and Revolutionary America*, Oxford University Press.

Wood, Gordon S. (2002), *The American Revolution: A History*, New York: Modern Library.

Nelson, Craig (2007), *Thomas Paine: Enlightenment, Revolution, and the Birth of Modern Nations*, New York: Penguin.

Internet References . . .

Correspondence and Other Writings of the Six Major Shapers of the United States

George Washington, Benjamin Franklin, John Adams (and family), Thomas Jefferson, Alexander Hamilton, and James Madison. Over 181,000 searchable documents, fully annotated, from the authoritative Founding Fathers Papers projects.

https://founders.archives.gov/

Rebellion: 1775–1776 Common Sense

http://americainclass.org/sources/makingrevolution/rebellion/text7/text7.htm

Thomas Paine National Historical Association

http://thomaspaine.org/

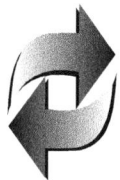

Unit 2

UNIT

Revolution and the New Nation

*T*he American Revolution led to independence from England and to the establishment of a new nation. As the United States matured, its people and leaders struggled to implement fully the ideals that had sparked the Revolution. What had been abstractions before the formation of the new government had to be applied and refined in day-to-day practice? A constitutional structure with protections against a potentially oppressive central government was developed to stabilize the new nation.

The emergence of political factionalism produced a two-party structure populated by Federalists and Democratic-Republicans in the 1790s and Whigs and Democrats by the 1830s. The expansion of democracy and educational institutions, applauded by many of the nation's leaders, promised new opportunities for "the common man" but had an ambiguous impact in the lives of women, African Americans, and Native Americans.

The historical questions in this unit of the volume speak to the political, economic, and social systems that emerged from the ideologies of the colonial period and became inextricable aspects of the democratic fabric of the United States. Equity, freedom, capitalism, and nationalism all played a historical role in the new nation, its foundation, and its evolution. Although the new nation emerged with great promise inspired by Enlightenment ideals those ideals were quickly overshadowed by pernicious traditions of bias and bigotry ensuring democracy would not truly be realized for the common man and women. Uniquely contrasted in this unity are the ideas of James Madison (Federalist No. 10) and Aristotle (Politics: Book VI) who offer perspectives that situate our comparisons and contrasts of the antecedents and subsequent ideas and ideals that formed and preserved a nation and its people. As the matters of establishing and sustaining a new nation took precedence over ideals of justice and equality, we see in the contrasting views of historians Donald F. Swansonk, Andrew P. Trout, Kori N. Schake, Donald Ratclifffe, and economist Edward Peter Stringham how it became apparent that the Revolution was likely as much about developing an economic sphere of influence as it was about creating a democratic nation. Through the diverse interpretive lenses that compare and contrast contemporary interpretation of the decisions that were made in the past, the authors in this epoch examine the complexities of the topics in ways not often considered in US History classes and curriculum. For example, what is the purpose of our political system—democracy or economic protectionism? What is the spirit of the Second Amendment? Did the economic legacy of Hamilton lead us on a path toward neoliberalism and was he this great man of history? What is the relationship between nationalism and reinvigorating our democracy? Each of these questions posed by characters of history in days gone by reverberate today in the debates taking place among contemporary actors in the halls of governments and the aisles of supermarkets across America.

ISSUE

Selected, Edited, and with Issue Framing Material by:
Kevin R. Magill and Tony L. Talbert, *Baylor University*

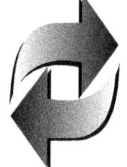

Did the Founding Fathers Create a Democratic System That Would Adequately Attend to the Problems of a Democracy?

YES: James Madison, from "Federalist No. 10," *The Federalist Papers No. 10* (1787)

NO: Aristotle, from "Politics: Book VI: A Treatise on Government," J. M. Dent & Sons (1912)

Learning Outcomes

After reading this issue, you will be able to:

- Understand the divergent ideas about control when conceptualizing democratic society.
- Discuss the extent to which the US government was expected to be democratic society.
- Nuance the philosophical aims of the founding fathers not commonly taught in the US History curriculum.
- Trouble the democratic relationship between people and government.
- Describe some of the theory and practice of democratic conceptualizations.

ISSUE SUMMARY

YES: In *Terms of the Senate 26 June*, Madison suggests the major problem with a new democratic system would be that it would require an egalitarian society. He believed those citizens without means would vote for policies that would lead to the redistribution of land and capital. Madison saw this as a problem, believing the country needed to be controlled by a certain class of men.

NO: In *Politics*, Aristotle also described inequality as a major problem in a democratic system. Taking the opposite approach to Madison, Aristotle argues a democratic society should be concerned with removing tyranny and oligarchy so communities of free and equal men are able to access its systems. He then believed that citizens could democratically work toward the common good for all in the society.

In this introduction, we utilize several principals outlined in Noam Chomsky's *Requiem for the American Dream: The 10 Principles of Concentration of Wealth & Power* to help readers examine the nature of Aristotelian and Madisonian democratic philosophies and more easily connect historically with these authors. Chomsky (2007) argues our democracy has become a mechanism for consolidating wealth and power achieved by: Reducing Democracy, Shaping Ideology, Redesigning the Economy, Overburdening the Poor, Attacking Solidarity, Controlling the Regulators, Engineering Elections, Keeping the Rabble in Line, Manufacturing Consent, and Marginalizing the Population. We encourage you to consider these principals as you examine contemporary democracy through its historical legacy.

Democratic thought and organization are inseparable parts of the American ethos. The political, philosophical, and social organization that unfolded from the revolutionary era has become perhaps the most prosperous, free, and open society in human history. However, extreme financial disparities existing have limited civic access for many. Subsequently, many citizens feel apathy and rage as they observe little democratic response to their participation (Carr, 2011; Magill, 2018). Our focal authors have much to say about the nature of wealth, power, and democracy. Each man understood that if a society were democratic, those without power and capital would naturally enact policies that would remove power and wealth from the most privileged class (Chomsky, 2017). Part of Madison's argument in *Terms of the Senate* is that the landowners should be protected against the possibility that the poor might transform society in this way (Chomsky, 2015a). It was in this spirit that Madison put forth that, "the primary purpose of government should be to protect the minority of opulent against the majority." Madison believed that authentic democratic power would lead to us now understand to be a welfare state or a socialist democracy. Conversely, Aristotle suggests in *Politics* that a democracy must "have equality according to number, not worth, and if this is the principle of justice prevailing, the multitude must of necessity be sovereign and the decision of the majority must be final and must constitute justice, for they say that each of the citizens ought to have an equal share; so that it results that in democracies the poor are more powerful than the rich, because there are more of them and whatever is decided by the majority is sovereign." We can see that in their responses to what they both understood as the problem of democracy, Aristotle suggested a society reduce inequity while Madison argued for reducing democracy (see Chomsky, 2017).

These factors are extremely relevant in a democratic society that now understands money as free speech (Citizens United) (see Chomsky, 2017). Each author, Aristotle and Madison, likely would have divergent opinions about this concept. Citizens United effectively ensures that corporate and wealthy will have more say than common citizens—a condition, which Aristotle vehemently opposed. The logic of the decision aligns with Madison's view and may have seen it as a means to ensure the republic he hoped to create. We suggest that this aristocratic and corporatocratic view of policy, law, organization, and civic agency has determined US democracy.

Though democratic access has risen and fallen throughout the history of the Republic, private, corporate, and capital influence on government in nothing new. However, current mechanisms limiting civic access have become increasingly insidious in response to the democratic demonstrations of the 1960s. This is no surprise since authentically democratic societies are threats to centralized power (Chomsky, 2015a). Following World War II, a new era emerged where middle-class jobs were relatively easy to find for white men. However, society began to change as activists responded to the sociopolitical inequalities experiences by other groups and people began to reject certain imposed social relations. People utilized their democratic agency in the 1960s to fight for a more egalitarian society (Freeman & Johnson, 1999; Newton & Seale, 1968) understanding democracy as Aristotle did. However, these democratic shows of unity were bad for big business and social control, so governmental terror group The Counter Intelligence Program (COINTELPRO) was developed to limit democratic involvement and organization (Blackstock, 1988; Chomsky, 2017). COINTELPRO tactics are alleged to have included discrediting targets through the use of psychological warfare, credibility smearing, document forging, and false media reporting. What is more, the program used violence and assassination—directed at groups who were largely fighting for more equitable access to democratic systems. Some of these groups included the Black Panthers, the Communist Party USA, the anti-Vietnam War organizers, the feminist movements, and the independence movements (i.e., Puerto Rico) (COINTELPRO also targeted hate groups such as the KKK) (Chomsky, 2015b; Newton & Seale, 1968). Many of these techniques are still used to limit the democratic participation in groups like Black Lives Matter (Craven, 2015).

While Aristotle would have naturally been in opposition to these practices, Madison may have seen these tactics as a necessary way to ensure the "minority of opulent." However, one could also argue that COINTELPRO is an example of the type of policy and practice that Madison would oppose as a so-called "anti-federalist" (see Hamilton, Madison, Jay, & Pole, 2005). That said, if we look more closely at Madison's "conditional anti-federalist," we might observe his rather inconsistent positions. James Madison the "Constitutionalist" applied Montesquieu's "Spirit of the Law" as he embraced the central significance of the separation of powers and checks and balances (Montesquieu & Nugent, 2011). In every circumstance where the Federal government fails to maintain proper checks and balances, Madison is in opposition to the very federal government he labored diligently to realize. Yet, when Madison was President, he enacted "War Hawk" policies during the War of 1812 (Stagg, 1976). We also see him exercising the power of "big government" in territory seizures of parts of Florida and Canada for example. That said, one might argue that his actions were in response to British incursions within disputed U.S. territory and that the British were enlisting the help of Native American tribes in Florida to fight against the United States. However, the so-called anti-federalist Madison, who opposed the Alien and Sedition Acts as enacted by Adams, seemed comfortable exercising federal powers when manipulating Constitutional protections when ordering the U.S. military to deny Native Americans, natural born and naturalized U.S. citizens, and noncitizens residing in the U.S. civil liberty protections.

It could be argued that the hawkish US government has played an active role in regulating world democracies and so-called "free markets" in all colonial and US wars. Often the government gained democratic consent through significant propaganda campaigns and false flag attacks. Consider too that since World War II, the government has imposed free market principals on small democratic, less wealthy, and dictatorial nations while manipulating markets to their benefit (Chang, 2010). The United States has propped several military dictatorships that in exchange provided the United States with exclusive rights to natural resources. Similarly, the privatization of publicly owned recourses has become another means of maintaining the "minority of opulent" among US citizens. Public funding, for example, has developed the foundational technologies for almost every major technological tool since World War II. The breakthroughs have paved the way for virtually all of the products that drive our modern economy. Private corporations then patent technologies that developed from the intellectual property that was created through taxpayer-funded initiatives (Chomsky, 2017; Furtado, 2016). Corporations then sell their products without including the public in profits. Those corporations take their surplus capital and use it to lobby politicians to provide their corporations with subsidies and tax breaks, while noncorporate taxpayers are asked to work within the so-called free market (Harrington, 1997). Wealthy business people and their stockholders own these companies and profit from this form of socialized capitalism (Baker, 2006). These business people then invest capital in more companies and stocks causing markets to artificially grow—further benefiting those wealthy enough to invest. The system gives the appearance of a healthy economy, however the natural inflation that occurs from the increased capital in circulation only creates further disparities between those who can invest and those who cannot. When, what Henry Giroux (2011) calls "casino capitalism," goes bust, most of the reckless players are bailed out by the taxpayers. This machine has already relegated the working class to nonfactors in US democracy and it appears that it is trying to do the same to the middle class.

Other measures have been taken in to ensure democracy would remain limited to a select few. How has this happened? Propaganda has effectively convinced American citizens to accept a government run by aristocrats and business interests and political parties who are in fact two sides of the same coin (also see Chomsky, 2017). In their civic ire, many citizens blame those perceived as "others" rather than the wealthy criminals who have lined their pockets by privatizing everything and using tax dollars to ensure free market capitalism is socialized for the wealthy and enforced for the poor (Furtado, 2016). Unsurprisingly, most in U.S. society even realize that the candidate with the most money wins the overwhelming majority of political elections. One notable exception was in the 2016 presidential election when then candidate Trump received free media attention because of his celebrity and outlandish behavior. Distracting the public with racist, classist, sexist, homophobic, and other comments became a successful political strategy (Douglas, 2018). Identity politics require address, but also distract people from the insidiousness of the political actions of the system at large. The Trump presidency became another way to keep citizens separated from their own political power, proving a new tool of austerity. He distracts the public by pointing the finger at the oppressed then helps the economic elite by giving them tax breaks, by privatizing, by removing environmental policies that limit profits, by defunding government programs for people, and by further pillaging the poor and middle class (Baker, 2006). Now consider that Clinton was the overwhelming choice of corporations (Waggaman, 2017).

Conversely, free Greek men were concerned with tyranny, oppressive power, and access to democracy for those counted as citizens. At least conceptually, they wanted everyone who participated to have reasonable access to all the rights of citizenship. Besides equitable access to voting, the Greeks had systems in place to ensure those things we have critiqued and tyranny would not be allowed to exist. They developed an "ostracon" (think ostracize from the Greek to banish) where citizens would have a vote to expel someone for 10 years if they were becoming too powerful or too tyrannical (Forsdyke, 2009). However, we can also critique these ancient Greeks because their often-lauded equitable democratic practices only extended to citizens who were landowning men.

The majority of U.S. policies are now largely in opposition to what the public claims they want when polled. For example, the majority of Americans support the policies of Bernie Sanders and his "radical leftist views," including tuition free higher education, environmental regulation, a single payer healthcare system, funding social security, and increasing the accountability of financial institutions, yet he was not elected (Muse, 2015). In the past, and in some western democracies, many of these policies are considered foundational to a democratic system, but currently, most people in the United States believe they would be impossible in the current political climate (Chomsky, 2015a).

Consider too that so-called conservatives in the United States use the phrase "welfare state" in derisive ways while conservatives elsewhere understand these social structures as basic human rights (Chomsky, 2017). What then is the nature of "United States democracy?"

Much of this introduction has been a critique of the conditions that have resulted from Madison's response to the problem of democracy. To be fair, Madison can be lauded for many of the positive aspects of the U.S. political system. The United States would likely have remained under colonial spheres of influence had they not developed systems that rejected status quo economic policies. It is also worth noting that Madison was living in a precapitalist society (as we now understand them). He could not have adequately understood how his views would exist in such a system. One could likely argue that as an anti-federalist, Madison would also not be in favor of many of the U.S. policies we have critiqued in the current economic climate. It may even be more appropriate to critique (and praise?) Alexander Hamilton for the inequitable economic systems, conditions, and philosophies that currently exist (Chang, 2003). Similarly, we can say that Aristotle's views of society existed in a time and place where direct democracy was more realistic. We must also note that Greeks only extended citizenship to certain people. Ultimately, we can at least say that people in the US system have some power in our democracy even though corporate, governmental, racist, classist, sexist, heterosexist, and other oppressive systems and ideology undoubtedly limit it in some way for most people.

We have much to learn from both Madison and Aristotle who each understood that a true and properly functioning democratic system would need to provide general egalitarianism (Chomsky, 2017). Each man also understood the need for supporting educated population to make democratic decisions. However, the two men were virtually, diametrically opposed in their theorizing of how to attend to inequality and education in a democratic society. Aristotle believed that a democratic society should be concerned with removing tyranny and oligarchy and promoting education among citizens so communities of free and equal men were able to access its systems. He believed that in an ideal democratic society, citizens could work toward the common good for all. If we are to believe Aristotle that the best form of democracy is one in which free men have reasonable access to its systems, society requires systems in place that will support such access. In Aristotle's view, the government would need to develop social welfare to achieve reasonable democratic access for all participants. Madison, on the other hand, believed that wealthy landowners should govern the United States and that those who were already educated should lead (at the time to be educated was to be wealthy or privileged) (Chomsky, 2015a). The United States has historically claimed its democratic tradition is second to none, however is this really the case when politicians consistently oppose the democratic will of the people? Did the Founding Fathers create a democratic system that would adequately attend to the problems of a democracy?

References

Baker, D. (2006). *The conservative Nanny State: How the wealthy use the government to stay rich and get richer*. Washington, DC: Center for Economic and Policy Research.

Blackstock, N. (2000). *Cointelpro: the FBI's secret war on political freedom*. New York: Pathfinder.

Carr, P. R. (2011). *Does your vote count?: critical pedagogy and democracy*. New York, NY: Peter Lang.

Chang, H. J. (2003). Kicking away the ladder: Neoliberals rewrite history. *Monthly Review, 54*(8), 10.

Chang, H. J. (2010). *Bad Samaritans: The myth of free trade and the secret history of capitalism*. New York, NY: Bloomsbury Publishing.

Chomsky, N. [Chomsky's Philosophy] (2015a, August 29). Noam Chomsky - Madison vs. Aristotle. [Video file] Retrieved from https://www.youtube.com/watch?v=gGfFXc0TwhU

Chomsky, N. [Chomsky's Philosophy] (2015b, February 24). Noam Chomsky on Watergate. [Video file] Retrieved from https://www.youtube.com/watch?v=IGIYam3p-Yc

Chomsky, N. (2017). *Requiem for the American dream: The 10 principles of concentration of wealth & power*. New York, NY: Seven Stories Press.

Craven, J. (2015). Surveillance of black lives matter movement recalls COINTELPRO. *The Huffington Post*. www.huffingtonpost.com/entry/surveillance-black-lives-matter-cointelpro_us_55d49dc6e4b055a6dab24008.

Douglas, L. (2018). Trump is a Twittertarian: a distraction despot in the age of social media | Lawrence Douglas. *The Guardian*, Guardian News and Media, Aug. 17, 2018. Retrieved from www.theguardian.com/commentisfree/2018/aug/17/trump-john-brennan-security-clearance-revoked-distraction-social-media

Forsdyke, S. (2009). *Exile, ostracism, and democracy: The politics of expulsion in ancient Greece*. Princeton, NJ: Princeton University Press.

Furtado, M. (2016). Socialism for the rich, capitalism for the poor: An interview with Noam Chomsky. *Truthout*, December 11, 2016. Retrieved from truthout.org/articles/socialism-for-the-rich-capitalism-for-the-poor-an-interview-with-noam-chomsky/

Freeman, J., & Johnson, V. (1999). *Waves of protest: social movements since the sixties*. Lanham: Rowman & Littlefield Publishers.

Giroux, H. A. (2011). *Zombie politics and culture in the age of Casino capitalism*. New York, NY: Peter Lang.

Hamilton, A., Madison, J., Jay, J., & Pole, J. R. (2005). *The Federalist*. Indianapolis, IN: Hackett Publishing.

Herman, E., & Chomsky, N. (2002). *Manufacturing consent: The political economy of the mass media*. New York: Pantheon Books.

Harrington, M. (1997). *The other America: Poverty in the United States*. New York: Simon & Schuster.

Magill, K. R. (2018). Critically civic teacher perception, posture and pedagogy: Negating civic archetypes. *The Journal of Social Studies Research*.

Montesquieu, B., & Nugent, T. (2011). *The spirit of Laws*. New York: Cosimo.

Muse, R. (2015). According to polls most Americans are socialists like Bernie Sanders. *POLITICUSUSA*, June 3, 2015. Retrieved from www.politicususa.com/2015/06/03/polls-americans-socialists-bernie-sanders.html

Newton, H., & Seale, R. (1968). The black panther ten-point program. *The North American Review, 253*(4), 16–17.

Rodriguez, A., & Magill, K. R. (2017). *Imagining education: Beyond the logic of global neoliberal capitalism*. Charlotte: Information Age.

Stagg, J. C. (1976). James Madison and the "Malcontents": The political origins of the war of 1812. *The William and Mary Quarterly: A Magazine of Early American History*, 557–585.

Waggaman, R. (2017). Hillary Clinton is the corporate greed candidate. *The Huffington Post*, April 20, 2017. Retrieved from www.huffingtonpost.com/riley-waggaman/hillary-clinton-is-the-corporate_b_9727998.html

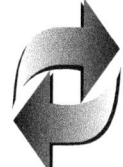

YES ↩ James Madison

The Federalist Number 10

Among the numerous advantages promised by a well constructed union, none deserves to be more accurately developed than its tendency to break and control the violence of faction. The friend of popular governments never finds himself so much alarmed for their character and fate, as when he contemplates their propensity to this dangerous vice. He will not fail therefore to set a due value on any plan which, without violating the principles to which he is attached, provides a proper cure for it. The instability, injustice, and confusion introduced into the public councils have in truth been the mortal diseases under which popular governments have everywhere perished, as they continue to be the favorite and fruitful topics from which the adversaries to liberty derive their most specious declamations. The valuable improvements made by the American constitutions on the popular models, both ancient and modern, cannot certainly be too much admired; but it would be an unwarrantable partiality, to contend that they have as effectually obviated the danger on this side as was wished and expected. Complaints are everywhere heard from our most considerate and virtuous citizens, equally the friends of public and private faith, and of public and personal liberty; that our governments are too unstable; that the public good is disregarded in the conflicts of rival parties; and that measures are too often decided, not according to the rules of justice, and the rights of the minor party; but by the superior force of an interested and overbearing majority. However anxiously we may wish that these complaints had no foundation, the evidence of known facts will not permit us to deny that they are in some degree true. It will be found indeed, on a candid review of our situation, that some of the distresses under which we labor have been erroneously charged on the operation of our governments; but it will be found at the same time that other causes will not alone account for many of our heaviest misfortunes; and particularly, for that prevailing and increasing distrust of public engagements and alarm for private rights, which are echoed from one end of the continent to the other. These must be chiefly, if not wholly, effects of the unsteadiness and injustice, with which a factious spirit has tainted our public administration.

By a faction, I understand a number of citizens, whether amounting to a majority or minority of the whole, who are united and actuated by some common impulse of passion, or of interest, adverse to the rights of other citizens, or to the permanent and aggregate interests of the community.

There are two methods of curing the mischiefs of faction: The one, by removing its causes; the other, by controlling its effects.

There are again two methods of removing the causes of faction: the one by destroying the liberty which is essential to its existence; the other, by giving to every citizen the same opinions, the same passions, and the same interests.

It could never be more truly said than of the first remedy, that it is worse than the disease. Liberty is to faction, what air is to fire, an aliment without which it instantly expires. But it could not be a less folly to abolish liberty, which is essential to political life, because it nourishes faction, than it would be to wish the annihilation of air, which is essential to animal life because it imparts to fire its destructive agency.

The second expedient is as impracticable, as the first would be unwise. As long as the reason of man continues fallible, and he is at liberty to exercise it, different opinions will be formed. As long as the connection subsists between his reason and his self-love, his opinions and his passions will have a reciprocal influence on each other; and the former will be objects to which the latter will attach themselves. The diversity in the faculties of men from which the rights of property originate is not less an insuperable obstacle to a uniformity of interests. The protection of these faculties is the first object of government. From the protection of different and unequal faculties of acquiring property, the possession of different degrees and kinds of property immediately results: and from the influence of these on the sentiments and views of the respective

Madison, James. "Federalist No. 10," *The Federalist Papers No. 10*, 1789.

proprietors ensues a division of the society into different interests and parties.

The latent causes of faction are thus sown in the nature of man; and we see them everywhere brought into different degrees of activity, according to the different circumstances of civil society. A zeal for different opinions concerning religion, concerning government, and many other points, as well of speculation as of practice; an attachment to different leaders ambitiously contending for preeminence and power; or to persons of other descriptions whose fortunes have been interesting to the human passions, have in turn divided mankind into parties, inflamed them with mutual animosity, and rendered them much more disposed to vex and oppress each other than to cooperate for their common good. So strong is this propensity of mankind to fall into mutual animosities, that where no substantial occasion presents itself, the most frivolous and fanciful distinctions have been sufficient to kindle their unfriendly passions and excite their most violent conflicts. But the most common and durable source of factions has been the various and unequal distribution of property. Those who hold, and those who are without property, have ever formed distinct interests in society. Those who are creditors, and those who are debtors, fall under a like discrimination. A landed interest, a manufacturing interest, a mercantile interest, a moneyed interest, with many lesser interests, grow up of necessity in civilized nations and divide them into different classes, actuated by different sentiments and views. The regulation of these various and interfering interests forms the principal task of modern legislation and involves the spirit of party and faction in the necessary and ordinary operations of government.

No man is allowed to be a judge in his own cause, because his interest would certainly bias his judgment and, not improbably, corrupt his integrity. With equal, nay with greater reason, a body of men are unfit to be both judges and parties, at the same time; yet, what are many of the most important acts of legislation, but so many judicial determinations, not indeed concerning the rights of single persons, but concerning the rights of large bodies of citizens; and what are the different classes of legislators, but advocates and parties to the causes which they determine? Is a law proposed concerning private debts? It is a question to which the creditors are parties on one side, and the debtors on the other. Justice ought to hold the balance between them. Yet the parties are and must be themselves the judges; and the most numerous party or, in other words, the most powerful faction must be expected to prevail. Shall domestic manufactures be encouraged, and in what degree, by restrictions on foreign manufactures? are questions which would be differently decided by the landed and the manufacturing classes; and probably by neither, with a sole regard to justice and the public good. The apportionment of taxes on the various descriptions of property is an act which seems to require the most exact impartiality, yet there is perhaps no legislative act in which greater opportunity and temptation are given to a predominant party, to trample on the rules of justice. Every shilling with which they overburden the inferior number is a shilling saved to their own pockets.

It is in vain to say that enlightened statesmen will be able to adjust these clashing interests and render them all subservient to the public good. Enlightened statesmen will not always be at the helm: nor, in many cases, can such an adjustment be made at all, without taking into view indirect and remote considerations, which will rarely prevail over the immediate interest which one party may find in disregarding the rights of another, or the good of the whole.

The inference to which we are brought is that the *causes* of faction cannot be removed and that relief is only to be sought in the means of controlling its *effects*.

If a faction consists of less than a majority, relief is supplied by the republican principle, which enables the majority to defeat its sinister views by regular vote: it may clog the administration, it may convulse the society; but it will be unable to execute and mask its violence under the forms of the constitution. When a majority is included in a faction, the form of popular government on the other hand enables it to sacrifice to its ruling passion or interest, both the public good and the rights of other citizens. To secure the public good and private rights against the danger of such a faction, and at the same time to preserve the spirit and the form of popular government, is then the great object to which our enquiries are directed. Let me add that it is the great desideratum, by which alone this form of government can be rescued from the opprobrium under which it has so long labored and be recommended to the esteem and adoption of mankind.

By what means is this object attainable? Evidently by one of two only. Either the existence of the same passion or interest in a majority at the same time must be prevented; or the majority, having such coexistent passion or interest, must be rendered, by their number and local situation, unable to concert and carry into effect schemes of oppression. If the impulse and the opportunity be suffered to coincide, we well know that neither moral nor religious motives can be relied on as an adequate control. They are not found to be such on the injustice and violence of individuals and lose their efficacy in proportion to the number combined together, that is, in proportion as their efficacy becomes needful.

From this view of the subject, it may be concluded that a pure democracy, by which I mean a society, consisting of a small number of citizens, who assemble and administer the government in person, can admit of no cure for the mischiefs of faction. A common passion or interest will, in almost every case, be felt by a majority of the whole; a communication and concert results from the form of government itself; and there is nothing to check the inducements to sacrifice the weaker party, or an obnoxious individual. Hence, it is that such democracies have ever been spectacles of turbulence and contention; have ever been found incompatible with personal security, or the rights of property; and have in general been as short in their lives, as they have been violent in their deaths. Theoretic politicians, who have patronized this species of government, have erroneously supposed, that by reducing mankind to a perfect equality in their political rights, they would, at the same time, be perfectly equalized and assimilated in their possessions, their opinions, and their passions.

A republic, by which I mean a government in which the scheme of representation takes place, opens a different prospect and promises the cure for which we are seeking. Let us examine the points in which it varies from pure democracy, and we shall comprehend both the nature of the cure and the efficacy which it must derive from the union.

The two great points of difference between a democracy and a republic are, first, the delegation of the government, in the latter, to a small number of citizens elected by the rest; secondly, the greater number of citizens and greater sphere of country, over which the latter may be extended.

The effect of the first difference is, on the one hand, to refine and enlarge the public views, by passing them through the medium of a chosen body of citizens, whose wisdom may best discern the true interest of their country and whose patriotism and love of justice will be least likely to sacrifice it to temporary or partial considerations. Under such a regulation, it may well happen that the public voice pronounced by the representatives of the people will be more consonant to the public good than if pronounced by the people themselves convened for the purpose. On the other hand, the effect may be inverted. Men of factious tempers, of local prejudices, or of sinister designs, may by intrigue, by corruption, or by other means, first obtain the suffrages, and then betray the interests of the people. The question resulting is, whether small or extensive republics are most favorable to the election of proper guardians of the public weal and it is clearly decided in favor of the latter by two obvious considerations.

In the first place, it is to be remarked that however small the republic may be, the representatives must be raised to a certain number, in order to guard against the cabals of a few; and that however large it may be, they must be limited to a certain number, in order to guard against the confusion of a multitude. Hence, the number of representatives in the two cases not being in proportion to that of the constituents and being proportionally greatest in the small republic, it follows that if the proportion of fit characters be not less in the large than in the small republic the former will present a greater option, and consequently a greater probability of a fit choice.

In the next place, as each representative will be chosen by a greater number of citizens in the large than in the small republic, it will be more difficult for unworthy candidates to practice with success the vicious arts, by which elections are too often carried; and the suffrages of the people being more free, will be more likely to center on men who possess the most attractive merit, and the most diffusive and established characters.

It must be confessed that in this, as in most other cases, there is a mean, on both sides of which inconveniencies will be found to lie. By enlarging too much the number of electors, you render the representative too little acquainted with all their local circumstances and lesser interests; as by reducing it too much, you render him unduly attached to these, and too little fit to comprehend and pursue great and national objects. The federal constitution forms a happy combination in this respect; the great and aggregate interests being referred to the national, the local, and particular to the state legislatures.

The other point of difference is the greater number of citizens and extent of territory which may be brought within the compass of republican than of democratic government; and it is this circumstance principally which renders factious combinations less to be dreaded in the former, than in the latter. The smaller the society, the fewer probably will be the distinct parties and interests composing it; the fewer the distinct parties and interests, the more frequently will a majority be found of the same party; and the smaller the number of individuals composing a majority and the smaller the compass within which they are placed, the more easily will they concert and execute their plans of oppression. Extend the sphere, and you take in a greater variety of parties and interests; you make it less probable that a majority of the whole will have a common motive to invade the rights of other citizens; or if such a common motive exists, it will be more difficult for all who feel it to discover their own strength and to act in unison with each other. Besides other impediments, it may be remarked that where there is a consciousness of unjust or dishonorable purposes, communication is always checked by distrust, in proportion to the number whose concurrence is necessary.

Hence, it clearly appears that the same advantage, which a republic has over a democracy, in controlling the effects of faction, is enjoyed by a large over a small republic—is enjoyed by the union over the states composing it. Does this advantage consist in the substitution of representatives, whose enlightened views and virtuous sentiments render them superior to local prejudices and to schemes of injustice? It will not be denied that the representation of the union will be most likely to possess these requisite endowments. Does it consist in the greater security afforded by a greater variety of parties, against the event of any one party being able to outnumber and oppress the rest? In an equal degree, does the increased variety of parties, comprised within the union, increase this security? Does it, in fine, consist in the greater obstacles opposed to the concert and accomplishment of the secret wishes of an unjust and interested majority? Here, again, the extent of the union gives it the most palpable advantage.

The influence of factious leaders may kindle a flame within their particular states, but will be unable to spread a general conflagration through the other states: a religious sect may degenerate into a political faction in a part of the confederacy; but the variety of sects dispersed over the entire face of it must secure the national councils against any danger from that source: a rage for paper money, for an abolition of debts, for an equal division of property, or for any other improper or wicked project will be less apt to pervade the whole body of the union than a particular member of it; in the same proportion as such, a malady is more likely to taint a particular county or district than an entire state.

In the extent and proper structure of the union, therefore, we behold a republican remedy for the diseases most incident to republican government. And according to the degree of pleasure and pride, we feel in being republicans, ought to be our zeal in cherishing the spirit and supporting the character of federalists.

Publius

Term of the Senate, [26 June] 1787
Term of the Senate

Read moved that the term be nine years.

Mr. Madison. In order to judge of the form to be given to this institution, it will be proper to take a view of the ends to be served by it. These were first to protect the people agst. their rulers: secondly to protect the people agst. the transient impressions into which they themselves might be led. A people deliberating in a temperate moment and with the experience of other nations before them, on the plan of Govt. most likely to secure their happiness, would first be aware, that those chargd. with the public happiness, might betray their trust. An obvious precaution agst. this danger wd. be to divide the trust between different bodies of men, who might watch & check each other. In this, they wd. be governed by the same prudence which has prevailed in organizing the subordinate departments of Govt., where all business liable to abuses is made to pass thro' separate hands, the one being a check on the other. It wd. next occur to such a people, that they themselves were liable to temporary errors, thro' want of information as to their true interest, and that men chosen for a short term, & employed but a small portion of that in public affairs, might err from the same cause. This reflection wd. naturally suggest that the Govt. be so constituted, as that one of its branches might have an oppy. of acquiring a competent knowledge of the public interests. Another reflection equally becoming a people on such an occasion, wd. be that they themselves, as well as a numerous body of Representatives, were liable to err also, from fickleness and passion. A necessary fence agst. this danger would be to select a portion of enlightened citizens, whose limited number and firmness might seasonably interpose agst. impetuous counsels. It ought finally to occur to a people deliberating on a Govt. for themselves, that as different interests necessarily result from the liberty meant to be secured, the major interest might under sudden impulses be tempted to commit injustice on the minority. In all civilized Countries, the people fall into different classes havg. a real or supposed difference of interests. There will be creditors & debtors, farmers, merchts. & manufacturers. There will be particularly the distinction of rich & poor. It was true as had been observd. (by Mr. Pinkney) we had not among us those hereditary distinctions, of rank which were a great source of the contests in the ancient Govts. as well as the modern States of Europe, nor those extremes of wealth or poverty which characterize the latter. We cannot however be regarded even at this time, as one homogeneous mass, in which everything that affects a part will affect in the same manner the whole. In framing a system which we wish to last for ages, we shd. not lose sight of the changes which ages will produce. An increase of population will of necessity increase the proportion of those who will labour under all the hardships of life, & secretly sigh for a more equal distribution of its blessings. These may in time outnumber those who are placed above the feelings of indigence. According to the equal laws of suffrage, the power will slide into the hands of the former. No agrarian attempts have yet been made in this Country, but symtoms, of a leveling spirit, as we have understood, have sufficiently appeared in a certain quarters to give notice of the future danger. How is this danger to be guarded agst. on republican principles? How is the danger in all cases of interested coalitions to oppress the minority to be guarded agst.? Among other means by the establishment of a body in the Govt. sufficiently respectable for its wisdom & virtue, to aid on such emergences, the preponderance of justice by throwing its weight into that scale. Such being the objects of the second branch in the proposed Govt. he thought a considerable duration ought to be given to it. He did not conceive that the term of nine years could threaten any real danger; but in pursuing his particular ideas on the subject, he should require that the long term allowed to the 2d. branch should not commence till such a period of life, as would render a perpetual disqualification to be reelected little inconvenient either in a public or private view. He observed that as it was more than probable we were now digesting a plan which in its operation wd. decide forever the fate of Republican Govt. we ought not only to provide every guard to liberty that its preservation cd. require, but be equally careful to supply the defects which our own experience had particularly pointed out.

JAMES MADISON was one of the founding fathers of the United States of America. He studied Latin, Greek, science, and philosophy at Princeton University and in his homeschooling experiences. He served as a Colonel in the Virginia Militia during the Revolutionary War. Madison was instrumental to the development of the philosophies that established the United States, particularly in his work as an author or coauthor of many important founding documents. These documents included the US Constitution, the Federalist Papers, and as sponsors of the US Bill of Rights. Madison served as the President of the United States from 1809 to 1817. He and Thomas Jefferson were considered to be cofounders of the Democratic Republican Party.

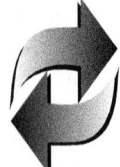

Aristotle

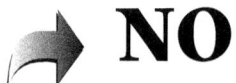

Politics Book VI: A Treatise on Government

Book VI

Chapter I

We have already shown what is the nature of the supreme council in the state, and wherein one may differ from another, and how the different magistrates should be regulated; and also the judicial department, and what is best suited to what state; and also to what causes both the destruction and preservation of governments are owing.

As there are very many species of democracies, as well as of other states, it will not be amiss to consider at the same time anything which we may have omitted to mention concerning either of them and to allot to each that mode of conduct which is peculiar to and advantageous for them; and also to inquire into the combinations of all these different modes of government which we [1317a] have mentioned; for as these are blended together the government is altered, as from an aristocracy to be an oligarchy, and from a free state to be a democracy. Now, I mean by those combinations of government (which I ought to examine into, but have not yet done), namely, whether the deliberative department and the election of magistrates is regulated in a manner correspondent to an oligarchy, or the judicial to an aristocracy, or the deliberative part only to an oligarchy, and the election of magistrates to an aristocracy, or whether, in any other manner, everything is not regulated according to the nature of the government. But we will first consider what particular sort of democracy is fitted to a particular city, and also what particular oligarchy to a particular people; and of other states, what is advantageous to what. It is also necessary to show clearly not only which of these governments is best for a state but also how it ought to be established there, and other things we will treat of briefly.

And first, we will speak of a democracy; and this will at the same time show clearly the nature of its opposite which some persons call an oligarchy; and in doing this, we must examine into all the parts of a democracy, and everything that is connected therewith; for from the manner in which these are compounded together different species of democracies arise: and hence, it is that they are more than one and of various natures. Now, there are two causes which occasion there being so many democracies; one of which is that which we have already mentioned; namely, there being different sorts of people; for in one country, the majority are husbandmen, in another mechanics, and hired servants; if the first of these is added to the second and the third to both of them, the democracy will not only differ in the particular of better or worse, but in this, that it will be no longer the same government; the other is that which we will now speak of. The different things which are connected with democracies and seem to make part of these states do, from their being joined to them, render them different from others: this attending a few, that more, and another all. It is necessary that he who would found any state which he may happen to approve of, or correct one, should be acquainted with all these particulars. All founders of states endeavor to comprehend within their own plan everything of nearly the same kind with it; but in doing this, they err, in the manner I have already described in treating of the preservation and destruction of governments. I will now speak of these first principles and manners, and whatever else a democratical state requires.

Chapter II

Now the foundation of a democratical state is liberty, and people have been accustomed to say this as if here only liberty was to be found; for they affirm that this is the end proposed by every democracy. But one part of liberty is to govern and be governed alternately; for, according to democratical justice, equality is measured by numbers, and not by worth: and this being just, it is necessary that the supreme power should be vested in the people at large; and that what the majority determine should be final: so that in a democracy, the poor ought to have more power than the rich, as being the greater number; for this is one mark of liberty which all framers of a democracy lay down as a criterion of that state; another is, to live as everyone likes; for this, they say, is a right which liberty gives, since he is a slave who must live as he likes not. This, then, is

From "A Treatise on Government" Translated From The Greek Of Aristotle By William Ellis, A.M., 1912. London : J.M. Dent & Sons, Ltd.; New York, E.P. Dutton & Co.

another criterion of a democracy. Hence arises the claim to be under no command whatsoever to any one, upon any account, any otherwise than by rotation, and that just as far only as that person is, in his turn, under his also. This also is conducive to that equality which liberty demands. These things being premised, and such being the government, it follows that such rules as the following should be observed in it that all the magistrates should be chosen out of all the people, and all to command each, and each in his turn all: that all the magistrates should be chosen by lot, except to those offices only which required some particular knowledge and skill: that no census, or a very small one, should be required to qualify a man for any office: that none should be in the same employment twice, or very few, and very seldom, except in the army: that all their appointments should be limited to a very short time, or at least as many as possible: that the whole community should be qualified to judge in all causes whatsoever, let the object be ever so extensive, ever so interesting, or of ever so high a nature; as at Athens, where the people at large judge the magistrates when they come out of office, and decide concerning public affairs as well as private contracts: that the supreme power should be in the public assembly; and that no magistrate should be allowed any discretionary power but in a few instances, and of no consequence to public business. Of all magistrates, a senate is best suited to a democracy, where the whole community is not paid for giving their attendance; for in that case, it loses its power; for then, the people will bring all causes before them, by appeal, as we have already mentioned in a former book. In the next place, there should, if possible, be a fund to pay all the citizens—who have any share in the management of public affairs, either as members of the assembly, judges, and magistrates; but if this cannot be done, at least the magistrates, the judges the senators, and members of the supreme assembly, and also those officers who are obliged to eat at a common table ought to be paid. Moreover, as an oligarchy is said to be a government of men of family, fortune, and education; so, on the contrary, a democracy is a government in the hands of men of no birth, indigent circumstances, and mechanical employments. In this state, also no office [1318a] should be for life; and, if any such should remain after the government has been long changed into a democracy, they should endeavor by degrees to diminish the power; and also elect by lot instead of vote. These things, then, appertain to all democracies; namely, to be established on that principle of justice which is homogeneous to those governments; that is, that all the members of the state, by number, should enjoy an equality, which seems chiefly to constitute a democracy, or government of the people: for it seems perfectly equal that the rich should have no more share in the government than the poor, nor be alone in power; but that all should be equal, according to number; for thus, they think, the equality and liberty of the state best preserved.

Chapter III

In the next place, we must inquire how this equality is to be procured. Shall the qualifications be divided so that 500 rich should be equal to 1000 poor, or shall the thousand have equal power with the 500? or shall we not establish our equality in this manner? but divide indeed thus, and afterward taking an equal number both out of the 500 and the 1,000, invest them with the power of creating the magistrates and judges. Is this state then established according to perfect democratical justice, or rather that which is guided by numbers only? For the defenders of a democracy say, that that is just which the majority approve of: but the favorers of an oligarchy say, that that is just which those who have most approve of; and that we ought to be directed by the value of property. Both the propositions are unjust; for if we agree with what the few propose we erect a tyranny: for if it should happen that an individual should have more than the rest who are rich, according to oligarchical justice, this man alone has a right to the supreme power; but if superiority of numbers is to prevail, injustice will then be done by confiscating the property of the rich, who are few, as we have already said. What then that equality is, which both parties will admit, must be collected from the definition of right which is common to them both; for they both say that what the majority of the state approves of ought to be established. Be it so; but not entirely: but since a city happens to be made up of two different ranks of people, the rich and the poor, let that be established which is approved of by both these, or the greater part: but should there be opposite sentiments, let that be established which shall be approved of by the greater part: but let this be according to the census; for instance, if there should be 10 of the rich and 20 of the poor, and 6 of the first and 15 of the last should agree upon any measure, and the remaining four of the rich should join with the remaining five of the poor in opposing it, that party whose census when added together should determine which opinion should be law, and should these happen to be equal, it should be regarded as a case similar to an assembly or court of justice dividing equally upon any question that comes before them, who either determine it by lot or some such method. But although, with [1318b] respect to what is equal and just, it may be very difficult to establish the truth, yet it is much easier to do than to persuade those who have it in their power to encroach upon others to be guided thereby; for the weak always desire what is equal and just, but the powerful pay no regard thereunto.

Chapter IV

There are four kinds of democracies. The best is that which is composed of those first in order, as we have already said, and this also is the most ancient of any. I call that the first which everyone would place so was he to divide the people; for the best part of these are the husbandmen. We see, then, that a democracy may be framed where the majority live by tillage or pasturage; for, as their property is but small, they will not be at leisure perpetually to hold public assemblies, but will be continually employed in following their own business, not having otherwise the means of living; nor will they be desirous of what another enjoys, but will rather like to follow their own business than meddle with state affairs and accept the offices of government, which will be attended with no great profit; for the major part of mankind are rather desirous of riches than honor (a proof of this is that they submitted to the tyrannies in ancient times and do now submit to the oligarchies, if no one hinders them in their usual occupations or deprives them of their property; for some of them soon get rich, others are removed from poverty); besides, their having the right of election and calling their magistrates to account for their conduct when they come out of office will satisfy their desire of honors, if any of them entertain that passion: for in some states, though the commonalty have not the right of electing the magistrates, yet it is vested in part of that body chosen to represent them: and it is sufficient for the people at large to possess the deliberative power: and this ought to be considered as a species of democracy; such was that formerly at Mantinsea: for which reason it is proper for the democracy we have been now treating of to have a power (and it has been usual for them to have it) of censuring their magistrates when out of office and sitting in judgment upon all causes: but that the chief magistrates should be elected, and according to a certain census, which should vary with the rank of their office, or else not by a census, but according to their abilities for their respective appointments. A state thus constituted must be well constituted; for the magistracies will be always filled with the best men with the approbation of the people; who will not envy their superiors: and these and the nobles should be content with this part in the administration; for they will not be governed by their inferiors. They will be also careful to use their power with moderation, as there are others to whom full power is delegated to censure their conduct; for it is very serviceable to the state to have them dependent upon others and not to be permitted to do whatsoever they choose; for with such a liberty, there would be no check to that evil particle there is in every one: therefore, it is [1319a] necessary and most for the benefit of the state that the offices thereof should be filled by the principal persons in it, whose characters are unblemished, and that the people are not oppressed. It is now evident that this is the best species of democracy, and on what account; because the people are such and have such powers as they ought to have. To establish a democracy of husbandmen some of those laws which were observed in many ancient states are universally useful; as, for instance, on no account to permit any one to possess more than a certain quantity of land, or within a certain distance from the city. Formerly also, in some states, no one was allowed to sell their original lot of land. They also mention a law of one Oxylus, which forbade any one to add to their patrimony by usury. We ought also to follow the law of the Aphutaeans, as useful to direct us in this particular we are now speaking of; for they having but very little ground, while they were a numerous people, and at the same time were all husbandmen, did not include all their lands within the census, but divided them in such a manner that, according to the census, the poor had more power than the rich. Next to the commonalty of husbandmen is one of shepherds and herdsmen; for they have many things in common with them, and, by their way of life, are excellently qualified to make good soldiers, stout in body, and able to continue in the open air all night. The generality of the people of whom other democracies are composed are much worse than these; for their lives are wretched nor have they any business with virtue in anything they do; these are your mechanics, your exchange-men, and hired servants; as all these sorts of men frequent the exchange and the citadel, they can readily attend the public assembly; whereas the husbandmen, being more dispersed in the country, cannot so easily meet together; nor are they equally desirous of doing it with these others! When a country happens to be so situated that a great part of the land lies at a distance from the city, there it is easy to establish a good democracy or a free state for the people in general will be obliged to live in the country; so that it will be necessary in such a democracy, though there may be an exchange-mob at hand, never to allow a legal assembly without the inhabitants of the country attend. We have shown in what manner the first and best democracy ought to be established, and it will be equally evident as to the rest, for from these we [1319b] should proceed as a guide, and always separate the meanest of the people from the rest. But the last and worst, which gives to every citizen without distinction a share in every part of the administration, is what few citizens can bear, nor is it easy to preserve for any long time, unless well supported by laws and manners. We have already noticed almost every cause that can destroy either this or any other state. Those who have taken the lead in such a democracy have endeavored to support it, and make the people powerful by collecting together as many persons as they could and giving them their freedom, not only legitimately but naturally born, and also if either of their parents were citizens, that is to say, if either their father or mother; and this method is better suited to this state than any other: and thus the demagogues have usually managed. They ought, however, to take care, and do this no longer than the common people are superior to the nobles and those of the middle rank, and then stop; for, if they proceed still further, they will make the state disorderly, and the nobles will ill brook the power of the common people, and be full of resentment against it; which was the cause of an insurrection at Cyrene: for a little evil is overlooked, but when it becomes a great one, it strikes the eye. It is, moreover, very useful in such a state to do as Clisthenes did at Athens, when he was desirous of increasing the power of the people, and as those did who established the democracy in Cyrene; that is, to institute many tribes and fraternities, and to make the religious rites of private persons few, and those common; and every means is to be contrived to associate and blend the people together as much as possible; and that all former customs be broken through. Moreover, whatsoever is practiced in a tyranny seems adapted to a democracy of this species; as, for instance, the licentiousness of the slaves, the women, and the children; for this to a certain degree is useful in such a state; and also to overlook every one's living as they choose; for many will support such a government: for it is more agreeable to many to live without any control than as prudence would direct.

Chapter V

It is also the business of the legislator and all those who would support a government of this sort not to make it too great a work, or too perfect; but to aim only to render it stable: for, let a state be constituted ever so badly, there is no difficulty in its continuing a few days: they should therefore endeavor to procure its safety by all those ways which we have described in assigning the causes of the preservation and destruction of governments; avoiding what is hurtful, and by framing such laws, written and unwritten, as contain those things which chiefly tend to the preservation of the state; nor to suppose that that is useful either for a democratic or [1320a] an oligarchic form of government which contributes to make them more purely so, but what will contribute to their duration: but our demagogues at present, to flatter the people, occasion frequent confiscations in the courts; for which reason those who have the welfare of the state really at heart should act directly opposite to what they do, and enact a law to prevent forfeitures from being divided among the people or paid into the treasury, but to have them set apart for sacred uses: for those who are of a bad disposition would not then be the less cautious, as their punishment would be the same; and the community would not be so ready to condemn those whom they sat in judgment on when they were to get nothing by it: they should also take care that the causes which are brought before the public should be as few as possible, and punish with the utmost severity those who rashly brought an action against any one; for it is not the commons but the nobles who are generally prosecuted: for in all things the citizens of the same state ought to be affectionate to each other, at least not to treat those who have the chief power in it as their enemies. Now, as the democracies which have been lately established are very numerous, and it is difficult to get the common people to attend the public assemblies without they are paid for it, this, when there is not a sufficient public revenue, is fatal to the nobles; for the deficiencies therein must be necessarily made up by taxes, confiscations, and fines imposed by corrupt courts of justice: which things have already destroyed many democracies. Whenever, then, the revenues of the state are small, there should be but few public assemblies and but few courts of justice: these, however, should have very extensive jurisdictions, but should continue sitting a few days only, for by this means the rich would not fear the expense, although they should receive nothing for their attendance, though the poor did; and judgment also would be given much better; for the rich will not choose to be long absent from their own affairs, but will willingly be so for a short time: and, when there are sufficient revenues, a different conduct ought to be pursued from what the demagogues at present follow; for now they divide the surplus of the public money among the poor; these receive it and again want the same supply, while the giving it is like pouring water into a sieve: but the true patriot in a democracy ought to take care that the majority of the community are not too poor, for this is the cause of rapacity in that government; he therefore should endeavor that they may enjoy perpetual plenty; and as this also is advantageous to the rich, what can be saved out of the public money should be put by, and then divided at once among the poor, if possible, in such a quantity as may enable every one of them to purchase a little field, and, if that cannot be done, at least to give each of them enough to procure the implements [1320b] of trade and husbandry; and if there is not enough for all to receive so much at once, then to divide it according to tribes or any other allotment. In the meantime, let the rich pay them for necessary services, but not be obliged to find them in useless amusements. And something like this was the manner in which they managed at Carthage, and preserved the affections of the people; for by continually sending some of their community into colonies they procured plenty. It is also worthy of a sensible and generous nobility to divide the poor among them, and supplying them with what is necessary, induce them to work; or to imitate the conduct of the people at Tarentum: for they, permitting the poor to partake in common of everything which is needful for them, gain the affections of the commonalty. They have also two different ways of electing their magistrates; for some are chosen by vote, others by lot; by the last, that the people at large may have some share in the administration; by the former, that the state may be well governed: the same may be accomplished if of the same magistrates you choose some by vote, others by lot. And thus much for the manner in which democracies ought to be established.

Chapter VI

What has been already said will almost of itself sufficiently show how an oligarchy ought to be founded; for he who would frame such a state should have in his view a democracy to oppose it; for every species of oligarchy should be founded on principles diametrically opposite to some species of democracy.

The first and best framed oligarchy is that which approaches near to what we call a free state; in which there ought to be two different census, the one high, the other low: from those who are within the latter the ordinary officers of the state ought to be chosen; from the former the supreme magistrates: nor should anyone be excluded from a part of the administration who was within the census; which should be so regulated that the commonalty who are included in it should by means thereof be superior to those who have no share in the government; for those who are to have the management of public affairs ought always to be chosen out of the better sort of the people. Much in the same manner ought that oligarchy to be established which is next in order: but as to that which is most opposite to a pure democracy, and approaches nearest to a dynasty and a tyranny, as it is of all others the worst, so it requires the greatest care and caution to preserve it: for as bodies of sound and healthy constitutions and ships which are well manned and well found for sailing can bear many injuries without perishing, while a diseased body or a leaky ship with an indifferent crew cannot support the [1321a] least shock; so the worst established governments want most looking after. A number of citizens is the preservation of a democracy; for these are opposed to those rights which are founded in rank: on the contrary, the preservation of an oligarchy depends upon the due regulation of the different orders in the society.

Chapter VII

As the greater part of the community are divided into four sorts of people; husbandmen, mechanics, traders, and hired servants; and as those who are employed in war may likewise be divided into four; the horsemen, the heavy-armed soldier, the light-armed, and the sailor, where the nature of the country can admit a great number of horse; there a powerful oligarchy may be easily established: for the safety of the inhabitants depends upon a force of that sort; but those who can support the expense of horsemen must be persons of some considerable fortune. Where the troops are chiefly heavy-armed, there an oligarchy, inferior in power to the other, may be established; for the heavy-armed are rather made up of men of substance than the poor: but the light-armed and the sailors always contribute to support a democracy: but where the number of these is very great and a sedition arises, the other parts of the community fight at a disadvantage; but a remedy for this evil is to be learned from skilful generals, who always mix a proper number of light-armed soldiers with their horse and heavy-armed: for it is with those that the populace get the better of the men of fortune in an insurrection; for these being lighter are easily a match for the horse and the heavy-armed: so that for an oligarchy to form a body of troops from these is to form it against itself: but as a city is composed of persons of different ages, some young and some old, the fathers should teach their sons, while they were very young, a light and easy exercise; but, when they are grown up, they should be perfect in every warlike exercise. Now, the admission of the people to any share in the government should either be (as I said before) regulated by a census, or else, as at Thebes, allowed to those who for a certain time have ceased from any mechanic employment, or as at Massalia, where they are chosen according to their worth, whether citizens or foreigners. With respect to the magistrates of the highest rank which it may be necessary to have in a state, the services they are bound to do the public should be expressly laid down, to prevent the common people from being desirous of accepting their employments, and also to induce them to regard their magistrates with favor when they know what a price they pay for their honors. It is also necessary that the magistrates, upon entering into their offices, should make magnificent sacrifices and erect some public structure, that the people partaking of the entertainment, and seeing the city ornamented with votive gifts in their temples and public structures, may see with pleasure the stability of the government: add to this also, that the nobles will have their generosity recorded: but now this is not the conduct which those who are at present at the head of an oligarchy pursue, but the contrary; for they are not more desirous of honor than of gain; for which reason such oligarchies may more properly be called little democracies. Thus [1321b] we have explained on what principles a democracy and an oligarchy ought to be established.

Chapter VIII

After what has been said I proceed next to treat particularly of the magistrates; of what nature they should be, how many, and for what purpose, as I have already mentioned: for without necessary magistrates, no state can exist, nor without those which contribute to its dignity and good order can exist happily: now it is necessary that in small states, the magistrates should be few; in a large one, many: also to know well what offices may be joined together, and what ought to be separated. The first thing necessary is to establish proper regulators in the markets; for which purpose a certain magistrate should be appointed to inspect their contracts and preserve good order; for of necessity, in almost every city there must be both buyers and sellers to supply each other's mutual wants: and this is what is most productive of the comforts of life; for the sake of which men seem to have joined together in one community. A second care, and nearly related to the first, is to have an eye both to the public and private edifices in the city, that they may be an ornament; and also to take care of all buildings which are likely to fall: and to see that the highways are kept in proper repair; and also that the landmarks between different estates are preserved, that there may be no disputes on that account; and all other business of the same nature. Now, this business may be divided into several branches, over each of which in populous cities they appoint a separate person; one to inspect the buildings, another the fountains, another the harbors; and they are called the inspectors of the city. A third, which is very like the last, and conversant nearly about the same objects, only in the country, is to take care of what is done out of the city. The officers who have this employment we call inspectors of the lands, or inspectors of the woods; but the business of all three of them is the same. There must also be other officers appointed to receive the public revenue and to deliver it out to those who are in the different departments of the state: these are called receivers or quaestors. There must also be another, before whom all private contracts and sentences of courts should be enrolled, as well as proceedings and declarations. Sometimes this employment is divided among many, but there is one supreme over the rest; these are called proctors, notaries, and the like. Next to these is an officer whose business is of all others the most necessary, and yet most difficult; namely, to take care that sentence is executed upon those who are condemned; and that everyone pays the fines laid on him; and also to have the charge of those who are in prison. [1322a] This office is very disagreeable on account of the odium attending it, so that no one will engage therein without it is made very profitable, or, if they do, will they be willing to execute it according to law; but it is most necessary, as it is of no service to pass judgment in any cause without that judgment is carried into execution: for without this, human society could not subsist: for which reason it is best that this office should not be executed by one person, but by some of the magistrates of the other courts. In like manner, the taking care that those fines which are ordered by the judges are levied should be divided among different persons. And as different magistrates judge different causes, let the causes of the young be heard by the young: and as to those which are already brought to a hearing, let one person pass sentence, and another see it executed: as, for instance, let the magistrates who have the care of the public buildings execute the sentence which the inspectors of the markets have passed, and the like in other cases: for by so much the less odium attends those who carry the laws into execution, by so much the easier will they be properly put in force: therefore for the same persons to pass the sentence and to execute it will subject them to general hatred; and if they pass it upon all, they will be considered as the enemies of all. Thus one person has often the custody of the prisoner's body, while another sees the sentence against him executed, as the eleven did at Athens: for which reason it is prudent to separate these offices, and to give great attention thereunto as equally necessary with anything we have already mentioned; for it will certainly happen that men of character will decline accepting this office, and worthless persons cannot properly be entrusted with it, as having themselves rather an occasion for a guard than being qualified to guard others. This, therefore, ought by no means to be a separate office from others; nor should it be continually allotted to any individuals, but the young men; where there is a city guard, the youths ought in turns to take these offices upon them. These, then, as the most necessary magistrates, ought to be first mentioned: next to these are others no less necessary, but of much higher rank, for they ought to be men of great skill and fidelity. These are they who have the guard of the city, and provide everything that is necessary for war; whose business it is, both in war and peace, to defend the walls and the gates, and to take care to muster and marshal the citizens. Over all these, there are sometimes more officers, sometimes fewer: thus, in little cities, there is only one whom they call either general or polemarch; but where there are horse and light-armed troops, and bowmen, and sailors, they sometimes put distinct commanders over each of these; who again have others under them, according to their different divisions; all of which join together to make one military body: and thus much for this department. Since some of the magistrates, if not all, have business with the public money, it is necessary that there should be other officers, whose employment should be nothing else than to take an account of what they have, and correct any mismanagement therein. But besides all these magistrates there is one who is supreme over them all, who very often has in his own power the disposal of the public revenue and taxes; who presides over the people when the supreme power is in them; for there must be some magistrate who has a power to summon them together, and to preside as head of the state. These are sometimes called preadvisers; but where there are many, more properly a council. These are nearly the civil magistrates which are requisite to a government: but there are other persons whose business is confined to religion; as the priests, and those who are to take care of the temples, that they are kept in proper repair, or, if they fall down, that they may be rebuilt; and whatever else belongs to public worship. This charge is sometimes entrusted to one person, as in very small cities: in others it is delegated to many, and these distinct from the priesthood, as the builders or keepers of holy places, and officers of the sacred revenue. Next to these are those who are appointed to have the general care of all those public sacrifices to the tutelar god of the state, which the laws do not entrust to the priests: and these in different states have different appellations. To enumerate in few words the different departments of all those magistrates who are necessary: these are either religion, war, taxes, expenditures, markets, public buildings, harbors, highways. Belonging to the courts of justice, there are scribes to enroll private contracts; and there must also be guards set over the prisoners, others to see the law is executed, council on either side, and also others to watch over the conduct of those who are to decide the causes. Among the magistrates also may finally be reckoned those who are to give their advice in public affairs. But separate states, who are peculiarly happy and have leisure to attend to more minute particulars, and are very attentive to good order, require particular magistrates for themselves; such as those who have the government of the women; who are to see the laws are executed; who take care of the boys and preside over their education. To these may be added those who have the care of their gymnastic exercises, [1323a] their theatres, and every other public spectacle which there may happen to be. Some of these, however, are not of general use; as the governors of the women: for the poor are obliged to employ their wives and children in servile offices for want of slaves. As there are three magistrates to whom some states entrust the supreme power; namely, guardians of the laws, preadvisers, and senators; guardians of the laws suit best to an aristocracy, preadvisers to an oligarchy, and a senate to a democracy. And thus much briefly concerning all magistrates.

ARISTOTLE was an Ancient Greek philosopher who studied at Plato's Academy in Athens for 20 years. After, he was called to be the tutor Alexander the Great. Later in life he Aristotle founded the Lyceum, where he spent most of the rest of his life studying, teaching, and writing. He is often considered one of the greatest political, psychological, and ethical thinkers in human history. Some of his most notable works include *Nichomachean Ethics*, *Politics*, *Metaphysics*, *Poetics*, and *Prior Analytics*. In *Politics*, Aristotle examined society and government as it related to human nature. He believed the purpose of government was to help citizens create the conditions by which they could achieve virtue and happiness.

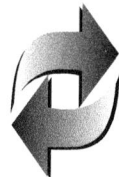

EXPLORING THE ISSUE

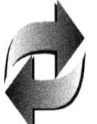

Did the Founding Fathers Create a Democratic System that Would Adequately Attend to the Problems of a Democracy?

Critical Thinking and Reflection

1. What is the essential nature of a democracy and do we have one?
2. Did Madison's approach to democracy adequately attend to the problems in a democracy?
3. Would Aristotle's visions for democracy work in modern US society?
4. What structures do you believe are vital for an authentic democracy?

Is There Common Ground?

On one hand, a functioning democracy requires an educated public, but on the other hand, can an educated public exist on the scale that the United States would require? Does this mean that the wealthy should be the only ones with political power and the middle class educated should be its stewards and managers? In other words, what is the responsibility of those who are educated, but who are not opulently wealthy? At what point do the middle class side with the poor and not the wealthy? Should a democracy focus on systems that perpetuate those things that the educated believe to be in the best interest of the people or are they beholden to the will of the people themselves? There is no doubt that the government currently functions as an arm of big business and that economic interests are maintained to ensure that capitalism works for those who already have capital. This systemic oppression has come at the detriment of the common man, but it has ensured that the United States has maintained its place atop the economic hierarchy. We can historically examine ways propaganda has caused citizens to betray their own interests and discard democratic conditions, though this type of targeted rhetoric is now more commonplace than ever in news programs where opinion and fact are comingled into a distracted a polarizing narrative. Like most democratic systems The Fourth Estate is also a tool of power rather that a tool for informing a democratic public. News systems are funded by clicks that are paid for by big business. Advertising dollars ensure news will be generally favorable to those paying for the programs. Subsequently, news aligns with business, existing systems, and existing power (Herman & Chomsky, 2002).

What is clear is that democracy must constantly be remade so the will of the people can exist. Both of these authors realize that democracy is a delicate thing—challenging to steward. The differences in the views of these authors likely speak to their unique purpose and context. Aristotle was writing about different types of democracies that did exist and might exist. He was conserved with describing a democratic ideal. Conversely, Madison was concerned with the actual establishment of a new democratic society after a revolution—a practical democracy (a republic). Both men lived in pseudoequitable societies that were faced with the question of citizenship. What does it mean to be a citizen, what are the rights of a citizen, and what are the responsibilities of a citizen? In Athens, democratic rights were afforded all citizens; however, citizenship meant that one was male and owned land. Similarly, in the young United States, the founding fathers were concerned with ensuring the government would help maintain the wealth of the ruling class. Where one falls on this issue represents the ways they understand the nature of democracy.

Additional Resources

Blaug, R. (Ed.). (2016). *Democracy: A reader*. Edinburgh: Edinburgh University Press.

Chomsky, N. (1977). The carter administration: Myth and reality. *Australian Left Review, 1*(62), 1–20.

Crick, B. (2002). *Democracy: A very short introduction*. Oxford: Oxford Paperbacks.

Internet References . . .

Democracy: US Department of State

https://www.state.gov/j/drl/democ/

Pembroke High School Primary Source Blog. "Democracy in America"

http://us1primarysources.blogspot.com/2009/08/in-america.html

Pew Research Center: Trust, Facts, and Democracy

http://www.people-press.org/2018/04/26/the-public-the-political-system-and-american-democracy/

Primary Documents in American History

https://www.loc.gov/rr/program/bib/ourdocs/index.html

The Power Cube

http://www.powercube.net/

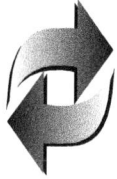

ISSUE

Selected, Edited, and with Issue Framing Material by:
Kevin R. Magill and Tony L. Talbert, *Baylor University*

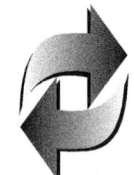

Was the Second Amendment Designed to Protect an Individual's Right to Own Guns?

YES: William W. Van Alstyne, from "The Second Amendment and the Personal Right to Arms," *Duke Law Journal* (1994)

NO: Lawrence Delbert Cress, from "A Well-Regulated Militia: The Origins and Meaning of the Second Amendment," Library of Virginia (1987)

Learning Outcomes

After reading this issue, you will be able to:

- Describe the historic and legal precedents of British common law that influenced the development and application of the Second Amendment of the U.S. Constitution.
- Understand the theoretical and applied roles of an individual's and state militia's access to guns during the pre-during-post Revolutionary War era in relationship to gun access during the late 20th and early 21st centuries.
- Compare and contrast the foundational arguments posited by legal scholars regarding the conflicting interpretations of the language of the Second Amendment to the U.S. Constitution.
- Research and discuss primary and secondary sources that address the philosophical, historical, legal, political, and social issues regarding the preservation and revision of the Second Amendment to the U.S. Constitution.

ISSUE SUMMARY

YES: William W. Van Alstyne contends that those who adhere to the belief that the Second Amendment to the U.S. Constitution protects an individual's right to own firearms is as historically and legally secure as those liberties guaranteed to individuals within the First Amendment to the U.S. Constitution. Van Alstyne therefore asserts that judicial and legislative mechanisms of interpretation of Second Amendment liberties have been put in place and to date those interpretations lean toward the protection of individual rights to gun ownership.

NO: Lawrence Delbert Cress suggests that a the Second Amendment refers to gun ownership for only to those participating in the "well-regulated militia," whose job it was to protect citizens from a tyrannical national government and other domestic incursions.

"A well regulated Militia, being necessary to the security of a free State, the right of the people to keep and bear Arms, shall not be infringed."—Amendment II, United States Constitution.

Twenty-seven words have been the source of legal and political debate and the impetus for philosophical divides among foes and friends for well over two centuries in America. The contemporary controversy over the interpretation of the Second Amendment of the U.S. Constitution is seemingly as bifurcated as the two dominant political parties in 21st century U.S. politics. Opponents of gun control believe that the section of the Second Amendment which states "the right of the people to keep and bear arms" means that individuals have a right to own guns without interference from the national government.

In contrast, supporters of gun control believe that the Second Amendment permits gun ownership only if you are a member of "a well-regulated militia."

So, whose interpretation of the Founder's intent in penning and adopting these twenty-seven words is most accurate? According to William W. Van Alstyne ". . . no provision in in the Constitution causes one to stumble quite so much on a first reading, or second, or third reading as this short provision in the Second Amendment of the Bill of Rights" (Van Alstyne, 1994). Although Lawrence Delbert Cress offers a different interpretation of the Second Amendment than Van Alstyne, he too concurs "we know little about the Second Amendment's reception in the States" during the 18th Century (Cress, 1984). There's no doubt that perspectives on gun access and ownership are complex when comparing 21st to 18th century societal realities. More so when comparing and contrasting recent United States Supreme Court decisions that have unsettled centuries of legal precedent by seemingly elevating the right individual ownership of guns (i.e., District of Columbia v. Heller, 554 U.S. 570, 2008; McDonald v. City of Chicago, 561 U.S. 3025, 2010) over the right of the state to regulate gun ownership (United States v. Cruikshank, 92 U.S. 542, 1875; Presser v. Illinois, 116 U.S. 252 1886; Miller v. Texas, 153 U.S./535/535, 894; Robertson v. Baldwin, 165 U.S. 275, 1897; United States v. Miller, 307 U.S. 174, 1939). Although the interpretation of Second Amendment liberties, protections, and restrictions is as complex as those found in any of the other twenty-five amendments to the U.S. Constitution, the arguments presented within this issue are offered within the confines of the two camps that have seemingly coalesced around individual vs. militia intent found within the ambiguity of the twenty-seven words that comprise this most contentious of amendments.

L. D. Cress provides a detailed description of 18th century American colonies' deliberate formation and implementation of militia organizations for the purpose of maintaining civil order and general protection of the welfare of all. Cress clearly articulates that when a crisis occurred, the part-time citizen-soldiers who formed the regulated militia would gather their arms and protect their respective communities and colonies from external and internal threats. Philosophically, the militia drew upon the heritage of the English political philosophers who argued that it was the virtuous yeoman farmers who formed militia units to protect themselves against a tyrannical king. Although the militias were militarily ineffective (e.g. George Washington and other military leaders were highly critical of the state units and formed a national army which was responsible for the major military victories at Saratoga and Yorktown), these citizen soldier militias were called into service prior to, during, and even after the Revolutionary War for the purpose of addressing domestic and international threats.

The Articles of Confederation, the first national government, was severely limited in its powers as evidenced by the formation of the 13 separate state governments, all maintaining significant control of their own societal and governmental interests. Amidst the formation and implementation of individual state governments as aligned with a central government, the influx of issues regarding taxation, regulation of commerce and trade, and engagement with foreign governments and corporate entities were matters of dispute among the competing individual state interests. However, as Cress notes, there seemed to be no significant disagreement among the state governments that a militia organized and maintained by the state was essential. Cress asserts, that in the 18th century, citizenship, which was defined in part by militia service. "No one argued that the individual had a right to bear arms outside the ranks of the militia. To the contrary, bearing arms outside the framework of the established militia structure immediately provoked fears for the constitutional stability of the Republic" (Cress, 1984).

Although Cress' assertion that there seemed to be little disagreement among the society at-large regarding the philosophical and operational role guns would play within the debate of individual liberties vs. collective governance William W. Van Alstyne offers a significant challenge to this notion based upon the 18th century, as well as the 21st century, debate among the general public about the merits and weaknesses of a decentralized vs. centralized government. While operationally speaking, this matter has largely been resolved by the existence of a large and powerful centralized United States government, the philosophical divides that defined the positions of the 18th century Federalists (i.e., nationalists) and the Antifederalists (i.e., localists) continue to be unresolved within the 21st century positions of Democrats and Republicans.

Van Alstyne frames his challenge to Cress' position based upon the historic and legal evidence of the Framer's intent when penning and proposing the Bill of Rights. The ratification of the new U.S. Constitution would not take place until a Virginia styled "declaration of rights" be incorporated for the purpose of protecting both states' powers and individuals' liberties from the potential hubris, if not tyranny, of a large centralized national government. It is within this historic context that W. W. Van Alstyne frames his argument contending that there is more evidence than not that the intent of the language found in the Second Amendment to the U.S. Constitution was and is to assert the philosophical and operational belief in the power of the individual over the state through the free exercise of individual liberties guaranteed by the U.S. Constitution. Van Alstyne posits, "Just as the Second Amendment declares that 'the right of the people to keep and bear Arms shall not be infringed' so, too the Fourth Amendment declares 'The right of the people to be secure in their persons, houses, papers, and effects, against unreasonable searches and seizures, shall not be violated. Here, in the familiar setting we are not at all confused in our take on the meaning" (Van Alstyne, 1994).

Van Alstyne's fundamental argument that the intent of the Framers of the U.S. Constitution and the understanding of a large contingent of the Anti-Federalist Founders and thus their constituencies residing in the individual states they represented was to promote and secure individual liberties. Van Alstyne's argument extends to evidence found in the language of the First, Sixth, and Seventh Amendments to the U.S. Constitution that clearly points to the Framers intent that "a right of the people to keep and bear Arms would make sense standing alone . . . even if it necessarily left some questions still to be settled" (Van Alstyne, 1994). Van Alstyne simply states, "That each of these rights—that all of these rights—are examples of personal rights protected by the Bill of Rights seems perfectly clear" (Van Alstyne, 1994).

While the structural nature of this text offers dueling positions on historical topics, like most complex issues, the "right to keep and bear Arms" cannot be considered from a singularly historical lens. Instead, bifocal, trifocal, and perhaps even a kaleidoscope of lens must be applied when attempting to sort out the notion of "Framers intent." For example, David Hemingway's book *Private Guns, Public Health* (2006) confronts the issue from a public health policy position as he argues that the high cost of gun deaths and injuries caused by firearms should not be tolerated by policy makers or the general public. Hemingway's well-developed and sensible arguments calling for a significant restriction on not only individual gun ownership but also gun manufacturing challenges the reader to embrace a social consciousness position that advocates for an evolving interpretation of the Second Amendment based in the contemporary context for the well-being of individuals and the society at-large. A contrasting lens is offered by Sanford Levinson whose seminal article "The Embarrassing Second Amendment," *Yale Law Journal* (vol. 99, December 1989) applies a legal lens that asserts the Second Amendment guarantees the individual's right of gun ownership. Levinson's application of the so-called "Standard Model" or "Originalist" interpretive lens contends that the most important precedent in determining contemporary policies and practices regarding the Second Amendment must always be consistent with the original when determining intent and application.

And here we are some 227 years since these 27 words that comprise the Second Amendment were ratified and still the shrill debate that historical, legal, public health, and a multitude of other scholars and practitioners have attempted to address rages on. What are we to do now that we find ourselves at this crossroads yet again? Perhaps, the answer exist explicitly and implicitly among the primary and secondary sources that students of history are called upon to continually examine in the quest for answers to the most pernicious and puzzling questions that comprise our human narrative.

YES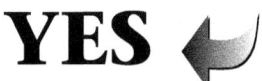

William W. Van Alstyne

The Second Amendment and the Personal Right to Arms

INTRODUCTION

Perhaps no provision in the Constitution causes one to stumble quite so much on a first reading, or second, or third reading, as the short provision in the Second Amendment of the Bill of Rights. No doubt this stumbling occurs because, despite the brevity of this amendment, as one reads, there is an apparent non sequitur—or disconnection of a sort—in midsentence. The amendment opens with a recitation about a need for "[a] well regulated Militia."[1] But having stipulated to the need for "[a] well regulated Militia," the amendment then declares that the right secured by the amendment—the described right that is to be free of "infringement"—is not (or not just) the right of a state, or of the United States, to provide a well regulated militia. Rather, it is "the right of the people to keep and bear Arms."

A well regulated Militia, being necessary to the security of a free State, the right of the people to keep and bear Arms, shall not be infringed.[2]

The postulation of a "right of the people to keep and bear Arms" would make sense standing alone, however, even if it necessarily left some questions still to be settled.[3] It would make sense in just the same unforced way we understand even upon a first reading of the neighboring clause in the Bill of Rights, which uses the exact same phrase in describing something as "the right of the people" that "shall not be violated" (or "infringed"). Just as the Second Amendment declares that "the right of the people to keep and bear Arms[] shall not be infringed." so, too, the Fourth Amendment declares:

> The right of the people to be secure in their persons, houses, papers, and effects, against unreasonable searches and seizures, shall not be violated. . . .[4]

Here, in the familiar setting of the Fourth Amendment, we are not at all confused in our take on the meaning of the amendment; it secures to each of us personally (as well as to all of us collectively) a certain right—even if we are also uncertain of its scope.[5] Nor are we confused in turning to other clauses. For example, the Sixth Amendment provides:

> In all criminal prosecutions, the accused shall enjoy the right to a speedy and public trial. . . .[6]

And so, too, the Seventh Amendment provides:

> In Suits at common law, where the value in controversy shall exceed twenty dollars, the right of trial by jury shall be preserved. . . .[7]

That each of these rights—that all of these rights—are examples of personal rights protected by the Bill of Rights seems perfectly clear. And, were it not for the opening clause in the Second Amendment, though there would still be much to thrash out, it is altogether likely the Second Amendment would be taken in the same way.

To be sure, as we have already once noted, were the Second Amendment taken in just this way, the scope of the right that *is* protected (namely, the right to keep and bear arms) would still remain to be defined.[8] But by itself, that sort of definitional determination would be of no unusual difficulty. For so much is true with respect to every right secured from government infringement, whether it be each person's freedom of speech (that freedom is not unbounded, either) or any other right specifically protected from infringement elsewhere in the Bill of Rights.[9] And in addressing this type of (merely general) problem, neither has the Supreme Court nor have other courts found it intractable and certainly none of these other clauses have been disparaged, much less have they been ignored. To the contrary, with respect to each, a strong, supportive case law has developed in the courts, albeit case law that has developed gradually, over quite a long time.

† William R. and Thomas L. Perkins Professor of Law, Duke University School of Law.

Van Alstyne, William W. "The Second Amendment and the Personal Right to Arms," *Duke Law Journal*, April 1994, pages 1236–1255. Copyright ©1994 by William Van Alstyne. Used with permission of the author.

In startling contrast, during this same time, however, the Second Amendment has generated almost no useful body of law. Indeed, it is substantially accurate to say that the useful case law of the Second Amendment, even in 1994, is mostly just missing in action. In its place, what we have is roughly of the same scanty and utterly underdeveloped nature[10] as was characteristic of the equally scanty and equally underdeveloped case law (such as it then was) of the First Amenament in 1904, as of which date there was still to issue from the Supreme Court a single decision establishing the First Amendment as an amendment of any genuine importance at all.[11] In short, what was true of the First Amendment as of 1904 remains true of the Second Amendment even now.

The reason for this failure of useful modem case law, moreover, is not that there has been no occasion to develop such law. So much is true only of the Third Amendment.[12] In contrast, it is no more true of the Second Amendment than of the First Amendment or the Fourth Amendment that we have lacked for appropriate occasions to join issue on these questions. The tendency in the twentieth century (though not earlier) of the federal government has been ever increasingly to tax, ever more greatly to regulate, and ever more substantially to prohibit various kinds of personal gun ownership and use.[13] This tendency, that is, is at least as commonplace as it was once equally the heavy tendency to tax, to regulate, and too often also to prohibit, various kinds of speech. The main reason there is such a vacuum of useful Second Amendment understanding, rather, is the arrested jurisprudence of the subject as such, a condition due substantially to the Supreme Court's own inertia—the same inertia that similarly afflicted the First Amendment virtually until the third decade of this twentieth century when Holmes and Brande is finally were moved personally to take the First Amendment seriously[14] (as previously it scarcely ever was).

With respect to the larger number of state and local regulations (many of these go far beyond the federal regulations), moreover, the case law of the Second Amendment is even more arrested; and this for the reason that the Supreme Court has simply declined to reconsider its otherwise discarded nineteenth-century decisions—decisions holding that the Fourteenth Amendment enacted little protection of anything, and none (i.e., *no* protection) drawn from the Bill of Rights.[15]

To trust to this arrested treatment of the Second Amendment—and of the Fourteenth Amendment—in 1994, in short, is as though one were inclined so to trust to the arrested treatment of the First Amendment in 1904. The difficulty in such a starting place is perfectly plain. No convincing jurisprudence is itself really possible under such circumstances. In the case of the First Amendment, we know quite well that such a jurisprudence effectively became possible only rather late, in the 1920s (but, one may add, better late than never). In the case of the Second Amendment, in an elementary sense, that jurisprudence is even now not possible until something more in the case law of the Second Amendment begins finally to fall into place. That "something more," I think, requires one to consider what one might be more willing to think about in the following way—that *perhaps the NRA is not wrong, after all, in its general Second Amendment stance*—a stance we turn here briefly to review.

I

The stance of those inclined to take the Second Amendment seriously reverts to the place we ourselves thought to be somewhat worthwhile to consult—namely, the express provisions of the Second Amendment—and it offers a series of suggestions fitting the respective clauses the amendment contains. Here is how these several propositions run:

1. The reference to a "well regulated *Militia*" is in the first as well as the last instance a reference to the ordinary citizenry. It is not at all a reference to regular armed soldiers as members of some standing army.[16] And quite obviously, neither is it a reference merely to the state or to the local police.

2. The very assumption of the clause, moreover, is that ordinary citizens (rather than merely soldiers, or merely the police) *may* themselves possess arms, for it is from these ordinary citizens who as citizens have a right to keep and bear arms (as the second clause provides) that such well regulated militia as a state may provide for, is itself to be drawn.

3. Indeed, it is more than merely an "assumption," however, precisely because "the right of the people to keep and bear Arms" is itself stipulated in the second clause. It is *this* right that is expressly identified as *"the* right" that is not to be *("shall not be")* infringed. That right is made the express guarantee of the clause.[17] There is thus no room left for a claim that, despite this language, the amendment actually means to reserve to Congress some power to contradict its very terms (e.g., that "the Congress may, if it thinks it proper, forbid the people to keep and bear arms to such extent Congress sees fit to do").[18]

4. Nor is there any basis so to read the Second Amendment as though it said anything like the following: "Congress may, if it thinks it proper,

forbid the people to keep and bear arms if, notwithstanding that these restrictions it may thus enact are inconsistent with the right of the people to keep and bear arms, they are not inconsistent with the right of each state to maintain some kind of militia as it may deem necessary to its security as a free state."[19]

Rather, the Second Amendment adheres to the guarantee of the right of the people to keep and bear arms as the predicate for the other provision to which it speaks, i.e., the provision respecting a militia, as distinct from a standing army separately subject to congressional regulation and control. Specifically, it looks to an ultimate reliance on the common citizen who has a right to keep and bear arms rather than only to some standing army, or only to some other politically separated, defined, and detached armed cadre, as an essential source of security of a free state.[20] In relating these propositions within one amendment, moreover, it does not disparage, much less does it subordinate, "the right of the people to keep and bear arms." To the contrary, it expressly *embraces* that right and indeed it erects the very scaffolding of a free state upon *that* guarantee. *It derives its definition of a well-regulated militia in just this way for a "free State"*: The militia to be well-regulated is a militia to be drawn from just such people (i.e., people with a right to keep and bear arms) rather than from some other source (i.e., from people without rights to keep and bear arms).

II

There is, to be sure, in the Second Amendment, an express reference to the security of a "free State."[21] It is not a reference to *the* security of THE STATE.[22] There are doubtless certain national constitutions that put a privileged emphasis on the security of "the state," but such as they are, they are all *unlike* our Constitution and the provisions they have respecting their security do not appear in a similarly phrased Bill of Rights. Accordingly, such constitutions make no reference to any right of the people to keep and bear arms, apart from state service.[23] And why do they not do so? Because, in contrast with the premises of constitutional government in this country, they reflect the belief that recognition of any such right "in the people" might well pose a threat to the security of "the state." In the view of these different constitutions, it is commonplace to find that no one within the state other than its own authorized personnel has any right to keep and bear arms[24]—a view emphatically rejected, rather than embraced, however, by the Second Amendment to the Constitution of the United States.

This rather fundamental difference among kinds of government was noted by James Madison in *The Federalist Papers,* even prior to the subsequent assurance expressly furnished by the Second Amendment in new and concrete terms. Thus, in *The Federalist* No. 46, Madison contrasted the "advantage . . . the Americans possess" (under the proposed constitution) with the circumstances in "several kingdoms of Europe . . . [where] the governments are afraid to trust the people with arms."[25] Here, in contrast, as Madison noted, they were, and no provision was entertained to empower Congress to abridge or to violate that trust, any more than, as Alexander Hamilton noted, there was any power proposed to enable government to abridge the freedom of the press.[26]

To be sure, in the course of the ratification debates, doubts were expressed respecting the adequacy of this kind of assurance (i.e., the assurance that no power was affirmatively proposed for Congress to provide any colorable claim of authority to take away or to abridge these rights of freedom of the press and of the right of the people to keep and bear arms).[27] And the quick resolve to add the Second Amendment, so to confirm that right more expressly, as not subject to infringement by Congress, is not difficult to understand.

The original constitutional provisions regarding the militia[28] placed major new powers in Congress beyond those previously conferred by the Articles of Confederation. These new powers not only included a wholly new power to provide for a regular, standing, national army even in peacetime,[29] but also powers for "calling forth the Militia,"[30] for "*organizing, arming, and disciplining*, the Militia,"[31] and for "governing such Part of them as may be employed in the Service of the United States."[32] Indeed, all that was *expressly* reserved from Congress's reach was "the Appointment of the officers" of this citizen militia, for even "the Authority of training the Militia," though reserved in the first instance from Congress, was itself subordinate to Congress in the important sense that such training was to be "according to the discipline prescribed by *Congress.*"[33]

These provisions were at once highly controversial, respecting their scope and possible implications of congressional power. In attempting to counter anti-ratification objections to the proposed constitution—objections that these lodgments of powers would concentrate excessive power in Congress in derogation of the rights of the people—Hamilton and Madison argued essentially three points:[34] (a) the appointment of militia officers was exclusively committed to state hands;[35] (b) the localized civilian-citizen nature of the militia would secure its loyalty to the rights of the people;[36] and (c) the people otherwise possessed a right to keep and bear arms—which right Congress was given no power whatever to regulate or to forbid.[37] And, as to the argument that the plan was defective insofar as it left the protection of the rights of the people insecure because no *express* prohibition on Congress was *separately* provided in respect to those rights (rather, the powerlessness of Congress to infringe them was solely a deduction from the doctrine of enumerated powers alone), Hamilton insisted that to specify anything further—to provide an *express* listing of particular prohibitions on Congress—was not only unnecessary but itself would be deeply problematic, because the implication of such a list would be that anything not named in the list might somehow be thought therefore in fact to be subject to regulation or prohibition by Congress though no enumerated power to affect any such subject was provided by the Constitution itself.[38] In brief, Hamilton maintained that to do anything in the nature of adding a Bill of Rights would cast doubt upon the doctrine of enumerated powers itself.

These several explanations were deemed insufficient, however, and to meet the objections of those in the state ratifying conventions unwilling to leave the protection of certain rights to mere inference from the doctrine of enumerated powers, objections raised in the course of several state ratification debates, the Bill of Rights, vas promptly produced by Madison, in the first Congress to assemble under the new Constitution, in 1789. Accordingly, as with "the freedom of the press," the protection of "the right of the people to keep and bear arms" was thus made *doubly* secure in the Bill of Rights.[39] Thomas Cooley quite accurately recapitulated the controlling circumstances in the leading nineteenth century treatise on constitutional law:

> The [Second] [A]mendment, like most other provisions in the Constitution, has a history. It was adopted with some modification and enlargement from the English Bill of Rights of 1688, where it stood as a protest against arbitrary action of the overturned dynasty in disarming the people, and as a pledge of the new rulers that this tyrannical action should cease. . . .
>
> *The Right is General.* . . . The meaning of the provision undoubtedly is, that the people, from whom the militia must be taken, shall have the right to keep and bear arms; and they need no permission or regulation of law for the purpose.[40]

Cooley's reference to English history, moreover, in illuminating the Second Amendment right (as personal to the citizen as such), is useful as well. For in this, he merely followed William Blackstone, from Blackstone's general treatise from 1765.

In chapter 1, appropriately captioned "Of The Rights of Persons," Blackstone divided what he called natural personal rights into two kinds: "primary" and "auxiliary."[41] The distinction was between those natural rights primary to each person intrinsically and those inseparable from their protection (thus themselves indispensable, "auxiliary" personal rights). Of the first kind, generically, are "the free enjoyment of personal security, of personal liberty, and of private property."[42] Of the latter are rights possessed "to vindicate" one's primary rights; and among these latter, Blackstone listed such things as access to "courts of law," and, so, too, "the right of petition[]," and *"the right of having and using arms for self-preservation and defence."*[43]

In contrast with all of this, the quite different view—the view of "the secure state" we were earlier considering—of countries *different* from the United States—assumes no right of the people to keep and bear arms. Rather, these differently constituted states put their own first stress on having a well regulated army (and also, of course, an internal state police). To be sure, such states also may provide for some kind of militia, but insofar as they may (and several do),[44] one can be quite certain that it will *not* be a militia drawn from the people with a "right to keep and bear Arms." For in these kinds of states, there is assuredly no such right. To the contrary, such a state is altogether likely to forbid the people to keep and bear arms unless and until they are conscripted into the militia, after which—to whatever extent they are deemed suitably "trustworthy" by the state—they might then (and only then) have arms fit for some assigned task.

But, again, the point to be made here is that the Second Amendment represented not an adoption, but a rejection, of this vision—a vision of the security state. It did not concede to any such state. Rather, it speaks to sources of security within a free state, within which (to quote the amendment itself still again) *"the right of the people to keep and bear Arms[] shall not be infringed."* The precautionary text of the amendment refutes the notion that the "well regulated Militia" the amendment contemplates is somehow a militia drawn from a people "who have no right to keep and bear arms." Rather, the opposite is what the amendment enacts.[45]

III

The Second Amendment of course does not assume that the right of the people to keep and bear arms will not be abused. Nor is the amendment insensible to the *many* forms which such abuses may take (e.g., as in robbing banks, in settling personal disputes, or in threatening varieties of force to secure one's will). But the Second Amendment's answer to the avoidance of abuse is to support such laws as are directed to those who threaten or demonstrate such abuse and to no one else. Accordingly, those who do neither—who neither commit crimes nor threaten such crimes—are entitled to be left alone.

To put the matter most simply, the governing principle here, in the Second Amendment, is not different from the same principle governing the First Amendment's provisions on freedom of speech and the freedom of the press. A person may be held to account for an abuse of that freedom (for example, by being held liable for using it to publish false claims with respect to the nutritional value of the food offered for public sale and consumption). Yet, no one today contends that just because the publication of such false statements is a danger one might in some measure reduce if, say, *licenses* also could be required as a condition of owning a newspaper or even a mimeograph machine, that therefore licensing can be made a requirement of owning either a newspaper or a mimeograph machine.[46]

The Second Amendment, like the First Amendment, is thus not mysterious. Nor is it equivocal. Least of all is it opaque. Rather, one may say, today it is simply unwelcome in any community that wants no one (save perhaps the police?) to keep or bear arms at all. But assuming it to be so, i.e., assuming this is how some now want matters to be, it is for them to seek a repeal of this amendment (and so the repeal of its guarantee), in order to have their way. Or so the Constitution itself assuredly appears to require, if that is the way things are to be.

IV

In the first instance, enacted as it was as part of the original Bill of Rights of 1791, the Second Amendment merely was addressed to Congress and not to the states. The mistrust and uncertainty of how *Congress* might presume to construe its new powers—powers newly enumerated in Article I of the Constitution—resulted in the Bill of Rights inclusive of the Second Amendment, proposed in the very first session of the new Congress in 1789. As it was then apprehended that although Congress was never given any power to preempt state constitutional provisions respecting freedom of speech or of the press, Congress might nonetheless presume to regulate those subjects to its own liking under pretext of some other authority if not barred from doing so by amendment, the Second Amendment—and the other amendments composing the original Bill of Rights—reflected the same mistrust and were adopted for the same reason as well. But, to be sure, neither the First nor the Second Amendment,[47] nor any of the other amendments in the Bill of Rights were addressed as limits on the states.[48]

In 1866, however, this original constitutional toleration of state differences with respect to their internal treatment of these rights came to an end, in the aftermath of the Civil War. The immunities of citizens with respect to rights previously secured only from abridging acts of Congress were recast in the Fourteenth Amendment as immunities secured also from any similar act by any state.[49] It was precisely in this manner that the citizen's right to keep and bear arms, formerly protected only from acts of Congress, came to be equally protected from abridging acts of the states as well.

So, in reporting the Fourteenth Amendment to the Senate on behalf of the Joint Committee on Reconstruction in 1866, Senator Jacob Meritt Howard of Michigan began by detailing the "first section" of that amendment, i.e., the section that "relates to the privileges and immunities of citizens."[50] He explained that the first clause of the amendment (the "first section"), once approved and ratified, would "restrain the power of the States"[51] even as Congress was already restrained (by the Bill of Rights) from abridging

> the personal rights guaranteed and secured by the first eight amendments of the Constitution; such as the freedom of speech and of the press; the right of the people peaceably to assemble and petition the Government for a redress of grievances, a right appertaining to each and all the people; *the right to keep and to bear arms;* the right to be exempted from the quartering of soldiers in a house without the consent of the owner; the right to be exempt from unreasonable searches and seizures[; etc., through the Eighth Amendment].[52]

In the end, Senator Howard concluded his remarks as follows:*"The great object of the first section of this amendment is, therefore, to restrain the power of the States and compel them at all times to respect these great fundamental guarantees."*[53] There was no dissent from this description of the clause.

Following ratification of the Fourteenth Amendment, therefore, some state constitutions might presume to provide even *more* protection of these same rights than the Fourteenth Amendment (and some continue even now to do so[54]), but none could thereafter presume to provide any less—whether the object of regulation was freedom of speech and of the press or of the personal right to arms. And it is quite clear that in the ratification debates of the Fourteenth Amendment, no distinction whatever was drawn between the "privileges and immunities" Congress was understood already to be bound to respect (pursuant to the Bill of Rights) and those now uniformly also to bind the states. Each was given the same constitutional immunity from abridging acts of state government as each was already recognized to possess from abridgment by Congress. What was previously forbidden only to Congress to do was, by the passage of the Fourteenth Amendment, made equally forbidden to any state. Moreover, the point was acknowledged to be particularly important in settling the Second Amendment right as a citizen's personal right, i.e., personal to each citizen as such.[55]

V

Again, however, one does not derive from these observations that each citizen has an uncircumscribable personal constitutional right to acquire, to own, and to employ any and all such arms as one might desire so to do, or necessarily to carry them into any place one might wish. To the contrary, restrictions generally consistent merely with safe usage, for example, or restrictions even of a particular "Arms" kind, are not all per se precluded by the two constitutional amendments and provisions we have briefly reviewed. There is a "rule of reason" applicable to the First Amendment, for example, and its equivalent will also be pertinent here. It is not the case that one may say whatever one wants and however one wants, wherever one wants, and whenever one likes—location, time, and associated circumstances do make a difference, consistent even with a very strong view of the freedom of speech and press accurately reflected in conscientious decisions of the Supreme Court. The freedoms of speech and of the press, it has been correctly said, are not absolute.

Neither is one's right to keep and bear arms absolute. It may fairly be questionable, for example, whether the type of arms one may have a "right to keep" consistent with the Second Amendment extend to a howitzer.[56] It may likewise be questionable whether the "arms" one *does* have a "right to keep" are necessarily arms one also may presume to "bear" wherever one wants, e.g., in courtrooms or in public schools. To be sure, each kind of example one might give will raise its own kind of question. And serious people are quite willing to confront serious problems in regulating "the right to keep and bear arms," as they are equally willing to confront serious problems in regulating "the freedom of speech and of the press."[57]

The difference between these serious people and others, however, was a large difference in the very beginning of this country and it remains as a large difference in the end. The difference is that such serious people begin with a constitutional understanding that declines to trivialize the Second Amendment or the Fourteenth Amendment, just as they likewise decline to trivialize any other right expressly identified elsewhere in the Bill of Rights. It is difficult to see why they are less than entirely right in this unremarkable view. That it has taken the NRA to speak for them, with respect to the Second Amendment, moreover, is merely interesting—perhaps far more as a comment on others, however, than on the NRA.

For the point to be made with respect to Congress and the Second Amendment[58] is that the essential claim (certainly not every claim—but the essential claim) advanced by the NRA with respect to the Second Amendment is extremely strong. Indeed, one may fairly declare, it is at least as well anchored in the Constitution in its own way as were the essential claims with respect to the First Amendment's protection of freedom of speech as first advanced on the Supreme Court by Holmes and Brandeis, seventy years ago.[59] And until the Supreme Court manages to express the central premise of the Second Amendment more fully and far more appropriately than it has done thus far, the constructive role of the NRA today, like the role of the ACLU in the 1920s with respect to the First Amendment (as it then was), ought itself not lightly to be dismissed.[60] Indeed, it is largely by the "unreasonable" persistence of just such organizations in this country that the Bill of Rights has endured.

Notes

1. The subject is that of "*A well regulated Militia*"—a militia the amendment declares to be "necessary to the security of a free State." U.S. CONST. amend. II. But it is hard to say on first reading whether the reference is to a well-regulated *national* militia or, instead, to a well-regulated *state* militia (i.e., a militia *in each state*). Perhaps, however, the reference is to both at once—a militia in each state, originally constituted under each state's authority, but subject to congressional authority to arm, to organize, and to make provision to call into national service, as a national militia. The possibility that this may be so tends to send one looking for other provisions in the Constitution that may help to clear this matter away. And a short search readily turns up several such provisions: Article I, section 8, clauses 15 and 16, and Article II, section 2, clause 1. *See infra* note 16.

2. U.S. CONST. amend. II.

3. For example, one might well still be uncertain of the breadth of the right to keep and bear arms (e.g., just what *kinds* of "Arms"?).

4. U.S. CONST. amend. IV.

5. For example, does the protection of "houses" and "effects" from unreasonable searches and seizures extend to trash one may have put outside in a garbage can? May it matter whether one has put the can itself outside one's garage or farther out, beside the street? *See* California v. Greenwood, 486 U.S. *35,* 37 (1988).

6. U.S. CONST. amend. VI.

7. *Id*. amend. VII.

8. For example, with respect to the kind of "Arms" one may have. Perhaps these include all arms as may be useful (though not exclusively so) as an incident of service in a militia—and indeed, this would make sense of the introductory portion of the amendment as well. *See* United States v. Miller, 307 U.S. 174, 178 (1939).

9. So, for example, though the Sixth Amendment provides a right to a *"speedy"* and *"public"* trial whenever one is accused of a (federal) crime, the amendment does not declare just *how* "speedy" the trial must be (i.e., exactly how soon following indictment the trial must be held) nor *how* "public" either (e.g., must it be televised to the world, or is an open courtroom, albeit with very limited seating, quite enough?). And the Fourth Amendment does not say there can be *no* searches and seizures—rather, only no "unreasonable" searches and seizures. Yet there is a very substantial body of highly developed case law that has given this genuine meaning and effect.

Likewise, when the Sixth and Seventh Amendments speak of the right to trial by "jury," then (even as is true of the Second Amendment in its reference to "Arms"?), though each of these amendments is silent as to what a jury means (a "jury" of how many people? a "jury" selected in what manner and by whom?), the provision means to be—and tends to be—given some real, some substantial, and some constitutionally significant effect. The point is, of course, that though there are questions of this sort with respect to *every* right furnished by the Bill of Rights, the expectation remains high that the right thus furnished will neither be ignored—treated as though it were not a right at all—nor so cynically misdefined or "qualified" in its ultimate description as to be reduced to an empty shell. It is only in the case of the Second Amendment that this is approximately the current state of the law. Indeed, it is only with respect to the Second Amendment that the current state of the law is roughly the same as was the state of the law with respect to the First Amendment's guarantees of freedom of speech and of the press as recently as 1904. As a restraint on the federal government, the First Amendment was deemed to be a restriction merely on certain kinds of prior restraint and hardly at all on what could be forbidden under threat of criminal sanction. *See, e.g.,* Patterson v. Colorado, 205 U.S. 454, 462 (1907). As to the states, the amendment was not known as necessarily furnishing any restraint at all. *See id.*

10. The most one can divine from the Supreme Court's scanty decisions ("scanty" is used advisedly-essentially there are only two) is that such right to keep and bear arms as may be secured by this amendment may extend to such "Arms" as would be serviceable within a militia but not otherwise (so a "sawed-off" shotgun may not qualify, though presumably-by *this* test-heavy duty automatic rifles assuredly would). *See* United States v. Miller, 307 U.S. 174, 178 (1939); *see also* Lewis v. United States, 445 U.S. 55, 65 n.8 (1980) (noting that legislative restrictions on the right of felons to possess firearms do not violate any constitutionally protected liberty); Robertson v. Baldwin, 165 U.S. 275, 282 (1897) (referring to "the right of the people to keep and bear Arms" as a personal right). These casual cases aside ("casual," because in *Miller,* for example, there was not even an appearance entered by the defendant-appellant in the Supreme Court), there are a few 19th-century decisions denying any relevance of the Second Amendment to the states: but these decisions, which have never been revisited by the Supreme Court, merely mimicked others of the same era in holding that *nope* of the rights or freedoms enumerated in the Bill of Rights were made applicable by the Fourteenth Amendment to the states. *See, e.g.,* Presser v. Illinois, 116 U.S. 252, 265 (1886) (citing United States v. Cruikshank, 92 U.S. 542. 553 (1875)). The shaky foundation of these cases ("shaky" because the effect was to eviscerate the Fourteenth Amendment itself) has long since been recognized—and long since repudiated by the Court in general. Notwithstanding, the lower

courts continue ritually to rely upon them, and the Supreme Court quite as regularly declines to find any suitable for review. *See, e.g.,* Quilici v. Village of Morton Grove, 695 F.2d 261, 269–70 (7th Cir. 1982) (holding that municipal handgun restrictions were constitutional), *cert. denied,* 464 U.S. 863 (1983). And why does one suppose that this is so?

11. *See supra* note 9.

12. Troops have not generally been quartered in private homes "in time of peace . . . without the consent of the Owner," nor even "in time of war," U.S. CONST. amend. III, for a very long time, and no Third Amendment case has ever been decided by the Supreme Court. Evidently, a Third Amendment case has arisen only once in a lower federal court. *See* Engblom v. Carey, 677 F.2d 957 (2d Cir. 1982) (holding that the Third Amendment protects the legitimate privacy interests of striking correction officers in keeping their housing from being used for quanering National Guard troops).

13. For a comprehensive review of congressional action since 1934, see United States v. Lopez. 2 F.3d 1342, 1348–60 (5th Cir. 1993).

14. *See, e.g.,* Whitney v. California, 274 U.S. 3S7. 372 (1927) (Brandeis and Holmes, JJ., concurring); Gitlow v. New York, 268 U.S. 652, 672 (1925) (Holmes and Brandeis, JJ., dissenting); United States *ex rel.* Milwaukee Social Democratic Publishing Co, v. Burleson, 255 U.S. 407, 417 (1921) (Holmes and Brandeis, JJ., dissenting); Abrams v. United States, 250 U.S. 616, 624 (1919) (Holmes and Brandeis, JJ., dissenting). *See generally* SAMUEL J. KONEFSKY, THE LEGACY OF HOLMES AND BRANDEIS 181–256 (1956) (reviewing the Holmes-Brandeis legacy of the First Amendment).

15. *See* Slaughter-House Cases, 83 U.S. (16 Wall.) 36 (1873); GERALD GUNTHER, CONSTITUTIONAL LAW 408-10 (12th ed. 1991). The *Slaughter-House Cases* denied that the Privileges and Immunities Clause of the Fourteenth Amendment extended any protection from the Bill of Rights against the states. Within three decades, however, the Court began the piecemeal abandonment of that position (albeit by relying on the Due Process Clause instead). *See* Chicago, B. & Q. R.R. v. Chicago, 166 U.S. 226 (1897) (applying the Fifth Amendment prohibition against the taking of private property for public use without just compensation and holding it to be equally a restraint against the states). In 1925, the Court proceeded in like fashion with respect to the Free Speech Clause of the First Amendment, *see Gitlow,* 268 U.S. at 666, and subsequently with respect to most of the rights enumerated in the Bill of Rights (exclusive, however, of the right to keep and bear arms). As already noted, the Court has declined to reexamine its 19th century cases (*Presser* and *Cruikshank*) that merely relied on the *Slaughter-House Cases* for their rationale. *Cf.* discussion *infra* Part IV.

16. Article I vests power in Congress "[t]o raise and support Armies," i.e., to provide for a national standing army as such, *see* U.S. CONST. art. I, § 8, cl. 12. It is pursuant to two different clauses that Congress is given certain powers with respect to the militia, such as the power "for *calling forth the Militia* to execute the Laws of the Union, suppress Insurrections and repel Invasions," *id.* cl. 15 (emphasis added), and the power "[t]o provide for organizing, arming, and disciplining, *tlie Militia,* and for governing such Part of them as may be employed in the Service of the United States, reserving to the States respectively, the Appointment of the Officers, and the Authority of *training lite Militia* according to the discipline prescribed by Congress," *id.* cl. 16 (emphasis added). So, too the description of the executive power carries over the distinction between the regular armed forces of the United States in a similar fashion. Accordingly, Article II, section 2 provides that "[t]he President shall be Commander in Chief of the Army and Navy of the United States, *and of the Militia* of the several States, when called into the actual Service of the United States," *Id.* art. II, § 2. cl. 1 (emphasis added).

17. And it is from the people, whose right this is, that such militia as the state may (as a free state) compose and regulate, shall be drawn—just as the amendment expressly declares.

18. Compare the utter incongruity of this suggestion with the actual provisions the Second Amendment enacts.

19. Compare this incompatible language and thought with the actual provisions of the amendment. Were the Second Amendment a mere federalism ("States' rights") provision, as it is not, it would assuredly appear in a place appropriate to that purpose (i.e., not in the same list with the First through the Eighth Amendments, but nearby the Tenth Amendment), and it would doubtless

reflect the same federalism style as the Tenth Amendment; for example, it might read: *"Congress shall make no law impairing the right of each state to maintain such well regulated militia as it may deem necessary to its security as a free state."* But it neither reads in any such fashion nor is it situated even to· imply such a thought. Instead. it is cast in terms that track the provisions in the neighboring personal rights clauses of the Bill of Rights. Just as the Fourth Amendment provides that *"[t]he right of the people to be secure in their persons, houses, papers, and effects. . . shall not be violated,"* U.S. CoNST. amend. IV (emphasis added), so, too, the Second Amendment matches that language and likewise provides that *"the right of the people to keep and bear Arms, shall not be infringed,"* id. amend. II (emphasis added); *see also* United States v. Verdugo-Urquidez, 494 U.S. 259, 265 (1990) ("The Second Amendment protects 'the right of the people to keep and bear Arms'. . . ."). In further response to the suggestion that the Second Amendment is a mere States' rights clause in analogy with the Tenth Amendment (by, e.g., Keith A. Ehrman & Dennis A. Henigan, *The Second Amendment in the Twentieth Century: Have You Seen Your Militia Lately?*, 15 U. DAYTON L REV. 5, 57 (1989)), see STEPHEN P. HALB OOK, THAT EVERY MAN BE ARMED: THE EVOLUTION OF A CONSTITUTIONAL RIGHT (1984). As Halbrook notes,

> In recent years it has been suggested that the Second Amendment protects the "collective" right of states to maintain militias, while it does not protect the right of "the people" to keep and bear arms. If anyone entertained this notion in the period during which the Constitution and Bill of Rights were debated and ratified, it remains one of the most closely guarded secrets of the eighteenth century, for *no known writing surviving from the period between 1787 and 1791 states such a thesis.*

Id. at 83 (emphasis added).

20. *See supra* note 16 and accompanying text.
21. U.S. CONST. amend. II (emphasis added). In James Madison's original draft of the amendment, moreover, the reference is to "a free country" (and not merely to "a free State"). *See* BERNARD ScHWARlZ, THE BILL OF RIGHTS: A DOCUMENTARY HISTORY 1026 (1971).
22. Once again, see the amendment and compare the difference in thought conveyed in these different wordings as they might appear, in contrast, in actual print.
23. *See, e.g.,* XIANFA (1982) [Constitution] art. 55. cl. 2 (P.R.C.), *translated in* THE CONSTITUTION OF THE PEOPLE'S REPUBLIC OF CHINA 41 (1983); *infra* note 44.
24. A position evidently preferred by many today in this country as well, with the apparent approval even of the ACLU. *See* AMERICAN CIVIL LIBERTIES UNION, POLICY GUIDE OF THE AMERICAN CIVIL LIBERTIES UNION 95 (1986) ("Except for lawful police and military purposes, the possession of weapons by individuals is not constitutionally protected.") It is quite beyond the scope of this brief Essay to attempt to account for the ACLU's stance—which may even now be undergoing some disagreement and internal review.
25. THE FEDERALIST No. 46, at 299 (James Madison) (Clinton Rossiter ed. 1961).
26. *Id*. No. 84 at 513–14 (Alexander Hamilton).
27. *See, e.g.,* Leonard W. Levy, *Bill of Rights (United States},* in 1 ENCYCLOPEDIA OF THE AMERICAN CONSTITUTION 113, 114–15 (Leonard w. Levy et al. eds., 1986).
28. *See supra* note 16.
29. U.S. CONST. art. I, § 8, els. 12–13.
30. *Id*. cl. 15.
31. *Id*. cl. 16 (emphasis added).
32. *Id.*
33. *Id*. (emphasis added).
34. *See* THE FEDERALIST Nos. 28, 29, 84 (Alexander Hamilton); *id*. No. 46 (James Madison) (Clinton Rossiter ed., 1961).
35. *Id*. No. 29 at 182, 186 (Alexander Hamilton) (emphasizing this point).
36. *See id*. at 185–87.
37. *See id*. No. 46 at 299–300 (James Madison).
38. *Id*. No. 84 at 512–14 (Alexander Hamilton).
39. *See* JOYCE L. MALCOLM, To KEEP AND BEAR ARMS 164 (1994). William Rawle, George Washington's candidate for the nation's first attorney general, made the same point. *See* WILLIAM RAWLE, A VIEW OF THE CONSTITUTION OF THE UNITED STATES OF AMERICA 125–26 (2d ed. 1829).

40. THOMAS M. COOLEY, THE GENERAL PRINCIPLES OF CONSTITUTIONAL LAW IN THE UNITED STATES OF AMERICA 270–71 (1880). To be sure, Cooley went on to note that the Second Amendment had, as a "further" purpose (not the chief purpose-which, as he says, was to confirm the citizen's personal right to keep and bear arms-but as a "further purpose"), the purpose to preclude any excuse of alleged need for a large standing army. *Id.; see also* PA. CONST of 1776, art. VIII ("That the people have a right to bear arms for the defence of themselves, and the state: and as standing armies in the time of peace, are dangerous to liberty, they ought not to be kept up: and that the military should be kept under strict subordination to and governed by the civil power.")

41. 1 WILLIAM BLACKSTONE, COMMENTARIES *129, *141.

42. *Id.* at *144.

43. *Id.* (emphasis added). Against this background, incidentally, the Supreme Court's decision in DeShaney v. Winnebago County Dep't of Social Servs., 489 U.S. 189 (1989), may be important to take into account in understanding the underpinnings of the personal right to keep and bear arms in the Blackstone minimal sense of the right to keep arms for self-preservation itself. To the extent that there is no enforceable constitutional obligation imposed on government in fact to protect every person from force or violence—and also no liability for a per se failure to come to any threatened person's aid or assistance (as *DeShaney* declares altogether emphatically)—the idea that the same government could nonetheless threaten one with criminal penalties merely "for having and using arms for self-preservation and defense" becomes impossibly difficult to sustain consistent with any plausible residual view of auxiliary natural rights. *See also* Nicholas Johnson, *Beyond the Second Amendment: An Individual Right to Arms Viewed Through, The Ninth Amendment,* 24 RUTGERS L.J. 1, 64–67 (1992) (collecting prior articles and references to the strong natural rights history of the personal right to possess essential means of self defense).

An impressive number of authors, whose work Nicholas Johnson reports (and to which he adds in this article), have sought to locate the right to keep and bear arms in the Ninth Amendment. They note that the Ninth Amendment provides precautionarily that "[t]he enumeration in the Constitution, of certain rights, shall not be construed to deny or disparage others retained by the people." U.S. CONST. amend. IX. And they go forward to show that the right to bear arms was a right of just this sort, i.e., that "the right to keep and bear Arms" was itself so utterly taken for granted, and so thoroughly accepted, that it fits the Ninth Amendment's description very aptly. *See* Johnson. *supra,* at 34–37. Unsurprisingly, however, the sources relied upon to show that this was so, strong as they are (and they are quite strong), are essentially just the very same sources that inform the Second Amendment with respect to the predicate clause on the right of the people to keep and bear arms. That is, they are the same materials that also show that there was a widespread understanding of a common right to keep and bear arms, which is itself the express right the Second Amendment expressly protects. Recourse to the same materials to fashion a Ninth Amendment ("unenumerated") right is not only largely replicative of the Second Amendment inquiry, but also singularly inappropriate under the circumstances—the right to bear arms is not left to the vagaries of Ninth Amendment disputes at all.

44. *E.g.,* XIANFA [Constitution] art. 55. cl.2 (P.R.C.), *translated in* THE CONSTITUTION OF THE PEOPLE'S REPUBLIC OF CHINA 41 (1983) ("It is the honourable duty of citizens of the People's Republic of China to perform military service and join the militia in accordance with the law.")

45. *See* MALCOLM, *supra* note 39, at 135–64 (tracing the English antecedents and reviewing the full original history of the Second Amendment). Professor Malcolm concludes, exactly as Thomas Cooley did a century earlier, *see supra* note 40, that

> [t]he Second Amendment was meant to accomplish two distinct goals, each perceived as crucial to the maintenance of liberty. First, it was meant to guarantee the individual's right to have arms for self-defence and self-preservation. Such an individual right was a legacy of the English Bill of Rights [broadened in scope in America from the English antecedent]. . . .
>
> . . . .

> The cause concerning the militia was not intended to limit ownership of arms to militia members or return control of the militia to the states, but rather to express the preference for a militia over a standing army.

MALCOM, *supra*, at 162–63. For other strongly confirming reviews, see, e.g., SUBCOMMITTEE ON THE CONSTITUTION OF THE COMM. ON THE JUDICIARY, THE RIGHT TO KEEP AND BEAR ARMS, 97th Cong., 2d Sess. (1982); HALBROOK, *supra* note 19, at 67–80: David I. Caplan, *Restoring the Balance: The Second Amendment Revisited*, 5 FORDHAM URB. L.J. 31, 33–34 (1976); Stephen P. Halbrook, *The Right of the People or the Power of the State: Bearing Arms, Arming Militias, and the Second Amendment*, 26 VAL U. L. REV. 131 (1991); David T. Hardy, *Armed Citizens, Citizen Armies: Toward a Jurisprudence of the Second Amendment*, 9 HARV. J.L. & PUB. POL'Y 559, 604–15 (1986); David T. Hardy, *The Second Amendment and the Historiography of the Bill of Rights*, 4 J.L & POL 1, 43–62 (1987); Don B. Kates, Jr., *Handgun Prohibition and the Original Meaning of the Second Amendment*, 82 MICH. L. REV. 204, 206, 211–45 (1983); Sanford Levinson, *The Embarrassing Second Amendment*, 99 YALE L.J. 637, 645–51 (1989); Robert E. Shalhope, *The Armed Citizen in the Early Republic*, 49 LAW & CONTEMP. PROBS., Winter 1986, at 125, 133–41. But see Ehrman & Henigan, *supra* note 19; Dennis A. Henigan, *Arms, Anarchy and the Second Amendment*, 26 VAL U. L. REV. 107, 111 n.17 (1991) (listing additional articles by others).

46. Compare the claim of a power in government to require "licensing" the right to keep arms.

47. The Second Amendment was originally the fourth amendment of twelve approved by the requisite two-thirds of both houses of Congress in 1789 and at once submitted for ratification by the state legislatures. Because only six states approved either the first or second of these twelve amendments during the ensuing two years (1789–1791), however, neither of these was adopted (since, unlike the others they failed to be confirmed by three-fourths of the states). So, what was originally proposed as the third amendment became the First Amendment and what was originally proposed as the fourth amendment became the Second Amendment in turn. (On May 22, 1992, however, the original proposed second amendment of 1789 was declared by Congress to have acquired sufficient state resolutions of ratification as of May 7, 1992, as also itself to have become effective as well. The result is that what was originally submitted as the second amendment has become the Twenty-Seventh Amendment instead.) *See* William Van Alstyne, *What Do You Think About the Twenty-Seventh Amendment?*, 10 CONST. COMMENTARY 9 (1993).

48. *See* Barron v. Mayor of Baltimore, 32 U.S. (7 Pet.) 243. 249 (1833) ("These amendments demanded security against the apprehended encroachments of the general government—not against those of the local governments.")

49. *See* U.S. CONST. amend. XIV.

50. CONG. GLOBE. 39th Cong., 1st Sess. 2765 (1866) (statement of Sen. Jacob Meritt Howard). Senator Howard is speaking here—and in his ensuing remarks—in explanation of the "first section" of the Fourteenth Amendment that provides: "No State shall make or enforce any law which shall abridge the privileges or immunities of citizens of the United States. . . ."

51. *Id.* at 2766.

52. *Id.* at 2765 (emphasis added).

53. *Id.* at 2766 (emphasis added). For the most recent review of this matter, with useful references to the previous scholarship on the same subject, and reaching the same conclusion still again, see Richard L. Aynes, *On Misreading John Bingham and the Fourteenth Amendment*, 103 YALE W. 57 (1993).

54. *See* Robert Dowlut. *Federal and State Constitutional Guarantees 10 Arms*, 1S U. DAYTON L. REV. 59, 79 (1989) ("State courts have on at least 20 reported occasions found arms laws to be unconstitutional."); Robert Dowlut & Janet A. Knoop, *State Constitutions and the Right to Keep and Bear Arms*, 7 OKLA, CITY U. L. REV. 177 (1982) (reviewing state constitutional clauses and the right to keep and bear arms).

55. The inclusion of this entitlement for personal protection is, in the Fourteenth Amendment, even more clear than as provided (as a premise) in the Second Amendment itself. It was, after all, the defenselessness of Negroes (denied legal rights to keep and bear arms by state law) from attack by night riders—even to protect their own lives, their own families, and their own homes—that made it imperative that they, as citizens,

could no longer be kept defenseless by a regime of state law denying them the common right to keep and bear arms. Note the description of the right as a personal right in the report by Senator Howard. *See supra* text accompanying note 52. For confirming references, see also the examples provided in MICHAEL K. CURTIS. No STATE SHALL ABRIDGE 24, 43, 56, 72, 138–41, 164, 203 (1986); HALBROOK, *supra* note 19, at 107–23: Skayoko Blodgett–Ford, *Do Battered Women Have a Right to Bear Arms?*, 11 YALE L. & POL'Y REV. 509, 513–24 (1993); Robert J. Cottrol & Raymond T. Diamond, *The Second Amendment: Toward an Afro-Americanist Reconsideration*, 80 GEO. L.J. 309 (1991); Kates, *supra* note 45, at 254–57. For an overall responsible general review, see also Levinson, *supra* note 45. For the most recent critical review, however, see Raoul Berger, *Constitutional Interpretation and Activist Famosies*, 82 KY. L.J. 1 (1993–1994) (with additional references to previous books and articles).

56. In contrast, the suggestion that it does not extend to handguns (in contrast to howitzers) is quite beyond the pale (i.e., it is wholly inconsistent with any sensible understanding of a meaningful right to keep arms as a personal right).

57. Such questions, moreover, are hardly on that account (merely as questions) necessarily hard or difficult to answer in reasonable ways, even fully conceding a strong view of the right to keep and bear arms (e.g., rules of tort or of statutory liability for careless storage endangering minors or others foreseeably put at unreasonable risk).

58. And equally with respect to the states, pursuant to the Fourteenth Amendment.

59. *See supra* notes 9–14 and accompanying text.

60. Unless, of course, one holds the view that it is really desirable after all that the Constitution should indeed be construed—the Second and Fourteenth Amendments to the contrary notwithstanding—to say that the right to keep and bear arms is the right to keep and bear arms as it is sometimes understood (i.e., as though it had the added words, "but only according to the sufferance of the state").

WILLIAM W. VAN ALSTYNE is a professor at Duke Law School and the Lee Professor of Law at the Marshall-Wythe Law School at the College of William and Mary. A scholar of constitutional law, Professor Van Alstyne's areas of specialization include U.S. Constitutional Law and Comparative Constitutional Systems. Professor Van Alstyne was named to Duke's William R. and Thomas S. Perkins Chair of Law in 1974. He holds a certificate from The Hague Academy of International Law and has been honored with LL.D. degrees by Wake Forest University and the College of William & Mary. Professor Van Alstyne's professional writings that address virtually every major subject in the field of constitutional law have appeared during four decades in the principal law journals in the United States, with frequent republication in foreign journals. His work has been cited in a large number of judicial opinions including those of the Supreme Court. The *Journal of Legal Studies* for January, 2000, named Professor Van Alstyne in the top 40 most frequently cited legal scholars in the United States of the preceding half-century. He has also appeared in numerous hearings before Senate and House Committees, on legislation affecting the separation of powers, war powers, constitutional amendments, impeachments, legislation affecting civil rights and civil liberties, and nominations to the Supreme Court. In 1987, Professor Van Alstyne was selected in a poll of federal judges, lawyers, and academics by the New York Law Journal as one of three academics among "the 10 most qualified" persons in the country for appointment to the Supreme Court, a distinction repeated in a similar poll by The American Lawyer, in 1991.

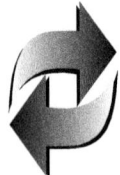

Lawrence Delbert Cress

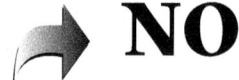

A Well-Regulated Militia: The Origins and Meaning of the Second Amendment

Unlike provisions of the Bill of Rights that guaranteed such individual rights as freedom of speech, due process, and religious choice, the Second Amendment to the United States Constitution was not written to assure private citizens the prerogative of carrying weapons. To the leaders of the American Revolution it meant something very different. The Second Amendment was intended to guarantee that the sovereign citizenry of the republic (armed, propertied, and able to vote) would always remain a vital force in America's constitutional order. Despite the militia's poor showing during the revolutionary war, Americans remained convinced that republican government would fail without a "well-regulated militia."

The lessons of history, they believed, were clear. Only a citizenry organized into local militia companies could deter ambitious tyrants or foreign invaders. Republics, whether ancient or modern, thrived only when their citizens were willing and able to leave the plow for the field of battle. When a professional army usurped the citizenry's role in national defense, especially as a consequence of political intrigue or moral decadence, republics withered and liberty fell victim to tyranny and oppression.

A well-regulated militia not only protected citizens against the intrigues of ambitious rulers, it also protected the body politic against civil disorder. Daniel Shays's Rebellion, an armed insurrection in western Massachusetts in 1786, had sent tremors through the nation. And, history suggested that republican governments were especially vulnerable to domestic turmoil. To the generation that wrote it, the Second Amendment was at once a declaration of a fundamental principle of good government and a means to protect the stability of republican institutions. It did not guarantee individuals, such as Daniel Shays and his followers, the right to stockpile armaments.

The Second Amendment had roots deep in Anglo-American political and constitutional theory. Since the mid-seventeenth century, English political theorists had linked the militia to the maintenance of a balanced, stable, and free constitution. James Harrington, whose *Commonwealth of Oceana* (London, 1656) was widely read by Americans of the revolutionary generation, recommended the militia both for national defense and to deter the misuse of political power. Political writers at the time of the Glorious Revolution of 1689 emphasized the militia's importance for constitutional stability. Algernon Sidney warned that tyranny arose whenever the militia was allowed to decay. John Trenchard, later popular in the colonies as the author with Thomas Gordon of *Cato's Letters,* began his career as a pamphleteer by chiding Parliament for providing William III with a standing army after the Treaty of Ryswick in 1697. Standing armies, he wrote, were the agents of political intrigue and corruption. Only a militia could be counted upon to protect both the territory and the liberties of free people.

Between 1763 and 1776, Americans felt the truth of Trenchard's indictment. The occupation of Boston by British soldiers in 1768 and again in 1774, to say nothing of the Boston Massacre of 1770, confirmed the belief that hired soldiers were agents of political oppression. Although America did resort to professional soldiers in the revolutionary war, the country emerged from the Revolution no less persuaded by Trenchard's condemnation of standing armies. When they framed the Bill of Rights with an eye to preserving the republican gains of the Revolution, both the danger of standing armies and the militia's positive role as the armed manifestation of the sovereign people were important considerations.

The statutory antecedents of the Second Amendment reached far into the Anglo-American past. Magna Carta, a feudal compact accepted by King John at Runnymede in 1215 in exchange for renewed pledges of loyalty from his rebellious nobles, outlined the prerogatives of the nobility and the limits of royal authority. As an agreement between the king and the politically articulate community of the realm, Magna Carta served as an important touchstone for the development of Anglo-American law. Chapter 29 guaranteed every knight the right to serve in the castle-guard

Cress, Lawrence Delbert, "A Well-Regulated Militia: The Origins and Meaning of the Second Amendment," *Virginia Calvalcade* 33 (Autumn 1983), 64–73. Copyright ©1983 by The Library of Virginia. Used with permission.

or to send someone of his own choosing to perform that duty and prohibited the king from forcing noblemen to pay taxes in lieu of personal service. The nobles in effect prevented King John from creating an army supported by their taxes but independent of their control. Magna Carta was the first step toward insuring the citizenry (then narrowly defined as the nobility) a role in the realm's defense.

Parliament grappled with similar matters during the Glorious Revolution. In the 1680s James II increased the number of Roman Catholic military officers and excluded Protestant officers in violation of the 1673 Test Act, and he imported Irish Catholics to fill the army's expanding ranks. Thus, as the English Bill of Rights phrased it, he "did endeavor to subvert and extirpate the Protestant religion, and the laws and liberties of this kingdom" by "raising and keeping a standing army . . . without consent of parliament" and by "causing several good subjects, being Protestants, to be disarmed, at the same time when papists were both armed and employed." To correct this, the Bill of Rights of 1689 prohibited the English monarchy from raising an army during peacetime without Parliament's consent and guaranteed that "subjects which are Protestants, may have arms for their defence suitable to their conditions, and as allowed by law." The English Bill of Rights did not create an unlimited right to bear arms, however, for Protestants were to "have arms for their defence" only as was "suitable to their conditions and as allowed by law." Arms were denied to men who did not own lands worth at least £100, unless they were the sons or heirs of an esquire, knight, or nobleman. Parliament also reserved the future option of restricting "by law" access to arms. These provisions were intended to ensure a stable government free from the threat of disruptions by Catholic Jacobites and the intrigues of future monarchs.

A century later, the framers of the American states' declarations of rights also sought to lay the foundations for constitutional stability. When Thomas Jefferson indicted George III in the Declaration of Independence for keeping "among us in time of peace, standing armies without the consent of our legislatures," he underscored the American concern about the relationship between liberty and citizen soldiers, but the militia tradition had more than just rhetorical significance. Patriot leaders in the colonies during the winter and spring of 1774–1775 adopted resolutions declaring "that a well-regulated Militia, composed of the gentlemen, freeholders, and other freemen, is the natural strength and only stable security of free Government." With independence at hand, the states' declarations of rights identified the militia as an institution necessary for the preservation of liberty.

Virginia's Declaration of Rights—adopted on 12 June 1776, nearly a month before the American colonies officially announced their independence—set the pattern. Article 13, drafted by George Mason and approved by a committee that included James Madison, declared "that a well regulated Militia, composed of the Body of the People, trained to Arms, is the proper, natural, and safe Defence of a free State." Two months later, Pennsylvania adopted in article 13 of its own declaration of rights the proposition that "the people have a right to bear arms for the defence of themselves and the state." The language was slightly different, but the meaning was the same. Only the trained, armed, and organized citizen militia could be depended upon to preserve republican liberties for "themselves" and to ensure the constitutional stability of the "state." Both Virginians and Pennsylvanians warned that standing armies were "dangerous to liberty" and stipulated that the military be kept "under strict subordination" to the civil government. Without a strong, popularly based militia, liberty would succumb to the dictates of tyrants.

Delaware, Maryland, and North Carolina adopted similar declarations during the first year of independence, the first two states by borrowing language from Virginia's article 13, and North Carolina following Pennsylvania's lead by declaring that "the people have a right to bear arms, for the defence of the state." Vermont, though not formally a state until 1792, quoted Pennsylvania's article 13 in its 1777 declaration of rights. In the same year, New York incorporated an equally clear statement in the body of its constitution. Announcing it to be "the duty of every man who enjoys the protection of society to be prepared and willing to defend it," New Yorkers proclaimed that the "militia . . . at all times . . . shall be armed and disciplined."

In Massachusetts, John Adams drafted the bill of rights that was ratified with the 1780 constitution. "The people," he wrote, "have a right to keep and bear arms for the common defence." New Hampshire's 1783 bill of rights made the same point, declaring "A well regulated militia is the proper, natural, and sure defence of a state." Both documents condemned standing armies and subordinated the military to civil authority, while affirming the citizen militia's collective role as the protector of personal liberty and constitutional stability against ambitious tyrants and uncontrolled mobs.

Several states put limits on citizens' militia obligation. Pennsylvania, Delaware, and Vermont provided that no "man who is consciencously scrupulous of bearing arms" could be "compeled" to serve in the militia, but they required that conscientious objectors meet their obligations with "equivalents," payments equal to the cost of their militia service. These clauses permitting conscientious objection to military service demonstrate yet again that for eighteenth-century Americans "to bear arms" meant militia service. State after state guaranteed a role in the common defense collectively to the "people" or the "militia." On the other hand, when describing individual rights such as freedom of conscience they used the terms "man" or "person." New Hampshire's bill of rights—the last written during the Confederation period and, as such, a compendium of previous thinking on the matter—is a case in point. It declared the importance of "a well regulated militia" to the defense of the state and exempted from service any "person . . . conscientiously scrupulous about the lawfulness of bearing arms." The individual right of conscience was asserted against the collective responsibility for the common defense. These same concerns surfaced in the debate about the Constitution.

During the last days of the Philadelphia convention, Virginia delegate George Mason, having failed to secure a separate bill of rights, sought an explicit statement of the militia's place in republican government. He wanted a clause explaining that the congressional power to arm, organize, and discipline the militia was intended to secure "the Liberties of the People . . . against the Dangers of regular Troops or standing Armies in time of Peace." When the Convention failed to agree, Mason refused to sign the Constitution. As he explained in his widely read "Objections to the Constitution of Government formed by the Convention," the document contained "no Declaration of Rights" and specifically lacked a "declaration of any kind . . . against the danger of standing armies." To correct this omission, Mason backed an amendment, drafted on the eve of Virginia's ratification convention, declaring that the "People have a Right to keep & bear Arms" because "a well regulated Militia [is] the proper natural and safe Defence of a free State." Mason's proposal also rehearsed the dangers of standing armies and the need for the "strict Subordination" of military to civil authority. A separate amendment would have provided that a person "religiously scrupulous of bearing Arms" be allowed "to employ another to bear Arms in his Stead." Never did Mason challenge the Constitution's failure to guarantee individual access to weapons.

During the debates over the Constitution, many critics worried that the proposed government threatened the militia's important role in the republic. Maryland Antifederalist Luther Martin challenged the proposed government's military prerogatives: "Instead of guarding against a standing army, . . . which has so often and so successfully been used for the subversion of freedom," Martin argued, the Constitution gave "it an express and constitutional sanction." Congress's authority over the state militias, he warned, could be used "even to disarm" them. Worse, the militia might be needlessly mobilized and sent marching to the far reaches of the Union so that the people would be glad to see a standing army raised in its stead. "When a government wishes to deprive its citizens of freedom," Martin noted, "it generally makes use of a standing army [while leaving] the militia in a situation as contemptible as possible, lest they might oppose its arbitrary designs." Pennsylvania's Antifederalists demanded that the states be given a veto over any call for militia service outside a state's borders.

Concern arose too over the Constitution's failure to protect conscientious objectors. Antifederalist candidates for the New York convention charged that the Constitution left "men conscientiously scrupulous of bearing arms . . . liable to perform military duty." Reflecting the sentiments of the state declarations of rights, the Antifederalists were determined to preserve the militia as a bulwark of republican government but also anxious to protect the individual's free exercise of conscience.

The notion that individual citizens should be guaranteed access to weapons surfaced several times during the debate over the Constitution. A minority report from the Pennsylvania ratifying convention borrowed language from the state's own declaration of rights to declare not only the people's right "to bear arms for the defence of themselves and their own State or the United States" but also the right to bear arms "for the purpose of killing game," while adding the proviso that "no law shall be passed for disarming the people or any of them." Samuel Adams, of Massachusetts, argued that the Constitution should never be construed "to authorize Congress to . . . prevent the people of the United States, who are peaceable citizens from keeping their own arms" but then renounced that position after reflecting on Shays's Rebellion in western Massachusetts. Finally, among a series of amendments recommended for consideration by the First Congress, New Hampshire proposed that "Congress shall never disarm any citizen unless such as are or have been in Actual Rebellion."

The principles of these resolutions were close to the classical republican understanding of the armed citizenry. In each case, bearing arms was linked to the citizenry's collective responsibility for defense, familiar warnings about the danger of standing armies, and affirmations, of the need to subordinate military to civil authority. Neither Pennsylvania's critics nor New Hampshire's cautious supporters of the Constitution had moved far, if at all, beyond the eighteenth-century notion that bearing arms meant militia service, and no other state followed their lead. Pennsylvania's Antifederalists provided for the disarming of criminals and conceded that further action would be appropriate if society faced "real danger of public injury from individuals." The order and safety of society always took precedence over the individual's claim to possess weapons, and constitutional stability remained the preeminent consideration. The only other hint that Americans may have viewed bearing arms as an individual right occurs in one of Thomas Jefferson's early draft proposals for Virginia's new state constitution. Jefferson's draft had a clause guaranteeing every freeman the use of arms "within his own lands or tenements," but this provision was not incorporated in the Constitution of 1776. Virginia's statesmen were satisfied that George Mason's thirteenth article of the Declaration of Rights protected the "Militia, composed of the body of the people, trained to arms" and accurately stated the armed citizenry's proper role in a republic.

The amendments proposed in the state ratifying conventions reflected the concerns about national military power and the republican principles embodied in the states' declarations of rights. New York and North Carolina wanted to limit congressional power to raise a peacetime army by requiring "the consent of two thirds" of the House and Senate. Maryland suggested limiting a soldier's enlistment to four years to prevent Congress from creating a permanent military force. More than half of the states advocated strong state militias to counter the tyrannical potential of the Constitution. Fearing that the militia would be purposely neglected, some states proposed guarantees that the states could organize, arm, and discipline their citizens if Congress failed to fulfill its responsibilities. Against the more common fear that Congress's right to call out the militia would prove detrimental to republican liberties, New Yorkers recommended that a state's militia not be allowed to serve outside its borders longer than six weeks "without the consent of the legislature thereof." Others worried that the subjection of the militia to martial law might lead to abuses. The Maryland and North Carolina conventions asked Congress to amend the Constitution so that the militia could be placed under martial law only "in time of war, invasion, or rebellion." Finally, several state conventions stated firmly that no person "religiously scrupulous of bearing arms" should be compelled to serve in the military.

Virginia's proposed amendments, which directly influenced Madison's draft of the Bill of Rights, bring into focus the concerns that ultimately produced the Second Amendment. Indeed, the changes proposed by the commonwealth's ratifying convention neatly defined the issues raised during later congressional debates. Declaring that "the people have a right to keep and bear arms," Virginians asked for constitutional recognition of the principle that "a well regulated Militia, composed of the Body of the People trained to Arms, is the proper, natural, and safe Defence of a free State." This proposition addressed the fear that the new government might disarm the citizenry while raising an oppressive standing army. To reinforce the point, the convention urged a constitutional declaration that standing armies "are dangerous to liberty, and therefore ought to be avoided, as far as the circumstances and protection of the community will admit." The Constitution was also found wanting for failing to pronounce the military "in all cases" subordinate to "civil power." The Virginia convention prepared a separate amendment "That any person religiously scrupulous of bearing arms ought to be exempted, upon payment of an equivalent to employ another to bear arms in his stead." No one expressed concern about an individual citizen's access to weapons.

Madison had Virginia's recommendations in mind when, on 8 June 1789, he proposed to Congress that the Constitution be amended to provide that "The right of the people to keep and bear arms shall not be infringed; a well armed and well regulated militia being the best security of a free country: but no person religiously scrupulous of bearing arms shall be compelled to render military service in person." Six weeks later, a committee composed of Madison and ten representatives (one from each of the other states that had ratified the Constitution), began preparing a formal state of amendments, using as a guide both Madison's recommendations and those proposed by the states. The committee revised Madison's original recommendation and stated more explicitly the armed citizenry's importance to the constitutional order.

Such doubts as were raised remind us of the militia's importance in the political theory of the day. The failure to link freedom of conscience with the obligation to find a substitute or pay an "equivalent" troubled many members of the House. Requiring one part of the population to provide for the defense of the other was simply "unjust," argued James Jackson, of Georgia. Others believed that matters of "religious persuasion" had no place in an amendment designed to guarantee a fundamental principle of republican government. "It is extremely injudicious," warned one congressman, "to intermix matters of doubt with fundamentals." Such concerns brought the House of Representatives within two votes of striking the conscientious objection clause from the proposed amendment.

Congressman Ædanus Burke, of South Carolina, proposed a clause declaring that a "standing army . . . in time of peace is dangerous to public liberty, and such shall not be raised . . . without the consent of two-thirds of the members present of both Houses" and an explicit statement of the subordination of military to civil authority. Burke's motion was defeated because some congressmen thought a simple majority vote was sufficient and other congressmen complained that the debate had already been closed. Nevertheless, Burke's amendment again demonstrates what Congress meant by the Second Amendment. The aim was to confirm a fundamental principle of republican government, that a well-regulated militia was "the best security of a free State."

Little is known about the Senate debate on the Second Amendment; it seems to have been similar to that in the House. The Senate joined the House in rejecting the proposal to restrict Congress's power to raise armies during peacetime but denied approval to the controversial conscientious objection clause. The Senate's changes were accepted by a joint conference committee of both houses, and on 24 and 25 September 1789, the House and Senate respectively voted their approval.

We also know little about debate on the Second Amendment in the states. No state legislature rejected it. As a statement of republican principles already commonplace in state declarations of rights, it probably evoked little discussion. If any doubts were raised, they might have focused on the amendment's failure explicitly to describe the dangers of a standing army.

When Virginia ratified the Second Amendment on 15 December 1791 the statement that "A well regulated militia, being necessary to the security of a free State, the right of the people to keep and bear arms, shall not be infringed," became a part of the United States Constitution. The militia had played an important role in stemming the tide of oppression that necessitated independence from Great Britain, and it alone offered a republican remedy to domestic disorders such as Shays's Rebellion. The Second Amendment gave constitutional sanction to the idea that the militia was the institutional expression of the citizenry's collective obligation to bear arms against the internal and external enemies of the state—"a well regulated militia" to defend the liberties of the people against a demagogue's armed mob or a tyrant's standing army.

LAWRENCE DELBERT CRESS was the former dean of the College of Liberal Arts at Willamette University where he served as professor of history. He is the author of *Citizens in Arms: The Army and Militia in American Society to the War of 1812* (University of North Carolina Press, 1982, 2010).

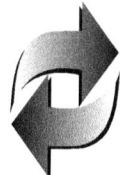

EXPLORING THE ISSUE

Was the Second Amendment Designed to Protect an Individual's Right to Own Guns?

Critical Thinking and Reflection

1. What right does the Second Amendment to the Constitution protect? Do you think this protection is necessary today? Why or why not?
2. Why did the Founders include the Second Amendment in the Bill of Rights? Do you think that their reasons are still valid today? Why or why not?
3. What are the two most convincing arguments made by W. W. Van Alstyne and L. D. Cress that support their respective positions? What are counter argument that you might offer to counter these convincing arguments by Van Alstyne and Cress?
4. You have been asked to offer your opinion on whether the Second Amendment to the U.S. Constitution should be interpreted and applied from an "originalist" perspective or a "living-evolving" perspective. What would your arguments be for one of these perspectives and how would that impact the application of the Second Amendment in the present?
5. "A well regulated militia, being necessary to the security of a free state, the right of the people to keep and bear arms, shall not be infringed."
   - Prefatory Clause: "A well regulated militia, being necessary to the security of a free state.
   - Operative Clause: "the right of the people to keep and bear arms, shall not be infringed."

   Instructions: Split the students into two groups a distribute copies of the Second Amendment to the U.S. Constitution (SAUSC). One group will examine the prefatory clause of the SAUSC and one group will examine the operative clause of the SAUSC. Have students read, analyze, and discuss in their groups the definition, meaning, and interpretive intent of their respective prefatory and operative clauses. As a group, the students will also determine their top one to three points of agreement and one to three points disagreement regarding the meaning and intent of their respective clauses. A group member should record the information (e.g., definition, meaning, interpretive intent, and agreement/disagreement points) and another group member should report the information when asked to do so. Upon completion of each group's reporting the instructor may choose to lead a discussion regarding areas of agreement and disagreement generated by the class as it compares and contrasts to historic and contemporary areas of agreement and disagreement.

Is There Common Ground?

Both William W. Van Alstyne and Lawrence Delbert Cress frame their positions within the philosophical, historical and legal language of English common law and Revolutionary American rhetoric. Though Van Alstyne and Cress offer distinctive interpretations of the "intent" of this language as applied within contemporary society both provide a well-reasoned examination of the explicit narrative and implicit nuance of the words and phrases that comprise the Second Amendment to the U.S. Constitution.

Van Alstyne and Cress also concur that it was America that remained an agrarian society where armed men would consider it their civic duty to join their state militia as armed citizens and protect themselves from the tyranny of our national government or any other external threat. Both use similar sources such as the debates at the Constitutional Convention of 1787 and the states' ratifying conventions to bolster their arguments, but they reach different conclusions on the liberties and limitations that were intended regarding gun rights among individuals as defined by the notion of a "militia." Cress believes that the Second Amendment meant that an individual could possess arms only if he were a member of the militia, while Van Alstyne maintains that there is no ambiguity in the language of the Second Amendment as evidenced by similar language and interpretation of the Fist, Fourth, Sixth, Seventh, et al. Amendments.

Additional Resources

Cress, L. D. 1984. "An Armed Community," *Journal of American History*. 71 (1).

Hemingway, D. 2006. Private Guns, Public Health. University of Michigan Press. Lansing, MI.

Levinson, S. 1989. The Embarrassing Second Amendment. *The Yale Law Journal*, 99 (3): 637-659.

Hemenway, David, Private Guns, Public Health, University of Michigan Press, 2004. A Harvard professor of health policy argues that the high cost of gun deaths and injuries caused by firearms should not be tolerated.

Van Alstyne, W.W. (1994). The Second Amendment and the Personal Right to Arms. *Duke Law Journal* vol. 43, Iss. 6. April pp. 1236-1255.

References

Cress, L.D. (1984). An Armed Community, Journal of American History. V. 71 No. 1.

Internet References . . .

American Civil Liberties Union—The Second Amendment

https://www.aclu.org/other/second-amendment

CQ Researcher—The Gun Control Debate

http://library.cqpress.com/cqresearcher/document.php?id=cqresrre2004111200

Teaching the Bill of Rights—The Second Amendment

https://billofrightsinstitute.org/educate/educator-resources/lessons-plans/bill-rights-institute-curricula-resources/teaching-complex-topics/teaching-bill-rights-second-amendment/

U.S. Constitution Center—The Second Amendment

https://constitutioncenter.org/interactive-constitution/amendments/amendment-ii

United States National Archives—The U.S. Constitution and The Bill of Rights

https://www.archives.gov/founding-docs/constitution-transcript

https://www.archives.gov/founding-docs/bill-of-rights

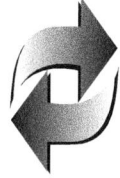

ISSUE

Selected, Edited, and with Issue Framing Material by:
Kevin R. Magill and Tony L. Talbert, *Baylor University*

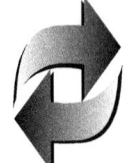

Was Alexander Hamilton an Economic Genius?

YES: Donald F. Swanson and Andrew P. Trout, from "Alexander Hamilton's Economic Policies After Two Centuries," *New York History* (1991)

NO: Edward Peter Stringham, from "Hamilton's Legacy and the Great Man Theory of Financial History," *Independent Review* (2017)

Learning Outcomes

After reading this issue, you will be able to:

- Explain the competing ideological positions supporting and refuting *The Great Man of History Theory* postulated in this chapter.
- Describe Swanson's and Trout's representation of Alexander Hamilton's influence on U.S. economic and politicial prowess as compared to Stringham's refutation of Hamilton's role in these economic and political outcomes.
- Compare and contrast the evidence offered in this chapter regarding the cause and effect impact of Alexander Hamilton and his contemporarires on the economic, political, and social philosophies, policies, and practices of the United States in the late 18th through mid-19th centuries.
- Develop a chain of evidence that either supports one of the positions represented in this chapter or propose an all-together counter position to the authors represented in this discussion.

ISSUE SUMMARY

YES: Donald F. Swanson and Andrew P. Trout contend that Alexander Hamilton's historic legacy is too often mischaracterized as one of financial interests alone. Swanson and Trout argue that Hamilton's legacy as America's greatest financial genius must encompass his commitment to supporting the development of a multi-institutional national system of governance that addressed both political and financial realities of the time. Hamilton's genius is founded in equal parts risk-taker and strategic pragmatist when enacting fiscal and philosophical policies that established America's national government on firm pathway to international prominence.

NO: Edward Peter Stringham argues against applying the "genius" (i.e., great man theory of history) to Alexander Hamilton, as has been done in the Hamilton musical, suggesting that Hamilton's primary philosophy was not grounded in a commitment to multi-institutional nationalism but primarily in developing a centralized economic system that should also not be solely credited to Hamilton but instead to the countless people who worked behind the scenes to make the historical and modern United States economy possible.

No great man lives in vain. The history of the world is but the biography of great men (Carlyle, 1907).

> I wrote my way out of hell. I wrote my way to revolution. I was louder than the crack in the bell. I wrote Eliza love letters until she fell. I wrote about The Constitution and defended it well. And in the face of ignorance and resistance, I wrote financial systems into existence. And when my prayers to God were met with indifference, I picked up a pen, I wrote my own deliverance. (Miranda, 2016, from *Hamilton—Act II "Hurricane"*)

The great man of history theory continues to find its place of prominence in the classrooms and barrooms across our nation. Are leaders made or are leaders born? What are the circumstances that give rise to great men (and women) of history? Is there a singularity of cause or an amalgam of antecedents that divulge the historic answers to these questions?

Donald F. Swanson, Andrew P. Trout, and Edward Peter Stringham take up this topic of debate on whether Hamilton qualifies as a *Great Man of History* based upon the attributes of genius not bound by an economic vision alone but a broader more complex nationalist ideal that saw nation building as an outcome of unified financial policies and an national economic system. While Swanson and Trout do not explicitly cite Thomas Carlyle's *Great Man of History* theory, they do offer a case supporting the notion that Alexander Hamilton qualifies as not simply an economic genius but also a visionary, if not a bit of a gambler, who can be credited for leading the new Amercian nation to eventual global dominance. Stringham's case against Hamilton as genius isn't founded on a rejection of the man's truly exceptional contributions to America's founding and perhaps eventual dominance, but instead is grounded in the notion that history is an amalgam of market forces where millions, if not billions, of competing actions and reactions lead to outcomes. Hamilton, Stringham might contend, is one of those actions and reactions that while important, perhaps even genius, is not necessarily evidence of singularity of cause. Taking a nontraditional approach, Stringham integrates the lyrics of the smash Broadway musical "Hamilton" into economic theory to make his case against Hamilton as a stand-alone economic genius.

Donald F. Swanson, Andrew P. Trout, and Edward Peter Stringham all agree that thousands of pages fill textbooks, curricula, historical biographies, and scholarly and popular culture articles depicting enumerable erroneous descriptions of Alexander Hamilton. Even with such name recognition deriving from voluminous pages in print, Hamilton, the constitutional signatory, founding father, and inaugural national treasury secretary, is seldom fully understood by the American public for his role in establishing a new national government. Simply put, Hamilton's legacy has become a mashup of American historical biography, heroic fables, and a popular culture Broadway hip-hop lyrics.

It is precisely this *mash-up* that Swanson and Trout seek to sort out with their argument that Alexander Hamilton's genius is founded in not simply his willingness to postulate economic theory as a means of establishing the new American nation on firm footing in a hostile global scene, but his visionary integration of established European debt to credit finance practices with a bold, if not risky, embrace of a nationalistic position which placed him at odds with many of his Founding Father contemporaries and certainly much of the rank and file populace from the southern and western colonies. The notion of Hamilton as anything more than a singularly focused economic policy strategist fails to take into account the full spectrum of his impact. Certainly, there's reason to believe that Hamilton viewed the world through economic lens' leading him to contribute to the structural development of the new American nation through financial mechanisms that would not only ensure a viable future for the nation but create a competitive stance within a hostile geopolitical market. Swanson and Trout assert to their readers that, "We shall understand Hamilton better if we remember that as secretary he was pursuing a policy whose purposes were fiscal as well as political" (Swanson & Trout, 1991, p. 289).

As we read Swanson's and Trout's supporting case for Alexander Hamilton as an economic genius, we must focus on their contention that the U.S. Constitution had not only formed a new government but also formed a new problem. That being, the U.S. Government was not responsible for the debts incurred to public and private sectors entities during the revolution. Therefore, the new nation's government could turn its back on the public and private interests that had extended credit for funding a risky revolution and thereby lose credibility and public confidence or take ownership of the debt and face public outcry that burdensome taxation policies from an intrusive federal government were soon to follow.

While George Washington can surely be credited with fending off all attackers and launching a new nation under his steady leadership, equal credit would have to be given to Alexander Hamilton for keeping the creditors at bay and keeping the fledgling nation solvent. Thomas

Jefferson and his contention pushed for debt retirement as the first economic step of the United States. Thus, ensuring the influence of the federal government continued to be restrained with the source of economic power firmly held by the competing interests of landowners and mercantilist of the states. Hamilton pushed back against this call for debt retirement and instead proposed that the U.S. government become a source of credit by assuming the debt. It is this grand wager with history that Swanson and Trout note as an example of Hamilton's genius and perhaps give a nod to Carlyle's *Great Man of History Theory* as applicable to Alexander Hamilton.

Reading the Hamiliton papers (Syrett, 1961–1987, Hamilton Papers, 6:106), one sees the genius, if not the madness, of Hamilton's daring wager. After seven years of hard scrabble fighting to win an unlikely victory over the most powerful nation in the world, the United States as a nation was about to enter into yet another risky campaign where debits and credits would replace bullets and canons as the means to victory. The Constitution had made these debts the debts of the new government, and unless the U.S. government was prepared to establish public credit, it would be forced to confront commercial depression and foreign ecnomic domination, and it seemed probably rebellion and collapse of the union. To assure confidence at home and abroad, Hamilton proposed a bold adoption of "Fair equivalents" and "Limited redeemability" economic policies derived from 1690s' England where creditors accept a lower interest rate than originally promised with the gurantee of having their contracts extended, thereby continuing to receive a portion of the increasing percentage of the principal each year. The result, domestic public confidence in their government increases, and international foreign confidence in the new U.S. economy sparks further investment and reciprocal trade relationships.

"Within a short space of time America went from a nation with no credit to one that could borrow in the major financial capitals of Europe on terms equal to those with the strongest credit" (Swanson & Trout, 1991, p. 293). Swanson and Trout cite the *Hamilton Papers* (Report on the Public Credit, 6: 106) "as a blueprint for a financial revolution" (Swanson & Trout, 1991, p. 297) that allowed Adams, Jefferson, Madison, Monroe, John Quincey Adams, and Jackson to strengthen nation's political, social, and economic influence both home and abroad. It is this and multiple other examples of Hamilton's innovative integration of historic public finance practices and his own blend of economic adventurism reflective of the spirit of the day that Swanson and Trout offer as evidence of Alexander Hamilton's economic genius and surely the right man rises to influence at the right time in history.

Given such fundamental historic evidence offered by Donald F. Swanson and Andrew P. Trout what possible refutation to Hamilton's genius and perhaps singularity of influence could Edward Peter Stringham possibly offer in refutation? It is in Swanson's and Trout's last assertion regarding the subsequent policies and practices of seven U.S. Presidents and the preceeding policies and practices of Washington, Jefferson, and numerous other individuals that speak to Stringham's counter argument of Hamilton's role as *singular genius* (i.e., *Great Man of* History) causation for America's economic and thus political rise on the global stage. Stringham notes that critics of Carlyle's *Great Man of History* notion (i.e., Leo Tolstoy and Herbert Spencer) affirm his own position that ". . . societal outcomes are determined by the totality of individuals in society, not just by a few great men. Using more modern economic language, market outcomes are a spontaneous or emergent order—a product of the choices and interactions of billions of people" (Stringham & Curott, 2015, pp. 324–340).

It is with this opening salvo of refutation that E. P. Stringham engages the reader with an innovative and intriguing integration of economic theory and lyrical renditions drawn from Stringham's economic scholarship and Lin-Manuel Miranda's musical showmanship. Stringham gives credit to an imaginative musical featuring the caricature of Hamilton but warns ". . . we must be careful not to ascribe too much importance to him or to any other one person for Founding America or American financial markets" (Stringham, 2017, p. 524). For example, Stringham directly confronts Swanson's and Trout's primary example of Hamilton's genius in creating a system national debt (i.e., "Fair equivalents" and "Limited redeemability"). Stringham asserts that far from genius, Hamilton simply applied the recognized "system of government debt in England" (i.e., distressed debt in contemporary parlance) to a new American nation context. While it certainly proved Hamilton's decision was fortuitous as an end result, it was less an act of genius and more of an act of one of many individuals engaged in the federalist vs. anti-federalist debate as contextualized by the pre and post revolutionary era.

Stringham extends this line of reasoning by offering an historical timeline that establishes a cause and effect chain of evidence to support his position that Alexander Hamilton is but one of many antecedents and actors in bringing about the economic systems that eventually propelled the new nation of the United States to prosperity. Stringham's multiple examples of interdependent historical characters and contexts draws from the traditional archives of history and the unlikely musical score of *Hamilton: An American Musical*. Stringham builds his argument against *The Great Man Theory* and Hamilton's singularity of influence by noting the multiple factors and faces that made up the Federalist v. Anti-federalist debates, the philosophical divide between northern and southern states/terriroties, and the competing domestic and international interests of public, private, and profiteering entitites in establishing a foothold of power in the new American nation. Stringham's contention that Hamilton, Jefferson, Adams, Madison, et al., were not singularly engaged in these debates but instead were a part of an historical cast made up of Constitutional celebrities to common citizenry (see Stringhams references to Miranda & McCarter, 2016; Wright, 2002; Wright & Cowen, 2008).

Constrasting the lyrical dialgoue of *"Hamilton: An American Musical"* to his own economic history scholarship, Stringham establishes his fundamental case against Hamilton's singular genius status by asserting that not unlike many readers of academic and popular culture texts that abbreviate and obfuscate the impact of multiple factors in historic and economic outcomes, "Viewers of the musical could come away with a pro-government message, and politicians might like the musical for making them look important. But economic analysis and economic history highlight how markets are not invented by one person. Despite what the great-man theory of history would have us believe, markets are the product of countless people's choices. Markets also evolve often in spite of what government officials desire" (Stringham, 2017, p. 529). Simply put, Stringham doesn't directly confirm nor contradict Hamilton "the man's" possible economic genius and Hamilton "the musical's" possible entertainment genius. However, he makes quite clear that Alexander Hamilton is but one of many antecedents and actors in bringing about the economic systems that eventually propelled the new nation of the United States to prosperity.

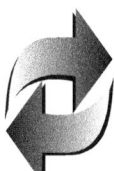

YES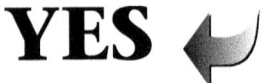

Donald F. Swanson and Andrew P. Trout

Alexander Hamilton's Economic Policies After Two Centuries

A commemorative examination of Hamilton's policies reveals and corrects a number of doubtful assumptions that have crept into the collective mind of American historians. Donald Swanson is Professor of Economics and Business Administration, and Andrew P. Trout is Professor of History, both at Indiana University Southeast in New Albany, Indiana.

Alexander Hamilton remains obscure to many Americans. Millions have seen his bronze statue at the foot of the south steps of the Treasury in Washington, DC, but how many know he lived his entire life as an American in New York? Yet, the name Alexander Hamilton is better known than that of many presidents of the United States. In fact, a recent survey found a large percentage of respondents believing he actually was a president![1] That misunderstanding is but the most obvious of several surrounding America's first secretary of the treasury. In the two centuries since he wrote his most famous reports to the U.S. Congress, one on public credit (1790) and the other on manufactures (1791), there has accumulated in textbooks and general histories a cluster of dubious assumptions about Hamilton. Few are entirely without foundation; a number are half-true or exaggerations. It is paradoxical that the name Hamilton is so widely known and yet his role in the new national government established by the U.S. Constitution is more obscure than it ought to be.

Among the most notable misunderstandings about Hamilton are: (1) that he favored the broad exercise of executive and congressional power, even to the point of being our first national planner; (2) that Hamilton's Bank of the United States was the capstone, the crowning point, of his economic policy; (3) that Hamilton was a protectionist who favored tariffs to aid manufacturers—some have even labeled him a mercantilist, a term suggesting not simply import restrictions but, among other things, statutes subsidizing or regulating business; (4) that Secretary Hamilton's policy was calculated to gain the support of the people who mattered by showing special regard for wealth as such; and (5) that to Hamilton a national debt was a good thing in itself—a "national blessing." A corollary of the last misunderstanding is that Hamilton, unlike Thomas Jefferson, never demonstrated much concern for a balanced budget.

Virtually every authority agrees that Hamilton was a nationalist in the sense of stressing the authority of the national rather than state governments—although inferences that historians draw from this will vary considerably. Born in the West Indies, Hamilton did not arrive in continental America until age 17 and never did develop a strong regional attachment; New York did not mean to him what Virginia meant to Thomas Jefferson or James Madison. In fact, he became highly suspicious of the power of the states, for he had seen that power used to excess, even in a manner that threatened to dissolve the "cement" of the union. No wonder he usually interpreted the powers of Congress more broadly than did "strict constructionists" like Madison and Jefferson.

Yet Hamilton's nationalism was selective, hardly amounting to a system. One of the few nationalistic measures that Hamilton actually did recommend was a Bank of the United States. But this he regarded mainly as a vehicle for administering treasury business rather than a foretaste of some economic grand plan.[2] He even opposed the bank's directors when they began establishing branches of the bank in states outside Pennsylvania.[3] But, as we shall see, there is undoubtedly a strong element of nationalism in his financial program in the sense that the national government would enhance its own importance by assuming responsibility not only for debts incurred by the United States but also for those of the several states.[4]

But if we stretch Hamiltonian nationalism much beyond this in the purely domestic sphere, we enter the realm of speculation. His other programs really did little to push forward the frontiers of national authority. Hamilton put forth no grandiose scheme to subsidize American commerce or manufacturing. He did not propose so much as a national system of roads or a rivers and harbors program to facilitate that commerce. Quite the contrary: in 1799, he contended that congressional legislation to provide internal improvements would be unconstitutional.[5] Although his famous Report on Manufactures abounds in fine words about a mixed economy of agriculture and manufacturing, it actually proposes very few government initiatives aside from a commission to apportion bounties on exports—the whole thing contingent on a treasury surplus.[6] The report not only failed to advocate a list of specific regulatory measures or subsidies—the cost might well have been prohibitive anyway—it stopped short of recommending even so much as a protective tariff.[7] For Hamilton, for reasons to be discussed, viewed a tariff strictly for revenue as far more compatible with his program to restore public credit.

Hamilton was an eighteenth-century man in an eighteenth-century environment. In that era, government was small by modern standards. European states, lacking modern means to tax their subjects' wealth, were usually pressed for revenues. The U.S.' tax resources were especially limited, for that government depended almost exclusively on the proceeds of import duties. There were no internal taxes when Hamilton became treasury secretary. Revenues from land sales and profits of the post office, neither of which were sizable, were the only other sources of money. Besides, the public normally expected that bolder initiatives, if any, would come from state or local administrations, not the national government. It was state and local government that chartered banks, subsidized and regulated what little industry there was, launched joint ventures with business to build roads or bridges, and more. Had the national government proposed ambitious programs, many in the Congress who were highly sensitive to the slightest encroachment on state autonomy would have objected.

We have observed that the secretary did not venture so far as to propose a protective tariff. Genuinely protective duties on imports would have interfered with his overall fiscal policy, which implied a brisk trade with England. Foreign trade brought in customs duties, and those revenues kept the U.S. government afloat in an age long before the income tax.[8]

If Hamilton's renown as nationalist or mercantilist is somewhat exaggerated, so too is his reputation as a partisan of the rich. Some recent historians have concluded that Hamilton's program was not tailored to the interests of a single class or to the wealthy in general.[9] Rather, the secretary held that without the support of moneyed men, government and the economy, both in their infancy, would falter. Undoubtedly, though, there were benefits for some holders of government securities and for those merchants that stood to profit from the commerce with England that Hamilton's fiscal program demanded.

We shall understand Hamilton better if we remember that as secretary he was pursuing a policy whose purposes were fiscal as well as political. Obvious as this may seem, it deserves emphasis. The fine points seem to have eluded many observers because understanding Hamilton means venturing into that thicket known as public finance. The 200th anniversary of his Report on the Public Credit recently passed almost unnoticed, but a look at this often cited but little read document is rewarding. It will help to answer the question: If Hamilton is widely conceded to have been a financial wizard, a genius, America's greatest finance minister, why?

One might begin by inquiring what was the most pressing problem facing the treasury secretary appointed (September 1789) by the recently inaugurated President George Washington. Hamilton—together with most contemporaries and subsequent historians—would surely have answered that it was to establish public credit. But the new finance minister faced what amounted to an enormous pile of unpaid bills; the "price of liberty" was not cheap.[10] Government securities issued during the revolutionary era were selling on the market at 10–20 cents on the dollar. The Constitution had made these debts the debts of the new government; one had to deal with them in order to establish public credit, or else face a threat to the life of the new nation. Commercial depression, foreign domination, rebellion, and a collapse of the union—all seemed possible. To assure confidence at home and abroad, something had to be done quickly, Hamilton reasoned, to put public credit on a solid foundation. The formula he proposed was quite bold.

Everything depended upon who was in charge of the treasury. Men like Jefferson believed that rapid debt retirement should have priority.[11] Hamilton thought otherwise and did the unexpected: he established credit within two years or less while, for all practical purposes, avoiding the use of tax revenues for immediate debt reduction. He knew that if the new nation dissipated its meager revenues on debt reduction at a time when simply meeting interest payments was a herculean task, the result would be neither substantial reduction of debt nor prompt payment of interest. The United States would continue to lack credit.

Hamilton's views on a national debt are widely misunderstood. For him debt was no unqualified blessing. There is no reason to assume that he would have created a debt had none existed. Rather, the debt he had inherited was an unpleasant fact that he had to deal with. To do so, he proposed to *fund* it—that is, to set aside, or mortgage, specific tax revenues for annual payment of interest. The idea can be found in his Report on the Public Credit although he explains it more clearly in later writings.[12] Creditors who had received past installments irregularly would, he hoped, regain confidence in government's commitment to pay its debts. Funding also meant indefinite postponement of repayment of principal. A government faced with no obligation to return principal on a fixed schedule could more easily use its sparse tax resources to pay interest in full. In other words, it would be easier to support the nation's debt if it were funded. It was a funded debt, and only a funded debt, that Hamilton considered a blessing![13]

More controversial than funding was the secretary's proposal not to discriminate between persons who had purchased securities directly from government and those who had obtained them from the original purchasers.[14] This struck Madison as highly unjust—a windfall for speculators who had bought up national government certificates cheaply at second hand. On its face, Madison's charge may seem well grounded. It is estimated that only 25 percent to 40 percent of security holders had acquired them at the time of issue; the others had bought them at depreciated prices. However, a closer look at the circumstances of original acquisitions may destroy one's illusions about the legions of widows and orphans who allegedly had paid good money for government paper, only to lose much in reselling the certificates to speculators. For example, before September 1777, loan office certificates with a face value of $200 were purchased with currency actually worth $65 to $100. In early 1778, it was possible to acquire 6 percent securities with notes worth no more than 25 cents on the dollar. Thus, the original holders of this government paper could draw interest perhaps as high as 25 percent—that is, as long as interest was paid. It is conceivable that some original holders profited as much in earlier years as did secondary holders who, later, benefited from Hamilton's plan.[15]

It was not simply the debts of the United States that were at stake; Hamilton further proposed to pay the debts incurred by the states during the Revolution, plus arrears of interest, on terms comparable to other debts.[16] There is no denying that assumption of state debts would add to annual interest charges owed by the treasury. How could a nation relying on little more than customs duties meet a heavy annual interest burden?

Hamilton's solution demonstrated audacity, to say the least. It amounted to reopening loan offices and inviting security holders to march in and trade (that is, to convert) their old 6 percent holdings for new annuities paying an average of 4 percent.[17] It should be stressed that the debt consisted largely of perpetual annuities—perpetual, that is, as long as the treasury chose not to redeem them by repaying principal. Conversion of these was possible, and legal, if the market rate of interest dropped. By redeeming old annuities bearing high interest rates and renegotiating them at lower rates, European governments had effected such conversions. Hamilton proposed to do so but with a difference: he would convert annuities not to the current market rate but to an anticipated lower market rate of around 4 percent (a rate he expected to prevail in 20 years). Thus, the secretary left himself vulnerable to the charge of partial repudiation.

Neither Hamilton nor the government creditors were fully in control. On the one hand, Hamilton lacked the leverage to insure their cooperation in accepting the lower rate. On the other hand, their depreciated securities might never increase in value unless Hamilton's plan worked. What is more, they lacked the numerous investment alternatives (such as certificates of deposit) available today. Hamilton was offering creditors less than they wanted, to be sure, but it was more than they were likely to recoup if his plan misfired. Besides, there is no way to assess accurately the impact of Hamilton's conversion on an individual annuity holder without knowing how much real money he had spent to purchase it.

To further complicate the picture, not all investors actually wanted the securities to increase in value. A number were engaged in short selling, trading depreciated government issues currently being accepted at par for public lands.[18] Hamilton could hardly count on these investors for assistance; their operations were more likely to undermine public credit than to enhance it.

What, then, did Hamilton have to trade for investors' cooperation? He devised several "fair equivalents" (to use his term) to appease them. Ordinarily, the holder of a perpetual annuity might worry about the government's canceling his contract (this was permissible) and repaying the principal at any time that the market rate of interest fell. However, in return for creditors' acceptance of the lower 4 percent interest rate, Hamilton assured them this would not happen—*except* for redemption of a small although ever increasing percentage of the principal each year. Limited redeemability was the "fair equivalent" that Congress eventually approved.[19] And, what was quite important, the secretary would assure public confidence by funding these new obligations.

Hamilton gambled that most public creditors would cooperate with the new regime. But the program was calculated to work only if it was accepted almost instantaneously. Drop the funding portion or the conversion and it might well collapse; without the former, there was far less assurance that interest would be paid regularly; without conversion, the government could ill afford to pay it. The tariff bill that Congress had passed a few months before Hamilton entered office—plus the small excises he persuaded it to enact—could hardly meet the nation's revenue needs if its creditors failed to agree to the conversion.

Hamilton was not only gambling on the voluntary cooperation of government creditors, he was also counting on support in Congress. Even at this early date in our nation's history, men cut political deals to gain the support of a congressional majority. Where assumption of the states' debts was concerned, nothing came cheaply. Special monetary considerations for Virginians financially interested in the settlement of state accounts and the eventual placement of the capital along the swampy banks of the Potomac river were the price of Virginia's assent to Hamilton's assumption proposal.

For Americans, Hamilton's program was novel. The very notion of funding a debt was derived from England of the 1690s.[20] Abroad, a legally imposed conversion was a familiar concept. But no one had ever combined all of Hamilton's proposals into one plan. There was no certainty that Congress would swallow the program whole; even if it did, there was still reason to wonder whether it would work.

The gamble worked. Congress did accept the scheme, enacting it into law on August 4, 1790, and so did the average public creditor. By July of the following year, the greater part of the funded debt was selling at par; by early 1792, it commanded a premium.[21] Within a short space of time, America went from a nation with no credit to one that could borrow in the major financial capitals of Europe on terms equal to those with the strongest credit.

There was no way to prevent speculators from benefiting from these rising security prices. But Hamilton's program was not designed to enrich either original or secondary holders of government debt; rather, he saw their profits as unavoidable results of stabilizing the market for U.S. securities, which for him was a precondition to establishing public credit. Hamilton in fact had no use for the speculators; their betting was destabilizing the securities market by driving it up and down.[22] He, for his part, was trying to raise and maintain the price of government debt instruments so that this paper could circulate as currency, adding to a money supply that he thought deficient. Nor did all speculators welcome the Hamilton funding program. Those who were bullish on government debt doubtless stood to benefit. But the short sellers who had contracted to buy national or state government land in the future by trading government securities at par were gambling on a low, if not lower, market price. Hamilton had no part in this; his concern was for stable public credit, not profiteering. Had his motives been so base as his opponents charged, the secretary might not have left office personally insolvent.

Alexander Hamilton and Thomas Jefferson, it is easy to assume, had to be on opposite sides of a given issue: if one plays this game, Hamilton must be tolerant of "special interests," high tariffs, and unbalanced budgets, among other things, while Jefferson is not. In practice, it is more difficult than is commonly believed to distinguish between a Hamiltonian and a Jeffersonian economic system. Occasionally, we see the partisans of each leader playing roles opposite those for which they are cast. It is not always easy to say whose system was better calculated to benefit the special interests Hamilton allegedly favored. Take the example of protective tariffs, which are almost bound to aid manufacturers. It was Hamilton who declined to recommend them. Higher tariffs eventually won approval from the Jefferson administration (1801–1809).[23] Finally, it was President James Madison who, in the words of a contemporary politician, "out-Hamiltons Alexander Hamilton."[24] In 1816, he signed America's first genuinely protective tariff. Even the Bank of the United States, proposed by Alexander Hamilton and deplored by the Jefferson–Madison faction, eventually won Madison's support; it was at his request that Congress rechartered the bank in 1816. Moreover, internal improvements that Hamilton did not endorse were recommended later by Jefferson's secretary of the treasury, Albert Gallatin, who in 1808 proposed a national system of roads and canals costing more than the Louisiana Purchase.

If Hamilton is widely viewed as one who believed that a national debt is a national blessing, he is at times cast as indifferent to, if not an advocate of, deficit spending. Neither view is tenable. Although the term deficit spending was not used in his day, we know what Hamilton thought about "currency finance": the term means that, following the lead of Massachusetts (1690), various colonial regimes spent more money than they collected in taxes and printed paper money to make up the difference.[25] In a number of instances, tax collections made it possible to withdraw the bills from circulation at a later date. But, unrestricted access to the printing press could spell disaster. From 1775 to 1779, the Continental Congress issued so many bills of credit that they eventually became "not worth a continental." In disillusionment, the authors of the Constitution specifically forbade states to print such bills. Hamilton not only endorsed this prohibition, he believed that it also applied to the federal government.[26] He was no friend of deficit spending.

Hamilton also rejected a commonplace English method of deficit spending. There, if a government suffered a shortfall in tax revenues, it could simply add that deficit to the funded debt. For the immediate future, the effect was to increase interest payable each year; principal repayment was indefinitely postponed. It is conventional to exaggerate Hamilton's dependence on the practices of English public finance, and here is one more example. Far from favoring this English approach, once Hamilton had funded the debt inherited from the Revolution, he refused to expand it—in fact, the funded debt held by the public declined between 1791 and 1795.[27]

It is clear that Hamilton wanted to repay that debt. And the limited redeemability clauses built into his conversion plan made it possible for government to liquidate the greater part of that debt in 34 years (reduced to 24 years by Congress).[28] Again, Hamilton is closer to Jefferson than is widely imagined; the latter advocated complete liquidation in 19 years. Meanwhile, any revenue deficiency incurred during Hamilton's years as secretary was covered by short-term loans (either in domestic markets or Amsterdam) requiring repayment of principal within the next few years. Hamilton's reports and letters make it quite clear that America's first head of the treasury strongly preferred to have all spending covered by tax revenues.

In this last respect, Hamilton's views were not far removed from Jefferson's. Although their reasoning differed, both men believed in balanced budgets. Jefferson was alarmed that each additional year of deficit meant a larger debt. It was a moral issue; one generation had no right to bind another.[29] Hamilton wanted to avoid deficits because the plan he chose for establishing public credit promised as much; he saw his funding system as basically a contract, a promise to the nation's creditors that revenues would be sufficient to cover all government spending, especially interest on the debt. The penalty for failure to live up to that promise was more than just passing a debt to one's children; it was tantamount to bequeathing them a nation lacking credit and financial and economic soundness.

This was not mere political rhetoric. During Hamilton's tenure as secretary, revenues were sufficient to establish public credit and to build a strong financial base. As might be expected, his halfdozen years in office saw both surpluses and deficits. Pursuing Hamiltonian financial practices, John Adams' administration (1797–1801) witnessed budgetary surpluses every year except one.[30]

The Report on the Public Credit can be seen as a blueprint for a financial revolution. At the time, the very idea of solvency was startling, to say the least. While other nations habitually got deeper in debt and expanded taxation, America did the reverse. Hamilton's policy was to limit spending and keep tax rates low; the economy would grow into debt reduction as tax revenues based on existing rates expanded. Jefferson went further. He abolished all internal taxes and reduced the debt simultaneously.[31] Revenues came primarily from import duties. Despite the costs of the Louisiana Purchase and the War of 1812, the national debt dropped to zero by 1835. America's fiscal experiment, both in its Hamiltonian and Jeffersonian versions, was truly revolutionary. Hamilton's maxim set the tone: "The creation of debt should always be accompanied with the means of extinguishment."[32]

Notes

1. The survey was of incoming freshmen at a major university in the mid-1980s.
2. Hamilton saw a national bank performing only an "auxiliary" role in the area of public credit. For the administration of the finances, he thought it essential; the routine chores this demanded could hardly make the bank the centerpiece of an economic planning mechanism. First Report on the Further Provision Necessary for Establishing Public Credit. 13 December 1790, Harold C. Syrett and others, eds., *The Papers of Alemnder Hamilton* (27 vols., New York, 1961–1987), 7: 235, hereafter cited as Hamilton Papers. Hamilton's ideas on a national bank changed over time. See Donald F. Swanson and Andrew P. Trout. "Alexander Hamilton, 'the Celebrated Mr. Neckar,' and Public Credit," *The William and Mary Quarterly* 47 (July 1990), 422–430.
3. Alexander Hamilton to William Seton. 25 November 1791, *Hamilton Papers*, 9: 538–539.
4. *Ibid.*, 6: 78.
5. Alexander Hamilton to Jonathan Dayton, October–November 1799, *Hamilton Papers*, 23: 603, and Report on the Subject of Manufactures, *ibid.*, 10: 310.
6. *Ibid.*, 10: 337–338.
7. Hamilton's report discussed theoretically or historically a number of ideas, including protectionism. The specific tariff rates he proposed, however, were significantly below those now considered protectionist. He recommended increasing ad valorem duties on items manufactured of iron to 10%; steel or brass products to 7½%. Other recommended rates included new highs of 7½% to 10%, even 15% for a few items. Still, the average tariff on goods taxed (many were untaxed),

if his recommendations had been accepted (they were not), would have been well below 15%. In other words, he did not propose anything close to a protective tariff. The tariff of 1816, considered America's first protective tariff, authorities estimate at anywhere from 15 percent to 20 percent on average.

8. The dependency of Hamilton's policies on import revenues was pointed out in Joseph Charles, *The Origins of the American Party System: Three Essays* (Williamsburg, VA, 1956), 13, 19. John R. Nelson, Jr. sees the timing of the presentation to Congress of Hamilton's Report on Manufactures as reflecting Hamilton's interest in promoting his pet project, the Society for the Encouragement of Manufuctures. This was a private manufacturing venture whose stock went on sale in late 1791. The report, requested by Congress nearly two years before, was presented on December 5, 1791. Nelson saw the issuance of the long-awaited report and the selling of stock in the society as more than a coincidence; had Hamilton been interested in promoting manufactures on a national scale he would not have delayed his report that long. *Liberty and Property: Political Economy and Policymaking in the New Nation, 1789–1812* (Baltimore, MD, 1987), 41 *and passim*.

9. Thomas P. Govan, "The Rich, the Well-born, and Alexander Hamilton," *The Mississippi Valley Historical Review 36* (March 1950), 675–680.

10. Report Relative to a Provision for the Support of Public Credit, 9 January 1790, *Hamilton Papers*, 6: 69.

11. Thomas Jefferson to George Washington, 9 September 1792, Paul Leicester Ford, ed., *The Writings of Thomas Jefferson* (10 vols., New York, 1892–1899), 6: 105.

12. *Hamilton Papers*, 6: 105–106, and The Defence of the Funding System, July 1795, *ibid.*, 19: 46, 50.

13. *Hamilton Papers*, 6: 106.

14. *Ibid.*, 78.

15. William G. Anderson, *The Price of Liberty: The Public Debt of the American Revolution* (Charlottesville, VA, 1983), 8–10, 37–38.

16. *Hamilton Papers*, 6: 78, 86–87.

17. *Ibid.*, 87–97, 109.

18. Forrest McDonald, *Alexnnder Hamilton: A Biography* (New York, 1979), 153–154.

19. Hamilton Papers, 6: 88, 90. Without assurance of limited redeemability, foreigners interested in U.S. domestic debt—burdened as they were with costs of insurance, brokerage, and the like—would find it uneconomical to hold those securities. So argued Fisher Ames, a Hamilton spokesman in the House of Representatives. March 13, 1790, Annals of the Congress of the United States: The Debates and Proceedings in the Congress of the United States (Washington, 1834), 2: 1441.

20. Donald F. Swanson, *The Origins of Hamilton's Fiscal Policies* (Gainesville, FL, 1963), 11–17, 85.

21. Joseph Stancliffe Davis, *Essays in the Earlier History of American Corporations* (2 vols., Cambridge, Mass., 1917), 1: 194–195 and John Watts Kearny, *Sketch of American Finances* (New York, 1887), 35.

22. *Hamilton Papers*, 6: 71.

23. Nelson, *Liberty and Property*, 153.

24. Cited in Irving Brant, *The Founh President: A Life of James Madison* (Indianapolis, 1970), 597.

25. E. James Ferguson, *The Power of the Purse* (Williamsburg, VA, 1961), 1–24 and *passim*.

26. *Hamilton Papers*, 7: 321–322.

27. Swanson, *Origins*, 57.

28. The 6 percent and 6 percent deferreds (the two types of limited redeemability securities) resulting from the conversion were liquidated in 1818 and 1824, respectively. Rafael Bayley, *The National Loans of the United States from July 4, 1776, to June 30, 1880* (2nd ed., New York, 1881), 110.

29. Jefferson to James Madison, 6 September 1789, Julian P. Boyd. ed., *The Papers of Thomas Jefferson* (22 vols. to date, Princeton, NJ, 1950–), 15: 392–393.

30. United States Bureau of the Census, Historical Statistics of the United States: Colonial Times to 1970 (Washington, 1975), 2: 1104.

31. Forrest McDonald, *The Presidency of Thomas Jefferson* (Lawrence, Kans., 1976), 52.

32. *Hamilton Papers*, 6: 106.

DONALD F. SWANSON, Professor of Economics and Business Administration, Indiana University Southeast, authored and coauthored dozens of books and journal articles that serve as influential works in the study of the public finance policies that impacted the founding and flourishing of the U.S. economic system(s) throughout the 18th and 19th centuries. From his early contributions "Orgins of Hamilton's Fiscal Policies" (1963) to his later works "Thomas Jefferson on Establishing Public Credit: The Debt Plans of a Would-be Secretary of the Treasury? (1993)," D. F. Swanson's impact on both academic and public discouse has been profound.

Andrew P. Trout, Professor of History, Indiana University, Southeast, authored and coauthored numerous journal articles examining both European (e.g., France) and North American (e.g., United States) social histories. Trout's works focusing on 17th and 19th centuries France (City of the seine: Paris in the time of Richelieu and Louis XIV, 1996) and his coauthored works with Donald F. Swanson examining U.S. economic and political histories in the 18th and 19th centuries have both informed academic and public policy conversations for the last two decades.

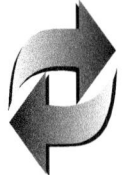

Edward Peter Stringham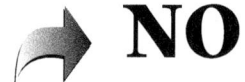

Hamilton's Legacy and the Great Man Theory of Financial History

Is Hamilton as important and visionary as most people say or an overrated mashup of often contradictory elements? It depends on whether we are talking about *Hamilton* the musical or Alexander Hamilton the politician. I must admit that I am not generally a fan of Broadway shows or anything related to hip-hop (Johann Strauss II is about as close to contemporary as I get), but I actually think *Hamilton* the musical is brilliant in multiple ways. It showcases the life and times of someone who was becoming an increasingly forgotten Founding Father, and it presents many details of his life and the history of America's Founding. As an art form, it is pathbreaking, and I can understand why it has won so many awards. In addition to its innovative musical form, I love its message about how an impoverished immigrant and an upstart nation can overcome barriers. In the words of the main character,

> I'm just like my country,
> I'm young, scrappy and hungry,
> And I am not throwing away my shot.
> ("My Shot" [Miranda and McCarter 2016, 26])

I also very much appreciate its assertion that the principles of the American Revolution can be inclusive to all groups: "And when I meet Thomas Jefferson . . . I'm 'a compel him to include women in the sequel!" (Angelica, "The Schuyler Sisters" [Miranda and McCarter 2016, 44]).

Even though I have no criticisms of this excellent work of theater, Alexander Hamilton, the politician, may not deserve as much praise. He was certainly an intriguing and important historical figure, but we must be careful not to ascribe too much importance to him or to any other one person for founding America or American financial markets specifically, as the *Economist* has done by calling Hamilton the "founder of 'Wall Street'" and a "visionary of capitalism" ("Hamiltonian America" 2011).

Although I believe that individuals, including Hamilton, have influenced historical outcomes, saying that a politician founded Wall Street is far off the mark and an unfortunate example of the great-man theory in action. In *Heroes, Hero-Worship, and the Heroic in History* ([1843] 2000), Thomas Carlyle advanced the theory that "the history of the world is but the biography of great men" (29). Early famous critics of the great-man theory included Leo Tolstoy ([1869] 2008) and Herbert Spencer (1873), who argued that societal outcomes are determined by the totality of individuals in society, not just by a few great men. Using more modern economic language, market outcomes are a spontaneous or emergent order—a product of the choices and interactions of billions of people (Stringham and Curott 2015). Each person makes conscious choices to advance his own wishes and desires; each person can influence outcomes; and some people can influence outcomes more than others. But societal or market outcomes are not the products or inventions of one great man or even of a few great men. To attribute modern American capitalism to Hamilton greatly exaggerates his importance. *Hamilton* is an amazingly creative adaptation of the life of an interesting person, but *Hamilton* mania should not be used to advance the narrative that politicians are responsible for inventing our financial system or American capitalism itself.

Does *Hamilton* Overemphasize the Importance of Politicians?

It would be unfair for a tweed-wearing professor to criticize a musical for lacking footnotes or the long meandering caveats found in academic journals or for containing rap battles with lines that are not 100 percent historically accurate. So nothing in this article should be interpreted as anything close to a critique of this excellent musical. But what people think about a particular topic or take away from a particular work of art is nevertheless important. *Hamilton* does not present the characters, including the lead, as flawless, and many characters, including George

Washington, James Madison, Thomas Jefferson, and Aaron Burr, advance good arguments at various points. Besides King George III—whom everyone should dislike—the musical does not come across as preachy about who is right or wrong in any debate. In certain ways, the musical takes the Socratic discussion of old ideas to a new level. Even if most of the audience is there for the musical experience and is unable to follow all of the fast-paced arguments, they will at least be exposed to some of the important debates that took place before, during, and after the American Revolution.

As an economist interested in the historical growth of financial markets, in watching *Hamilton*, I was most focused on the debates between Hamilton and Jefferson regarding Hamilton's plan to create a system of national debt.[1] During the American Revolution, many colonies issued bonds to finance the efforts to break free from England. After the revolution, although many state bonds seemed likely to be repaid, others were in a tenuous situation. Many holders of these bonds, who anticipated a lower probability of being paid, ended up selling them to speculators, who would assume the risk of default or the potential gain of any repayment. In modern times, we would call such bonds "distressed debt." A market for distressed debt exists because some people want to cash out now, whereas others are willing to assume more risk. At the time, Hamilton believed that having the federal government buy all state debt and redeem it at par would strengthen the federal government by enabling it to borrow more in the future. Much of this idea was based on the system of government debt in England, which was controversial to many who had just fought a revolution against such a relatively large centralized government. Hamilton presents this economic debate in a way that I and most others never would have predicted: through a high-speed rap battle. After the musical's first half depicts the American Revolution, it then moves to a discussion of governance and Hamilton's financial plans, among other things. With Jefferson still basking in victory, singing, "Lookin' at the rolling fields/I can't believe that we are free," Madison gives a wake-up call:

> Thomas, we are engaged in a battle for our nation's very soul. Can you get us out of the mess we're in?
> . . . .
> Hamilton's new financial plan is nothing less
> Than government control.
> . . . .
> Where have you been?
> ("What'd I Miss?" [Miranda and McCarter 2016, 152–53])

In the scene "Cabinet Battle #1," Washington sets the stage: "The issue on the table: Secretary Hamilton's plan to assume state debt and establish a national bank. Secretary Jefferson, you have the floor." Jefferson then begins the debate:

> JEFFERSON: "Life, liberty and the pursuit of happiness." We fought for these ideals; we shouldn't settle for less.
> These are wise words, enterprising men quote 'em.
> Don't act surprised, you guys, cuz I wrote 'em.
> JEFFERSON/MADISON: Oww.
> JEFFERSON: But Hamilton forgets
> His plan would have the government assume states' debts.

Now, place your bets as to who that benefits:

the very seat of government where Hamilton sits.

Jefferson then goes on to state:

> Ooh, if the shoe fits, wear it.
> If New York's in debt—
> Why should Virginia bear it? Uh! Our debts are paid, I'm afraid.
> Don't tax the South cuz we got it made in the shade.
> In Virginia, we plant seeds in the ground.
> We create. You just wanna move our money around.
>
> This financial plan is an outrageous demand,
> And it's too many damn pages for any man to understand.
> Stand with me in the land of the free
> And pray to God we never see Hamilton's candidacy.
> Look, when Britain taxed our tea, we got frisky.
> Imagine what gon' happen when you try to tax our whisky.
> ("Cabinet Battle #1" [Miranda and McCarter 2016, 161])

Here, we see two possible strands of criticism in Jefferson's arguments: one against central government and central debt and one possibly against banking in general. The Hamilton biography by Ron Chernow (2004), on which the musical is based, sometimes lumps these two positions together or at least does not get into the finer distinctions for future playwrights. As Jefferson suggests, having the federal government assume state debts would mean that the federal government would need to start collecting taxes from all. Those who bought New York bonds essentially lent that state money with the hope of being repaid. Default risk is built into the interest rate on any loan in case the borrower will not pay. As Murray Rothbard (1992) and Jeffrey Rogers Hummel (2012) describe, any time government creates debt, it creates a claim on future taxpayers' money, and the natural question is: Why should federal taxpayers pay for the losses incurred by investors who voluntarily assumed the risks of lending the government money?

Jefferson's next debate point can be interpreted in a libertarian or possibly not libertarian way, as condemning centralized government debt in particular or finance in general. Jefferson suggests that Virginians actually create, whereas northeasterners just move money around.[2] The musical later contains some anti–Wall Street sentiment from Jefferson and Burr. Describing Hamilton, Jefferson says:

> I get no satisfaction witnessing his fits of passion.
> The way he primps and preens and dresses like the pits of fashion.
> Our poorest citizens, our farmers, live ration to ration
> As Wall Street robs 'em blind in search of chips to cash in.
> ("Washington on Your Side" [Miranda and McCarter 2016, 199])

And at another point in the play, Burr criticizes Hamilton:

> Oh, Wall Street thinks you're great.
> You'll always be adored by the things you create.
> But upstate—
> . . . .
> —people think you're crooked!
> ("Schuyler Defeated" [Miranda and McCarter 2016, 191])

This exchange likely puts many Broadway showgoers in a difficult position. Although a *Rolling Stone* writer such as Matt Taibbi (2011) would likely reject the idea that we need to be farmers to create value, he argues at the same time that Wall Street finance is nothing more than "bubble machines, vampire squids, and the long con that is breaking America." The proper libertarian position, I believe, is to condemn a system of government bailouts where some people or corporations voluntarily assume risks and then discharge those risks onto unwilling taxpayers when things turn sour. Bailouts indeed shift money around without creating anything of value. But that does not mean we should condemn financial intermediation and Wall Street in general. Helping companies raise money from the general public expands the pool of available finance to help companies expand, and it lets regular people share in large corporations' success by giving them a small ownership stake and claim to some of the company's profits. Such financial intermediation is voluntary for all parties involved, and it puts the little guy on the same side as big business. Helping companies grow benefits consumers, too. Without a basic understanding of economics, any Occupy Wall Street–leaning viewer will miss this point and not know whom to root for in this debate.

> Back in "Cabinet Battle #1," Hamilton responds:
> Thomas. That was a real nice declaration.
> Welcome to the present, we're running a real nation.
> Would you like to join us, or stay mellow,
> Doin' whatever the hell it is you do in Monticello?
> If we assume the debts, the union gets
> A new line of credit, a financial diuretic.
> How do you not get it? If we're aggressive and competitive.
> The union gets a boost. You'd rather give it a sedative?
> (Miranda and McCarter 2016 161)

Hamilton goes on to discuss how the Virginians' debts are paid because they "don't pay for labor" and then speaks some lines best left out of an academic article.

The main character does not get into the importance of manufacturing or trade (whether free market or mercantilist),[3] but he definitely appears to be on the side of economic progress. But at what cost, and who is the driver? To many, economic progress depends on government expansion. Jefferson later criticizes Hamilton for being power hungry but still suggests he is advancing the economy: "Have you an ounce of regret?/You accumulate debt, you accumulate power" ("Cabinet Battle #2" [Miranda and McCarter 2016, 193]).

> And the others complain about Hamilton:
> MADISON: So, he's doubled the size of the government.
> Wasn't the trouble with much of our previous government size?
> BURR: Look in his eyes!
> JEFFERSON: See how he lies.
> MADISON: Follow the scent of his enterprise.
> JEFFERSON: Centralizing national credit
> And making American credit competitive.
> ("Washington on Your Side" [Miranda and McCarter 2016, 199])

After this, a great deal of drama happens—I will leave out any spoilers about whether anyone dies in a duel in Weehawken, NJ—but many people, including Hamilton's former adversaries, end up praising him. In a moment of reflection, Hamilton talks about what he has achieved:

I wrote about The Constitution and defended it well.
And in the face of ignorance and resistance,
I wrote financial systems into existence.
("Hurricane" [Miranda and McCarter 2016, 232]).

In the end, his former critics sing:

JEFFERSON: I'll give him this: his financial system is a
Work of genius. I couldn't undo it if I tried.
And I tried.
. . . .
MADISON: He took our country from bankruptcy to prosperity.
I hate to admit it, but he doesn't get enough credit
For all the credit he gave us.
("Who Lives, Who Dies, Who Tells Your Story?" [Miranda and McCarter 2016, 280])

Markets: A Creation of an Invisible Hand or of Politicians?

Viewers of the musical could come away with a pro-Hamilton and pro-government message, and politicians might like the musical for making them look important.[4] But economic analysis and economic history highlight how markets are not invented by one person. Describing the origins of the London Stock Exchange, the historian Harold Wincott writes, "It would be nice to start this book with a satisfyingly round sentence: 'on the –th day of —— in the year of our Lord ——, the Stock Exchange, London, came into being.' Alas for those with tidy minds, the Stock Exchange is a typically British institution. No one can say with any certainty exactly when it started. Like Topsy, it almost seems it never was born, but just 'grow'd'" (1946, 1).[5]

Despite what the great-man theory of history would have us believe, markets are the product of countless people's choices. Markets also evolve often in spite of what government officials desire. In Amsterdam, London, and New York, stockbrokers saw the opportunity to make money and started conducting business hundreds of years before government gave them the official go ahead. One thus cannot attribute the invention of these markets to government or to any one politician.

People who have state-centric views of markets would argue that such contracts can exist only when government enforces them. It turns out, however, that from very early on government looked down on these types of contracts and refused to enforce them, but people engaged in them anyway. Since the earliest financial markets, political authorities have not understood them and have considered many transactions associated with the stock market as wasteful, manipulative, and immoral (De Vries and Ad Van Der Woude 1997, 150; Garber 2000, 34). The first major stock market emerged in Amsterdam around 1600, but within a few years, government officials started passing laws against much of the speculative trading that they called "trading in wind" (Kellenbenz [1957] 1996, 34–35). Even though brokers' contracts were now illegal, brokers were not punished for engaging in them, so people ignored the prohibitions. Not only did market participants engage in these forward contracts where one party had a long position and the other had a short position but they also developed many other advanced contracts, including hypothetication (pledging securities as collateral for a loan), options, and derivatives. All of these contracts were complex, and none was enforceable in court.

How did unregulated markets work? Rather than relying on law, brokers relied on market mechanisms, including the discipline of continuous dealings to induce contractual performance (Smith [1766] 1982; Klein 1997). One seventeenth-century stockbroker, Josef Penso de la Vega ([1688] 1996), describes how trade, repeat dealings, and reputation mechanisms work. Although anyone could show up to the market, he could not necessarily find trading counterparts. De la Vega outlines the consequences of building a reputation (201). People who were new to the market had to start off small and gradually build up their reputation before they could engage in larger transactions. Anyone who defaulted, whether intentionally or by accident, would be badmouthed and boycotted by others.[6] The market became wildly successful, and the Dutch East India Company and the Dutch West India Company helped create capitalism for the masses. The Dutch Golden Age was made possible by companies that were not even intended to be around for more than a few years. Henry Hudson's voyage in 1609 to what is now known as the Hudson River in New York was financed by the Dutch East India Company, and New Amsterdam (New York) was a trading post of the Dutch West India Company.

Almost a century later in England, the government was also hardly supportive of the stock market and passed various rules and regulations interfering with it. In 1696, officials passed an act "To Restrain the Number and the Practice of Brokers and Stockjobbers" and effectively banned stockbrokers from trading at the Royal Exchange (Harris 2000, 225). In the Bubble Act of 1720, officials all but outlawed the formation of new joint stock companies,[7] and a bill in 1734 intended "to prevent the infamous Practice of Stock-jobbing" also banned options, futures, and margin trading. Government animosity toward stock traders persisted for well more than a century (Harris 2000, 225).

Despite the law, stock markets persisted, and stockbrokers continued trading. Although much of their trading was illegal, government did not actively punish them and essentially left them alone. Without an official home, stockbrokers met around Change Alley and in Jonathan's and Garraway's Coffee Houses. Intentional or unintentional default is bad for business, so brokers decided to transform coffee houses into private clubs to create and enforce rules and exclude defaulters. At first, they put defaulters' names on a chalkboard, and later they had stricter membership requirements. By excluding unreliable parties, the market became more dependable. As Thomas Mortimer wrote in 1761, "The gentlemen at this very period of time . . . have taken it into their heads that some of the fraternity are not so good as themselves . . . and have entered into an association to exclude them from [Jonathan's] coffee-house" (quoted in Smith 1929, 215). The name of their trading venue evolved from "Jonathan's Coffee House" to "New Jonathan's" to "Stock Subscription Room" to "Stock Exchange," and it is now known as the London Stock Exchange. So who "designed" the London Stock Exchange? Many people and the market itself.

Financial markets in America have a similar history, with no one party creating them. When Hamilton was 22 years old, in 1779, George Washington wrote, "Stock jobbing, speculating, engrossing, &ca. &ca., seems to be the great business of the day" (1939, 73), and when Hamilton was around 34, in 1791, James Madison wrote, "[S]tock jobbing drowns every other subject. The coffee house is an eternal buzz with the gamblers" (1865, 538). The precursor to the New York Stock and Exchange Board and later the New York Stock Exchange was the Tontine Tavern and Coffee House, created by merchants in 1792.

As much as one might admire Hamilton's singing or rap-battle prowess, he did not invent financial markets. At best, he helped issue new government debt. Libertarians and others can debate whether issuing this new debt was good or bad. But looking at an issuer of debt and concluding that this person created financial markets would be equivalent to looking at Anheuser-Busch's recent large bond issue and saying that the company invented the first bonds or beer itself. The great-man view of history tends to overlook the actions of the multitude and to say that markets were created by one man or a particular set of men. But that is not how markets work.

Conclusion

Although I think *Hamilton* is great, it should not be used to advance a great-man theory of history or let politicians claim that modern markets are attributable to their forebears. At a time when most people hold politicians in such low regard (Kessler 2013), I can easily envision politicians watching the musical and projecting their own importance onto the main character. I do not fault the musical for having a main character and focusing on his achievements. A musical starring an invisible hand would not be popular. Nevertheless, we can question enablers of politicians who want to overstate their importance in the creation of positive outcomes in the economy.

In contrast to the line that states Hamilton "doesn't get enough credit/For all the credit he gave us" ("Who Lives, Who Dies, Who Tells Your Story?" [Miranda and McCarter 2016, 280]), I think the credit should go to the countless people who worked behind the scenes to make modern markets possible and whom history has forgotten. Whereas government debt truly shifts money around and does not create value, financial markets help funnel money from investors to productive companies, which benefits all parties. Such outcomes are not the invention of one man, such as Hamilton, but instead are made possible by the 450,000 New Yorkers currently working in finance and their countless contemporaries and precursors around the world.

Notes

1. For a detailed history of Hamilton's role in creating national debt, see Wright (2002, 2008) and Wright and Cowen (2006).

2. In subsequent commentary, Miranda writes, "The fun in writing these debates is of course articulating the perspectives of these men in a way that feels contemporary. Jefferson echoes the feelings of many critics of Wall Street when he says, 'We create. You just move our money around.' If I were watching that in a rap battle, I'd nod my head" (Miranda and McCarter 2016, 161).

3. For an insight into Hamilton's pro-industry but not necessarily pro-free-market perspective, see

Hamilton (1791). Lawrence White (2016) describes Hamilton as "a second-hand dealer in retrograde mercantilist ideas."

4. This section draws from Stringham (2015) and Stringham and Curott (2015).

5. The stock exchange had various rules, and it documented them in its first written rulebook in 1812. The rulebook stated that although many disputes could be settled with existing rules, "many others (which, from their nature and extent, preclude the possibility of forming any general laws on the subject, so as to meet every contingency) may also be adjusted by the known custom and practice of the market" (Committee for General Purposes of the Stock-Exchange 1812, 10). The stock exchange had rules about admissions and membership and what would happen if someone defaulted or got into a dispute. The rules stated that "all disputes between individuals (not affecting the general interests of the Stock-Exchange) shall be referred to arbitration" (20). Defaulters would have their membership suspended and could have their membership renewed only if they made good on their debts and petitioned to have their membership reinstated. By excluding most of the unreliable people to begin with and kicking out anyone else who violated the rules, the London Stock Exchange created a system of privately generated order. It later adopted as its motto "My word is my bond."

6. De la Vega writes, "Since the status, the insignificant capital, the low reputation, and the limited trustworthiness of such people are well known, they do not dare attempt to carry on any considerable business" (1688, 201). For more illustrations about the importance of reputation, see also de la Vega (1688, 150, 172, 176).

7. The Bubble Act was passed in the midst of a government scheme to convert government debts into ssshares of the South Sea Company. Shortly thereafter, the price of South Sea Company stock plummeted, and, of course, government blamed the market for this bubble.

References

Carlyle, Thomas. [1843] 2010. *On Heroes, Hero-Worship, and the Heroic in History*. Cambridge: Cambridge University Press.

Chernow, Ron. 2004. *Alexander Hamilton*. New York: Penguin.

Committee for General Purposes of the Stock-Exchange. 1812. *Rules and Regulations Adopted by the Committee for General Purposes of the Stock-Exchange*. London: Stephen Couchman Printers.

De la Vega, Josef Penso. [1688] 1996. *Confusion de confusiones*. New York: Wiley.

De Vries, Jan, and Ad Van Der Woude. 1997. *The First Modern Economy: Success, Failure, and Perseverance of the Dutch Economy, 1500–1815*. Cambridge: Cambridge University Press.

Garber, Peter. 2000. *Famous First Bubbles: The Fundamentals of Early Manias*. Cambridge, Mass.: MIT Press.

Hamilton, Alexander. 1791. *Report on the Manufacturers*. Submitted to the U.S. Congress, December 5. http://www.constitution.org/ah/rpt_manufactures.pdf.

Hamiltonian America. 2011. *Economist*, April 8.

Harris, Ron. 2000. *Industrializing English Law: Entrepreneurship and Business Organization, 1720–1844*. New York: Cambridge University Press.

Hummel, Jeffrey Rogers. 2012. Some Possible Consequences of a U.S. Government Default. *Econ Journal Watch* 9, no. 1: 24–40.

Kellenbenz, Hermann. [1957] 1996. Introduction to Josef Penso de la Vega, *Confusion de confusiones*, edited by Martin Fridson, 25–46. New York: Wiley.

Kessler, Glenn. 2013. Harry Reid's Claim That Congress Ranks Lower Than North Korea. *Washington Post*, July 15.

Klein, Daniel B., ed. 1997. *Reputation: Studies in the Voluntary Elicitation of Good Conduct*. Ann Arbor, MI: University of Michigan Press.

Madison, James. 1865. *Letters and Other Writings of James Madison*. Vol. 1: 1769–1793. Philadelphia, PA: Lippincott.

Miranda, Lin-Manuel, and Jeremy McCarter. 2016. *Hamilton: The Revolution. Being the Complete Libretto of the Broadway Musical with a True Account of Its Creation and Concise Remarks on Hip-Hop, the Power of Stories, and the New America*. New York: Grand Central.

Mortimer, Thomas. 1761. *Every Man His Own Broker: Or, a Guide to Exchange-Alley*. London: Hooper.

Rothbard, Murray. 1992. Repudiating the National Debt. *Chronicles*, June, 49–52.

Smith, Adam. [1766] 1982. *Lectures on Jurisprudence*. Indianapolis, Ind.: Liberty Classics.

Smith, C. F. 1929. The Early History of the London Stock Exchange. *American Economic Review* 19, no. 2: 206–16.

Spencer, Herbert. 1873. *The Study of Sociology*. London: King.

Stringham, Edward Peter. 2015. *Private Governance: Creating Order in Economic and Social Life*. New York: Oxford University Press.

Stringham, Edward Peter, and Nicholas A. Curott. 2015. On the Origins of Stock Markets. In *The Oxford Handbook of Austrian Economics*, edited by Peter Boettke and Christopher Coyne, 324–40. Oxford: Oxford University Press.

Taibbi, Matt. 2011. *Griftopia: Bubble Machines, Vampire Squids, and the Long Con That Is Breaking America. A Story of Bankers, Politicians, and the Most Audacious Power Grab in American History*. New York: Spiegel & Grau.

Tolstoy, Leo. [1869] 2008. *War and Peace*. New York: Vintage Classics.

Washington, George. 1939. *The Writings of George Washington from the Original Manuscript Sources, 1745–1799*. Washington, DC: Library of Congress.

White, Lawrence. 2016. Alexander Hamilton, a Second-Hand Dealer in Retrograde Mercantilist Ideas. *Foundation for Economic Education Daily Articles*, September 6.

Wincott, Harold. 1946. *The Stock Exchange*. London: Sampson Low, Marston.

Wright, Robert E. 2002. *Hamilton Unbound: Finance and the Creation of the American Republic*. Westport, Conn.: Greenwood Press.

Wright, Robert E. 2008. *One Nation under Debt: Hamilton, Jefferson, and the History of What We Owe*. New York, NY: McGraw-Hill.

Wright, Robert E., and David J. Cowen. 2006. *Financial Founding Fathers: The Men Who Made America Rich*. Chicago, IL: University of Chicago Press.

EDWARD PETER STRINGHAM is President of the American Institute for Economic Research, Davis Professor of Economic Organizations and Innovation at Trinity College, and editor of the *Journal of Private Enterprise*. Stringham is the editor of two books ("*Anarchy, State, and Public Choice*", 2005; "*Anarchy and the Law: The Political Economy of Choice*," 2007) and author of more than 70 journal articles, book chapters, and policy studies. His work has been discussed on more than 100 broadcast stations, including CBS, CNBC, CNN, Headline News, NPR, and MTV. A frequent guest on Fox and a regular contributor to the Wall Street Journal. In 2016, Rise Global ranked Stringham as the 77th most influential economist. His first single authored book, *Private Governance: Creating Order in Economic and Social Life* (2018) is published by Oxford University Press.

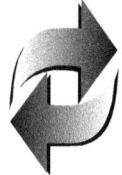

EXPLORING THE ISSUE

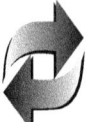

Was Alexander Hamilton an Economic Genius?

Critical Thinking and Reflection

1. What are the ideological positions offered by Swanson and Trout supporting Carlyle's *Great Man of History Theory* as contrasted to Stringham's ideological positions refuting this popular historical theory?
2. From most important to least important what would be your rank order of examples offered by Swanson and Trout regarding Alexander Hamilton's dominant influence on the economic and politicial polcity/practice decisions of the United States?
3. Reviweing your responses in question 2, what do you believe would be Stringham's evidence of refutation to these examples of Hamilton's dominant influence in these economic and political policies/practices of the United States?
4. Drs. Swanson, Trout, and Stringham have invited you to join them for dinner. At the conclusion of dinner, each have asked you to offer them your critique of their position presented in this chapter. What would be your critique of one supporting and one opposing evidenciary argument that the authors offered in this chapter?

Is There Common Ground?

Who Lives, Who Dies, Who Tells Your Story? (Miranda& McCarter, 2016, p. 280)

Edward P. Stringham's opening sentence succinctly inquires, "Is Hamilton an important and visionary as most people say or an overrated mashup of often contradictory elements?" (Stringham, 2017, p. 523). It is at this inquisitive juncture that Swanson, Trout, and Stringham seem to draw their dividing line with little apparent common ground to be shared. Yet, with a closer look, we find two areas where our opinining authors my intersect, if ever so slightly, in agreement.

Even amidst the unqualified dispute regarding the application and even the legitimacy of the so-called *Great Man of History Theory*, Donald F. Swanson, Andrew P. Trout, and Edward Peter Stringham concur that multiple volumes of textbooks, competing historical biographies, hundreds of pages of grade school and university curricula, plus countless scholarly and popular culture articles all seem to have failed to depict a cogent and accurate representation of the impact of Alexander Hamilton on U.S. and world histories. From this common ground, Swanson, Trout, and Stringham find another position with which they can *somewhat agree*. *Somewhat agree* in italics is intended to denote that while Swanson, Trout, and Stringham each concur that most scholars ascribe Hamilton's operational bearings rooted in a nationalist (i.e., Federalist) philosophy (Stringham, 2017, pp. 525–528; Swanson-Trout, 1991, p. 286), it is entirely too simplistic a categorization to fully explain the full complement of economic and political implications being debated.

For Swanson and Trout, the notion of Hamilton as anything more than a nationalistic economic policy strategist fails to take into account the full spectrum of his impact. Certainly, there's reason to believe that Hamilton viewed the world through economic lens' leading him to contribute to the structural development of the new American nation through financial mechanisms that would not only ensure a viable future for the nation but create a competitive stance within a hostile geopolitical market. Yet, there's no evidence of Hamilton the myopic economic wonk who fails to recognize the symbiotic relationship of the economic, political, and social factors that make up the whole of nation building and governance. Swanson and Trout assert that the nuances of Hamilton are best realized when ". . . we remember that as secretary he was pursuing a policy whose purposes were fiscal as well as political" (Swanson & Trout, p. 289).

Stringham would seemingly concur that placing Hamilton in a simplistic category fails to account for the complexities of the multiple historical factors that comprise the contents of the debate regarding Hamilton's role as singular influencer or standard instigater. Drawing from his integration of resources from the historical record and the musical score Stringham asserts, "As much as one might admire Hamilton's singing or rap-battle prowess, he did not invent financial markets. At best, he helped issue new government debt. . . . [L]ooking at an issuer of debt and concluding that this person created financial markets would be equivalent to looking at Anheuser-Busch's recent large bond issue and saying that the company invented the first bonds or beer itself. The great-man view of history tends to overlook the actions of the multitude and to say that markets were created by one man or a particular set of men. But that is not how markets work" (Stringham, 2018, p. 531).

Beyond these two points of agreement (i.e., the historical and popular culture record has poorly represented an accurate representation of Alexander Hamilton's impact on U.S. and World history; categorization of Hamilton as simply a nationalistic economic policy wonk fails to either recognize the nuances of the man's greatness and/or the complexities of the multiple competing factors that serve as tipping points in history), Robert F. Swanson, Andrew P. Trout, and Edward P. Stringham draw the line of disagreement rather boldly when debating the question *Was Alexander Hamilton an Economic Genius?* Thus, we are left with the evidence as presented by our represented scholars or perhaps evidence hypothesized and tested by you the reader in answering the question at hand. Perhaps, it is most fitting to end this discussion with with a lyric from the hit Broadway musical, *"Hamilton: An American Musical"* as we, like Alexander Hamilton himself ponders, "Legacy. What is a legacy? It's planting seeds in a garden you never get to see"(Miranda, 2016, p. 77).

Additional Resources

Carlyle, T., & Adams, J.C. (1907). *On heroes, hero-worship, and the heroic in history.* Boston, MA: Houghton, Miffline and Company.

Miranda, L. (2016). Hamilton: An American musical. In J. McCarter (Ed.), *Hamilton: Hurricane* (pp. 46–47). New York: Grand Central Publishing.

Miranda, L.M., & McCarter, J. (2016). *Hamilton: The revolution. being the complete libretto of the Broadway musical with a true account of its creation and concise remarks on hip-hop, the power of stories, and the new America.* New York: Grand Central Publishing.

Stringham, E.P., & Curott, N.A. (2015). On the origins of stock Markets. In P. Boettke & C. Coyne (Eds.), *The Oxford handbook of Austrian economics.* Oxford: Oxford University Press. 324–40.

Swanson, D.F. (1963). *The origins of Hamilton's fiscal policies.* Gainsville, FL: University of Florida Press.

Syrett, H.C., & other editors. (1790, December 13). Report on the further provision necessary for establishing public credit. The papers of Alexander Hamilton (27 vols). New York, 1961–1987.

Wright, R.E. (2002). *One nation under debt: Hamilton, Jefferson, and the history of what we owe.* New York: McGraw-Hill.

Wright, R.E., & Cowen, D.J. (2008). *Financial founding fathers: The men who made America rich.* Chicago, IL: University of Chicago Press.

Internet References . . .

Alexander Hamilton—The Man Who Made Modern America

https://www.loc.gov/rr/program/bib/hamilton/related.html

Library of Congress—Alexander Hamilton Resource Guide

https://www.loc.gov/rr/program/bib/hamilton/related.html

Online Library of Liberty—Alexander Hamilton

https://www.loc.gov/rr/program/bib/hamilton/related.html

The Founders Online—The Papers of Alexander Hamilton

https://www.loc.gov/rr/program/bib/hamilton/related.html

The Gildere Lehrman Institute of American History—Alexander Hamilton Search

https://www.loc.gov/rr/program/bib/hamilton/related.html

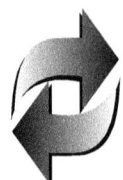

ISSUE

Selected, Edited, and with Issue Framing Material by:
Kevin R. Magill and Tony L. Talbert, *Baylor University*

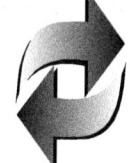

Were Jackson's Anti-Politics and Nationalism Beneficial for Increased Democratic Participation?

YES: Kori N. Schake, from "Trump and the 'New Nationalism': It's Not New at All," *Hoover Digest* (2017)

NO: Donald Ratcliffe, from "The Right to Vote and the Rise of Democracy, 1787–1828," *Journal of the Early Republic* (2013)

Learning Outcomes

After reading this issue, you will be able to:

- Identify the role of anti-politics and nationalism in Andrew Jackson's presidency.
- Assess the type and level of impact of the executive branch on sociopolitical change and democratic participation.
- Evaluate the concept of democratic participation as intended by the founding fathers.
- Consider the connection between past and present populist movements in American democracy.

ISSUE SUMMARY

YES: Kori N. Schake suggests that Andrew Jackson and Donald Trump both champion a populist style, which did and will strengthen American democracy by "activat[ing] antibodies in opposition to [their] policies, mobilizing the civic powers that undergird our democracy into greater activism." She offers comparisons in the presidential approaches of both men suggesting that their elections represent the United States people's routine disenfranchisement with the governmental status quo.

NO: Donald Ratcliffe argues that despite the fact that it is often understood as a golden age for democracy, the Jacksonian Era was not a social revolution. He claims, "suffrage had significantly expanded" in the "United States [and it] had, in many ways, become a functioning democracy long before 1815." However, he contends that the Jackson presidency affected the radial ideology of the Democratic Party.

Issue Framing with Victoria A. Davis

Andrew Jackson embodies the complexity of the American democratic experiment. At times, he seems a champion of liberalism in its most classical form and at other moments a tyrant himself working to diminish the rights of our most marginalized communities and to wield singular political authority. Jackson's presidency causes us to take a closer look at our founding fathers' beliefs and to consider the context in which they wrote the Constitution. A presidency such as Jackson's brings into question the original design of our democratic experiment, its parameters, and how it ought to be implemented.

Jackson, for better or worse, was an extremist. He took stances from which others shied away, often centering himself among the warring sides of public opinion. He is known as the champion of "the common man" for his efforts to expand political recognition to a community that had been left behind as non-landholders and therefore incapable of genuine and sustainable public contribution. In pursing an expansion of suffrage to all white men, Jackson helped form the foundational beliefs of the Democratic Party. But, not without his opponents forming a countermovement in the form of the Whig Party. As Feller (n.d.) notes, "The Democratic Party was Jackson's child; the national two-party system his legacy." To people both past and present, Jackson represents either the ideals of democracy or a threat to our founding principles.

In considering Jackson's impact on democratic participation, it is prudent to first consider two questions—how should we interpret democratic participation and why use a presidency as a lens with which to analyze American civic life? Democratic participation is often reduced to voting. At an early age, people are taught that the principal act of citizenship is voting. In American history courses, legislation on increased suffrage is taught as a hallmark of democratic progress with the 15th and 19th amendments often serving as evidence of such progress. Although democratic participation may far too often be simplified to the single act of voting, it remains true that widespread access to voting is what makes our country uniquely democratic. Voting is the space where the voice of the people materializes. Jackson understood how extending the vote could capitalize on the symbolic power offered to poorer whites, allowing him to become the champion of "the common man."

Presidencies and presidential elections serve as a useful hermeneutic for analyzing democratic participation and a gauge of political feeling for larger national and global occurrences. Akin to simplifying democratic participation to the vote, presidencies are often stamped with general characterizations and turned into icons of the time in which they serve. However, presidents and presidential campaigns ought not be understood to operate in isolation. Historical interpretations must be scrutinized according to the ways they are embedded within larger national and global sociopolitical currents. Current political analysis, for example, requires situating political action within the context of globalization. Some of the extreme nationalist rhetoric, in its contemporary form, is a reaction to the negative externalities associated with globalization. In the United States and Britain, we see the common man reacting to the inequities within the current geopolitical climate by turning to Donald Trump and by calling for a Brexit which are superficial reactions to a much more complex issue. Similarly, during the Jacksonian Era, the country was experiencing the epoch of westward expansion and a pivotal moment of tyrannical suspicion of the upper class by the common man. American life was pushing beyond its cradle and the sociocultural confines of the original colonies. Landownership was on the rise, and voter identity was becoming something new. Additionally, America was experiencing economic growth, and tensions were beginning to rise between the industrial North and agrarian South.

The issue at hand centers on the notion of populism and one president's use of populism during his time in office. In considering the various interpretations of populism within the history of the presidency, Brimes and Mulroy (2004, p. 137) "argue that populism is linked to the state-building goals of presidents and their parties." Additionally, the authors identify two components of presidential populism: (1) the role of the populace in legitimizing presidential action and (2) the use of contrasting the interest of the people with special interests. Throughout his presidency, Jackson made clear his intentions to use the people to legitimize his choices and actions. As Brimes and Mulroy (2004, p. 143) note, "In his first and second annual messages, Jackson followed up [his mandate to reform the electoral process], calling for a constitutional amendment to eliminate both the Electoral College and the run-off election in the House of Representatives. Jackson contended that these intervening institutions distorted the choice of the people." During his presidency, Jackson also vetoed 12 bills (Feller, n.d.), an outward sign of his anti-political sentiment and a sign of skepticism that Congress genuinely served the needs of the common man.

In leading during a time of national change and expansion, Jackson also showed a desire to maintain and further define and unify American identity. He refused to allow South Carolina to threaten this national identity during the nullification crisis. This determination to protect national interest during a time of significant change can be compared to the current trade war of the Trump presidency. Both presidents stop at nothing to protect what they perceive, or claim to be, America's economic interests. Jackson's approach to the nullification crisis carried with it a religious level of devotion to a unified nation. As Gannon (2013, p. 387) notes regarding Jackson during the nullification crisis, "This morally-tinged nationalism—where there was no ambiguity about who the 'right' and 'wrong' parties were—was a prominent feature of Andrew Jackson's political worldview." Of further note on Jackson's nationalistic interest is the Indian Removal Act of 1830. Indigenous peoples served as a threat to American identity which was now closely linked with Manifest Destiny. By passing the Indian Removal Act, Jackson helped to unify the country behind the dream of westward expansion thereby using nationalism as a means to *trump* controversial threats to growing nation.

So, did Andrew Jackson increase democratic participation? Were his anti-politics and nationalistic positions beneficial to civic life? Ratcliffe (2013) brings Jackson's rally for "the common man" into question by examining the numbers. Historical documentation of voting policies shows widespread expansion of voting rights to the nonelite male prior to 1815. Ratcliffe demonstrates that Jackson's actions did not make a quantifiable difference in voting rights and brings into question his status as the champion for increased democratic participation. What Jackson did indeed do is help to establish the defining, anti-classist tenants of the Democratic Party.

Schake (2017) argues that anti-political populist movements such as Jackson's and the modern Trump presidency are representative of the core element of democratic participation in a liberal democracy—the voice of the people to hold the government accountable. To Schake, Jackson and Trump, because of their extreme actions, also bring those in opposition of their leadership to the center of civic debate. It is argued, therefore, that by bringing contested issues to the people through public civic debate, Jackson and Trump champion democratic participation in its most authentic form.

Again, we must consider what democratic participation *is* to adequately answer the question were Jackson's anti-politics and nationalism beneficial for democratic participation? Is democracy about uniting a majority of the nation around particular versions of democratic ideology? Or, is democracy the plurality of thought that helps citizens reconsider their positions in relation to the common good? Does democracy require being knocked from its equilibrium when political thought and action becomes stagnant? How much can we attribute to presidents who act to destabilize this equilibrium? Are the actions of these politicians' authentic responses to the political will of the common man, or are they simply rejections of status quo politics that have not worked for them? It's clear that men like Trump and Jackson are men of their time—changing times, which represent the common people's struggle for increased democracy. Both men claim the system is rigged, scapegoat groups of people as an internal "other," claim to be champions of the common man, appeal to poor Whites, and impose protectionist tariffs. However, it is unclear if what these presidents offer, or if what they truly represent, is an increase in democratic participation and more rights for the common man or the appearance of representation for a portion of the population who feels disenfranchised in an unsure political climate.

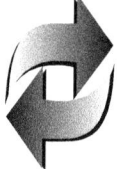

YES

Kori N. Schake

Trump and the "New Nationalism"

It's Not New at All

Andrew Jackson, almost two centuries ago, also championed a populist style—and, in the end, strengthened American democracy.

President Trump has cultivated comparisons between himself and Andrew Jackson by hanging a portrait of Jackson in the White House, making a pilgrimage to Jackson's grave, and pointedly emphasizing that he, like Jackson, "fought to defend forgotten men and women from the arrogant elite of his day." It is a choice distressing to those who associate Jackson with illiberal policies of slavery, Indian removal, and refusing to enforce Supreme Court verdicts. It also has fueled an avalanche of journalism about "new nationalism," which is thought to be somehow more virulent and dangerous than previous iterations.

This is deeply unfair to President Trump and his supporters—and a key to the bitterness many of them feel at the political establishment, which has tended to ignore their concerns and stigmatize their beliefs.

Nationalism as an idea grew out of the Enlightenment. Before that, monarchs held power by force. Nationalism was the belief that government could have an attractive power. It reduced the demand for the state to enforce its hold on people living within territory claimed by the sovereign.

The United States has always had a particularly resonant nationalism, relying as it does on association with our creed rather than ethnicity or territory as the basis for our nationalism. This is what Mexican historian Edmundo O'Gorman called the "invention of America." Abraham Lincoln described our political values as "the electric cord in that Declaration that links the hearts of patriotic and liberty-loving men together."

The Pendulum Swings

The idea of a "new nationalism" precedes the conflating of nationalism with despotism in the twentieth century; the phrase comes from Theodore Roosevelt who in 1910 urged an expansion of government activism to better protect human welfare. In our current fevered political climate, however, the new nationalism is flipped on its head, defined by what it opposes: immigration, trade, globalization, and political correctness.

The *Economist* is more restrained than most in its pejorative caricature: "Reagan's America was optimistic: Mr. Trump's is angry." Trump is said to represent a dangerous force if not new in American history then at least new in its repudiation of the post–World War II order.

Jackson governed erratically, brutally, and in many ways unsuccessfully. But he revivified American democracy.

What Trump actually represents is a routine disaffection by American voters with our government, a willingness to experiment with a new direction, a pendular correction from what exasperated voters in the previous administration, and a high degree of trust in the constraining benefits of our political institutions.

The work of sociologists Bart Bonikowski and Paul DiMaggio shows that the American public is divided in a fairly stable fashion over time into four groups, with the largest—about 30 percent—exhibiting what Bonikowski calls "ethnocultural exclusion, along with a low level of pride in the state." Their preferred definition of *American* is a Christian who speaks English and was born in the United States. Journalists have characterized this group as low-education and low-income white males. In fact, Bonikowski and DiMaggio's data suggest that 68 percent of blacks, 55 percent of Hispanics, and more Democrats than Republicans hold those views. They are also more likely to be women. The new nationalism, then, is not some backlash of the white working poor, but—as President Trump has asserted—a broad movement of people fed up with the direction they perceive our country taking.

A Vibrant Strand

Nor does the "America first" ideology of Trump's foreign policies represent a new nationalism. Its main thrusts—economic protectionism, the belief that allies are taking advantage of the United States, and concern about immigration changing the character of America—have long, bipartisan pedigrees in American politics.

If Robert Taft had beaten Dwight Eisenhower for the Republican nomination for president in 1952, that might well have been mainstream conservative policy. At the height of the Cold War, American administrations had to devote an enormous amount of effort to beating back legislation sponsored by Senator Mike Mansfield that would have forced withdrawal of US forces from Europe because allies paid too little. Thomas Jefferson's purchase of Louisiana was criticized in its time for admitting to citizenship Catholics who were believed, because of their religion, to lack the independent thought necessary in a democracy. Every wave of immigrants to America has created concern about dilution of the country's essence.

The American political system is particularly susceptible to nationalism in both its positive and nasty forms—which is simply to say that our political system is tied more tightly in accountability to the public than are even most other democracies. US allies quail at our routine willingness to elect inexperienced or rough-hewn presidents, our tolerance for the risks in throwing aside inherited dogma or established policies, and our national penchant for sounding our "barbaric yawp over the roofs of the world" (as Walt Whitman phrased it in "Song of Myself").

That responsiveness to the public will is, however, also the great vibrancy of American democracy. Andrew Jackson spoke for the aspirations of frontier communities thirsty for land and security and access to capital, for slaveholders adamant at preserving their way of life, for a population restive under political dominance by educated elites. Jackson governed erratically, brutally, and in many ways unsuccessfully. But he revivified American democracy, passing the torch from an East Coast establishment living in safety and cultural superiority to the harder life, rougher mentality, and challenges of the frontier. In his excesses, Jackson also activated antibodies in opposition to his policies, mobilizing the civic powers that undergird our democracy into greater activism.

Nationalism originated in the Enlightenment as the belief that government could have an attractive power.

Donald Trump is likely to give American democracy another such civics lesson—appreciation for limited government, the power of the courts and civil society to rein in the executive, reminders of obscure but important concerns of the founders (who knew about the emoluments clause six months ago?)—stimulated by his actions.

Trump represents a routine disaffection by American voters with our government, a willingness to experiment, and a high degree of trust in our political institutions.

KORI N. SCHAKE is the deputy director-general of the International Institute for Strategic Studies. She was previously a research fellow at Stanford University's Hoover Institution. Schake has served in several influential political positions including at the Pentagon, on the National Security Council, at The State Department and in academia holding positions at West Point, The University of Maryland, and National Defense University.

Donald Ratcliffe

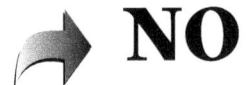

The Right to Vote and the Rise of Democracy, 1787–1828

A long tradition in American political history associates the presidency of Andrew Jackson with the achievement of universal suffrage and the coming of democracy, at least for adult white males. There is some justification for this view, but only in limited senses; for the most part, this interpretation has had a deleterious effect on our understanding of political development in the early republic. In particular, it has created the belief that relatively few people possessed the right to vote in the early republic, and that therefore mass participation was postponed to the years after 1815. As recently as September 2008, the distinguished historian Jill Lepore could write in the *New Yorker* that during Washington's presidency only 6 percent of Americans could vote—which admittedly translates into about 15 percent of the free adult population. Sean Wilentz's prizewinning *Rise of American Democracy* (2005) recognizes that the suffrage was much more widely spread before 1815, but he still builds his interpretation around the assumption that politics did not involve the public at large until *The Age of Jackson*. Even Alexander Keyssar's illuminating *The Right to Vote* (2000) and Daniel Walker Howe's excellent *What Hath God Wrought* (2007) assume that the practice of politics became more democratic in the 1820s because of recent fundamental changes in electoral rules. Such views are explicitly contradicted by the voting data that Philip Lampi has gathered that are now available on the A New Nation Votes website, which confirm the huge expansion of popular participation within two decades or so of the adoption of the U.S. Constitution.[1]

This expansion was possible because the right to vote had always been extraordinarily widespread—at least among adult white males—even before the country gained its independence. During the colonial period, the right to vote for the lower house of colonial legislatures had been defined in traditional British terms: only people who had freehold landed property sufficient to ensure that they were personally independent and had a vested interest in the welfare of their communities could vote. That qualification normally applied to men who were heads of households, since women were almost by definition dependent, but the right could extend to widows who had become responsible for the family property. Some colonies excluded propertied people whose civic commitment they suspected—recent arrivals, members of minority religious sects, and racial groups deemed unacceptable. But those most generally excluded were laborers, tenant farmers, unskilled workers, and indentured servants, all of whom were considered to lack a "stake in society," a permanent interest in the community, and the wherewithal to withstand corruption.[2]

In Britain, property qualifications increasingly restricted the number qualified to vote. Whereas over 20 percent of adult males had enjoyed the franchise, around 1700, population growth and the increasing concentration of wealth reduced the proportion to 17.2 percent by 1754, continuing down to 12.7 percent in England and Wales by the 1820s.[3]

By contrast, the abundance and availability of land in North America meant that large numbers of colonists satisfied similarly defined requirements. This was especially true where the requirement was expressed in terms of acreage rather than value, as was customarily the case in the southern colonies: it was much easier to acquire (and to measure) 50 acres than land worth £50 either at sale or in annual rents. Six colonies also allowed alternative qualifications to freehold ownership in the form of personal property or payment of taxes, opening the suffrage to owners of urban property, and even to those prosperous farmers who rented their land or held it on some form of leasehold.[4]

Consequently, as early as the 1720s, the suffrage was uniquely wide in the colonies. Virginia reputedly had the most restrictive franchise with fewer than ½ the free white males qualified to vote but a recent calculation raises the figure to ⅔ at mid-century declining slightly thereafter. In some New England colonies and in the great northeastern seaports about ¾ of adult males met the requirement.

Ratcliffe, Donald. "The Right to Vote and the Rise of Democracy, 1787–1828," *Journal of the Early Republic*, 2013. Copyright ©2013 by Society for Historians of the Early American Republic. Used with permission of University of Pennsylvania Press.

Already before the Revolution an unprecedentedly large proportion of the adult free male population could vote, though historians have been uncertain in their calculation of just how many. Chilton Williamson and Robert Dinkin estimated that in the late Colonial Era the proportion of freehold owners ranged between 50 percent and 75 (or even 80) percent in the various communities and states, while Alexander Keyssar suggests that overall nearly 60 percent of adult white males were eligible to vote.[5]

***

The Revolution established the pattern of voting rights that determined American politics in the generation after 1787. The years from 1774 to 1787 did not see a drastic qualitative change, but they did see the proportion of eligible voters expand, probably by significantly more than 10 percent.[6]

On the one hand, the controversy with Britain after 1763 over political rights stimulated democratic sentiment in both the colonies and the metropolis, and radicals began to argue that the right to vote was inherent within individual manhood. In the revolutionary crisis of 1775 and 1776, the need to ensure popular support encouraged several states to allow men—especially militia men—who did not meet the formal requirements to vote at critical moments, while the Declaration of Independence resoundingly based the legitimacy of the new nation on the consent of the governed. Radicals began to insist that every adult male deserved the right to vote, and that individual citizens needed the vote to protect them against the possible tyranny of lawmakers.[7]

On the other hand, many leading patriots remained committed to the idea that voting was a privilege open to those who were tied to the community's long-term welfare and had a sufficient tangible measure of that commitment. As a result, the new state constitutions generally established a more conservative electoral system than the democrats wanted. In 1776, the most radical state, Pennsylvania, enfranchised all taxpaying adult males and so broadened the electorate markedly, especially in older eastern areas where no more than 50–60 percent of adult males had previously qualified. In 1787, it was estimated that, in the state as a whole, upward of 87.5 percent of adult white males could now vote.[8]

But, significantly, even the Pennsylvania radicals of 1776 still associated representation with taxation: only "free men having a sufficient evident common interest with and attachment to the community" deserved the privilege of voting in a republican polity. There was no desire to enfranchise the poor, who were commonly identified as profligate or idle. As J. R. Pole suggested, what was significant was not that lots of men could vote but that it was still thought necessary to exclude some, however few, from the polls.[9]

The determination to maintain meaningful tests arose from the awareness that broader social and economic trends were actually reducing the proportion of men who owned property. In newly settled areas where land was cheap, 70 or 80 percent of adult white males held enough property to be enfranchised. But in some older areas, notably New England, the limited availability of land and the practice of subdividing family plots among children reduced the number who possessed the minimum estate. Kenneth Lockridge found a 30 percent decline in eastern Massachusetts between mid-century and 1790, and the situation may have been worse in the middle states. In cities, the crowds of poor men swelled, as economic tendencies made rich and poor ever more distinct. Such developments raised fears that in the near future a large propertyless proletariat might appear in the United States, and statesmen were apprehensive of the effects a class that lacked true moral independence might have on the politics of the growing republic.[10]

Virginia and New York are the prime instances of states that marginally eased their property requirements but essentially maintained a restrictive regime intact. Virginia in 1776 held to its basic freehold qualification of 25 acres of improved land, but then in 1785 lowered the alternative requirement for freehold owners of unimproved land from 100 to 50 acres. Calculations as to how many men possessed this level of property have ranged widely, but since long-term leaseholders and some residents of the few towns could also vote, most authorities have accepted that between ½ and ⅔ of adult white males could vote in the 1780s. Certainly most adult sons, tenants, laborers, artisans, merchants, professional men, and their employees did not legally qualify, but, as Pole observed of the years before the revolution, suffrage in Virginia "was often exercised in fact by persons to whom it did not belong as a right under the law." As a result, he calculated, the "effective voting force" in revolutionary Virginia "could rise to over 60 percent of the white male population of adults"—and sometimes even higher.[11]

New York's revolutionary reforms were, if anything, more restrictive. The 1777 constitution opened the qualification to vote for the house to both those who owned a £20 freehold (previously £50) and tenants who paid 40 shillings annual rent and state taxes, as well as to those merchants, artisans, and professionals who had previously become freemen of the cities of New York and Albany. These terms continued to exclude many of New York's tenant farmers and laborers (and their adult sons), but less completely than might be imagined since long-term tenancies were treated as freeholds, which enfranchised many tenants on the great feudal estates of the Hudson valley. In the New York of 1790, about 58 percent of adult white males—that is, 70.7 percent of heads of households—could vote for the assembly.[12]

Four other states that retained their colonial restrictions intact already allowed fairly broad access to the suffrage. Delaware retained both its old 50-acre freehold requirement and its traditional alternative of £40 personal property, which in colonial days had enabled about 80 percent of adult white males to vote. South Carolina is normally regarded as preserving a conservative establishment in 1778: it did keep its existing 50-acre freehold rule, but it also lowered its previous alternative of paying 20 shillings in taxes to paying taxes equal to the tax on 50 acres. Yet this tax concession seems to have been of little significance since the acquisition of a £50 freehold continued to be relatively easy in South Carolina, where tax records reveal that over 80 percent of adult white males owned qualifying freeholds in the 1780s.[13]

Rhode Island and Connecticut retained intact their colonial charters and ancient suffrage rules: both states required those who could meet the property qualifications to take the freeman's oath before they could vote. The Rhode Island charter restricted the oath to those who owned real estate valued at £40 or rented for 40 shillings per annum (and their eldest sons), a qualification that about 74 percent of adult males could meet in 1778. However, only about ⅘ of them took the freeman's oath so that in 1788 only about 60–70 percent of adult males were *bona fide* freemen. The same was true in Connecticut, where the qualifications for the oath were described as "maturity in years, quiet and peaceable behavior, a civil conversation, and forty shillings freehold." In practice, probably no more than 60 percent of adult males took the freeman's oath in the 1780s. Yet in both cases, the oath should surely be seen as a sort of registration process: as Joel Cohen has suggested, failure to take the oath can be considered as voluntarily choosing not to vote rather than being ineligible. Dinkin calculated that those eligible to take the oath in 1789 amounted to about 75 percent in each state, though other evidence suggests that the qualification was becoming harder to meet, and 65 percent would be nearer the mark.[14]

Of the other six states, five deliberately eased the qualifications required for voting for their legislative assemblies, even while rejecting the principle of universal manhood suffrage. Eager to attach more social groups to the republic, they decisively broadened their view of what could constitute a "stake in society" and accepted various forms of wealth and evidences of social contribution as alternatives to property. New Jersey in 1776 gave the vote to all possessing £50 of personal estate. Pennsylvania included the adult sons of freeholders even when not taxpayers. Georgia in 1777 retained its old qualification of £10 in any sort of property but now also accepted non-property owners who paid taxes or pursued a "mechanic trade." In a few states, relaxing the rules meant introducing residence requirements—usually one year in the state—in order to ensure voter commitment to the community or locality.[15]

Three states—North Carolina, New Hampshire, and Pennsylvania—gave up landed property qualifications entirely for elections to the assembly and adopted taxpaying as the essential sign of contribution to the maintenance of the republic. Like Georgia, these three also introduced light, compulsory poll taxes which transformed the taxpaying requirement into a broad adult white male suffrage. In North Carolina, for example, the poll tax enfranchised all adult males, except "sons living under the paternal roof, apprentices, slaves, and indentured servants." In all four states, taxables represented about 90 percent of the adult white male population.[16]

Changes in the value of money markedly affected the restrictive power of qualifications, as seven states issued their own paper money and inflation became rampant during and after the war. Maryland may have retained its 50-acre freehold qualification in 1776, but it changed its alternative qualification from £40 in other forms of property to £30 in current money, which cut the amount needed in ½. This opened the suffrage to most freemen, with inflation expanding the proportion of Maryland's adult white males who could meet that standard from 64 percent in 1783 to over 70 percent by 1789.[17]

In New Jersey after 1776 the necessary £50 was to be measured not in sterling but in currency or proclamation money, which reduced the level by ⅓. As Richard P. McCormick remarked, "The percentage of men who could not swear to being worth 50 pounds, lawful money, must have been extremely small, especially when the currency depreciation of the times is taken into consideration." In New Jersey, this meant that "the potential electorate included all but a small fraction of the white males over 21."[18]

Notoriously, Massachusetts in 1780 was the one state to raise the level of its qualification for state elections—from £40 to £60 of personal property, while the freehold alternative increased from £2 to £3 annual value. However, it is doubtful whether this move actually disfranchised many people, since the old requirement was in sterling while new one was in paper currency. According to one estimate, between 60 percent and 70 percent of adult males in Massachusetts seaboard towns could vote, and as many as 80–90 percent in most rural sections. But in any case within a few years, the property qualifications were being ignored: by 1786, according to some witnesses, everyone with settled residence or who paid a poll tax was admitted to the polls, and the alternative requirement of an estate worth £3 per annum was commonly construed to mean any man who earned £3 per annum could vote, which enfranchised common laborers! According to one Bay State politician, "so small are the qualifications of voters that scarce a single man is excluded," which allowed the upsurge of rural voters in 1787 to overthrow the conservatives whose fiscal policies had provoked Shays's rebellion.[19]

This growing electorate was not restricted to voting for the lower houses of the legislature. In colonial times, governors had normally been appointed by higher authority, by the king or a proprietor, but in Rhode Island and Connecticut, the local electorate could elect the governor even before the Revolution. After 1776, the four New England states and New York allowed their voters to choose the governor, but elsewhere—and especially in the South—governors continued to be appointed, but now by the legislature. Similarly, the upper chamber had usually been appointed by the governor in colonial days, except in Rhode Island, Connecticut, and Massachusetts. Now the upper house too became elective, though on slightly different terms from the lower house: the districts were larger, the terms longer, and usually the officeholder had to meet more stringent requirements on age, residence, and wealth. In North Carolina and New York, the franchise was also more restricted. Both states lowered the requirements to vote in a house election but retained the earlier property qualification for the upper house: 50 acres in the former, £100 freehold in the latter. In New York, under this provision, only 28.9 percent of adult white males could vote for the state senate in 1790, ½ the number that could vote for the house. In most states, though, the senates of the 1790s were fairly reflective of popular opinion and, in any case, power was concentrated more in the lower houses.[20]

The broadening of the suffrage and the attraction of the equal-rights ideology raised awkward questions about the rights of those whose exclusion from the suffrage had previously been taken for granted. After the Revolution, most states specifically disfranchised women, even when property holders, though Rhode Island, Connecticut, and Delaware did not; only New Jersey explicitly enfranchised "all inhabitants" who could meet the residence and property qualifications.[21]

For male minorities, the new state constitutions were more favorable. The five provinces that had traditionally disfranchised Roman Catholics now admitted them, though New York's constitution called for new immigrants to take an oath renouncing all foreign ecclesiastical allegiances. Jews were now allowed to vote (though not hold office) in almost every state, though Maryland continued to require the voter to be a "Christian." The three states that had previously prohibited free African Americans from voting (Virginia, South Carolina, and Georgia) maintained their bans, and Maryland in 1783 limited the right to vote to those manumitted before that year. Otherwise, at the Revolution, free black adult males were enfranchised in every other state, mainly through silence and ignoring of the issue, subject of course to property or tax requirements. Only New York, New Jersey, Pennsylvania, and North Carolina explicitly enfranchised black males on the same terms as white men.[22]

So how many adult males could vote for the most popular branch of their state government by 1790? Fewer than half of adult white men, as the latest version of the *Guide to U.S. Elections* issued by the *Congressional Quarterly* asserted in 2010. Alexander Keyssar has claimed that, "according to most estimates, roughly 60–70 percent of adult white males (and very few others) could vote." This calculation is, however, not justified by the sources he cites: influenced no doubt by the evidence that the proportion of property owners was declining, Keyssar neglects the alternative routes to qualification that appeared even in the more conservative states, as well as the impact of currency changes and inflation. Yet even Keyssar's 60–70 percent figure suggests an eligible adult male electorate incomparably larger than many historians continue to assume.[23]

A more careful examination of the same sources made earlier by Robert Dinkin calculated that by the end of the 1780s the qualified electorate in the 13 states probably fell in the range from about 60 percent to 90 percent of adult white males, with most states toward the upper end. When some of his figures for individual states have been slightly adjusted to conform to revised figures given above, his tabulation places six states at around 90 percent (New Hampshire, New Jersey, Pennsylvania, North Carolina, and Georgia), and three states above 80 percent (Massachusetts, Delaware, and South Carolina); Rhode Island, Connecticut, and Maryland stand between 65 percent and 70 percent, followed by Virginia and New York at about 60 percent, or just below. Revised or not, Dinkin's survey suggests that, across the nation as a whole, about 80 percent of adult white males were eligible to vote in the late 1780s.[24]

Certainly, many leading figures of the time believed that the country had become too democratic. The view that an overly powerful popular will was corrupting politics in the states was commonly expressed among those who by the late 1780s were working to strengthen the Union. In the Northwest Ordinance of 1787, the Congress, worried about the loyalty of western settlers, laid down a 50-acre freehold requirement for voting in the new territory that was more stringent than in any of the states. In the Philadelphia constitutional convention of 1787, several delegates blamed the nation's weaknesses on the excessive democracy within too many states. Conservatives such as Gouvernor Morris and John Dickinson wanted the new instrument of government to introduce a freehold qualification across the country, but their arguments were effectively countered by the need to secure ratification in the several states. As Oliver Ellsworth of Connecticut pointed out, the people would "not readily subscribe to the national constitution if it should subject them to be disfranchised."[25]

In the end, the United States Constitution neither limited nor broadened the suffrage anywhere, since it left the issue to the individual states. Its sole requirement was that, in elections to the federal House of Representatives, the states must use the same franchise as they used for "the most numerous Branch of the State Legislature" (article 1, section 2). Thus the Constitution underwrote the expansion of the suffrage since 1776. Moreover, the belief that the new instrument of government must be grounded in popular consent ensured that ratification would be the responsibility of popularly elected ratifying conventions. The suffrage for those elections was left to the states, which universally adopted the broadest franchise used in state elections, except that New York and Connecticut enfranchised all free adult males especially for the occasion. The new Constitution might offset the power of the popularly elected federal House of Representatives with the balancing power of a president and senate that were both indirectly elected; but, as James Madison pointed out, election to these two bodies depended upon the very state legislatures that some Founders considered too dependent on the broad popular electorate that had emerged from the Revolution.

The United States Constitution may have reflected a desire for a more republican, less democratic way of organizing governments, but those states that rewrote their constitutions between 1789 and 1791 never reduced the right to vote for adult white males. In 1789, Georgia confirmed that all free white males who paid tax during the previous year could vote. In 1790, South Carolina broadened the suffrage slightly by admitting all free white males who owned a 50-acre freehold, *or* who owned a town lot, *or* who had been resident for six months and paid a tax of at least 3 shillings sterling. In 1790, Pennsylvania rejected the radicalism of 1776 and introduced a more balanced constitution based on bicameralism and a stronger executive, but no change was made to the suffrage in state elections and the governor was now to be popularly elected. Most drastically, in 1791–1792, Delaware at last dropped its freehold qualification and enfranchised adult white male residents who had paid a state or county tax. Together with New Hampshire (which in 1791 also chose to retain its taxpaying qualification) and North Carolina, these states all maintained tax systems that made qualification easy. Prevailing attitudes may have wished to restrict the right to vote to freeholders, householders, taxpayers, and settled residents, but there could now be no question of withdrawing the vote from any group of white men that already possessed it.[26]

Thus by the time of George Washington's reelection in 1792, after the admission of Vermont and Kentucky, 7 of the 15 states had given up property qualifications in voting for their lower house of assembly. In at least three others, inflation had made existing property requirements relatively unrestrictive. Taxpaying requirements too provided little obstacle: as in Pennsylvania, a small property tax or county road tax was enough to establish what historian Philip Klein described as "almost universal manhood suffrage." Across the nation as a whole, at least 80 percent of adult white males could vote. And in the states where the legislature did not reserve the privilege to itself, that was the electorate that chose the state's presidential electors.[27]

***

The mere fact that so many adult white males could vote for the lower houses of both state and federal government did not make the United States of 1790 a democracy. Not only were women largely excluded from the political process, but contemporaries still did not think that all adult white males deserved the vote even when citizens. The assumption that the poor, the idle, and the profligate had to be prevented from corrupting the electoral process remained strong, and the principle of universal manhood suffrage made only slow headway. Yet, in practice, in most states the opportunity to vote was gradually extended, so that by 1812 very few adult white males outside Rhode Island, Virginia, and the new, unusual state of Louisiana were denied access to the polls in elections for state and federal legislatures. The process by which that happened— and the timing of the process—are too frequently slipped over by recent historians who remain fixated with the notion of Jacksonian Democracy.[28]

Immediately after the acceptance of the Constitution there was little demand for greater democracy. Most voters proved reluctant to use their vote, and not all electoral units actually claimed their right of representation. Those who did vote commonly preferred their traditional leaders, gentry in the country, and merchants in the cities, though the social sources of legislators were broadening considerably. The formal criteria for membership of legislatures were much stiffer than for voters, requiring of the representative not just maturity in years, citizenship, and residence but also in many states significant levels of property ownership, especially for state senators. Moreover, the principle that elected bodies should represent persons rather than interests was still not generally accepted: in Virginia, South Carolina (till 1819), and some parts of Kentucky, the principle of plural voting persisted, allowing wealthy men to vote in every county in which they owned sufficient property. In many states, the house reflected the distribution of persons, while the senate represented property and established interests. Representation was commonly skewed to give dominance to the seaboard areas, especially through state senates; in the South Atlantic states, in particular, this device provided extra protection for the interests of slavery. The protection of property also encouraged the retention of higher qualifications (including stricter residency and citizenship rules) for voting in local elections where men of property feared discriminatory local taxation. In most southern states, local government remained essentially appointive, notably in Virginia through the county court system, and continued so in the 1820s.[29]

Yet elite control did not generally extend to the electoral process. Historians have commonly assumed that in the early republic the voters exercised their electoral privilege under the close supervision of their social superiors. Certainly in Virginia, Kentucky, Maryland, and for a time in some parts of other states, voting continued to be done publicly *viva voce*, with "living voice": the voters, one by one, had to swear that they were qualified and then publicly declare the names of those they were voting for. This was a slow process and open to abuse, especially where less wealthy men had to announce their vote in the presence of those to whom they were beholden-landlords, employers (possibly of family members), and local officials with real authority.[30]

But even in colonial days, paper ballots, discreetly folded and deposited in a sealed box, were used to protect the voter's integrity throughout New England and the Carolinas, and in parts of Pennsylvania. With the Revolution, the practice became obligatory in those places. New York, New Jersey, and other parts of Pennsylvania experimented further with paper ballots during the Revolutionary War, so that by 1787–1788 nine states had substantially adopted the practice.[31]

As a result—and contrary to common historical opinion—the secret ballot was the norm in the early republic. Other jurisdictions soon adopted it: Georgia in 1789, Delaware in 1791, the Northwest Territory in 1800, New York City in 1804, and Maryland in 1802 for state elections and 1810 for all elections. When the Federalists of Connecticut introduced the Stand Up law in 1801, which replaced the existing secret ballot with a public declaration in congressional elections (though not in elections for governor or town representative), it served only to enhance the Republican claim that Federalists scorned the ordinary voter, and the Republicans repealed it in 1817.[32]

Only in Virginia and Kentucky did the old-fashioned English mode of elections continue, lasting throughout the antebellum period. Oral voting, added to the persisting power of local sheriffs and county courts in parts of the Upper South, gave local elites some control over elections. Interestingly, one southern-influenced western state, Illinois, adopted the ballot in 1819, moved to oral voting in 1821, back to the ballot in 1823, and readopted oral voting again in 1829, all in an effort to combat secret intrigues during elections.[33]

Otherwise, the polling place was a less closely supervised place than historians have sometimes assumed. Even in the North, it has been argued, voters were traditionally subject to close scrutiny in the act of voting, essentially to ensure that they were duly qualified members of the local community. Some of the evidence for such scrutiny is stronger, however, at the height of the Second Party System in the 1840s than in the early republic. About the turn of the century enforcement of voting qualifications was generally very lax. In disputed election cases, the complaint was normally that too many people had been allowed to vote, not that arguably qualified voters had been turned away. When disappointed candidates did appeal to the legislature, they generally stopped short of courting unpopularity by appearing to favor a restricted franchise.[34]

Voter-qualification laws concerning the ownership of property were difficult to enforce in newly opened areas where titles had not yet been confirmed, which is why most frontier states avoided property qualifications. Election judges could not rule authoritatively on land ownership in any areas—like New England and Pennsylvania—where small amounts of land were frequently bought and sold or taken into joint ownership. In these circumstances, the old practice of handing over title deeds for a day, and so creating "fagot votes" as a temporary qualification could not be effectively policed. Where other forms of property were acceptable, the practice grew of accepting any evidence the voter brought forward: in Massachusetts, some voters brought the tools of their trade, a couple of cattle, and even credit notes as proof that they possessed enough substance to satisfy the law. Even bankrupts could qualify since the law allowed them to keep, free of distrait, household effects that happened to be worth enough to meet the property requirement. In theory, tax qualifications ought to have been easier to enforce. Yet official records were not readily available, and voters were asked to self-certify that they had paid sufficient taxes, which simply encouraged perjury. In any case, the onus of proof was on the objector to prove nonqualification, not the voter to prove his eligibility. This helps to explain the comparative lack of public demand for the extension of franchise—because the legal limitations did not have much effect, at least not for anyone who wished to vote.[35]

Many voters simply assumed that they could vote because they could not conceive why they should not be able to. War veterans, in particular, turned up to vote, as in South Carolina in the 1790s, regardless of the suffrage rules. In New York, Vermonters settling on the Holland Purchase in western New York presumed that they could not be deprived of a right they had enjoyed in Vermont and used their fists at the polls in 1807 to enforce that right. Cultural attitudes were shifting in the wake of the Revolution, so that the suffrage franchise was seen as the natural right of men who supported government, did their civic duty, risked their lives for the republic, or worked hard to become property owners, regardless of their current wealth. By 1801, as the Federalist George Cabot recognized, "The spirit of our country is doubtless more democratic than the *form* of our government."[36]

The shift in attitude was most obvious in those states that had occasion to write or rewrite their rules. Six of the 10 new states that established their political institutions from scratch before 1821 instituted universal manhood suffrage, at least for whites. In 1777, Vermont had accepted this revolutionary principle at its first organization, though it did not become a state of the Union till 1791. Kentucky followed suit in 1792, as did almost all the states admitted between 1816 and 1821. Tennessee, in 1796, was the only frontier state to introduce a property qualification, but it applied only to those who had not lived in the county concerned for more than six months.[37]

In the territories, Congress initially tried to maintain a freehold franchise but finally conceded a taxpaying qualification for the Indiana, Illinois, and Mississippi territories between 1811 and 1814. Three of the new states adopted taxpaying qualifications, but these were not always a great restriction. Certainly, Louisiana, dominated by a Gallic population determined to retain its control, imposed in 1812 a tax requirement that effectively excluded over ½ the state's adult white males from voting, despite exempting from the qualification for five years those who had bought land from the United States government. By contrast, Mississippi in 1817 exempted from its own taxpaying requirements all those who were enrolled in the local militia—or who were exempt from militia service! Earlier, in 1802, Ohio had given the franchise to taxpayers and those who worked on the roads, but since all adult males were obliged to work on the roads, this amounted to a thoroughly democratic franchise (for white males) that, without amendment, would make possible the huge turnouts there in the Jacksonian period.[38]

In the older states, where existing property qualifications had long existed, elites were understandably concerned that their interests might be jeopardized if power was transferred to a popular majority. Accordingly, they resisted the demand for liberalization, but with limited success. In New York City, the charter of 1730, which restricted voting to property owners, was reformed in 1804 by a Republican state legislature that extended the suffrage also to taxpayers who paid rent of twenty-five dollars or more a year. In Maryland, a broad bipartisan movement for universal white male suffrage appeared after 1797, with huge backing from the landless residents of rapidly growing Baltimore. In the face of diehards in the state senate, a reform bill finally passed the legislature in 1801 and was confirmed in 1802 (thus making it a constitutional amendment), admitting all free white adult males, 12-month resident in a county, to vote in elections for sheriffs, delegates, and other state officials. In 1810, a constitutional amendment confirmed that this privilege extended also to voting for congressmen and presidential electors, but the state senate and governor continued to be indirectly elected. Similarly, South Carolina, after a three-year struggle over the suffrage, confirmed in 1810 that all free white males with two years' residence could vote, though only for the lower house and congressmen. By 1810, three of the southeastern states—the exceptions were Virginia and North Carolina—had achieved a thoroughly democratic suffrage for white adult males, at least in elections for the lower house of assembly and for congressmen.[39]

In most states, new constitutional provisions did not result from widespread popular demands for a wider suffrage. Usually, constitutional conventions were called to settle other problems, especially the basis of regional representation within the states, and the opportunity was taken to introduce reforms of the suffrage. As representation was made fairer, so, too, the restrictions on voting for upper houses were democratized, though in a piecemeal way. Property qualifications for appointive and elective officeholders were also made less restrictive, as in Maryland in 1809. Local government opened up in many states, as, for example, in Massachusetts in 1811, and the franchise made more generous. The most restrictive systems of local government survived in New York and in seven southern states where county courts, either appointed by the legislature (as in South Carolina) or co-optive and self-perpetuating (as in Virginia and Kentucky), remained the fulcrum of local government.[40]

Pressure for a change in the franchise rules came simply from the increase in the number of people voting. Before 1790, voters had not used the right to vote in large numbers even when they possessed it; in a routine election like that for governor of Connecticut in 1793 only 5 percent of eligibles turned out. But much greater numbers were possible if exciting or important matters seemed at stake, and, as in England between 1694 and 1716, shorter terms and more frequent elections served to stimulate interest. In this respect, the introduction of popular elections for Congress provided an important stimulus, especially in states like South Carolina that otherwise did not have many popular elections. In practical terms, the most effective way of encouraging voter turnout was to make voting places more accessible, and the introduction of smaller election districts, notably in New Jersey, Maryland, and Ohio, greatly stimulated voting.[41]

The greatest incentive to rouse popular participation came in the 1790s with the development of two-party conflict. As the governing elite divided, so each side recognized that the existence of a huge pool of uncommitted potential voters could decide the outcome of the struggle, and each appealed downward for support among the mass electorate. As a consequence, two-party conflict created in many areas a close competition that stimulated interest and brought large numbers to the polls in 1798–1800, including even in Virginia.[42]

After 1800, the Jeffersonians for some years enjoyed an easy predominance that made voting seem less necessary, but after 1807 party competition revived north of the Potomac, creating electoral excitement in ⅔ of the states for the next eight years. As David Fischer argued in 1965, this was a major democratizing experience for the New England, Middle Atlantic, and coastal border states.[43]

One important consequence was a decline in the habit of deference as politicians used issues to rouse popular support in their opponents' traditional areas of strength. Significantly, between 1800 and 1810, delegate nominating conventions were introduced at the local level in the middle states, and even in Ohio, to reassure voters that the candidates they voted for were indeed the people's choice.[44]

A further stimulus to voter participation came with the extension of statewide elections. Though party conflict aroused interest, there was little motivation to vote in the many counties and districts, where opinion was overwhelmingly one-sided. But a statewide contest made every vote potentially critical: politicians had every reason to mobilize isolated supporters in hostile areas and to persuade voters in areas of strength of the need to offset hostile votes elsewhere in the state. Overall, the popular election of governors operated to stimulate higher turnouts after 1790 in most states north of the Potomac; where repeated annually, as in New England, it had an even more powerful democratizing effect.[45]

Similarly, before 1842, some states, usually smaller ones, chose their congressmen by a general-ticket election, as of course did those allowed only one congressman. Such statewide elections were in general less common in the South, but the biennial statewide contest for congressmen brought democratic agitation to Delaware, Georgia, and Louisiana before 1815, and Alabama and Mississippi thereafter.[46]

Half a century ago, J. R. Pole and Richard P. McCormick demonstrated that during the presidencies of Jefferson and Madison voters began turning up to the polls in huge numbers. Between 1808 and 1816, statewide turnouts in Massachusetts, New Hampshire, and New Jersey commonly passed 60 percent. As Pole pointed out, a higher proportion of adult males in Massachusetts voted in these years than at any subsequent time down to the Civil War. In some Maryland counties, turnout reached heights of over 80 percent between 1808 and 1812. Moreover, in many states, these high levels of turnout did not entirely disappear after 1816. Partisan conflicts continued to raise their heads from time to time, and the Panic of 1819 brought a degree of popular distress that roused high turnouts in the early 1820s in some states. The gist of these figures is now being confirmed by scholars using Lampi's much more extensive, precise, and authoritative data for 1787–1825.[47]

These returns confirm that close party conflict at the state level drew to the polls many men who were not qualified to vote. Candidates and parties that were determined to win had little scruple in encouraging the unqualified to vote, as they did, for example, by creating "fagot votes" and encouraging aliens to vote. In New York, where severe restrictions supposedly applied, even conservative Federalist landlords encouraged tenants to vote, paying their traveling expenses and offering financial inducements to vote appropriately. In turn, New York Republicans used some ingenious devices, from at least 1807 onward, to bring every man over the age of 21 to the polls. Several counties between 1807 and 1814 cast more votes than they had eligible voters: Martin Van Buren claimed there were 600 illegal voters in his county in 1810. Though the suffrage rules considerably reduced the numbers voting in New York, electoral frauds, according to historian Harvey Strum, "created a de facto lowering of property qualifications for voting in gubernatorial and senatorial races . . . and significantly enlarged the potential electorate."[48]

The high turnouts of 1808–1812 confirmed, as J. R. Pole remarked, that "constitutional limitations [on voting] were not only slight in themselves but were seldom enforced by local authorities and did little to prevent the exercise of the suffrage franchise by almost any member of the adult male population." In his view, New England (outside Rhode Island) had not known an effective freehold rule, or much enforcement of the suffrage laws, since the Revolution. Even the Massachusetts constitution of 1780 could not prevent the existence by 1809 of what Chilton Williamson described as "a condition bordering on universal suffrage."[49]

In New Jersey, all serious thought about enforcing property qualifications disappeared long before the constitutional reform of 1807; as in Maryland in 1801, that apparently fundamental change simply confirmed what had been previously been common and regular though unconstitutional, and turnout scarcely increased as a result of the reforms. Lax interpretation of the rules not only served the parties but also solved the problem of established voters whose deteriorating socioeconomic condition meant that they could no longer meet the formal requirements, even though they remained worthy citizens.[50]

The open disregard of suffrage rules, encouraged by political parties that flagrantly breached the law at election time, made it clear that the only way to secure honesty in elections was to remove property restrictions. As one Connecticut legislator in effect said in 1801, the state's property tests should be abolished because they were treated as meaningless in many towns. In addition, many appreciated that electoral fraud, especially as practiced in New York, allowed party politicians to control who voted and when they voted, a control that could be broken by introducing a universal suffrage (for white males) either legally or *de facto*. Though in some states, Federalists sometimes argued for tightening up the rules and feared that Republicans would be the main beneficiaries of extension, many other Federalists came to feel they could not oppose a popular demand and in any case recognized the need to reform rules that could not be enforced. Thus, movements to broaden the suffrage rules arose in the 1810s as much as a consequence of high voter participation as in hope of creating it.[51]

Even so, much resistance persisted to the abandonment of the principle of a "stake in society" from those who feared the growth of an unreliable and ill-equipped population. Republicans were on the whole more sympathetic to reform, especially in the northern states, but they were far from united on the issue: in New York, in particular, a significant minority of Republicans helped to obstruct reform in the legislature. In general, upper houses were more conservative, regardless of party control, and lower houses more aware of the disadvantage of seeming to oppose a widespread right to vote. Before 1812, such internal divisions ensured that contests for reform failed in Massachusetts, Rhode Island, Connecticut, and New York. The one exception was New Jersey, where anxiety about corrupt practices in elections—and about the number of aliens, blacks, and women voting—led to a major reform in 1807. This placed suffrage on a clear taxpaying basis, creating a very broad franchise for white men but disfranchising women and African Americans. As a mark of white male hegemony, apparently neither group protested.[52]

The demand for reform affected New England in the years immediately following the party passions of 1807–1815 and the War of 1812. As in Mississippi, veterans in particular were widely thought to have earned the right to vote, regardless of all other considerations. In Connecticut, the postwar union of Republicans and dissenters brought about a new constitution in 1818 that gave the vote to adult white males of "good character" and six months' residence who were $7 freeholders or state taxpayers or militiamen. Here, as in many other states, a taxpaying qualification amounted, in Williamson's judgment, to "almost manhood suffrage, so long as males of voting age were almost all polled."[53]

In 1819, the new state of Maine adopted the principle of universal manhood suffrage that had in fact existed in previous years when it conducted its politics as part of Massachusetts. So too in 1821 Massachusetts at last adopted taxpaying in place of its property qualification, but this probably did not make the Massachusetts electoral system significantly more democratic in its operation than before the Revolution. Constitutional reform in New England basically sanctioned voting practices that had previously been common but irregular unconstitutional and possibly producing results that were subject to challenge in the legislature.[54]

A real change did take place in New York, where constitutional reform was an extension of recent reform movements in New England. The flood of Yankee settlers into New York in the years since 1800 prompted demands for liberalization that the regular Democratic Republicans could not resist. The new constitution of 1821 abolished the severely restrictive franchise for the state senate and extended the right to vote for the assembly to all male taxpayers and militia men. This formally increased the proportion of adult white males able to vote for the assembly, it is estimated, from 78 percent to 90 percent. However, as elsewhere, interpretation of the taxpaying qualification proved complex and difficult. The search for simplification produced a noncontentious shift in 1826 from taxpaying to a qualification based simply on citizenship, age, and residence—which increased the electorate by 1 percent! Far more significant than the franchise changes was the abolition, in 1821, of the Council of Appointment, which had controlled 15,000 officeholders at all levels of government, and the consequent increase in the number of offices open to popular election.[55]

New York was the only state where a constitutional convention held in the 1820s effectively extended the democratization of politics. Although the process of constitutional change here was deeply affected by party hostilities, the issue of the suffrage did not reflect unbridgeable differences. The main argument was not over the principle of extending the right to vote, but whether a higher qualification should be retained for the senate. Most of the Democratic Republican Party favored manhood suffrage, but their leaders, notably Martin Van Buren, preferred a more limited franchise because they recognized that the new constitution had to be approved by a referendum among the old restricted electorate. Though arguing in favor of retaining some restrictions, many Federalists saw little danger in broadening the franchise, as long as the judiciary remained independent. As the old Federalist standard-bearer Rufus King pointedly remarked, "I have not observed that the States in which a property qualification is established, either choose wiser men or are less democratic than those where the property qualification for electors does not exist. We are so nearly alike, and have so much intercourse, that it has appeared to me pretty certain that the popular claim would prevail over that of property." His main concern was to stop potentially corrupt party managers from perverting the popular will: "We must choose the [presidential] electors by the people or the public liberties will be lost. . . . They cannot be bribed, they are safe against corruption."[56]

The widespread acceptance of manhood as the essential qualification for enfranchisement had carried with it a definition of those who could be trusted to preserve property and liberty, and that in turn required a definition of those not to be trusted. Paupers were seen as unworthy, criminals as dangerous, and women as inherently dependent, while attitudes to aliens fluctuated, often being viewed as acceptable voters but not officeholders.

The shift to recognizing civic contributions (such as military service and road work) that were then essentially male activities inevitably undermined the claim of women to the vote, as did the gradual replacement of Enlightenment environmentalism by biological determinism.[57]

It has become almost a commonplace that "As the Anglo-American political system became more 'democratic,' it also became even more racist and sexist as women and blacks were stripped of rights." The growing cultural belief in inherent racial differences ensured that African Americans, even when free, would increasingly be considered unworthy of citizenship, and so suffered disfranchisement as socioeconomic barriers to voting disappeared between 1790 and 1821. This process of marking out blacks as an unacceptable *racial* group began in the South, where the three seaboard states that already had prohibitions in place were joined by three border states—Delaware in 1792, Kentucky in 1799, and Maryland in 1801—that had large and growing free black communities.[58]

Ohio, in 1802, was the first free state to ban African Americans from the polls; every new state to join the Union thereafter, whether slave or free, followed Ohio's precedent, with the exception of Maine in 1819–1820. New Jersey in 1807, Connecticut (by statute in 1811 and by constitution in 1818), and Rhode Island in 1822 instituted their own bans, while New York in 1821 allowed free black voting only if a heightened property qualification could be met. Though racial intolerance would deepen further in the 1820s, disfranchisement temporarily halted. In 1828, eight states still officially allowed voting by free blacks: four in New England where their numbers were low, plus New York (in its limited way), Pennsylvania, North Carolina, and Tennessee.[59]

The suffrage was therefore not entirely restricted to men who could pass as white, but it was undoubtedly the preserve of adult males. The principle of universal manhood suffrage (at least for whites) had been formally established in only eight states by 1828, while, in Virginia and Rhode Island, social and economic change was making traditional legal restrictions actually reduce the size of the legal electorate. But that did not alter the fact that overall the United States was already a functioning mass democracy for white males, and in many states substantially had been for some considerable time before the rise to political prominence of Andrew Jackson.

***

The assumption that there was a connection between enlarging the franchise and the election of Andrew Jackson to the presidency rests upon rather fuzzy assumptions.

It is not always clear whether Jackson supposedly owed his rise to power to a prior expansion of the voting public or whether he himself somehow contributed toward the process of democratizing the franchise. Either way, there is a presumption that in the early nineteenth century the franchise was—as Keyssar claimed—"generally granted... only to property holders," even though the evidence widely available in authoritative monographs suggests, as we have seen, that many nonproperty holders already enjoyed the privilege, both in theory and practice. As a result, it is simply not true that political parties of the 1820s and 1830s "often campaigned on the promise of eliminating property requirements." It is also frequently said that the destruction of property tests in "the constitutional conventions of the 1820s" prepared the way for Jackson's presidential victories, even though there was only one decisive reforming state constitutional convention (New York) between 1815 and 1832. If there were a connection between Jackson's victory and an expanded voter universe, it was surely that Jackson was the first presidential candidate to win a clear popular majority in a competitive presidential election in which the popular voice directly determined the final outcome in the Electoral College.[60]

In the 1820s, voters began to act in presidential elections as they had previously, in many states, at the state and local levels. Presidential elections had been bitterly fought in 1796 and 1800, but thereafter the electoral predominance and caucus nominations of the Jeffersonian Republican Party made the outcome of these contests predictable. Only in 1812, when the Federalists exploited the Republican factional split in New York, might the nominee of the congressional caucus have failed. After the Republican walkovers of 1816 and 1820, it became clear by 1823 that the party could no longer agree upon a single candidate, and the resort to a congressional caucus in 1824 was essentially a maneuver by the Republican faction most confident of winning the plurality needed to lay claim to the traditional party label. The uncertainties of the early 1820s, when economic breakdown stimulated voter turnout to new levels in a number of (mainly Western) states, created a situation in which ambitious leading national politicians could be challenged by an outsider, especially one who, like Jackson, was an acclaimed national hero. By 1827–1828, two new political formations had appeared, each campaigning to attract popular support, and the contest to win the White House became the central driving force behind political mobilization.[61]

It is misleading to assume that, before then, traditional aristocratic attitudes had previously placed the selection of the Electoral College in the hands of the state legislatures, or that its members exercised their judgment independent of the ticket upon which they were elected. In 1792, the New York legislature apologetically explained that it gave itself the privilege of choosing the state's presidential electors only because there was not sufficient time to organize a popular election for that year. By the time of the first contested election in 1796, respect for popular sentiment had persuaded eight states—half of them—to allow all those people who could vote for the assembly and congressmen to choose the state's electors. By 1800, four states had moved the decision away from the people back to the assembly, but the demand for popular participation ensured that in 1804 and 1808 only 7 legislatures of 17 kept the electoral vote in their own hands. Those Jeffersonian elections—not that of 1824, as often asserted—were probably the first in which a majority of adult white males had the opportunity to participate in a presidential election.[62]

The retraction, in some states, of the choice of electors from the people arose from the majority party's determination to ensure that it won every one of the state's electoral votes, a necessity that its own intensely partisan supporters could readily accept. Such partisanship underlay the resort to legislative control in some states in 1800; again in 1812, the New Jersey and North Carolina legislatures reclaimed the privilege in order to ensure that all the state's electoral votes went to Madison. Still in 1816, the states were evenly divided between legislative and popular elections for president, but the growing irrelevance of the old party fight at the federal level undermined the argument against giving the choice of electors to the people. Of the 24 states, by 1820 only nine state legislatures still kept the decision in their own hands and by 1824 only six. In New York, the regular Republican leadership under Van Buren persisted in preserving the legislature's privilege gained in 1792 and uniquely clung to it in 1824 because they wished to elect as president a man who was unpopular with the state's voters. The voter uprising in New York that temporarily overthrew Van Buren's control in 1824 finally discredited the legitimacy of legislative prerogative, so that in 1828 only Delaware and South Carolina retained it—and from 1832 until the Civil War only South Carolina.

In rousing popular participation, it was not enough to give the voters the power to choose members of the state's branch of the Electoral College: the election had also to be organized on an at-large, winner-take-all basis. The district system may have seemed more democratic because it gave greater representation to minority interests, but in districts possessing overwhelming partisan agreement, it could instill apathy in comparison with a statewide election. Only if an easy statewide majority existed, as it did in Virginia, did the at-large election undermine participation in the relatively few evenly divided districts. In the first four presidential elections, only three or four states used the general-ticket system at any one time—most commonly, New Hampshire and Pennsylvania. After 1800, Rhode Island, New Jersey, Virginia, and Ohio joined them on a regular basis. Not until 1824 did half the states choose their electors in a statewide election, with 9 of those 12 in the North. The originality of 1828 lay in the fact that 18 states (of 24) used the general-ticket system, eight of them slave states. In that sense, certainly, agitation of the electorate across the nation became possible in a presidential election as never before.[63]

In securing his great popular victory in 1828, Jackson did not owe his success to new states admitted since 1815 or to the suffrage extensions of 1818–1821 in the East. New Western states carried little weight in presidential elections, while older, larger states like Ohio and Kentucky were closely divided between the parties. Of the states in which recent constitutional reform had been concentrated, those in New England overwhelmingly preferred John Quincy Adams in both 1824 and 1828, while New York virtually ignored Jackson in 1824 and in 1828 split its Electoral College votes between him and Adams, 20 to 16. Nationwide, the total numbers voting for Jackson in 1824, 1828, and 1832 were not unprecedented in state elections, though renewed competition for the presidency now encouraged men to vote in large numbers in presidential as well as in congressional and state elections. The great increase in turnout came after Jackson had left the White House, with the sharpening of two-party conflict in 1840.[64]

Indeed, the heart of Jackson's support lay in the least democratic section of the Union. Whereas there had been nothing to choose between North and South in 1790 in terms of allowing an extensive franchise; by the 1820s, the older South was remarkable for the barriers it retained to the full operation of democratic choice. Throughout the southern seaboard states, voters could not vote for governor, except in Delaware and in Georgia from 1824 onward, and contrived representation systems ensured that eastern voters counted for more than western. Voters continued to be excluded from control of county government in 7 of the 10 southern states. South Carolina, in particular, stood out as a state that allowed a broad electorate to choose the legislature and then gave that legislature absolute centralized power to elect other officers and run both the state and local government. Far from demanding greater democracy, the Southeast's Jacksonian Democrats were often distinguished by their support of the *status quo*: in Virginia, for example, they supported the 1829 state constitutional convention's decision to relax only marginally the state's complex property qualifications.[65]

Significant reform began in the South with Mississippi in 1832 and Tennessee in 1834. Both states adopted universal white male suffrage, opened up a wide range of offices to local election, and democratized county governments. Traditional obstacles persisted elsewhere in the South but did not prevent the development of two party conflict in most of the older southern states after 1834. As a result, the South Atlantic region at last experienced the democratizing effects of an upsurge of popular participation such as the states north of the Potomac had experienced before 1815.[66]

Although Jackson's presidency had almost no direct influence on the few state constitutional reforms that did take place between 1829 and 1837, it did have one important lasting effect. Largely as a result of his controversial financial policies, national party competition rose to new levels after 1836 and the Democratic Party developed a more pronounced and radical ideology. Among other things, it committed itself to the doctrine that the suffrage must be based on the civic equality inherent in all adult white males. Thereafter, whenever a state constitution came to be revised, Democrats pressed for universal white manhood suffrage, even though in practice the existing situation did not seriously disfranchise any adult white males. In a series of state constitutional conventions between 1832 and 1851, Jacksonian Democrats would abolish property and taxpaying rules and extend the principle of universal white manhood suffrage in six states, half of them in the South. Even so, in 1855, some form of property requirement would still survive in three states and the principle of taxpaying in six others.[67]

Jacksonian reforms were usually accomplished without great popular demand or pressure, and without great resistance; in many cases, the new constitutions (as Pole said of New Jersey in 1844) simply enshrined the practice of the last 40 years. In only one state, Rhode Island, would this demand lead to a serious political conflagration? Here an antiquated suffrage, dating back to 1662, proved increasingly restrictive as the growth of industry proletarianized the state's lower classes, sparking fears of the effects of admitting such people to the electoral process. The Dorr War of 1842 underlines the fact that, in the rest of the United States, the suffrage had been democratized before industrialization occurred.[68]

As Tocqueville famously remarked in the 1830s, the Americans had "arrived at a state of democracy without having to endure a democratic revolution." The early creation of a mass democracy had its origins in the inheritance of British representative systems, the wide availability of land, and the liberalizing impact of the Revolution's equal-rights ideology. In a situation in which a large proportion of adult white males could already vote, it proved difficult to refuse the vote to other white men, especially when they were adult sons of property owners, or tenant farmers, or pioneers buying on credit, or self-employed artisans—men difficult to see as unworthy, potentially subversive, or lacking moral integrity. The exclusion of other people on gender and racial grounds is highly invidious in retrospect, but the fact remains that a system that admitted women and racial minorities could have been just as constraining for the future of democracy if at the same time it had limited the suffrage to an exclusive socioeconomic elite. The expansion of the active electorate between 1787 and 1828 incorporated an unattractive belief in essential biological differences that denied political equality, but in practice, it also created a structure and situation out of which a more open and broadly democratic system might emerge.[69]

Notes

1. Jill Lepore, "Rock, Paper, Scissors: How We Used to Vote," *The New Yorker*, October 13, 2008, 2, consulted at http://www.newyorker.com/reporting/2008/10/13/081013fa_fact_lepore?currentPage=2; Sean Wilentz, *The Rise of American Democracy: Jefferson to Lincoln* (New York, 2005); Alexander Keyssar, *The Right to Vote: The Contested History of Democracy in the United States* (New York, 2000); Daniel Walker Howe, *What Hath God Wrought: The Transformation of America, 1815–1848* (New York, 2007). See also Charles Sellers, *The Market Revolution: Jacksonian America, 1815–1846* (New York, 1991). The A New Nation Votes: American Election Returns 1787–1825 website may be found at http://elections.lib.tufts.edue faas_portalfindex.xq.

2. The best overall study of the evolution of the suffrage before the Civil War remains Chilton Williamson, *American Suffrage from Property to Democracy, 1760–1860* (Princeton, NJ, 1960). For colonial attitudes, see ibid., 1–61; Jack P. Greene, *All Men Are Created Equal: Some Reflections on the Character of the American Revolution* (Oxford, UK, 1976), reprinted in his *Imperatives, Behaviors, and Identities: Essays in Early American Cultural History* (Charlottesville, VA, 1992), esp. 246–59; Robert J. Steinfeld, "Property and Suffrage in the Early American Republic" *Stanford Law Review* 41 (*January* 1989), 335–76, esp. 339–48.

3. The Great Reform Act of 1832 would increase the potential electorate to only 18.4 percent in England and Wales. Frank O'Gorman, *The Long Eighteenth Century: British Political and Social History, 1688–1832* (London, 1997) 49, 140, 369.

4. Robert J. Dinkin, *Voting in Provincial America: A Study of Elections in the Thirteen Colonies, 1689–1776* (Westport, CT, 1977), 39.

5. Williamson, *American Suffrage*, 20–39, esp. 38; Dinkin, *Voting in Provincial America*, 49; Keyssar, *The Right to Vote*, 7. See also Richard R. Beeman, *The Varieties of Political Experience in Eighteenth-Century America* (Philadelphia, PA, 2004), 75, 105–106, 250, 293–94, 310. The calculation that 85 percent of free white males could vote, made by Robert E. Brown and B. Katherine Brown, Virginia, 1707–1786: *Democracy or Aristocracy* (East Lansing, MI, 1964), has generally been regarded as too high. Historians have tended to follow Charles S. Sydnor, *Gentlemen Freeholders: Political Practices in Washington's Virginia* (Chapel Hill, NC, 1952), 34–43, in preferring a figure below 50 percent. The more recent midway calculation was made by John Kolp, *Gentlemen and Freeholders: Electoral Politics in Colonial Virginia* (Baltimore, 1998), 38–49.

6. Robert J. Dinkin, *Voting in Revolutionary America: A Study of Elections in the Original Thirteen States, 1776–1789* (Westport, CT, 1982), 39.

7. Marc W. Kruman, *Between Authority and Liberty: State Constitution Making in Revolutionary America* (Chapel Hill, NC, 1997), 87–108; Elisha P. Douglass, *Rebels and Democrats: The Struggle for Equal Political Rights and Majority Rule during the American Revolution* (Chapel Hill, NC, 1955); Edmund S. Morgan, *Inventing the People: The Rise of Popular Sovereignty in England and America* (New York, 1988); Wilentz, *Rise of American Democracy*, 13–39.

8. Dinkin, *Voting in Revolutionary America*, 36. See also Willi Paul Adams, *The First American Constitutions: Republican Ideology and the Making of the State Constitutions in the Revolutionary Era* (Chapel Hill, NC, 1980).

9. Quotation from the 1776 constitution, in Greene, *Imperatives*, 260; J. R. Pole, "Historians and the Problem of Early American Democracy," *American Historical Review* 67 (April 1962), 626–46, and reprinted in his *Paths to the American Past* (New York, 1979), 223–49. Pole's important pioneering

contributions to the subject came in a series of still valuable articles, listed here by state: "Suffrage and Representation in Massachusetts: A Statistical Note," *William and Mary Quarterly* 14 (October 1957), 560–92, as corrected by Richard P. McCormick, "Letters to the Editors," *William and Mary Quarterly* 15 (July 1958), 412–16; Pole, "The Suffrage in New Jersey, 1790–1807," *Proceedings of the New Jersey Historical Society* 71 (1953), 39–61; Pole, "Suffrage Reform and the American Revolution in New Jersey," *Proceedings of the New Jersey Historical Society* 74 (1956), 173–94; Pole, "Jeffersonian Democracy and the Federalist Dilemma in New Jersey," *Proceedings of the New Jersey Historical Society* 74 (1956), 260–92; Pole, "Election Statistics in Pennsylvania, 1790–1840," *Pennsylvania Magazine of History and Biography* 82 (April 1958), 217–19; Pole, "Suffrage and Representation in Maryland from 1776 to 1810: A Statistical Note and Some Reflections," *Journal of Southern History* 24 (May 1958), 218–25; Pole, "Constitutional Reform and Election Statistics in Maryland, 1790–1812," *Maryland Historical Magazine* 55 (December 1960), 278–92; Pole, "Representation and Authority in Virginia from the Revolution to Reform," *Journal of Southern History* 24 (February 1958), 16–50, reprinted in his *Paths to the American Past*, 3–40; Pole, "Election Statistics in North Carolina, To 1861,"*Journal of Southern History* 24 (May 1958), 225–28; all resulting in his magisterial *Political Representation in England and the Origins of the American Republic* (New York, 1966).

10. Kenneth Lockridge, "Land, Population, and the Evolution of New England Society, 1630–1790," *Past and Present* 39 (April 1968), 62–80; Allan Kulikoff, "The Progress of Inequality in Revolutionary Boston," *William and Mary Quarterly* 28 (July 1971), 375–412.

11. Pole, *Political Representation*, 146–47. For the debate over the size of Virginia's electorate in the mid-eighteenth century, see note 5 above. For the postrevolutionary period, Jackson Turner Main, *The Antifederalists: Critics of the Constitution, 1781–1788* (Chapel Hill, NC, 1961), 31, found that in most counties about half the adult white males could meet the requirements, a view accepted by Richard P. McCormick, *The Second American Party System: Party Formation in the Jacksonian Era* (Chapel Hill, NC, 1966), 179. The suggestion of Dinkin, *Voting in Revolutionary America*, 38, that 70–75 percent of adult white males in Virginia were qualified in the 1780s seems to go beyond the evidence he cites. Later writers see 60–65 percent as close to the mark. Kolp, *Gentlemen and Freeholders*, 38–49; William G. Shade, *Democratizing the Old Dominion: Virginia and the Second Party System, 1824–1861* (Charlottesville, VA, 1996), 4.

12. New York's figures are not beyond dispute. Linda DePauw estimated that 92 percent of adult white males could vote in 1790, but Alfred Young's careful analysis argues convincingly that she and other historians (including himself) had misunderstood contemporary tabulations and that the figure was closer to 58 percent. Linda Grant De Pauw, *The Eleventh Pillar: New York State and the Federal Constitution* (Ithaca, NY, 1966), 141–46; Alfred F. Young, *The Democratic Republicans of New York: The Origins, 1763–1797* (Chapel Hill, NC, 1967), 83–84, 585–87. See also John Brooke, "King George Has Issued Too many Patents for Us": Property and Democracy in Jeffersonian New York," in this issue of JER.

13. Dinkin, *Voting in Revolutionary America*, 35–36, 37.

14. The description of the Connecticut qualifications comes from the *Pennsylvania Magazine* (1776), quoted in Marchette Chute, *The First Liberty: A History of the Right to Vote in America, 1619–1850* (London, 1969), 286. See also Joel A. Cohen, "Democracy in Revolutionary Rhode Island: A Statistical Analysis," *Rhode Island History* 29 (Winter/Spring 1970), 5; Dinkin, *Voting in Revolutionary America*, 39; Williamson, *American Suffrage*, 165–66, 243–47; Charles S. Grant, *Democracy in the Connecticut Frontier Town of Kent* (New York, 1961).

15. Dinkin, *Voting in Revolutionary America*, 32–33, 42–43; James H. Kettner, *The Development of American Citizenship, 1608–1870* (Chapel Hill, NC, 1978), 102–103; Kruman, *Between Authority and Liberty*, 98.

16. Dinkin, *Voting in Revolutionary America*, 32–33, 36–37; Williamson, *American Suffrage*, 135–36.

17. Williamson, *American Suffrage*, 108–10, 121. Conversely, Pole could detect no indication that the improvement in the currency after 1789 disfranchised any voters in New Jersey or Maryland. Pole, "Suffrage and Representation in Maryland," 220–21; Thornton Anderson, "Eighteenth-Century Suffrage: The Case of Maryland," *Maryland Historical Magazine* 76 (Summer 1981), 141–58, esp. 149; Dinkin, *Voting in Revolutionary America*, 38.

18. Richard P. McCormick, *The History of Voting in New Jersey: A Study of the Development of Election Machinery, 1664–1911* (New Brunswick, NJ, 1953), 77, 85.
19. George Minot, in 1788, quoted in Dinkin, *Voting in Revolutionary America*, 37; Pole, "Suffrage and Representation in Massachusetts," 567, 569, 570, 577–78, 580.
20. Pole, *Political Representation*, "Suffrage and Representation in Massachusetts," 571, and "Constitutional Reform in Maryland," 275–76; Young, *Democratic Republicans of New York*, 83–84, 585–87; Jackson Turner Main, *The Upper House in Revolutionary America, 1763–1788* (Madison, WI, 1967).
21. Rosemarie Zagarri, *Revolutionary Backlash: Women and Politics in the Early American Republic* (Philadelphia, 2007).
22. Dinkin, *Voting in Revolutionary America*, 41–42; Williamson, *American Suffrage*, 115.
23. Jon P. Preimesberger, ed., *Congressional Quarterly's Guide to U.S. Elections*, 6th ed. (2 vols., Washington, DC, 2010), 1:23; Keyssar, *The Right to Vote*, 24.
24. Dinkin, *Voting in Revolutionary America*, 39.
25. Williamson, *American Suffrage*, 117–18, 124–31; Ellsworth, quoted in Dinkin, *Voting in Revolutionary America*, 40.
26. Williamson, *American Suffrage*, 131–37.
27. Philip S. Klein, *Pennsylvania Politics, 1817–1832: A Game without Rules* (Philadelphia, PA, 1940), 34. See also Pole, "Election Statistics in Pennsylvania," 217–19.
28. Keyssar's *Right to Vote* is particularly disappointing in its overly generalized treatment of the changes from 1790 to the 1850s, though his tabulations of constitutional changes relating to voting, 340–61, are invaluable and relied upon here. Likewise, Wilentz's *Rise of Democracy*, 40–178, misses the significance of the developments of 1790–1815. If democratization had substantially taken place by 1815, it becomes inappropriate to explain it in terms of changes that occurred after 1815, as in Sean Wilentz, "Property and Power: Suffrage Reform in the United States, 1787–1860," in *Voting and the Spirit of American Democracy: Essays on the History of Voting and Voting Rights in America*, ed. Donald W. Rogers and Christine B. Scriabine (Urbana, IL, 1990), 31–42. One consequence of recent disregard of the earlier period is that much of the best secondary literature on the subject is now half a century old.
29. Pole, *Political Representation;* Jackson Turner Main, "Government by the People: The American Revolution and the Democratization of the Legislatures," *William and Mary Quarterly* 23 (July 1966), 391–407; Pole, "Suffrage and Representation in Massachusetts," 561–62; Charles S. Sydnor, *The Development of Southern Sectionalism, 1819–1848* (Baton Rouge, LA, 1948), 33–53.
30. Sydnor, *Gentlemen Freeholders*, 27–31; Donald J. Ratcliffe, *Party Spirit in a Frontier Republic: Democratic Politics in Ohio, 1793–1821* (Columbus, OH, 1998), 34–35.
31. Keyssar, *Right to Vote*, 5–6, 17; Williamson, *American Suffrage*, 104, 108, 121–22; Dinkin, *Voting in Revolutionary America*, 101–104. See also Morgan, *Inventing the People*, 174–233, esp. 183; and Eldon Cobb Evans, "A History of the Australian Ballot System in the United States" (Chicago, 1917), chapter 1, available at http:Jfen.wikisource.orgfwiki/A_History_of_the_Australian_Ballot_System_in_the_United_States.
32. Williamson, *American Suffrage*, 135, 149, 169–70, 183–84, 212. See also Thomas P. Abernethy, *The South in the New Nation, 1789–1819* (Baton Rouge, LA, 1961), 31; John T. Willis, *Presidential Elections in Maryland* (Mount Airy, MD, 1984), 3; Richard J. Purcell, *Connecticut in Transition, 1775–1818* (Washington, DC, 1918), 139–40, 156, 252.
33. Sydnor, *Development*, 48–49, 49–52; Robert M. Ireland, "Aristocrats All: The Politics of County Government in Ante-bellum Kentucky," *Review of Politics* 32 (July 1970), 365–83. For Illinois, see Theodore C. Pease, *The Frontier State, 1818–1848* (Springfield, IL, 1918), 39; Thomas Ford, *A History of Illinois, From Its Commencement as a State in 1818 to 1847* (1854; repr., Urbana, IL, 1995), Similarly, Kentucky had adopted the secret ballot in 1792 and then reverted to publicly recorded voice voting in 1799, mainly because of fraud surrounding the ballot system. Joan Wells Coward, *Kentucky in the New Republic: The Process of Constitution Making* (Lexington, KY, 1979), 143.
34. Compare Kenneth J. Winkle, *The Politics of Community: Migration and Politics in Antebellum Ohio* (New York, 1988), with Ratcliffe, *Party Spirit*, 11, 105–106, 163. See also Pole, "Suffrage in Maryland," 221–22, and "Representation and Authority in Virginia," in Pole's *Paths to the American Past*, 20.

35. Pole, "Suffrage in Massachusetts," 572–74, 576; Williamson, *American Suffrage*, 210–13, 134.

36. Cabot quoted in Williamson, *American Suffrage*, 174. See also ibid., 152–53; Harvey Strum, "Property Qualifications and Voting Behavior in New York, 1807–1816," *Journal of the Early Republic* 1 (Winter 1981), 347–71, esp. 364–65.

37. The states admitted between 1816 and 1821 were Indiana (1816), Mississippi (1817, the only one to adopt a taxpaying qualification), Alabama (1819), Illinois (1819), Maine (1820), and Missouri (1821).

38. Williamson, *American Suffrage*, 97–99, 208–209, 213–14; Donald J. Ratcliffe, "Voter Turnout in Early Ohio," *Journal of the Early Republic* 7 (Autumn 1987), 233–34, 246–50. For Louisiana, see Joseph G. Tregle, *Louisiana in the Age of Jackson: A Clash of Cultures and Personalities* (Baton Rouge, LA, 1999), 65, 68; Samuel C. Hyde, Jr., *Pistols and Politics: The Dilemma of Democracy in Louisiana's Florida Parishes, 1810–1899* (Baton Rouge, LA, 1996), 47; and John M. Sacher, *A Perfect War of Politics: Parties, Politicians, and Democracy in Louisiana, 1824–1861* (Baton Rouge, LA, 2003), 12, 205–207.

39. Pole, "Constitutional Reform in Maryland," 278–81; Williamson, *American Suffrage*, 138–57, 162–64.

40. Pole, "Constitutional Reform in Maryland," 281–82, and "Suffrage in Massachusetts," 564; Williamson, *American Suffrage*, 133–34; Sydnor, *Development*, 33–43, 287; Ireland, "Aristocrats All." For reform of local government elections, see Keyssar, *The Right to Vote*, 30–31, 50.

41. McCormick, *Voting in New Jersey*, 80–81, 84, 95–97, 119–20; Ratcliffe, *Party Spirit*, 34, 48–49; Pole, "Constitutional Reform in Maryland," 278; Williamson, *American Suffrage*, 166, 180.

42. Pole, *Political Representation*; Andrew W. Robertson, "Voting Rites and Voting Acts: Electioneering Ritual, 1790–1820," in *Beyond the Founders: New Approaches to the Political History of the Early American Republic*, ed. Jeffrey L. Pasley, Andrew W. Robertson, and David Waldstreicher (Chapel Hill, NC, 2004), 73–74.

43. David Hackett Fischer, *The Revolution of American Conservatism: The Federalist Party in the Era of Jeffersonian Democracy* (New York, 1965). It is a sly mark of Wilentz's rejection of Fischer's thesis that he entitles his section on the Whig Party in the mid-1830s "The Revolution of American Conservatism." Wilentz, *Rise of American Democracy*, 483.

44. For the decline of deference, see also Strum, "Property Qualifications," 366–69, and Donald J. Ratcliffe, "The Changing Political World of Thomas Worthington," in *The Center of a Great Empire: The Ohio Country in the Early American Republic*, ed. Andrew R. L. Cayton and Stuart D. Hobbs (Athens, OH, 2005), 36–61. For the significance of delegate nominating conventions, see Noble E. Cunningham, *The Jeffersonian Republicans in Power: Party Operations, 1801–1809* (Chapel Hill, NC, 1963), 196–200; Pole, "Jeffersonian Democracy and the Federalist Dilemma in New Jersey," 263–70; Carl Prince, *New Jersey's Jeffersonian Republicans: The Genesis of an Early Party Machine*, 1789–1817 (Chapel Hill, NC, 1967), 71ff.; Ratcliffe, *Party Spirit*, 45–57, 101–13, 125–35, 161–65, 185, 210–17, 235–38.

45. By 1792, seven states allowed popular statewide election of their governor, including Pennsylvania (from 1790) and Delaware (from 1792), both of which, like New York, held their election every three years. The exception among the free states, New Jersey, did not give the election to the people until 1844. All the states admitted after 1789 had direct popular elections for governor, except Louisiana. *Gubernatorial Elections, 1787–1997* (Washington, DC, 1998).

46. Rosemarie Zagarri, The Politics of Size: Representation in the United States, 1776–1850 (Ithaca, NY, 1987), 125–31, 154–59. For a debate over the party advantages of statewide as opposed to district elections, see Pole, "Jeffersonian Democracy and the Federalist Dilemma in New Jersey." Congress mandated compulsory district voting for the House in 1842.

47. J. R. Pole, "Letters to the Editor," 414. See also his "Suffrage in Maryland," 222, and "Constitutional Reform in Maryland," 280–81. The voting data that appeared in Pole's articles (cited fully in note 9) were reprinted in Pole, *Political Representation*, 543–64. See also McCormick, *Voting in New Jersey*, 119–20, and "New Perspectives," 292; Fischer, *Revolution of American Conservatism*, 188–90. Even in ostensibly one-party Ohio, the few counties that experienced close two-party conflict saw turnouts exceeding 60 percent of adult white males between 1808 and 1815. Statewide, turnout remained constant, 1808–1818. Ratcliffe, "Voter

Turnout in Early Ohio," 237, 239, 245, 247. See also Ratcliffe, Party Spirit, passim, and "Changing Political World"; Jeffrey L. Pasley, "The Cheese and the Words: Popular Political Culture and Participatory Democracy in the Early American Republic," in *Beyond the Founders*, ed. Pasley, Robertson, and Waldstreicher, 46–48; and Robertson, "Voting Rites," ibid., 73–74. The significance of close party competition and high turnouts before 1815 is missed by Keyssar, *The Right to Vote*, 40.

48. Williamson, *American Suffrage*, 159–63; Strum, "Property Qualifications," 360–66 (quotation at 366); Keyssar, *The Right to Vote*, 34–35. McCormick calculated that 41.8 percent of adult white males could legally vote for governor and state senator in New York in 1807 and 36.6 percent in 1814. Turnout for governor reached 93 percent of eligibles in 1807 and 95 percent in 1814, surely reflecting considerable intervention by illegal voters. McCormick, "Suffrage Classes and Party Alignments: A Study in Voter Behavior," *Mississippi Valley Historical Review* 46 (December 1959), 397–410; Strum, "Property Qualifications," 362.

49. Pole, "Suffrage and Representation in Massachusetts," 561; Williamson, *American Suffrage*, 169, 176, 177 (quotation), 178. See also Paul Goodman, *The Democratic-Republicans of Massachusetts: Politics in a Young Republic* (Cambridge, MA, 1964), 136–45; Ronald P. Formisano, *The Transformation of Political Culture: Massachusetts Parties, 1790s–1840s* (New York, 1983), 408–409.

50. Williamson, *American Suffrage*, 176–77, 209; Pole, "Suffrage in Maryland," 220–23. See also Pole, "Election Statistics in Pennsylvania," 217–19.

51. Williamson, *American Suffrage*, 171, 188–90, 192–94; Strum, "Property Qualifications," 360, 366.

52. Pole, "Constitutional Reform in Maryland," 282–84; Strum, "Property Qualifications," 358–59; Williamson, *American Suffrage*, 158–64, 177; McCormick, *Voting in New Jersey*, 97–101; Zagarri, *Revolutionary Backlash*, 36. See also Judith Apter Klinghoffer and Lois Elkis, "'The Petticoat Electors': Women's Suffrage in New Jersey, 1776–1807," *Journal of the Early Republic* 12 (Summer 1992), 159–94.

53. That is, so long as they had to pay a poll tax. Williamson, *American Suffrage*, 190. See also ibid., 182–90; Purcell, *Connecticut in Transition*, 399.

54. Williamson, *American Suffrage*, 190–95. Maine followed the precedent of Vermont in 1777, which Williamson argued, had simply legalized the loose practices of Connecticut electoral politics before the Revolution. Ibid., 97–99, 190.

55. Williamson, *American Suffrage* 204, 207. For the significance of the 1821 convention, see Jabez D. Hammond, *The History of Political Parties in the State of New York, From the Ratification of the Constitution to December, 1840* (2 vols., Albany, NY, 1842), esp. 2: 1–85.

56. Rufus King to Charles Gore, December 18, 1820, in *The Life and Correspondence of Rufns King, Comprising his Letters, Private and Official, His Public Documents, and his Speeches*, ed. Charles R. King (6 vols., New York, 1894–1900), 6: 365, 519–20, 532–33. For a different but perceptive perspective on voting reform after 1815, see Wilentz, *Rise of American Democracy*, 181–202.

57. Keyssar, *The Right to Vote*, 32–33, 54–59, 61–63; Kettner, *Development of American Citizenship*, 102–103, 122–24, 214–18, 231; Zagarri, *Revolutionary Backlash*, 164–73. For the limitation of democratic rights by racial, ethnic and gender hierarchies, see Rogers M. Smith, *Civic Ideals: Conflicting Visions of Citizenship in U.S. History* (New Haven, CT, 1997). Paupers were disfranchised before 1828 in only New Hampshire (1792), South Carolina (1810), Maine (1819), and Massachusetts (1821), though in most seaboard states after 1828. Steinfeld, "Property and Suffrage," 335–36, 353.

58. Richard Young and Jeffrey Meiser, "Race and the Dual State in the Early American Republic," in *Race and American Political Development*, ed. Joseph Lowndes, Julie Novkov, and Dorian T. Warren (New York, 2008), 43; Smith, *Civic Ideals*, 165–232. Virginia, South Carolina, and Georgia already prohibited black voting.

59. Keyssar, *The Right to Vote*, 349–53; for Connecticut, see Pole, "Suffrage in Massachusetts," 581. The new states banning free black voting were Louisiana (1812), Indiana (1816), Mississippi (1817), Illinois (1818), Alabama (1819), and Missouri (1820–1821). Bans were later introduced in Tennessee in 1834, North Carolina in 1835, and Pennsylvania in 1838; Rhode Island reversed its ban in 1842. For an interesting discussion of these different outcomes, see Christopher Malone, *Between Freedom and Bondage: Race, Party, and Voting Rights in the Antebellum North* (New York, 2008). For the "racialization" of politics, see David Waldstreicher, "The Nationalization and Racialization

of American Politics: Before, Beneath, and Between Parties, 1790–1840," in *Contesting Democracy: Substance and Structure in American Political History, 1775–2000*, ed. Byron E. Shafer and Anthony J. Badger (Lawrence, KS, 2001), 37–63, and the literature cited therein; and for the process in the 1820s, see Donald J. Ratcliffe, "The Decline of Antislavery Politics, 1815–1840," in *Contesting Slavery: The Politics of Bondage and Freedom in the New American Nation*, ed. John Craig Hammond and Matthew Mason (Charlottesville, VA, 2011), 267–90, esp. 282–84, 302–303.

60. Keyssar, *The Right to Vote*, xvi; Rogers, ed., *Voting and the Spirit of American Democracy*, 11–12. These common assumptions have been expressed in, for example, Waldstreicher, "The Nationalization and Racialization of American Politics," 51; Howe, *What Hath God Wrought*, 231, 269, 281, 489–91; and the *Congressional Quarterly's Guide to U.S. Elections*, 1: 5. The idea of the 1820s as an age of constitutional reform owes much to the title of Merrill D. Peterson's valuable anthology, *Democracy, Liberty, and Property: The State Constitutional Conventions of the 1820's* (Indianapolis, IN, 1966), which reprints part of the debates of the Massachusetts (1820–1821), New York (1821), and Virginia (1829–1830) conventions.

61. For the rise in voter turnout at the state level since 1818, see Richard P. McCormick, "New Perspectives on Jacksonian Politics," *American Historical Review* 65 (January 1960), 288–301, esp. table 1; Ratcliffe, "Voter Turnout," 245–46; and especially Daniel Peart, "Popular Engagement with Politics in the United States during the Early 1820s" (PhD diss., University of London, 2011). For the priority of presidential politics over state issues by 1828, see Donald J. Ratcliffe, "Antimasonry and Partisanship in Greater New England, 1826–1836," *Journal of the Early Republic* 15 (Summer 1995), 199–239.

62. C. H. Rammelkamp, "The Campaign of 1824 in New York," in *Annual Report of the American Historical Association for 1904* (Washington, DC, 1905), 181–82. Methods of choosing presidential electors are tabulated in *Historical Statistics of the United States: Colonial Times to 1970* (2 vols., Washington, DC, 1975), 2: 1071. The assertion about 1824 has most recently been made in Lynn Hudson Parsons, *The Birth of Modern Politics: Andrew Jackson, John Quincy Adams, and the Election of 1828* (New York, 2009), 69. The belief that members of the Electoral College often disregarded the ticket they were elected on is expressed, for example, in Howe, *What Hath God Wrought*, 207–208, 231. In fact, between 1789 and 1820 only five (at most) out of nearly 1,500 electors ignored their implied pledges—one (but arguably four) in 1796, and one (famously) in 1820. *Congressional Quarterly's Guide to U.S. Elections*, 1: 819.

63. The shift to at-large, winner-take-all voting came from the desire to maximize the electoral weight of the state. It surely stretches things a little to claim that larger states as a class initially preferred the district system, in view of the adoption of the general ticket in presidential elections by Pennsylvania and Virginia from an early date. Cf. Zagarri, *Politics of Size*, 131–33.

64. McCormick, "New Perspectives."

65. Sydnor, *Development*, 275–89; Fletcher M. Green, *Constitutional Development in the South Atlantic States, 1776–1860: A Study in the Evolution of Democracy* (1930; repr., Clark, NJ, 2008). After 1831 about ⅓ of Virginia's adult white males were disfranchised: McCormick, *Second American Party System*, 180–81; Shade, *Democratizing the Old Dominion*, 4. Jackson's dependence on the South has been emphasized in recent times by William W. Freehling, *The Road to Disunion: Secessionists at Bay, 1776–1854* (New York, 1990); Donald J. Ratcliffe, "The Nullification Crisis, Southern Discontents, and the American Political Process," *American Nineteenth Century History* 1, no. 2 (2000), 1–30; and Howe, *What Hath God Wrought*, 279–84, 328–445.

66. Shade, *Democratizing the Old Dominion*; Fletcher M. Green, "Democracy in the Old South," *Journal of Southern History* 12 (February 1946), 3–23. Even South Carolina experienced an invigorating internal conflict in 1830–1832: James B. Stewart, "'A Great Talking and Eating Machine': Patriarchy, Mobilization and the Dynamics of Nullification in South Carolina," *Civil War History* 27 (September 1981), 197–220. North Carolina and Maryland threw open their gubernatorial elections to popular voting in 1835 and 1837, respectively.

67. John Ashworth, *"Agrarians" and "Aristocrats": Party Political Ideology in the United States, 1837–1846* (London, 1983); Keyssar, *The Right to Vote*, 29. An important aspect of this later spell of con-

stitutional reform was the opening of more offices to popular election: for example, whereas in 1833 judges were elected in only 5 of 25 states, the practice had extended by 1844 to 12 of 29 states and by 1853 to 25 of 31. Tax qualifications for voting were abandoned in Mississippi in 1832, Tennessee in 1834, New Jersey in 1844, Connecticut in 1844–1845, Louisiana in 1845, and Ohio in 1850–1851. They were retained in Pennsylvania (1838), New Hampshire, and Massachusetts (1851). Massachusetts did not recognize universal manhood suffrage constitutionally until 1891.

68. Pole, "Suffrage in New Jersey," 39; Howe, *What Hath God Wrought*, 599–603. For debates after 1820 over the political status of propertyless wage earners, and the distinction between the self-supporting and the dependent, see Steinfeld, "Property and Suffrage," 353–74.

69. Alexis De Tocqueville, *Democracy in America*, 2 vols. (1835, 1840), many editions, vol. 2, Book 2, chapter 3.

DONALD RATCLIFFE was a professor of United States History at the University of Durham and held an instructor position at Oxford. He is currently chair of the Hook Norton Local History Group. His most recent book, *The One-Party Presidential Contest: Adams, Jackson, and 1824's Five-Horse Race*, has been awarded the Lasky Prize for the best book on American political history.

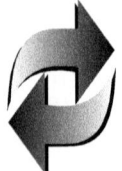

EXPLORING THE ISSUE

Were Jackson's Anti-Politics and Nationalism Beneficial for Increased Democratic Participation?

Critical Thinking and Reflection

1. During the Jacksonian Era, what did it look like to democratically participate? Who got to democratically participate?
2. Compare and contrast Ratcliffe and Schake's understanding of democratic participation and the role of Andrew Jackson in the civic life of the people.
3. Is a strong public authority in politics a sign of civic participation or civic chaos?
4. What was the cause(s) of an increase in civic participation during Andrew Jackson's presidency?
5. What causes a rise in nationalism and what is the goal of nationalism? Is nationalism always warranted?

Is There Common Ground?

In some ways, these two authors argue something similar. Ratcliffe suggests Jackson's common man reputation is overstated, just as Schake suggests those calling Trump undemocratic are overstating the situation because of the existing political climate. President Trump and President Jackson represent men of their times, responding to the anguish living beneath the superficial political surface. The elections of both men represent referendums of the non-elite, and both men were unquestionably elected based on their popularity for things other than pure politics.

Ratcliffe and Schake understand the symbolic significance of Andrew Jackson. It is also clear to both writers that America was experiencing dramatic shifts in all realms—social, political, economic, and geographic—at the time of Jackson's presidency. The voice of the people was getting louder whether we can credit this to Jackson or not. American identity was shifting, and Jackson was at the center of this shift.

Given the context of the time in which Jackson was leading the country, both authors would likely acknowledge the complex, perhaps divisive, nature of Jackson. Where Ratcliffe points to his influence on the two-party system, Schake acknowledges his influence on public debate, but both authors acknowledge the impact of Jackson. Where the two would find themselves in disagreement is in the extent to which Jackson benefited American civic life. Jackson is a complex historical figure of intrigue to many. These authors are no exception as they try to make sense of this strong-willed, multifaceted man.

Additional Resources

Adams, S. P. (Ed.). (2013). *A companion to the era of Andrew Jackson*. Chichester: John Wiley & Sons.

Bimes, T., & Mulroy, Q. (2004). The rise and decline of presidential populism. *Studies in American Political Development, 18*(2), 136–159.

Wilentz, S. (2007). *Andrew Jackson: The American Presidents Series: The 7th President, 1829–1837*. Macmillan.

Internet References . . .

Andrew Jackson: Impact and Legacy

https://millercenter.org/president/jackson/impact-and-legacy

Hermitage: Home of the People's President

https://thehermitage.com/learn/andrew-jackson/

Library of Congress: Andrew Jackson Papers

https://www.loc.gov/collections/andrew-jackson-papers/about-this-collection/

The Gilder Lehrman Institute of American History

https://www.gilderlehrman.org/site-search?keys=Andrew+Jackson

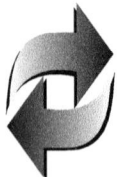

Unit 3

UNIT

Antebellum America

Pressures and trends that began building in the early years of the American nation continued to gather momentum until conflict was almost inevitable. The institution of slavery persisted in 15 states, and population growth and territorial expansion brought the country into conflict with other nations under the banner of "Manifest Destiny."

The twin beliefs in democracy and progress produced an era of reform to address a variety of challenges that confronted a rapidly changing society. A dedicated group of activists, motivated by both intellectual and religious principle, determined that the ideals of human rights and democratic participation that guided the founding of the nation had been applied only to selected segments of the population and set out to eliminate social evils where they found them.

How do we distinguish between a terrorist and a freedom fighter? When do we label an action imperialistic or nationalistic? What are the criteria for determining when social justice activists become members of a meddling mob? Implicit and at times explicit are questions that emerge from the spirited debates presented by the authors of the documents in this unit. The young American nation began to wrestle with a deeper understanding of herself and her citizens while elected and would be leaders continued to make choices that would establish an American presence in global affairs for the foreseeable future. As the political and economic policies and practices of the United States were asserted more frequently on the international stage, we see the perspicuous emergence of the notion of American Exceptionalism as evidenced through the vast land acquisitions and cultural appropriations that occurred with such events and edicts as the Louisiana Purchase, the War of 1812, and the Monroe Doctrine.

Debated throughout this unit are the risks and rewards of the free exercise of US imperialism that saw the size of the nation double in a matter of decades (Ramón Eduardo Ruiz and Norman A. Graebner, Manifest Destiny and the Mexican American War). In the midst of what appeared to be a meteoric expansion of American ascendency were the pernicious cracks in the very ideals that would serve as the foundation for the so-called American Exceptionalism. Access to equality of opportunities for human rights, citizenship, education, and well-being are debated by James N. Gilbert, Scott John Hammond, Mary Kelly, Lucia McMahon, Laura A. Schmidt, and John J. Rumbarger. Inherent in these debates are the cause and effect triggers that lure us into believing in the linear repetitive phenomenological interpretation of history. Yet upon closer examination we are able to see through the writings of the authors selected for this unit's topics of debate that there is not so much a linearity of cause and effect relationships among the issues presented but perhaps multiple branches, some twisting others turning back onto themselves. It is through this closer examination of the nuances of the issues presented that we begin to see emerge the milieu of political, economic, religious, social, intellectual, and area (PERSIA) themes that provide a fascinating juxtaposition of traditional positivist historic cause and effect (linear-repetitive) versus a nontraditional post-positivist correlation and choice (multi-directional-rhyming) interpretation of clashing views in United States history.

ISSUE

Selected, Edited, and with Issue Framing Material by:
Kevin R. Magill and Tony L. Talbert, *Baylor University*

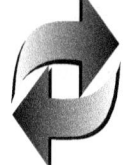

Did Improved Educational Opportunities for Women in the New Nation Significantly Expand Their Participation in Antebellum Society?

YES: Mary Kelley, from "Learning to Stand and Speak: Women, Education, and Public Life in America's Republic," University of North Carolina Press (2006)

NO: Lucia McMahon, from "Between Cupid and Minerva" and "Education, Equality, or Difference," Cornell University Press (2012)

Learning Outcomes
After reading this issue, you will be able to: • Explain the role of social and cultural capital in Antebellum society. • Compare and contrast feminine public and private spheres. • Evaluate the benefit or cost to women in pursuing education and an expanded role in society. • Draw connections and comparisons of the public life of women in Antebellum and modern society. • Evaluate the effect of prescriptive literature on gender performance.

ISSUE SUMMARY

YES: Mary Kelley describes how expanding educational opportunities encouraged women to redefine themselves by opening doors to careers beyond the domestic sphere, economic self-support, and public participation in civil society that transformed their understanding of the rights of citizenship in the post-revolutionary and antebellum United States.

NO: Lucia McMahon concludes that the unprecedented access to education afforded women in the early national period fostered recognition of women's intellectual capacity, but she argues that most educated women confronted a limited range of opportunities in a society that remained largely committed to a social and political order rooted in notions of sexual difference and male hierarchy.

Issue Framing with H. Scottie Johnson, Ph.D

If we were to document the histories of our own families with a focus on the women in our lineage, it is likely that the core of the historical narrative would remain the same across time. This picture was one of women as domestics whose role is to care for the family. However, we are at an exciting historical moment. Perhaps our own mothers and grandmother's stories have demonstrated shifts in the ways we understand woman's historical roles. Similarly, we have seen shifts new frameworks by which can understand women, gender, and agency. If we take a deeper historical look into the lives of the women we are likely to discover more than docile housewives.

Until the late 1960s, the serious student of American women's history could store all the important scholarly studies of women on one shelf of a bookcase. These works typically fell into two categories: broad surveys based upon the limited sources available, such as Eleanor Flexner's *Century of Struggle: The Woman's Rights Movement in the United States* (Harvard University Press, 1959) and Andrew Sinclair's *The Better Half: The Emancipation of the American Woman* (Harper & Row, 1965); and "great women" biographies, studies of pioneering women in the fields of abolitionism, education, and the suffrage movement. The official literature on American women's history for the majority of time has remained passive (Flexner, 1959 & Sinclair, 1965) or only highlighting particular, exceptional women. Women's studies were forever changed in the 1960s. In 1963, journalist Betty Friedan published *The Feminine Mystique*, a stinging indictment of sex inequality in the United States in which she characterized the traditional domestic sphere for women as "a comfortable concentration camp" that infantilized its female inhabitants. Friedan helped brake the normalized historiography of American women. However, what remained absent from the historical discourse was the agency of the everyday woman. Keber (1988) notes that the women writing in the wake of Friedan "argued that American women's history had to be understood not only by way of events but through a prism of ideology as well" (p.11). When we look at the history of American women through a prism of ideology, a richer story emerges; one that allows us to consider if improved educational opportunities for women in the new nation significantly expanded their participation in Antebellum society.

Therefore, in the 1960's and 1970's, the waves of feminist activism carried historical study into territories that had largely been ignored. Prior to this, the field of historical study, like society at large, had almost exclusively focused on the work of men. The very arenas where women were denied participation were practically the only topics considered worthy of serious historical investigation. When women had appeared in the historical narrative, it was almost always in terms of their binary relationship to men. Other pioneers such as Mabel Newcomer, Janice Law Trecker, and Barbara Miller Solomon uncovered the lives of women who had been erased and forgotten in history. They searched for glimpses of women in unexpected, nontraditional and indirect ways, expanding the boundaries of historical sources as well as creating new frameworks for understanding women's experiences.

However, much of the first work focused on White women while presenting their experiences as indicative of those of the rest of their gender. This generation of women's history filled in gaps to the dominant narrative and amplified some silenced voices, but it did not challenge the economic, racial or social structures of what was valued as topics of mainstream history. In the field of educational history, most attention was paid to the hard-won progress women made in establishing their right to an education and acknowledgement of their intellectual abilities. Milestones were celebrated such as the founding of the exclusive women's seminaries, academies, and colleges such as Vassar and Smith. Meanwhile, stories that did not fit into the framework of achievement seemed not to be heard amidst the celebration of great women. The strongest voices in the past have louder echoes through time, and, as such, historical study can replicate the same inequalities it is trying to investigate.

However as the field progressed, women's history has expanded to include more perspectives. The lives of "ordinary" women, distant from seats of power, from a myriad of regions, classes, races and experiences have now been legitimized as holding a valid place in the historical narrative. Historians such as Gilda Lerner, Linda Kerber, and Laurel Thatcher Ulrich examined the past from the bottom up, highlighting commonplace women such as midwives, farmers, nurses, and servants. In pursuing this approach of uncovering the history of women, Lerner (1982) notes the value of asking appropriate questions for historical analysis – questions that consider the work of women reaching beyond the confines of a male-centric interpretation. Women become a hermeneutic for interpreting the past.

Lerner suggested that scholars of women's history should (1) search for women whose experiences deserve to be well known; (2) identify women associated with topics and issues deemed important to the American mainstream; (3) test familiar narratives and revise generalizations when they appear to be wrong; and (4) understand gender as a social construct, and rewrite and develop new frameworks and concepts to understand women's history. Joan Scott's work similarly helped create theories of the role gender plays in forming hierarchies and positions of power. Specifically, in the field of women's education, literature drew attention to who was included or excluded from education, what institutions were founded, succeeded, failed or were never built and, most importantly, why and for what purpose. This shift in perspective is critical to understanding the experiences of a broader range of women, not just a few.

Frameworks for analyzing women's historical essence now rejected the traditional binary view of gender and power. Informed by the ideas of Judith Butler and Joan Scott, gender is now understood as something performed, which shifts based on the needs of a society. The subjectivity and invalidity of essential definitions of gender and patriarchy can be observed in the historic variation with which they manifest. Women are not all the same, their goals and definitions differ and their intersectionality with race and class position them in various ways in respect to voice and agency. These examinations of race, and class have troubled expansionist and progressive narration of women's opportunities by investigating the absences and exclusions within women's education. From this perspective, the story is not simply one of women gaining power in relation to men, but troubling the reality that White middle- and upper-class women gained power while ignoring or denying the oppression of other races and other classes of women. As Michel Foucault suggests, clear binaries of oppressed and oppressor do not always exist, as is the case when we examine the history of women. Historians taking this approach have opened up new opportunities for recognition, disruption, and agency forever transforming the master narrative.

In this issue, historians Mary Kelley and Lucia McMahon use these more nuanced frameworks to examine the causes and effects of the expanding opportunities for female education in post-revolutionary and Antebellum American society. Utilizing prescriptive works and cautionary tales from male and female authors, McMahon notes that educational curriculum for women was restricted and its main function was to "improve" women for their role as wives and mothers. Education became a vehicle for linking and limiting women's contribution by maintaining the boundaries of womanhood while minimizing their intellectual, rational or civic participation. Female academies were quick to reassure young women's parents that their educational model would reinforce rather than challenge traditional roles and duties.

Mary Kelly suggests that by the 1850s, women were understood to be the intellectual equals to men. Educated women gained leadership skills for activities outside their households by experiencing a course of study that, in many cases, matched their male colleagues. Women contributed to the national discourse on religious, political, sexual and racial matters. Kelley writes that, acceptance of traditional gender models became in and of themselves a form of agency for women; for how could women, left in their "natural" state, engage in republican values or teach them to their children? Kelley argues that the feminine sphere was not isolated, nor simply a foil to the state, but that it played a critical civic role. To her, the education of women is an indicator of the progress of a civilization. Importantly, no educational system could completely control what was learned or how that learning was applied and enacted. Just as expansion of White men's suffrage spread past the elitist classical republican vision of many of the founding fathers, so too did ideas about women's power and role extend past a servile vision of true womanhood. In their homes, schools, salons, voluntary associations, and benevolence societies, most women remained part of what society understood to be acceptable feminine roles, but women also created their own roles, for their own purposes. These women slowly expanded rather than shattered traditional spheres of influence. Lucia McMahon suggests that the increased educational opportunities for women were largely designed to help them better serve men, rather than to provide increased opportunity for women. McMahon argues most supporters for the improved educational opportunities still demanded male hierarchy, and, as a result, American women did not achieve substantial equality or emancipation. For McMahon, women remained the victims of society's continued ambivalence.

It is from this perspective that we examine the impact of education on the status of women during a moment when common school education expanded throughout the United States. At this time, middle-class families began to understand the need for more advanced training for their daughters. However, many disagreed on what the curriculum would look like. Some felt the training should increase moral influence in society and women's performance in the domestic sphere. Others felt Women needed to be taught a wider range of social roles. Women were certainly limited to certain jobs, however there is no doubt that the common school movement helped to open a significant number of new professional opportunities for women, particularly as teachers. We therefore ask, to what extent did improved educational opportunities for women in the Antebellum period improve their status in the public sphere?

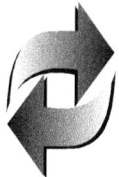

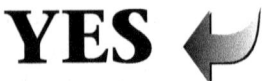

Mary Kelley

Learning to Stand and Speak: Women, Education, and Public Life in America's Republic

In an essay that appeared in the *School Gazette*, which students published at Hartford Female Seminary in the 1820s, one student took stock of the aspirations generated in becoming a learned woman and of the risks in claiming that mantle in post-Revolutionary and antebellum America. The author, who chose to remain anonymous, asked her classmates to consider an "Enigma." She introduces herself as "both the feminine and neuter gender." There are those who disdain her as a deviant, as "a good for nothing weed growing out of doors." Uneasy in her presence, they "would be glad to be rid of me." But she is not so easily dismissed and instead is always present in the hours devoted to schooling in the seminary's Study Hall. In those hours and in that setting, she reckons, "my company is welcome to all." Students reading their classmate's "Enigma" might have looked around the Study Hall to try to identify the author. Was she the current editor? Or was she instead one of the other contributors to the *Gazette*? Then they might have turned to an equally important project—deciphering the code and solving the riddle. Did the author's subject symbolize the promise of an advanced education for women? Did that education challenge conventional gender relations? Still playful and still elusive, the anonymous author might have answered both of these questions in the affirmative, telling her classmates that this was the "Enigma."

The student who calculated the potential benefits and costs was an actor in one of the most profound changes in gender relations in the course of the nation's history—the movement of women into public life. In asking how and why post-Revolutionary and antebellum women shaped their lives anew, *Learning to Stand and Speak* measures the significance of this transformation in individual and social identities. As the subtitle, *Women, Education, and Public Life*, suggests, it looks to the role schooling at female academies and seminaries played in mediating this process. In recasting women's subjectivity and the felt reality of their collective experience, that education was decisive. Employing the benefits of their schooling, women redefined themselves and their relationship to civil society. As educators, as writers, as editors, and as reformers, they entered the "public sphere," or the social space situated between the institutions of the family and the nation-state. The large majority of the women who claimed these careers and who led the movement of women into the world beyond their households were schooled at these institutions.

Consider Harriet Beecher Stowe. Stowe's parents, Lyman and Roxana Foote Beecher, had relatively little economic capital. The minister of the Congregational church at Litchfield, Connecticut, Lyman relied upon his parishioners for a modest salary, which included a yearly supply of firewood. But what Lyman and Roxana did command had a telling salience. The descendants of families who had migrated to New England in the seventeenth century, both had a large network of social connections. The skillful deployment of this form of capital accomplished its purpose for the Yale-trained minister, who was called from an isolated parsonage in East Hampton, Long Island, to Litchfield's prestigious Congregational church in 1810. Now at the center of a powerful network, Lyman and Roxana claimed the privileges of families long accustomed to leadership in their communities. Lyman substituted social capital for the economic resources typically needed to educate his daughter, Harriet, who was born the year after the family had moved to Connecticut. In return for pastoral services at Litchfield Female Academy, he was able to barter the costs of her education at one of the nation's most prominent academies. Harriet's schooling did not end at Litchfield. Having attended Sarah

From EMPIRE OF REASON: THE MAKING OF LEARNED WOMEN IN AMERICA'S REPUBLIC by Mary Kelley. Published for the Omohundro Institute of Early American History and Culture. Copyright ©2006 by the University of North Carolina Press. Used by permission of the publisher. www.uncpress.unc.edu

Pierce's Academy for the four years between 1819 and 1824, Harriet was then sent to Hartford Female Seminary, which her sister, Catharine, had founded in 1821.

Educated at institutions that took the lead in providing a course of study that matched that of male colleges, Stowe was schooled in the competencies post-Revolutionary and antebellum Americans identified as the basis for cultural capital. Pierce and her nephew John Brace provided an education that certified Stowe's command of the canon of Western literature Alexis de Tocqueville identified as necessary for "remain[ing] civilized or to becom[ing] so." Familiarity with this canon was central to Stowe's education, both formal and informal. Well before she was sent to Litchfield Female Academy, Stowe had received from her family a cultural inheritance that predisposed her to books and ideas. She took to the printed page from the moment she was able to make meaning of the words and read widely in history, fiction, and poetry. As the child of a minister enthralled with his Calvinist predecessors, Cotton Mather's *Magnalia Christi Americana* was an obvious choice. Harriet leavened Mather's millennial visions with the novels of Scott and the poetry of Byron. The education did not stop there. Roxana and her sister, the beloved Harriet Foote, with whom the younger Harriet spent a year after her mother's death, disciplined her in the manners and bearing displayed by members of post-Revolutionary America's elite and aspiring middling classes. Six decades later, Stowe would inscribe this training on the pages of *My Wife and I* and its sequel, *We and Our Neighbors*, two novels that doubled as conduct manuals for the middling classes.

Was Stowe representative? No more nor less than other women schooled at a female academy or seminary. Some had more economic capital at their disposal. Others had less opportunity than Stowe to acquire cultural capital before they began their education at one of these schools. Still others came from families well supplied with both social and economic capital. However, if one compares them with other women of their generation, these differences matter relatively little. Two factors set these women apart, first, their parents' access to resources needed for the accumulation of capital in one or more of its forms and, second, their decision to commit that capital to the education of daughters.

Although there were a host of variables that shaped the decisions individual families made, certain patterns can be discerned. The convergence of a market revolution fueled by innovations in transportation and communication, capital accumulation, and increasing shortages in available land transformed the lives of all Americans. Nowhere was the impact more profound than in rural America, where 80 percent of the nation's population resided between the American Revolution and the Civil War. Once able to provide sons with farms and daughters with dowries, parents found it increasingly difficult to sustain these traditions. Those who looked to education as an alternative endowment made the same commitment as Lyman and Roxana Beecher, contributing their economic, social, and cultural capital to the education of children. Some sons and daughters took their schooling at local academies that instructed men and women together. Others, whose families invested more of their capital in education, attended male colleges or female academies and seminaries. Some who attended these schools returned to their local communities. Many more populated the two migrations that marked these decades, one from East to West and the other from countryside to town or city.

Perhaps the most important article in the baggage these generations took with them, an advanced education opened the door to economic self-support. Men entered traditional professions as lawyers, doctors, and ministers or market-oriented careers as merchants, bankers, retailers, and manufacturers. Women, with these possibilities closed to them, took advantage of newly emerging opportunities to be writers and editors. An unprecedented number also embarked on careers as teachers. Many women pursued these opportunities simultaneously. Stowe's sister, Catharine Beecher, is emblematic in this regard. Not only did she establish three female seminaries, but she also published influential volumes on moral philosophy, physical health, and domestic economy. Compared with other women who attended a female academy or seminary, Stowe ranked as perhaps the most influential in the making of public opinion. But this difference matters not at all if compared with the influence wielded by these women as a whole. Thousands of women who had access to sufficient resources and who were educated at one of these schools followed the same trajectory as Stowe, entering civil society and taking its practice and discourse in an unprecedented direction.

Civil Society

... To the degree that this project is a study of social roles and institutions, it challenges the familiar model that divides the nineteenth century into private and public, feminine and masculine, household and marketplace. Teachers and students at female academies and seminaries simultaneously deployed and dismantled these binaries as they linked them to the reciprocal rights and obligations of citizenship inscribed in the nation's Constitution.

Women boldly entered civil society beginning in the 1790s and in increasingly large numbers in later decades. Sarah Josepha Hale, editor of the *Lady's Book* (later, *Godey's Lady's Book*), spoke to the importance of the institutional and discursive spaces in which they exercised influence. In the aptly titled "Conversazione," which she published in January 1837, Hale called the public broadly conceived "civil society." In its most inclusive form, antebellum Americans defined civil society as a national public in which citizens were secured in basic freedoms before the law. Embodied in the Constitution's Bill of Rights, these freedoms included speech, press, and assembly. Hale and her contemporaries also invested civil society with a more specific meaning, marking it as a public inhabited by private persons. In addition, they set the boundaries of this public, excluding the operations of the market economy from its domain. If the post-Revolutionary compromise denied women access to participation in the public sphere of organized politics, it left civil society fully open as a public sphere in which first white and then black women were able to flourish as never before. Instead of restricting them to the household, the Republic's establishment facilitated the entry of women into this rapidly expanding social space.

Post-Revolutionary and antebellum European Americans constituted civil society at a series of sites, each of which emerged in a specific historical context. Free African Americans in the North and to a lesser extent in the South acted in parallel settings, challenging discriminatory premises and practices of European Americans. Despite differences in temporal identity and emphasis, European and African American sites were all linked in a common understanding of civil society as composed of private citizens meeting together. These discursive and institutional spaces emerged in the middle of the eighteenth century as institutions of sociability where the propertied gathered for conversation; they were transformed in the post-Revolutionary decades into entities more explicitly engaged in the making of public opinion; and they came to the fore yet again in the 1830s in the voluntary associations Tocqueville identified as the key medium for articulation of the citizenry's concern with cultural uplift and moral reform. From the post-Revolutionary academies to the antebellum seminaries, students prepared themselves for engagement in civil society. Most notably, they fashioned a subjectivity in which rights and obligations of citizenship were fundamental to their sense of self.

Elite white women took their places at tea tables and salons, institutions of sociability that along with male clubs, taverns, and coffeehouses were dedicated to making public opinion. The sociability the eighteenth-century elite practiced not only separated European Americans from multiple others but also marked them as privileged relative to their counterparts in the lower ranks. Post-Revolutionary and antebellum European Americans established a host of institutions, ranging from organizations dedicated to benevolence to movements for social reform—including white women's rights and black people's emancipation—to institutions variously called literary societies, reading circles, and mutual improvement associations. Described by Tocqueville as "intellectual and moral" in their orientation, these voluntary associations were a powerful resource in the making of public opinion. Like their eighteenth-century predecessors, antebellum European Americans who engaged in organized benevolence demarcated the elite and the emerging "middling classes" from the multiple others whom they defined as "uncivilized" objects of reform. European Americans and African Americans enlisted in movements calling for the rights of white women and the end of slavery took the opposite tack. In contrast to those who insisted upon conformity to the prevailing order, they protested sexual and racial discrimination.

In addition to editing *Godey's Lady's Book*, Hale published *Woman's Record; or, Sketches of All Distinguished Women, from "the Beginning" till A.D.* 1850, a compilation of sixteen hundred individual biographies. In a volume that spanned the centuries from the birth of Christ to 1850, she devoted more than a third of the pages to women still living. Herself one of the nation's powerful makers of public opinion, Hale introduced readers to post-Revolutionary and antebellum America's most visible contributors to civil society. Although *Woman's Record* purported to sketch all women who had distinguished themselves in voluntary associations, it celebrated elite and middle-class Protestants with whom Hale shared social status and religious inclinations. African American and white working-class women were excluded, although these women were also prominent in associational life. The approaches taken by all these women illustrate the importance of class and race in defining an individual's engagement in organized benevolence, social reform, and associations devoted to reading and writing. In contrast to their elite and middle-class counterparts, white working-class women concentrated their energies on mutual aid societies. Free African American women in the North were likely to link mutual aid not only with benevolence but also with self-improvement and social reform. Free women of color in Savannah, Georgia, began to organize church-based benevolent societies in the 1830s. In the same decade, free African American women in the North organized literary societies. Doubling as acts of resistance, the collective acts of interpretation they produced in these societies took as their subjects slavery and racial prejudice, both of which were excoriated in essays, stories, and poems that members published in antislavery newspapers.

Hale also introduced readers of *Woman's Record* to founders of female academies and seminaries, whom she celebrated as exemplars. Columns and articles in *Godey's Lady's Book*, which Hale edited for four decades, praised their counterparts, the teachers in the nation's common schools. In the decades before the Civil War, the proportion of women in the classroom was higher in urban than in rural America. By 1860, women constituted between 65 and 80 percent of the teachers in the towns and cities of every region. In rural America, where 80 percent of the population lived, the proportions of women teaching varied considerably. In New England, fully 84 percent of the region's rural teachers were female. The proportions were lower in the Middle Atlantic and in the South, 59 percent and 36 percent, respectively. In Michigan and Minnesota, 86 percent of the teachers were women. In the other seven states of the Middle West, the proportion was a significantly lower 58 percent. Regional differences aside, the trend was unmistakably clear: America's classrooms were rapidly becoming a woman's domain. The women who embarked on careers as teachers were largely responsible for the rapid increase in literacy between the American Revolution and the Civil War. The students whom they taught entered a world of print that enlarged the horizon of a reader's imagination and encouraged a reflective consciousness, both of which were crucial to participation in civil society. Conversely, readers shaped that world, not only by advancing the circulation of print but also by claiming careers as writers and editors.

Woman's Record included these writers and editors whom Hale presented as an increasingly influential presence in the literary marketplace. In terms of their social and cultural importance, she was right. Between the American Revolution and the Civil War, women in the North and the South emerged as leaders in the nation's lively trade in texts. The number of genres in which they wrote expanded rapidly, as did the role they took in shaping a distinctively American literature. In the novels, histories, poems, and biographies they published and in the magazines they edited, these women contributed to national discourses on religious doctrine and denominationalism, on politics and political parties, on women and domesticity, and on the nation and its potential as the world's redeemer. By the 1840s and the 1850s, the most successful of these writers and editors could expect to make a livelihood with their pen.

Remaining Civilized or Becoming So

Like Hale's "Conversazione," which appeared three years before the publication of *Democracy in America* in 1840, Tocqueville's foundational text in American exceptionalism focused on voluntary associations that were designed to cultivate an individual's intellectual and moral potential. Indeed, these organizations stood at the center of the civil society Tocqueville described in the second volume of his treatise. In contrast to associations devoted to commerce and politics, Tocqueville told readers, voluntary associations had received relatively little consideration. And yet for him, as for Hale, they were as critical, indeed "perhaps more so," to the success of the political democracy constituted by antebellum white males. Grounded in networks of social interaction, these associations were, according to Tocqueville, the key to "remain[ing] civilized or to becom[ing] so."

In ascribing this double purpose to voluntary societies, Tocqueville went to the crux of antebellum associational life. Like those who had led the institutions of sociability that preceded them, members of voluntary organizations aligned themselves with social and cultural values they insisted were required for "remain[ing]" a "civilized" people. In women's literary societies, reading circles, and mutual improvement associations, members engaged the culturally privileged knowledge European Americans had defined as the possession of "civilized" peoples. British American women established the precedent. Gathering in reading circles a decade before the American Revolution and dedicating themselves to reading and writing, they pursued history, biography, poetry, and fiction. Through conversation and presentation of essays, they disciplined their minds and sharpened their analytical faculties. Not least, they applied the knowledge they had garnered to social and political issues. In all, they laid the basis for women's claim to the public voice and intellectual authority necessary for the making of public opinion. Students at female academies and seminaries engaged in the same critical thought and cultural production in literary societies, which were designed to intersect with and serve as a supplement to classroom instruction. These institutions were a crucial resource as students crafted subjectivities inflected by the advanced education they were learning to command. Women whose schooling had been completed extended their education in the hundreds of organizations dedicated to reading and writing they founded in villages, towns, and cities in the nation. In these settings, as in literary societies at female academies and seminaries, women addressed the larger meanings of the knowledge they were pursuing, practiced the art of persuasive self-presentation, and instructed themselves in the values and vocabularies of civil society.

Women in organized benevolence embarked on the project that Tocqueville had considered as critical as remaining "civilized"—schooling others in becoming "civilized," which they identified as the basis for citizenship. Those whom they marked as the other, or the yet-to-be elevated intellectually and morally, were expected to yield their principles to the values of reformers who claimed the right to define what it meant to be "civilized." That peoples as diverse as immigrant Catholics and native Americans resisted what we now label "cultural imperialism" should surprise no one. Others, if they suspected the motives of those who sought to impose their values, nonetheless welcomed the aid provided by evangelical Protestants, who rallied their communities on behalf of support for the indigent, education for the less privileged, aid for the widowed, and homes for the orphaned. Social reformers in the North, some evangelical, some not, took on the much more controversial issues of white women's rights and black people's emancipation.

The assemblage of associations that so impressed Hale and Tocqueville has long fascinated scholars investigating the foundations of political democracy in the nineteenth and twentieth centuries. Leading neo-Tocquevillean Robert Putnam has argued that voluntary associations are a liberal society's linchpin in "making democracy work." Envisioned as socializing agents in the nation's communities, these associations reflect and reinforce a public-spiritedness akin to the republican virtue celebrated by the post-Revolutionary elite. In creating and consolidating shared values, these organizations also serve as a counterweight to the divisiveness of antebellum America's conventional politics. However, nineteenth-century voluntary associations also played an opposite role in relation to consensus, bringing individuals together to interrogate the dominant social and political order. Whether they defended or called into question dominant values, the thousands of women who participated in voluntary associations forged lives at the intersection of newly available educational opportunities and engagement with civil society in local, regional, and national communities.

If the neo-Tocquevillean model sees voluntary associations as providing support for the masculine state, the model presented here has as its center a civil society in which women and men engaged in individual action and critical thought. In its female voluntary associations, civil society was constructed as the feminine other of the masculine state. Of course, feminist scholars, and I include myself here, have been taught to beware of binary oppositions. I am introducing this opposition, however, not as an exclusive or limiting binary, but as one among others. The household has been proposed as the binary opposite of the state, for example, and its counterpart domesticity as the feminine other to the masculine state. Introducing the concept of civil society as an additional complement to the state opens more possibilities. It also helps us to see that exclusion from one sphere of action does not necessarily imply confinement to another. The presence of women in the public sphere of civil society dismantles the false binary that identifies women exclusively with the household, even as it calls into question the symbiotic relationship between this institutional and discursive space and the masculine state. Not all women constituted this site any more than all men constituted the state. That certain women came to play leading roles in this public sphere and to shape the course it took in post-Revolutionary and antebellum America highlights the significance of education as the key both to women's entering civil society and to the influence they exercised as makers of public opinion. . . .

In the letter in which Lucy Stone recalled that she and Antoinette Brown Blackwell had "learned to stand and speak" as members of literary societies, she herself was speaking from the perspective of more than five decades of activism on behalf of women's rights. Stone, one of the movement's most influential leaders and a graduate of Mount Holyoke Seminary, understood the transformative potential of these societies and the schools that housed them. In cultivating reasoning and rhetorical faculties, modeling persuasive self-presentation, and disciplining the mind, literary societies reinforced the formal instruction provided in the classrooms of female academies and seminaries. We can be certain that Antoinette Brown Blackwell agreed with her friend. In an exchange of letters some forty years earlier, she told Stone about the impact of one such society. In the winter of 1847, the fifty members, including Brown, had organized themselves in typical fashion. In a weekly rotation, six submitted compositions for all to read and then led the debate at the meeting. "*All take a deep* interest in the exercises," Brown declared. Brown herself had "never before improved so rapidly in my life in the use of the tongue." The experience led her to repeat the claim that champion of female education Judith Sargent Murray had made a half-century earlier. With no little confidence, Brown predicted, "There is soon to be a new era in womans history." In 1798, when Murray told the *Gleaner*'s readers that women who were attending the newly emerging female academies would inaugurate "a new era in female history," she looked forward to an exponential increase in women's influence in civil society. By the 1850s, women had transformed the face of civil society, and Brown was ready to extend that influence to suffrage.

The subjectivities of thousands of women were shaped by their experience as students at a female academy or seminary. Educated at institutions created exclusively for women, they attended schools with a clearly articulated mission, a faculty that offered inspiring role models, and a curriculum that introduced them to female exemplars. In educational practices ranging from classroom instruction to literary societies to reading protocols to emulation of intellectually accomplished women, students were schooled in a curriculum that matched the course of study at male colleges. Embracing the convictions of principals and teachers who held that an improved mind was a woman's greatest treasure, they committed themselves to earning the mantle of learned women.

. . . Contributors to this discourse made advanced education integral to the role they projected for women in civil society. From the Judith Sargent Murrays to the Antoinette Brown Blackwells, post-Revolutionary and antebellum women asked themselves what it meant to be a learned woman. Initially, there were those who saw little reason for a female education that went beyond reading, writing, and ciphering. Ranking women as inferior to men in matters of the mind, they doubted that a woman could be truly learned. With the establishment of female academies in the 1780s, the issue of women's intellectual potential was debated for the next three decades. In catalogs, circulars, and plans of study that highlighted schooling in reason as a primary objective, educators asserted that women were fully able to engage in critical thinking and cultural production. They also called on the women who were attending these schools to "vindicate the equality of female intellect," as Sarah Pierce charged her students in 1818. Beginning in the 1820s, the introduction of a curriculum as rigorous as that in male colleges and the performance of students at hundreds of female academies and seminaries settled the question. There were exceptions, of course. But, in most circles, women were now regarded as the intellectual equals of men.

A second and related issue generated a debate that has yet to be fully resolved. More than two centuries ago, newly independent Americans asked themselves: What should a woman do with her learning? In linking the right to an advanced education to the fulfillment of gendered social and political obligations, post-Revolutionary Americans forged an enduring compromise. Instead of claiming that women had the right to pursue knowledge for individual ends, those who were constituting gendered republicanism debated the boundaries of the domain within which women ought to meet obligations to the larger social good. Those who subscribed to the more conservative model insisted that they deploy their influence only as wives and mothers. Others pressed those boundaries. Although they acknowledged that responsibilities to one's family remained primary, they asked that women take the lead in instructing their nation in republican virtue. Even as women claimed the moral authority sanctioning their roles in the household and in the larger society and as the impact of their presence and power became increasingly visible in the latter domain, most chose not to challenge a social and political system that still rendered them subordinate to men. Instead, they proclaimed their loyalty to deference, one of the fundamental principles in systems of gender relations in which women are not accorded the same standing as men. "Woman," as Catharine Beecher declared in *Suggestions respecting Improvements in Education, Presented to the Trustees of the Hartford Female Seminary* in 1829, was "bound to 'honor and obey' those on whom she depends for protection and support." Claims to deference such as Beecher's masked women's newly acquired agency with the rhetoric of subordination. Behind this rhetoric existed a larger social reality in which thousands of women were steadily enlarging upon the power they wielded in civil society. By the middle of the 1850s, Beecher, who was founding her third and final seminary, could proclaim confidently that women had the mandate to "civilize the world." Mandate or not, women who had focused initially on their local communities were now claiming responsibility for schooling native American, South Asian, and Eastern European peoples in the tenets of republican virtue and its corollary, American exceptionalism.

The women who attended a female academy or seminary were white, and whatever their status in terms of property or income they had access to one or more forms of economic, social, and cultural capital. As its title indicates, *Notable American Women* recovers women who are "notable" in terms of social, intellectual, political, and cultural leadership. The three volumes of entries show that the large majority of the leaders of post-Revolutionary and antebellum America's organized benevolence and social reform attended a female academy or seminary. The same can be said for the educational reformers, who not only attended women's schools but also became founders and teachers. The correlation between being educated at a female academy or seminary and becoming a member of the nation's community of letters is equally strong for the writers and editors who came to maturity between 1790 and 1860. The combined privileges of skin color, social standing, and advanced education provided these women with an unparalleled opportunity to set the terms of women's engagement with public life. In elaborating an increasingly expansive gendered republicanism and in calling women to the role they projected, they did exactly that.

. . . These schools institutionalized women's access to higher education. They established the foundations of a collegiate course of study. They provided models for negotiating between the aspirations generated by higher education and the feminine conventions women were expected to practice. And they extended to generations of women the rights and obligations of citizenship.

Let me return to the riddle with which we began. For the thousands of women whose subjectivities had been shaped at female academies and seminaries, the "Enigma" the student presented to her classmates was a deeply felt reality. With little or no hesitation, these women embraced an education wrapped in the values and vocabularies of gendered republicanism. In puzzling through the challenge to the prevailing system of gender relations entailed in that education, they tacked back and forth between personal aspiration and social constraint. The paths they fashioned and the strategies they invented were multiple and complex. Decade by decade, they revised and elaborated the choices they had made. Acting on local, regional, and national stages, they became influential makers of public opinion. In all this they enacted a transformation in women's relationship to public life that has proved an enduring legacy.

MARY KELLEY is the Ruth Bordin Collegiate Professor of History, American Culture, and Woman's Studies at the University of Michigan. She has held academic appointments at the City University of New York, the University of North Carolina at Charlotte, and Dartmouth College. She is the author of *Woman's Being, Woman's Place: Female Identity and Vocation in American History* and *The Limits of Sisterhood: The Beecher Sisters on Woman's Rights and Woman's Sphere*, and has edited *The Power of Her Sympathy: The Autobiography and Journal of Catherine Maria Sedgewick.*

Lucia McMahon

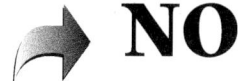

Between Cupid and Minerva

In an 1802 essay provocatively titled, "Plan for the Emancipation of the Female Sex," an anonymous author suggested that women "would willingly relinquish that authority which they have so long enjoyed by courtesy, in order to appear formally on the theatre of the world merely as the equals of man." To achieve mere equality, women could "petition the legislature to sanction their emancipation by law." To gain equality, women needed only to ask for it—equality was, in essence, already theirs for the taking because no "gallant man" would allow his wife or mother to "sue in vain." This author recognized the law as one road to female emancipation, but he also underscored the early national connection between education and equality. As part of his "Plan for Emancipation," he proposed that the nation "found a college for the instruction of females in the arts and sciences." The faculty at this college would be women devoted entirely to their careers. "For the better preservation of female rights," he insisted, "the professors should all be enjoined celibacy." In addition to teaching, these "fair sages" would publish works on "the nobler subjects of civil polity or philosophy." Yet female students would be trained not to emulate their professors' public careers but to assume traditional domestic roles: "Young women entrusted to the tuition of female philosophers in this university, may when they become mothers, instruct their children; . . . and thus a gradual increase of wisdom, and consequently, of happiness, will be diffused throughout the community."

By 1802, when this essay was published, scores of female academies were being established throughout the young nation, yet the idea of a college for women was still outside serious consideration. Indeed, it is difficult to discern if the essay's author was principally serious or sarcastic. If the "Plan for Emancipation" was meant as a parody, its stance on women's education did not contain enough true derision. The author presented the female college and its students in largely positive terms and failed, unlike most critics, to disparage educated women as pedants or bluestockings. As another author noted, "Few men would (I imagine) wish their wives and daughters to prefer Horace and Virgil to the care of their families." Whatever the intentions of this 1802 "Plan for Emancipation," the fluid, nebulous nature of early national ideas about women's education and gender roles made it difficult to distinguish where possibility ended and parody began.

In 1819, less than two decades after the publication of the "Plan for Emancipation," Emma Willard, educator, echoed many of its suggestions and strategies in her "Plan for Improving Female Education." Willard petitioned the New York legislature not for female emancipation as such but, rather, for official improvements in and government support of women's education. Willard insisted that schools for women needed the same "respectability, permanency, and uniformity of operation" that characterized male institutions. As Willard argued, "It is the duty of a government, to do all in its power to promote the present and future prosperity of the nation, over which it is placed. This prosperity will depend on the character of its citizens." Women were citizens, and their proper education was vital to the success of the nation. Yet, according to her nineteenth-century biographer, Willard struggled "to find a suitable name for her ideal institution," and reportedly asserted, "It would never do to call it a 'college,' for the proposal to send young ladies to college would strike everyone as an absurdity." She instead decided upon the term "female seminary," hopeful that such naming "will not create a jealousy that we mean to intrude upon the province of the men." Willard was careful to insist that she had no desire to offer "a masculine education," stressing that education needed to reflect men and women's "difference of characters and duties."

Whether presented as parody or possibility, early national articulations of women's education were marked by this persistent tension between intellectual equality and sexual difference. In essence, proponents of women's education insisted that women were at once equal to and

---

McMahon, Lucia. "Between Cupid and Minerva" and *"Education, Equality, or Difference," Mere Equals: The Paradox of Educated Women in the Early American Republic*, 2012. Copyright ©2012 by Cornell University. Used by permission of the author and the publisher, Cornell University Press.

different from men. This paradox found expression in Willard's rejection of "masculine education" for women, as well as in the assertion in the 1802 "Plan for Emancipation" that education would put women in positions *merely* as the equals of man. Yet it is also striking that both plans proposed legal and educational measures as paths to women's equality. Women in post-Revolutionary America did not achieve substantial measures of equality or emancipation through legal channels. Early national women could not vote or hold office; and once married, women were subject to the doctrine of coverture, which made it challenging for them to hold property or acquire independent wealth. Within the educational landscape, however, progress was well underway. The period from approximately 1785 to 1825 represented a watershed moment in women's institutional access to education. Although colleges remained closed to them, women enjoyed unprecedented access to a variety of new educational opportunities.

As the institutional landscape changed, so did representations of educated women within the literary public sphere. Through a variety of forms—including engravings, poetry, essays, anecdotes, character sketches, and novels—prescriptive writers explored the place of educated women in early national America. Although many supported advancements in women's education, early national Americans were troubled by the idea that women's intellectual equality might disrupt the social, economic, and political frameworks that were sustained by the notion of sexual difference. Understanding how prescriptive writings articulated the tensions between education, equality, and difference is a crucial first step that will inform subsequent explorations of how individual women understood and experienced the boundaries of mere equality within their own lives.

"The Female Mind Shall Equal Prove"

Prior to the American Revolution, as one 1810 essayist recalled, women were "systemically shut out of Minerva's Temple." The young nation sought to expand women's access to education: "Thanks to the liberal and aspiring spirit of the age and country, the genius and education of women are not shamefully neglected." Educators established scores of new academies and seminaries for both women and men, insisting that education was an essential component of nation building. "It must therefore be a pleasure to all who wish for the prosperity and glory of this rising nation," the *Pennsylvania Gazette* reported in 1786, "to observe the zealous and liberal exertions of its citizens, in promoting the cause of literature, and providing for the instruction of youth in every useful and ornamental science." The need for well-educated men reflected political and social ideals about well-informed citizens who would take the lead in matters concerning the political, economic, and literary spheres of the nation. Yet many early national Americans asserted that the proper education of women was equally important. As advocates insisted, women's education involved nothing less than "the most effectual means of establishing, promoting, and securing, on the most solid foundation, the domestic and social happiness of the present and future ages." Education was both a symptom and cause of the commitment of the young nation to liberty, freedom, and independence.

Such enlightened faith in the powers of education was accompanied by an optimistic, and potentially radical, belief in the equality of women's and men's intellectual capacities. Educators asserted that women "were beings endowed with reason," who possessed intellectual capacity and "an equality of mind" with men. As one author contended, women "possess a strength of reason equal to ours . . . and can attain the knowledge of every thing they are required to do, with at least, an equal facility." Another essay on female education began with a poem that captured the era's optimistic faith in women's intellectual potential: "When'er the female mind shall equal prove . . . No longer shall it vauntingly be said /*Her's is inferior to the mind of man.*" This widespread belief in women's intellectual equality had promising potential, suggesting that women could perhaps live merely as the equals of man. As John Burton, author of *Lectures on Female Education and Manners*, argued, "it cannot be denied, that your sex have given equal proofs with the men, of genius, judgment, taste, and imagination." Burton tantalizingly intimated that women were, in theory, as capable of receiving the same education as men, perhaps for the same ends: "It is not necessary, neither it is expedient for the purpose of civil society, that girls should be educated in the same manner as boys: but were a similar plan to be adopted, the women, without doubt, would be as well informed in the system of human knowledge, as the men." As Burton suggested, women's station in society was a matter of custom and access to education, not due to any lack of intellectual ability. Yet, because it was deemed neither "necessary" nor "expedient" for women to be granted full access to political and economic equality, writers such as Burton repeatedly tempered their celebratory remarks about women's intellectual capacities by evoking prescribed gender roles: "The respective employments of the male and female sex being different, a different mode of education is consequently required. For whatever equality there may be in the natural powers of their minds, which I shall not consider at present, yet the female sex, from their situation in life, and from the duties corresponding with it, must evidently be instructed in a manner suitable to their destination, and to the tasks which they will have to perform."

Despite their enlightened faith in women's intellectual equality, early national Americans continued to believe that men and women were dissimilar beings with contrasting manners, morals, and dispositions—and duties. Although the female mind was capable of intellectual equality, the female body apparently was not fitted for political equality: "'Tis Nature herself that prescribes for them a sedentary life, and devotes them to domestic occupations;' tis Nature herself that secludes from public offices, the functions of which could not be combined with the duties of a mother and a nurse." The enthusiasm for women's educational accomplishments stopped well short of extending the rights of suffrage and direct political power to women. This tension produced the notion of mere equality that dominated early national discussions of women's education.

The belief that women were indeed mere equals of men, at least intellectually and socially, while at the same time profoundly different in body and station, generated conflicting models of womanhood. To negotiate this thorny realm of equality and difference, early national Americans explored complementary gender roles that celebrated certain elements of equality (intellectual and social) while simultaneously insisting that "natural" distinctions (gender and race) defined the parameters of full political citizenship. Stressing the mutuality of relations between the sexes, writers urged women to find contentment in a model of gender identity that remained inherently hierarchical. "Do not these facts justify the order of society, and render some difference in rank between the sexes, necessary to the happiness of both?" This complementary model of gender relations attempted to square the overriding insistence on prescribed gender roles with a positive characterization of women's intellectual capacities. In the process, the prescriptive literature obscured questions of power and authority inherent in this model of social organization. Although granting women intellectual capacity equal to that of men, prescriptive writers ultimately focused on maintaining a social and political order rooted in sexual difference and male hierarchy.

Discussions of women's education thus revealed a persistent contradiction between women's intellectual capacity (which many agreed was equal to that of men), and the decidedly different uses intended for education in their everyday lives. In essence, once having agreed that women could learn, proponents of women's education could not agree about what women should learn because their universal faith in the capacity of women's intellectual abilities came into conflict with their adherence to conventional gender roles. As one author insisted, "A *good* education is that which renders the ladies correct in their manners, respectable in their families, and agreeable in society. That education is always *wrong*, which raises a woman above the duties of her station." Instead of selfishly acquiring knowledge for their own sakes, women were asked to educate themselves for the benefit of early republican society. "How much better it would be then, were females educated, in order to make useful and ornamental members of society." As John Burton stressed, "the accomplishments, therefore, which you should acquire, are those that will contribute to render you serviceable in domestic, and agreeable in social life."The main purpose of women's education, then, was not to provide women with the means to develop personal autonomy and ambition but, rather, to enable them to serve men and society. . . . [A]ccess to education dramatically affected how individual women made sense of themselves and the world around them. But such changes in women's identity formation were of little interest to most prescriptive writers. Instead, educated women's roles were defined almost exclusively in relationship to men; they were to exercise moral influence, to provide pleasing conversation, and to serve as attractive companions. Prescriptive writers expressed little regard for the individual aspirations of educated women; rather, they worried about how women's pursuit of education would affect men.

Thus, while recognizing that the acquisition of education could enable women to live as mere equals to men, writers repeatedly warned that too much intellectual "sameness" between men and women would jeopardize domestic and social harmony by creating rivalry and competition. Prescriptive writings asserted that there was "a line of character between the sexes, which neither can pass without becoming contemptible." Women overly interested in the "masculine attainments" associated with certain forms of education and knowledge were accused of selfishness, pedantry, and affectation, traits considered "repugnant to female delicacy, so derogatory to the natural characteristic of her sex." As another author, identified as "Alphonzo," insisted, "A strong attachment to books in a lady, often deters a man from approaching her with the offer of his heart. This is ascribed to the pride of our sex." Implicitly, men did not want women who were smarter than they were, women who would disagree with them, or women who would seek opportunities in the spheres of government and business:

> When a woman quits her own department, she offends her husband, not merely because she obtrudes herself upon *his* business, but because she departs from that sphere which is assigned *her* in the order of society—because she neglects *her* duties and leaves *her own* department vacant. . . . The same principle which excludes a man from an attention to domestic business, excludes a woman from law, mathematics, and astronomy. Each sex feels a degree of pride in being best qualified for a particular station, and a degree of resentment when the other encroaches upon their privilege. This is acting conformably to the constitution of society.

In promoting a separate spheres model, writers insisted that women could not occupy themselves with "masculine" concerns without necessarily neglecting their domesticity and desirability. Accordingly, the prescriptive literature urged women to make themselves "lovely" to men, and as Alphonzo insisted, "to be *lovely* you must be content to be *women*; to be mild, social and sentimental—to be acquainted with all that belongs to your department—and leave the masculine virtues, and the profound researches of study to the province of the other sex." Prescriptive writings stressed the need for educated women to retain their feminine attractiveness and desirability to men, fearful of what might occur if educated women were no longer "content to be *women*"—in other words, if they sought to live *merely* as the equals of man.

"Knowledge, Combined with Beauty"

Part celebratory, part cautionary, prescriptive representations were important tools by which social commentators attempted to teach particular lessons about the proper content, forms, and effects of women's education. The frontispiece of the 1791 volume of the *Massachusetts Magazine* presented an inspirational model of womanhood meant to guide educated women. Surrounded by mythological and material embodiments of education, this representative woman exhibited an aura of intellectual seriousness *and* attractive femininity. The editors offered an "Explanation of the Frontispiece":

> The Fair Daughters of Massachusetts, are collectively represented by the symbolic figure of an elegant and accomplished young Lady, seated in her study, contemplating the various pages of the Magazine. Their general acquaintance with the necessary branches of reading and writing, and the more ornamental ones, of History and Geography, is happily depicted, by those instruments of Science, which adorn the Hall of Meditation. *Minerva*, the Goddess of Wisdom, assisted by *Cupid*, crowns her with a chaplet of Laurel: *Hymen*'s burning Torch is displayed aloft— a delicate intimation, that knowledge, combined with beauty, enkindles the purest flames of love.

In this representation, love and learning were coupled seamlessly in that both Cupid and Minerva crowned the achievements of this symbolic figure. "Knowledge, combined with beauty," enabled women to spread happiness and harmony throughout the young nation. As Daniel Bryan, educator, insisted, "the influence of enlightened Beauty" was "inconceivable." An attractive and intelligent woman, as a student at a female academy remarked, represented the ideal form of womanhood: "I do not know any thing which so nearly approaches the *acme* of human excellence, as a young female of an enlightened understanding, a well-informed mind, and a pure and virtuous heart, united in a fair-proportioned and beautiful form."

An "enlightened beauty" presented no apparent contradiction between love and learning, yet prescriptive thinkers frequently expressed concern about the potentially negative effects of women's education. In an 1809 essay titled, "On Female Education," James Milnor, a trustee of the Philadelphia Academy, aptly described the merits, as well as the possible dangers, inherent in women's pursuit of education. Milnor noted, "that as a polite and well-informed woman is the most welcome companion of the intelligent of our sex, a female pedant is in all respects the reverse." By failing to acquire "useful" knowledge, a pedant was given to affectation and the "ostentatious display of the decorations of her mind." But Milnor also recognized that in the effort to avoid pedantry, educators "may err on the contrary extreme." Young women also had to fear the consequences of a poor education, produced most often by reading novels. "Instead of the evil of pedantry, these are calculated to seduce the unsetted minds of young persons into the adoption of erroneous and immoral principles." Such women entertained "frivolity" and "false views of life" that often led to "disastrous course of conduct."

In his essay, Milnor identified two extremes on a spectrum of ideas about educated women. Education and knowledge were presented as important antidotes to frivolity and coquetry (symptoms of undereducation), but the danger of overeducation (specifically, pedantry) was ever-present. In effect, educated women were asked to perform a delicate balancing act. They constantly risked falling into one or the other of these perceived extremes—extremes that can be thought of as representing either too much love or too much learning. A poorly educated woman was in danger of becoming too coquettish, too sexualized, and too susceptible to seduction. On the other end of the spectrum was the woman with too much education, or more precisely, one who had gained knowledge considered inappropriate for women. Both the undereducated coquette and the overeducated pedant let their level of education interfere with their attractiveness to men—thus threatening compatibility between the sexes. The figures of the pedant and the coquette served as foils against which model republican wives and mothers were measured.

On one end of the spectrum was the pedant. Both supporters and critics of women's education agreed that the pedant was a dangerous figure—a woman who selfishly pursued knowledge to the detriment of her domestic and social duties. "Female pedantry is the object of my ridicule," one author remarked with obvious disdain. When a woman "applied herself to her study" too much, her actions resulted not in "that deference and respect which she had vainly expected" but, rather, "desertion and contempion." Instead of properly preparing herself for participation in early national society, the pedant exhibited behavior that was antisocial, selfish, and vain. It was best, as *The American Lady's Preceptor* recommended, for women to avoid "all abstract learning, all difficult researches, which may blunt the finer edges of their wit, and change the delicacy in which they excel into pedantic coarseness." Even the strongest proponents of women's education were careful to warn about the dangers of overeducating women. As Susanna Rowson, author of several books and founder of a female academy, underscored, "many are the prejudices entertained, and the witticisms thrown out against what are called learned women." Rowson summarized this mindset in her *Present for Young Ladies:* "The mind of a female is certainly as capable of acquiring knowledge, as that of the other sex; but if an enlightened mind must consequently be a conceited one it were better to remain in ignorance, since pedantry and presumption in a woman is more disgusting than an entire want of literary information, the one often awakens compassion, the other invariably excites contempt."

Pedantry was rooted in conceit and vanity. As John Burton warned, young women needed to avoid becoming "vain enough to imagine, that your boasted merit is held in the same estimation by others." Such affectation, he asserted, implied that women were "so full of their own importance" as to exhibit an "egotism" that was "intolerable." Samuel Whiting, author of *Elegant Lessons*, agreed, remarking, "affectation of learning and authorship, in a woman with very little merit, draws upon itself the contempt and hatred of both sexes." . . .

"The Arts of Coquetry"

If a woman was too engrossed with education, she risked being labeled a pedant. Yet, if a woman's attention to education was too superficial, she could be criticized for that as well. Samuel Whiting, author, warned about the dangers awaiting any "utterly uncultivated" young woman: "What is there to correct her passions, or to govern her practice? What is there to direct her in the choice of companions and diversions; to guard her against the follies of her own sex, and the arts of ours?" As critics warned, the path to coquetry was most often laid "by a false Education, the folly of parents, or the flattery of a corrupted world." Unlike the pedant, who was preoccupied with learning, the coquette neglected her education, afraid that any overexertion might interfere with her beauty and charm. As one author quipped, "useful studies must by no means be attended to, as possibly it might damp Miss's vivacity."

Neglecting useful studies, coquettes instead were more likely to spend countless hours engaged in reading novels. Indeed, novel reading was perhaps the surest path to coquetry. Prone to coquettish behavior, novel readers were ill prepared for the realities of courtship and marriage, preferring instead to inhabit a dreamlike world of their own imagination. Such was the case for "Melissa," a young woman whose "invincible attachment to novels" turned her into a coquette. Melissa felt herself "well qualified for a heroine, as any, who shine in the page of romance. . . . Indeed she had charms, and her mind was well stored with modern female erudition; (for she had perused numberless novels)." Melissa replaced real education with romantic fancies, and through her voracious novel reading, "the arts of coquetry were. . . . carefully studied." Given to affectation and flirting, Melissa rejected many sound marriage proposals, "knowing that once sacrificed at the altar of Hymen, she could no longer enjoy the felicity of coquetry." Instead, Melissa spent her entire life an unmarried woman, and when her charms no longer worked, "she professed herself a *man hater.*"

Whereas the pedant was cast as an unattractive, masculine figure, the coquette represented disorder in the form of excessive female sexuality. The "ultimate aim" of the coquette was to gain "power" over male admirers and the surrounding social scene. Ultimately, however, this power was chimerical: "However flattering it may be to the vanity of the female sex, to make conquests, or to have many admirers, yet it betrays a kind of coquetry by no means admirable." Although coquettes reveled in their ability to attract men, they represented a disruptive form of desirability—one that ultimately led to rejection and embarrassment for men. Expecting to meet heroic men who resembled characters from novels, coquettes hesitated to accept "several offers that would otherwise have appeared highly advantageous and proper." By rejecting marriage proposals from respectable men, coquettes eventually found themselves alone and unwanted. As critics repeatedly warned, any worthy man would come to recognize the insincere flirtations of a coquette and would refuse to consider her as an ideal mate. "How faint and spiritless are the charms of a coquet [sic], with the real loveliness of . . . innocence, piety, good-humour, and truth." By disrupting marital models, coquettes were as problematic as pedants. . . .

"On an Equal Footing"

Through myriad warnings and cautionary tales, the literary public sphere revealed a continued sense of ambivalence about educated women's roles in society. Rather than clarifying the relationship among education, equality, and difference, such prescriptive models may have created confusion for any woman who was relying on them to guide her behavior. As one proponent of women's education rhetorically asked, "How can a pretty woman fail to be ignorant, when the first lesson she is taught, is that beauty supersedes and dispenses with every other quality; . . . [and] that to be intelligent is to be pedantic?" Women recognized that the charge of pedantry could be used to discredit their intellectual pursuits. Yet, by stressing the need for women to remain desirable and attractive to men, prescriptive writers could be guilty of encouraging coquettish practices. "Shall we blame her for being a coquette," this author continued, "when the indiscriminate flattery of every man teaches her that the homage of one is as good as that of another?"

The censure of both coquettish and pedantic behavior reflected two extremes on a spectrum of fears about the implications of women's education. . . . Both the pedant and coquette challenged gender roles by insisting on living merely as the equals of man on their own misguide terms.

. . . [I]t was not educated women themselves but rather early national society as a whole that was unready for woman to explore the possibilities of mere equality. . . . Early national woman eagerly embraced opportunities to acquire education and put it to good use. As a student at a female academy in New York insisted, "Since we have the same natural abilities as themselves, why should we not have the same opportunity of polishing and displaying them by the principles of an independent and virtuous education." This young woman rejoiced that enlightened Americans "wish to see the fair sex on an equal footing with themselves, enjoying all the blessings of freedom."

Inspired by this equal footing, educated women began to imagine what it would be like to live merely as the equals of man—at least in their personal and social relationships. . . . Female academies inspired women to develop identities that celebrated their intellectual ambitions. Enthusiastic about their studies, young women were determined to defend their ardent interest in education against prescriptive warnings about both coquettish and pedantic behavior.

When they left the safe, nurturing space of the female academy, educated women searched for new ways to enact identities founded in the promise of mere equality. . . . In all stages of their lives, women self-consciously crafted personal and social relationships in which their intellectual achievements were valued, appreciated, and celebrated. Through relationships with like-minded individuals, educated women searched for mere equality, inextricably linking their intellectual, emotional, and social aspirations. In particular, women believed that egalitarian relationships between men and women *were* possible, and to their credit, they found men willing and eager to enact relationships that emphasized shared intellectual and emotional interests.

Despite prescriptive fears about masculine, pedantic women, early national men did not seem troubled by the intellectual women in their lives, nor did early national women reject their domestic roles after acquiring education. In fact, we could argue that most educated women faced the inverse of the disruptive scenarios envisioned by prescriptive writers: Could they sustain the promise of mere equality when faced with the increasing demands of family life and domesticity? That is, could individual women enact identities and relationships rooted in expressions of mere equality *within* their assigned gender roles? The first generation of educated women did not, as a whole, make larger claims for political equality—they asked primarily for the right to be educated. Accepting the constraints of prescribed gender roles with respect to the law and politics, women who acquired education channeled those energies primarily toward their individual identities and relationships. "Ask those gentlemen of this assembly whose wives have been the best educated whether they find them to be less attentive to domestic concerns," Anna Harrington suggested to the audience of a Ladies' Exhibition held at an academy in Lincoln, Massachusetts. "May not more women be trusted with knowledge, as well as these. Or is there any fear that women shall gain too much influence; and become mistresses of the world in spite of man?" The fear that intellectual equality would lead women to seek "too much influence" was not borne out by the everyday lives of educated women. "When we shall quit our domestic employments, put on offensive armor, and become fond of the art of war," Anna asserted, "then such an event may be feared." While accepting (for the time being) the limited range of such efforts, educated women began to explore—and without "offensive armor"—what the promises of mere equality might entail in their individual lives....

Education, Equality, or Difference

> Pray you excuse me, if I have gone too far
> In telling you what we've learnt: and what we are
> We'll strive to show, if you will deign to hear us;
> If worthy, let your approbation cheer us.

Miss A. M. Burton read this poem at commencement exercises held at Susanna Rowson's Female Academy in October 1803. The poem was published in the *Boston Weekly Magazine*, making Burton's acquisition of education at once a lived experience and a literary representation. The interplay between the personal and prescriptive was also reflected in the poem itself, which asserted women's steadfast determination to acquire and demonstrate knowledge ("we'll strive to show"), along with persistent concerns about male reception ("if you will deign to hear us"). Such worries about male criticism were not unfounded, but the story is more complicated than that. As early national women acquired education, many advocates expressed confidence that women would easily achieve a state of near, or mere, equality with men. "By giving *mind* to the fair sex," as one author asserted, "we shall make them equal to any thing that is attainable by rational beings." Another essayist proudly noted that human qualifications, "when properly cultivated and exerted, put men and women nearly on an equal footing with each other, and share the advantages and disadvantages of life impartially between them."

Left unresolved were more precise discussions of what it meant for women to live merely as the equals of man—how near an equal footing was possible, given the legal, political, and economic realities of early American life? Many women succeeded, as one essayist noted, in achieving "moments of transient equality," demonstrating intellectual "ability equal to ours." But those moments remained transient. After promoting women's intellectual capacities and celebrating their importance to civic society, prescriptive writers failed to advocate for women's legal, political, and professional equality with men. Unable to concede the possibility of women's full participation in political and economic spheres, social and political thinkers instead relied on the murky notion of mere equality in an effort to contain the potentially liberating aspects of their own rhetoric. Educated women learned to settle for social and cultural expressions of "approbation" rather than more expansive opportunities to fully utilize their intellectual capacities.

Despite these tensions, early national Americans clearly recognized that women's acquisition of education represented a critical step in their path to equality. Yet more than fifty years later, the subject of women's intellectual equality remained open to debate. In an 1840 essay published in *Godey's Lady Book*, author Mary Hale echoed sentiments expressed half a century earlier, insisting, "with proper cultivation, with the enjoyment of equal advantages, the intellectual attainments of women may equal those of men." Over the course of fifty years, educated women had proven their intellectual capacities in ever-increasing number and in an ever-expanding variety of subjects. "Has the short space of a half century given woman new powers," Hale wondered, "or is the spirit of our institutions more favourable to an enlarged cultivation of those she already possessed?" According to Hale, the answer was obvious: expanded access to educational opportunities had clearly led to women's increased attainment of knowledge and understanding.

Women had repeatedly demonstrated that they possessed intellectual capacity equal to that of men; why, then, did Hale still have to defend this assertion? Moreover, why had expanded access to education not led to even more expansive opportunities for women? In 1840, when Hale's article was published, only a handful of colleges admitted women. The clergy, law, and legislature all remained closed to women. Women continued to occupy "a less *public* station" than men, not from lack of intellectual capacity but from lack of access and opportunity. Despite her ardent support of women's educational capacities, Hale largely accepted these constraints as the will of Providence. Yet her essay also pointed to a more secular explanation—the continued criticism leveled against "a literary lady." Any woman who appeared too interested in education risked being tainted with the stain of "pedantry, self-sufficiency and insipidity." Nineteenth-century Americans remained deeply suspicious of women's intellectual accomplishments.

Reading Hale's essay, we may wonder whether little had actually changed in the course of fifty years. Fears of educated women continued to proliferate in the literary public sphere, perhaps in part because women's access to education continued to expand exponentially. By 1840, scores of academies, seminaries, and collegiate institutes existed, offering a variety of advanced educational opportunities for women. Schools such as the Troy Female Seminary (founded by Emma Willard in 1821), the Hartford Female Seminary (founded by Catherine Beecher in 1823), and Mount Holyoke (founded by Mary Lyon in 1837) offered women the equivalent of a college education—although without explicitly referring to it as such. In 1837, Oberlin College admitted its first female students, paving the way for women's admission to other colleges in the decades to follow. Well-educated women filled the ranks of teachers, authors, missionaries, and reformers. In essence, educated women attended institutions and engaged in the types of activities proposed in the 1802 "Plan for the Emancipation of the Female Sex"—yet without resolving the thorny issue of mere equality.

As women's access to education expanded, nineteenth-century Americans remained at once celebratory and cautious about educated women's influence in society. Articles proudly boasted that the United States "can vie with any nation on earth in a good proportion of intelligent and pious females." To those skeptics who doubted the need for women's education, one author suggested that such critics undoubtedly held "very limited views" of the importance of education or that they had conflated education with affectation: "Perhaps their idea of an 'educated lady' is associated in their mind with nothing better than some starched nun, or round-mouthed pedant." Despite impressive institutional advancements and individual achievements in women's education, prescriptive writers still relied on the figure of the pedant to discredit women's intellectual ambitions. Improperly educated women could still be dismissed as "triflers and silly women," as one female essayist noted, "but if any of us have resolution enough to soar beyond those narrow limits, . . . we are called critics, wits, female pedants, &c." For over half a century, women steadfastly acquired education, but the potential uses of their intellectual capacities remained constrained by custom, law, and prejudice. Accordingly, the prescriptive literature continued to define women's education through a series of contradictions—between capacity and utilization, between learning and desirability, between coquetry and pedantry.

In their everyday lives, educated women attempted to sort through competing sets of discourses, resisting negative representations while favoring models that validated their intellectual interests. Skeptical of both the pedant and the coquette, women refashioned narrow representations of womanhood into more expansive models. Women experimented with personal interpretations of print, reshaping discourses to suit their individual needs and aspirations. At every stage of their lives, women explored the boundaries of mere equality. In particular, educated women sought relationships with like-minded individuals willing to accept them as their intellectual and social equals. Women such as Eunice Callender, Sarah Ripley Stearns, Elizabeth and Margaret Shippen, Linda Raymond Ward, Jane Bowne Haines, and Jane Bayard Kirkpatrick all enjoyed platonic or romantic relationships with men who valued their intellectual attainments. Shared intellectual interests became a key means by which men and women crafted fulfilling relationships that celebrated areas of affinity and mutuality, in contrast to prescriptive ideas that insisted on models of gender difference and hierarchy. These women's efforts remind us that prescriptive literature can tell us only part of the history of an era, and they illustrate the continued interplay between prescriptive literature and lived experience that informed women's emotional and intellectual lives.

It is important to underscore, and tempting to celebrate, how early national women achieved some measures of mere equality in their everyday lives and relationships, even as we recognize that their efforts failed to challenge structural systems of inequality and inequity. That early national women did not advocate more fully for political rights may be seen as a lost opportunity, yet the paradoxical nature of mere equality offered them few avenues to pursue such broad goals. The narrow expressions of mere equality that educated women achieved reflected not just their own individual limitations but also larger cultural and prescriptive constraints. Despite their enlightened faith in women's intellectual capacity, early national Americans struggled to sustain the malleable and elusive concept of mere equality. Ultimately, when faced with the fundamental question of whether women could be simultaneously equal to and different from men, nineteenth-century Americans could not square the search for mere equality with their overriding belief in sexual difference. In their own lives, women accepted these constraints even as they bristled against them. "I think if we had the advantages of the other sex, we should be equally as reasonable and orderly a set of beings as they are." Elizabeth Lindsay mused to her friend Apphia Rouzee in 1806. Yet, like most of her contemporaries, Elizabeth stopped short of articulating a more radical call for equality: "but enough on the superiority of the sexes, for after all, I believe it is the best way to content ourselves with the station of life in which we have been placed." To best serve society, Elizabeth reflected, educated women needed to learn a final lesson—to "bend all our ambition on becoming as useful as we can." It can be argued that the women of this study bent their ambition, living quiet lives that until recently warranted little historical inquiry. They were well educated and determined to enact useful lives as learned women, but they had few avenues to directly challenge patriarchal systems of inequity.

The more well-known stories in women's history often revolve around those women who were able to express their desires for equality in more ambitious ways. These women, it should be noted, typically enjoyed access to educational opportunities pioneered by the early national generation. In 1848, Elizabeth Cady Stanton—a graduate of Emma Willard's Troy Seminary—presented her *Declaration of Sentiments* at the Seneca Falls convention. Recognizing the link between knowledge and power, Stanton argued that women's educational status contributed to their subordinated place in American society: "He has denied her the facilities for obtaining a thorough education, all colleges being closed against her." Women's rights activists understood that the franchise was only one path to equality; thus, they sought not only the right to vote but further access to education, reforms to divorce and property rights legislation, and expanded economic opportunities, including "an equal participation with men in the various trades, professions and commerce." Women's rights activists called for something greater than mere equality—they sought a comprehensive vision of gender equality largely unconstrained by narrow representations of difference. Perhaps it was, in part, the limits of mere equality that inspired these activists to develop a more expansive women's rights agenda.

We know that most nineteenth-century Americans sharply resisted women's efforts to claim a more fundamental equality with men, as they evoked reformulated arguments about separate spheres and sexual difference in their efforts to maintain patriarchal systems of power. As the idea of mere equality evolved into struggles for wide-ranging forms of equality, the reactions against women became more vigorous. Indeed, the doctrine of separate spheres found its fullest expression in the prescriptive literature *after* women began to assert larger claims for political and economic equality. Writers articulated a narrowly defined private sphere of domesticity at the very time that numerous women were carving out public roles for themselves and making demands for equal access to educational and economic opportunities. Thus, the notion of separate spheres that has dominated the historiography for decades can be better understood as a *reaction* to early national women's experiments with mere equality rather than as an accurate depiction of women's lives during this time period. The sharp emphasis of the antebellum era on difference came to dominate after women had attempted to live merely—and then more fully—as the equals of man.

Perhaps most worthy of future study are the thorny questions of how and why so many women learned to adopt the rhetoric of difference and, indeed, often did so as a conscious, deliberate strategy to justify their public roles. "On the whole, (even if fame be the object of pursuit)," Hannah More, author, argued, "is it not better to succeed as women, than to fail as men?" A leading advocate of women's education, More promoted a model of female excellence sustained not by mere equality but by sharp delineations of difference. She asked women to consider whether it was better "to shine, by walking honorably in the road which nature, custom, and education seem to have marked out, rather than to counteract them all, by moving awkwardly in a path diametrically opposite?" Like other prescriptive writers, More urged women to find cultural authority by seeking "to be excellent women, rather than indifferent men." Such arguments proved persuasive, and as the nineteenth century progressed, many women rejected the complex challenges of mere equality for such clear articulations of difference.

Why did women retreat from the idea of becoming merely the equals of man and embrace a social order rooted in sexual difference? What did the rhetoric of difference offer women that mere equality failed to provide or sustain? As scholars have shown, the prescriptive rhetoric promoting women's "sphere of influence" enabled women to enact a number of expanded roles for themselves as reformers, missionaries, educators, and authors. "There is an influence spread abroad in society," wrote M. H. S. Brown, a member of the Young Ladies' Association of the New Hampton Female Seminary, in 1840. "It is felt, though it may be unacknowledged, in the halls of legislation, as well as in the drawing room, and exerts itself powerfully upon the most gifted as upon the most unintellectual of men. . . . This influence is woman's." Yet such influence came at a price—it was sustained by the explicit notion that women were acting in these influential roles as *women*, not as the mere equals of men.

The abandonment of mere equality was perhaps inevitable, in that it represented a paradoxical expression of gender identity that simultaneously reified sexual difference even as it promoted intellectual equality. Faced with this contradiction, . . . educated women often experienced a sense of ambivalence that complicated their understandings of the connections among education, equality, and difference. Although their efforts met with only limited success, the stories of how individual women attempted to live merely as the equals of man raise fundamental questions about the place of difference in a nation dedicated to the proposition that all men are created equal. Such questions have resonance today, as we consider the ways in which women continue to achieve certain measures of equality that have not required men to cede significant power or privilege. At stake, then and now, has been nothing less than (mere) equality.

LUCIA MCMAHON is an associate professor and assistant chair in the Department of History at William Paterson University. A specialist in U.S. early national and women's and gender history, she earned her PhD from Rutgers University in 2004.

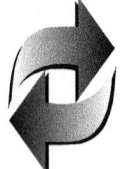

EXPLORING THE ISSUE

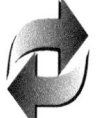

Did Improved Educational Opportunities for Women in the New Nation Significantly Expand Their Participation in Antebellum Society?

Critical Thinking and Reflection

1. What impact did female education have on women's status in antebellum American public life?
2. In what specific ways were American women able to use their education to participate in civil society?
3. In what ways were the ideals of the New Republic reflected in the educational opportunities for women?
4. Explain the difference class and race had on antebellum women's public participation. Compare and contrast the ways these same factors impact the civic involvement of women today.
5. Consider what women were left out of higher education as well as who was let in. In what ways does this reinforce society's ideas of gender, race and class?

Is There Common Ground?

In both studies, Kelley and McMahon recognize the forms of subtle or compliant resistance utilized by women while acknowledging that progress was predicated on and restricted by entrenched views of gender. For while education of all citizens was recognized in the early 19th century as critical component of an effective democracy and republic, the ways in which men and women were allowed to act upon their knowledge was strictly prescribed. Both authors cite references to women couching their desires for greater educational and intellectual opportunities in non-competitive and service-oriented language. In doing so, these educated women helped usher in the Second Great Awakening and the subsequent period of social reform and change. They applied themselves to a variety of fields such as abolition, temperance, sufferance, and to expanding educational and employment opportunities for women.

Angelica Grimke, for example used her position within Southern genteel society and later her authority as a wife of prominent abolitionist Theodore Weld as a platform for her work to end slavery. Catherine Beecher, daughter of minister Lyman Beecher and sister to author Harriet Beecher Stowe, championed women being educated for teaching by utilizing interest intersection and working within frameworks of feminine gender norms even while tacitly acknowledging that many used teaching to escape the prescribed and normed path of marriage and motherhood. Teachers and other educated women may have had less status or power than their male counterparts, but their professions and work were a source of satisfaction and public identity. Founder of the American women's suffrage movement Elizabeth Cady Stanton was very careful of, and made much use of, her image as a happy and contented mother and wife to pursue of her goals. By pushing from within the accepted feminine sphere, she was able to maneuver around her critic's claims of the unnaturalness of her demands for emancipation, suffrage and self-sovereignty.

Kelley and McMahon's works also bring us pause for reflection of our own time and society. Women continue to work mainly in areas of service to others and these feminized professions are still less respected and valued. While the 19th Amendment approaches its centennial anniversary, women still have yet to achieve political parity in representation. Indeed, in what ways are women still pressured to appear non-confrontational, non-competitive and to put others at ease? Is compliant resistance a source of unrecognized strength that simply does not fit with masculinized views of power and agency, or is it a symptom of the continuing patriarchal gender bifurcation hierarchy and oppression?

Additional Resources

Eastman, Carolynn. "The female Cicero: Young women's oratory and gendered public participation in the early American republic." Gender and History 19, no. 2 (August 2007): 260-283.

Kerber, Linda. Women of the republic: Intellect and ideology in revolutionary America. Chapel Hill: The University of North Carolina Press, 1980.

Lerner, Gerda. The Grimke sisters from South Carolina: Pioneers for woman's rights and abolition. New York: Oxford University Press, 1998.

Nash, Margaret. "The Historiography of Education for Girls and Women in the United States." In Rethinking the History of American Education, edited by William J. Reese and John L. Rury, 143-161. New York: Palgrave MacMillan, 2008.

Schloesser, P. E. The fair sex: White women and the racial patriarchy in the early republic. New York: NYU Press, 2002.

Internet References . . .

History of Women's Education

https://www.bustle.com/p/heres-how-women-fought-for-the-right-to-be-educated-throughout-history-53150

National Women's History Museum

https://www.womenshistory.org/womens-history

The United States House of Representatives: The Women's Rights Movement, 1848–1920

http://history.house.gov/Exhibitions-and-Publications/WIC/Historical-Essays/No-Lady/Womens-Rights/

Women and Reform

https://www.loc.gov/teachers/classroommaterials/connections/time-capsule/history5.html

Education in Early America

https://study.com/academy/lesson/education-in-early-america-birth-of-public-schools-and-universities.html

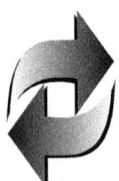

ISSUE

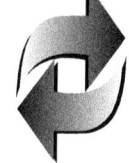

Selected, Edited, and with Issue Framing Material by:
Kevin R. Magill and Tony L. Talbert, *Baylor University*

Was Antebellum Temperance Reform Driven by Theological Doctrine?

YES: Laura A. Schmidt, from "'A Battle Not Man's but God's': Origins of the American Temperance Crusade in the Struggle for Religious Authority," *Journal of Studies on Alcohol* (1995)

NO: John J. Rumbarger, from "The Social and Ideological Origins of Drink Reform, 1800–1836," State University of New York Press (1989)

Learning Outcomes

After reading this issue, you will be able to:

- Discuss the connections between religion, politics, industrialization, and social reform in the early nineteenth century.
- Evaluate the economic arguments that promoted attacks on American drinking habits.
- Analyze ways in which temperance reform represented a mechanism of social control over undesirable individual behavior.

ISSUE SUMMARY

YES: Laura A. Schmidt argues that the temperance movement was developed primarily to offer clergymen a solution to those who contested their authority at a time of social transformation. Many believed religious salvation occurred through the suppression of vice, which allowed the clergymen an additional avenue to win souls to God, guard collective salvation, and petition the government to promote religious obedience.

NO: John J. Rumbarger believes temperance was directed by men of power who "defined, directed, and controlled" the movement to feed the expansionist tendencies of the American economy by encouraging a more productive and reliable workforce.

Issue Framing with Neil Graham Shanks, PhD

In the aftermath of the 2016 presidential election, political science was replete with analyses of the unexpected victory of Donald Trump. Was his victory due to the anxieties of economically disadvantaged folks in the rust belt (Thompson, 2016)? Was it a clash of generations, with older folks yearning to return to the America of their youth (Milbank, 2016)? Or, was it a split along gender lines, with men more comfortable with the unsavory "locker-room talk" demonstrated by the president prior to the election (Enten & Casteel, 2018)? While race and racism were among the most statistically significant predictors of support for the Republican candidate (McElwee & McDaniel, 2017), within the White electorate, it was not income, nor age, nor gender, nor geographic region, nor education that best predicted support for Trump prior to the election. In fact, it was religion (specifically religious attendance) that most closely tracked white vote share (Beckman, 2016), and this support has kicked off a wave of inquiry among thinkers and writers about religion and politics who question the fervent support for a thrice-married serial adulterer by culturally conservative voters (Bacon Jr., 2018; Cox, 2018; Newport, 2018; Stern, 2018; Worthen, 2017). Twenty-five years ago, the Christian Coalition identified the Republican Party as a vehicle through which they could further their political interests. Reverend D. James Kennedy's address to the Christian Coalition in 2005 is an example of the values of this strong voting block and their leader's calls to political power, "Our job is to reclaim America for Christ, whatever the cost. As the vice regents of God, we are to exercise godly dominion and influence over our neighborhoods, our schools, our government, our literature and arts, our sports arenas, our entertainment media, our news media, our scientific endeavors—in short, over every aspect and institution of human society." Much like temperance, political power often precedes certain foundational Christian values such as service to the poor. Exercising domination over others is hardly loving our neighbor as ourselves. Therefore, perhaps we should examine the multiple intersecting relationships between what we understand to be our spiritual–social values and our political acting. Keep or remove?

What then, are we to make of the relationship between faith, politics, and policy? Does the relationship between Trump and his supporters signal a marriage of convenience or a consignment by white people of faith in the president's signature achievements thus far? While evidence exists that white evangelical protestants are among the most likely to support the hardline immigration policies (Thomson-DeVeaux, 2018) that have been implemented under the Trump administration, there are economic questions at stake as well, particularly the signature tax policy that will overwhelmingly benefit the wealthiest Americans (Thompson, 2017). Have evangelicals pushed their candidate into office on a wave of support for a Supreme Court nominee (or nominees) that align with their reform agenda? Or, have the wealthy coopted the religious right to ensure that tax policies will preserve and protect their fortune? This embroilment of Christianity and capitalism is nothing new in America, and yet as a nation we continue to grapple with the consequences of the myriad entanglements of piety, politics, economic growth, and social policy.

To begin to sort out this tangled web and consider its ramifications for understanding the temperance movement and support for prohibition, it is imperative to consider the landscape of early 19th-century America and the specific place Protestantism held in that landscape. The Jacksonian democracy of the early 1800s was accompanied by Jacksonian attitudes toward Native Americans and the subsequent brutality of removal policies. Newly opened territories were cleared and access was expanded through new transportation networks. The growth of the nation's borders coincided with a growth in the economy, but this early industrialization brought its ubiquitous companions: poverty, greed, and vice. In response, a spirit of reform sprung up from the citizenry that was channeled through a variety of mediums.

As the nation changed, the role of the church was shifting as well. Rather than holding sway over local communities and bodies politic, clergy and laymen alike had to reconsider their relationship to the evolving and ever-expansive secular government. Additionally, the church needed to respond to the social changes brought about by the extreme geographic distance between communities and the increasing concentrations of poverty and diversity in growing cities. Finally, the religious fervor engendered by the "long Great Awakening" was establishing fundamental tenets of American Christianity while setting up fault lines that would continue as evangelicalism began to grow throughout this time period (Kidd, 2008).

Historians of the era have considered several interpretations of what caused reform to permeate this time of rapid expansion and ecclesiastical restructuring. Early attempts to explain this spirit dwelled on traits considered to be interwoven in the American spirit, a general humanitarianism engendered by democratic ideals and Christian faith (Tyler, 2013). Later, scholars seized upon explanations that specifically outlined the manner by which reform efforts enhanced the control of the middle- and upper classes by way of punitively denying freedom to the lower classes and enforcing a specific way of being that accorded with their ideal habitus (Bourdieu, 1977). Finally, there are those who attempt to find middle ground between these humanitarian and social control perspectives, emphasizing the utility of the outcome for promoting a social hierarchy while recognizing that reformers genuinely believed they were making the world a better place (Walters, 1997).

While reform took many directions during this era, including the introduction of the common school, prison reform, care for the mentally ill, and women's rights, no issue better highlights the way that organized religion, business interests, and political influence were intertwined than the state control of alcohol production or consumption. The following essays explore two distinct interpretations of the impetus for this particular reform in the early nineteenth century.

Alice Felt Tyler offers the analysis that Antebellum reformers were primarily motivated by ideals in service to the American Republic. She claims that temperance reform was the natural evolution of America's democratic and evangelical spirit. David Donnald suggests that the reform movements emerged, in part, from the "status revolts" against a society in which power had shifted to slave owners and industrialists. Still other historians suggest that the movement was an effort of the haves to further their own interests over the have-nots. The upper- and middle-class reformers in the eyes of these historians tried to impose morality on the lower class, denying their freedoms as means of control. Some take umbrage with claims to social control, suggesting instead that the reformers were simply imposing their sense of morality on others.

The following pieces consider varying interpretations of historical efforts to moderate or abolish the consumption of alcohol in the United States in the first half of the nineteenth century. Laura Schmidt contextualizes the vital role that religion played in stimulating calls for reform. Specifically, she considers the pressures plaguing Protestant churches at the time who grappled with the "crisis of contested authority." Campaigns to end vice among individuals and throughout society via the state lent organized religion a new authority, and reasserted its vitality in a changing world. Reform then asserted the role of religion in political affairs as a response to the specific challenges facing the church. John Rumbarger conversely makes the case for market forces driving temperance reforms. Specifically, the employers of the growing industrial and agricultural economy sought ways to curb the drinking practices of their employees in order to promote efficiency. Therefore, reform was a tool of the capitalist class to assert political control in an effort to maximize profitability.

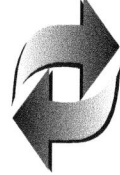

YES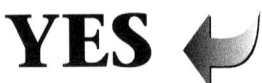

Laura A. Schmidt

"A Battle Not Man's but God's": Origins of the American Temperance Crusade in the Struggle for Religious Authority

To all . . . in antagonism to this great evil, I would say, THE BATTLE IS NOT YOUR'S BUT GOD'S. And yet, that I may not be misapprehended, and that none may be lulled into inaction, I would .first observe, Your's most rightly and properly it is. . . . In a word, your's it is as living in an age when the ravages of intemperance are most deeply felt, and when it can be expelled only by agency and instrumentality;—your's, for God has made it such and will hold you responsible for the vigorous and exterminating warfare. And yet, it is not your's. This is a paradox which the men of this world will not understand.

–John Marsh (1788–1868)
The Temperance Battle Not Man's But God's

Major theories of the origins of American temperance have emphasized materialist explanations without taking seriously enough the independent role of ideas—and, in particular, religious ideas—in stimulating the reform. Joseph Gusfield's (1965) classic study, for example, interpreted early temperance mobilization as a battle between shifting status groups, emphasizing the political cleavage between Federalists and Republicans as a crucial dimension. Harry Levine's (1978a, 1978b) studies locate sources of temperance reform in changing class structure and in new demands for inner-discipline arising from maturing entrepreneurial capitalism; consistent with this, temperance ideology is secularized as a "modem" and "bourgeois" ideology of self-control. Rorabaugh's analysis (1979) focuses on republican dimensions in the rhetoric of reformers; he locates sources of the movement in rising spirits consumption and in growing demands for controls on heavy drinking in the early republic. These studies have illuminated important facets of the movement. However, the implication of much current theoretical analysis of temperance is that the religious ideas which preoccupied its early proponents were of little consequence to the ultimate origins of the movement. Rather, they suggest that what was *really* important were deeper and more tangible developments at the levels of the social structure, economic and political systems. These developments, it is implied, were far more important than what contemporaries had to say about the reasons for instigating temperance reform. Consequently, current theories have tended to cast temperance ideology as an epiphenomenon related to material factors rather than as a direct cause of the reform and may have overemphasized its secular and political dimensions.

In viewing early temperance from the vantage point of our so-called "modem," "postindustrial," and "secular" society, we are prone to dismiss the significance of reformers' claims that their crusade was a "battle not man's but God's." But to its early advocates in America, temperance was a domestic holy war of social significance equaling that of the then recently concluded War for Independence—a war that would this time be fought for independence from an internal and spiritual foe of the republic. The early movement's goals extended well beyond a strictly political agenda to encompass loftier and less worldly ambitions. These included a spiritual regeneration within the masses and the moral transformation of seemingly corrupt government institutions. Through persuasive argument and the practice of "moral education," early temperance reformers believed they could assist in the transformation of depraved and irreligious sinners into virtuous citizens. Through the political activism and organized suffrage of that spiritually regenerated citizenry, they ultimately sought to cleanse corrupt government institutions of vice and irreligion, and to institute a new "moral government" modeled on divine institutions.

The religious origins of the American temperance movement and its ideology lie in what I will call a "crisis of contested authority" that befell the Protestant denominations descended from Puritanism during the early years of the 19th century. Here I refer to the fact that most ideologues, including American religious leaders in the Puritan tradition, stand in a tradition of inherited ideas not of their own creation. And as a result, from time to time they must face the problem of maintaining the relevance of these traditional views as historical events and social circumstances unfold in unpredictable ways. Such are the difficulties currently faced by orthodox Marxists in the aftermath of the Eastern European revolutions of 1989, and by leaders of the Mormon church as their doctrinal predictions of the coming of the millennium at precise dates and times have failed to materialize. As events in history challenge the credibility of traditional views, there is often only one solution available to ideologues of the old regime of ideas. That is to preserve their own authority and the authority of their beliefs by introducing revisions or "making adjustments," thus bringing traditional ideas more into line with a changing social order.[1]

It was precisely such "adjustments" to traditional Puritan ideas, made in response to a crisis of contested religious authority, that would ultimately become the ideology of the temperance movement. One outgrowth of the crisis that afflicted the churches during the early years of the 19th century was a new kind of religious ideology and strategy for winning converts *en masse*. The new approach offered interested clergymen innovative and more effective tools for promoting the public observance of religious obligations and moral standards, and thus for ensuring the salvation of souls. Around the mid-1810s, this new vision and strategy coalesced into a voluntary campaign to rid the American republic of vice and irreligion. While still linked to the churches in its ideology, goals, and leadership, the campaign against vice retained formal autonomy from the denominational hierarchy through the creation of independent and voluntary "moral societies." It was this religiously inspired anti-vice crusade that would contribute an infrastructure and core of beliefs for an abiding movement to suppress intemperance in America.

This article will trace back these religious sources of American temperance and its ideology of reform by examining the movement's formative years, between 1800 and 1825. I shall begin by examining the sources of a crisis in the authority of traditional Puritan doctrine apparent after 1800, and the predicament this vacuum created for religious leaders attached to these doctrine, especially those in the Presbyterian and Congregational churches. The second section of this article traces in the public addresses and personal writings of clergymen in these churches the development of a response to this ideological crisis, in a new theology focused on religious salvation through the suppression of vice. Third, I show how this new ideology provided the symbolic resources for organizing an independent crusade against vice, and how, when put into practice, it naturally led followers to focus their reform efforts more narrowly on the vice of intemperance. Finally, this article considers how temperance ideology and voluntary moral societies provided clergymen with a platform outside the churches, and a new approach for reestablishing the influence of religious ideas over individual moral conduct, as well as for leveraging government reform. Thus, the focus of this historical narrative will be on developing an alternative interpretation of the role of temperance in America, and one that will hold implications for how we understand the meaning of the movement's unique ideology: at least initially, temperance was part of a new kind of effort to assert the authority of religious ideas in the public sphere, and to regroup religious forces under auspices outside the church.

Sources

There has been some scholarly debate about exactly when and by whom a temperance movement was instigated in America. Some historians have de-emphasized the continuity between church-based action against vice in the 1810s and the national temperance campaign of the latter 1820s and 1830s (for a critique of these studies, see Rohrer, 1990). However, newer studies have shown how early anti-vice reforms by Presbyterian and Congregational leaders were linked to the fully flowered national temperance crusade (e.g., Bernard, 1991; Rohrer, 1990), suggesting that these were "the same movement at different stages of development" (Rohrer, 1990, p. 235). They have also urged further research into the role of reform efforts during the 1810s in providing an ideological and organizational infrastructure for a national temperance campaign. This issue, in turn, has served as a focus for this study in selecting sources from the abundant materials on early temperance.

Sources for this study thus involve a review of historical materials on relationships between the Protestant churches and the early temperance movement, emphasizing biographical materials on those men who shared significant roles in both, such as the Reverends Timothy Dwight and Lyman Beecher. In particular, Beecher has been noted both for his central role in founding early moral societies and for his leadership in the national temperance crusade, being credited by historians inside the movement as temperance reform's "great pioneer" (Cherrington, 1920, p. 66; see also Dorchester, 1886, p. 119). Sources selected for this study concentrated on the New England Presbyterian and Congregational churches where early leaders were based, and on the temperance movement's formative period between 1800 and 1825. This period begins with the emergence of an active public dialogue about vice and intemperance and ends with the emergence of a national temperance campaign, signified in the founding of the American Temperance Society in 1826.

Within these boundaries of time and place, a variety of types of sources were consulted, including both primary and secondary historical materials. The latter included histories of early temperance and biographies of early reformers, as well as similar materials on the early 19th-century churches and revival movement, sometimes called the "Second Great Awakening." Accounts of historians from both inside (e.g., Cherrington, 1920; Dorchester, 1886, 1888) and outside (e.g., Clark, 1976; Krout, 1925; Tyrrell, 1979) the temperance movement were consulted. Primary sources include the diaries, autobiographies, religious writings, and personal correspondence available on early church-based movement organizers.[2] Also consulted were compilations of sermons, tracts, and the recorded minutes of national temperance society meetings from the earliest years that these are available, that is, from the 1820s.

Religious Origins of American Temperance

A Crisis of Contested Religious Authority

We begin by considering the position of church leaders in the denominations descended from Puritanism—in particular, Presbyterians and Congregationalists—during the first two decades of the 19th century. Religious leadership at this time faced a crisis of legitimacy that affected not only the political power and influence enjoyed by members of the clergy but also, more importantly, the very meaning and relevance of its traditional belief system. This involved a crisis over the authority of traditional religious ideas, brought about by historic change during the period of nation building that followed the American Revolution.

As established in the colonial period, the traditional role of the Puritan clergy granted religious leadership and religiously defined collective goals a central place in civic affairs. The public mandate of clergymen had been to move the colonies toward closer approximation of Calvinism's central political ideal, the "godly commonwealth."[3] In the Puritan tradition of Calvinism in America, a tradition often referred to as "covenant theology," salvation was a public good shared by a whole community of the "elect," who were linked together and to God by a "national covenant"; just as the individual convert made an "internal covenant" with God, the whole community pledged adherence to a religiously inspired, but politically binding, moral code that dictated its shared fate (Bellah, 1975). As a result, religious leaders aspired to a central role in governing the collectivity according to religious precepts. In New England townships, ideally, clergymen forged political alliances with "godly magistrates," thus allowing civic and religious authorities to enforce public piety together and "from above," which ensured the observance of religious obligations specified by the national covenant. Through repressive measures prohibiting vice, such as Sabbath-breaking, profanity, drunkenness, and even "idle tippling" on Sundays, they could ensure religious compliance and, ultimately, collective salvation (Blocker, 1989; Lender, 1973; Lender and Martin, 1982). Thus, when in the 1690s Puritan divine Cotton Mather perceived a "flood of excess drinking" to be "drowning Christianity," he joined with other men of the cloth to influence civil authorities to carry out stricter enforcement of legal controls on tavern licensing (Krout, 1925, pp. 53–54). Indeed, in many New England townships, the process of licensing taverns routinely involved consultation with local clergy as to the social standing of prospective tavern-keepers (Conroy, 1991).

However, by the end of the Revolution, it had become evident that religious leaders in the tradition of covenant theology would face new and discernable challenges to their capacity to enforce piety and religious practices through legal mandate. The ministries' problems were most tangibly evident in rising church disestablishment that progressed on a state by state basis during the first decades of the 19th century. They were also evident in the institution of a new secular regime which, after 1800, proved highly unsympathetic to the clergyman's concerns. In the years immediately following the war, the clergy had grown more sensitive to what one described as "a monopolizing spirit in some politicians, who would exclude clergymen from all attention to matters of state and government" (Jeremy Belknap quoted in Banner, 1970, p. 157). However, it was institution of the Jefferson regime in 1800 that produced undeniable evidence of flagrant "irreligion" at even the highest ranks of government (Dwight, 1801, p. 532). As a deist and admirer of French secular philosophies, Thomas Jefferson embodied the growing threat to religious authority. An active critic of traditional revealed religion, he had once described Calvinist dogma as the "deliria of crazed imaginations" (Jefferson, 1822, p. 516). Perhaps more alarming to the clergy was the fact that, as a statesman in Virginia, Jefferson had played a central role in that state's disestablishment movement (Smith et al., 1960).

Disestablishment and the growing influence of secular authorities unsympathetic to religious concerns posed clear challenges to the practical authority of the clergy in carrying out their divine mandate. However, these developments also raised a more tacit challenge to the authority of the traditional doctrine to which the clergy was attached. For leaders in the tradition of covenant theology, there was first the problem of how to reconcile their own worldly failure and declining influence with a traditional view of the clergy as privileged leaders of God's "elect." Moreover, it was in the early decades of the republic that religious leaders first faced the problem of how they were to coexist with the nation's first fully legitimate and secular government—and one that with Jefferson had grown visibly hostile. In this new context, how would men of the cloth now fulfill their theocratic vision of a "holy commonwealth" cooperatively administered along religious lines by clergy and the "godly magistrates" of government?

Concern about the challenged authority of traditional beliefs manifested in a growing preoccupation among clergymen with the waning influence of religion over individual moral conduct and with the apparent growing popularity of vice and "irreligion." Thus, in 1798, the Presbyterian General Assembly called for a national day of fasting and atonement, so that the public might "heed its ecclesiastical 'watchmen,' cease backsliding, and return to ancestral piety" (Berk, 1974, p. 124). Congregational leaders such a Timothy Dwight publicly expressed concern over the more acquisitive lifestyle and growing immorality of a "backsliding generation," attributable to postwar economic boom and the war experience itself. Exposure to British and French "infidel philosophies" of the Enlightenment and the "loose opinions and loose practices" of foreign soldiers were claimed to have fostered irreligion among the American public (Dwight, 1801, pp. 531–532). Other clergymen blamed the unholy transformation in public morality on the apparent indifference of secular officials (no longer "godly magistrates") to moral misconduct, and their abandonment of colonial laws prohibiting vice:

> Our institutions, civil and religious have outlived that domestic discipline and official vigilance in magistrates which rendered obedience easy and habitual. The laws are now beginning to operate extensively upon necks unaccustomed to the yoke, and when they shall become irksome to the majority, their execution will become impracticable. . . . Drunkards reel through the streets day after day, and year after year, with entire impunity. Profane swearing is heard, and even by magistrates as though they heard it not. Efforts to stop traveling on the Sabbath have in all places become feeble, and in many places have wholly ceased. . . . The mass is changing. We are becoming another people. (Beecher, pub. 1866, vol. 1, p. 192; see also Beecher, 1814)

Geographic expansion in the early years of the 19th century raised additional logistical problems for clergymen who hoped to sustain religious enthusiasm among populations on the newly settled frontier—or to fulfill what they perceived to be an urgent need for "disciplining the West" (Sweet, 1936). Because the Presbyterian and Congregational churches were highly centralized with hierarchies yoked to colleges in New England, it proved difficult for them to effectively reach out to dispersed populations in the settlement regions (Berk, 1974). Moreover, high educational standards for clergymen led to a significant shortage of preachers to meet the demand for new churches on the frontier (Cross, 1950). These problems appeared particularly acute in light of the highly effective missionary approach of the fast-growing revival movement and evangelical churches of Methodists, Quakers, and Baptists. The latter had evolved more decentralized organizations that catered their ministries to the frontier situation. They used camp meetings, mobile tent churches, as well as circuit-riding and lay preachers to deliver religious inspiration to scattered populations in an efficient manner (Keller, 1942; Niebuhr, 1929; Norwood, 1974; Nottingham, 1944).

These practical problems for the Presbyterian and Congregational ministries also corresponded to deeper problems with the legitimacy and appeal of traditional doctrine in a changing nation. Liberty, of course, was the "great theme" of the early republic, enshrined in the public sentiment by the revolutionaries' success against British tyranny (Hatch, 1977; Heimert, 1966); under the Jeffersonian Republicans, democratic enthusiasm had been translated into an egalitarian emphasis on the governing power of the "common man." In the face of this growing republican optimism, traditional Puritan doctrine of predestination, election and original sin imposed a harsh alternative focused on a characterization of humans as essentially depraved, and completely impotent with regard to their own salvation for instance, their pessimistic world view was summarized in the Presbyterians' confession of faith declaring all men to be "utterly indisposed, disabled, and made opposite to all good." Even more dissonant was the clergy's theocratic vision of a holy commonwealth that emphasized mass obedience to religious authority in the face of a growing republican emphasis on the authority of the "common man." Again, the contrast with the rising evangelical churches and revival movement was stark, as these faiths proselytized a "democratized theology" emphasizing the spiritual "inner light" within all believers, lay authority to preach, and human agency in spiritual matters (McLoughlin, 1978; Niebuhr, 1929).

The threat to religious leadership deepened when doctrinal disputes erupted within the Presbyterian and Congregational churches. After 1800, a liberal faction began to unify and strengthen, adopting a gentler and more optimistic interpretation of traditional views (Haroutunian, 1932; Keller, 1942; Youngs, 1990). In opposition, an increasingly recalcitrant cleavage of "Old School" and "Consistent Calvinists" accused liberals of fomenting a "dark conspiracy" to subvert Puritanism (McLoughlin, 1959, p. 15) and held steadfastly to the traditional vision of human depravity and impotence in salvation—a view that their liberal critics came to call a "willingness-to-be-damned" notion of salvation (McLoughlin, 1978, p. 101). By the 1830s, this doctrinal controversy would devolve into a schism within the Presbyterian church, at which time the conservative-dominated hierarchy would exscind nearly half of its churches and ministers (McLoughlin, 1959; Sweet, 1936).

To summarize, at the turn of the 18th century, religious leaders in the Presbyterian and Congregational churches found themselves in a new, postcolonial nation where their capacity to enforce religious obligations and public piety "from above" had been significantly curtailed. Disestablishment and a new secular government of nonsympathizers limited the practical authority of clergymen, while westward expansion raised new logistical problems in spreading their brand of religion to the frontier. However, beneath these more tangible aspects of their predicament lay a deeper, tacit challenge to the very meaning and legitimacy of traditional beliefs. The Jefferson regime offered a valid alternative to the traditional religious ideal of America as a holy commonwealth. This was an alternative and secular ideology focused on personal freedom and human self-reliance whose growing authority deeply undermined the Puritan tradition's view of a depraved and helpless human condition. Among the ranks of the clergy, these difficulties gave rise to growing concerns about how they would promote public compliance with religious dictates and thus ensure collective salvation under the national covenant. And within the denominational hierarchy, the challenge to traditional ideas surfaced in internal conflicts between doctrinal liberals and conservatives.

The Clergy's Response in a Crusade against Vice

It was from the liberal side of the doctrinal cleavage that a response to the ministry's problems of contested authority was organized. The crisis of religious belief had left an opening for new ideas to take hold. After 1800, theologian and president of Yale College Timothy Dwight, assisted by students and followers such as Lyman Beecher and Nathaniel Taylor,[4] began to fill the breech with a series of revisions to Puritan ideas. Their doctrinal interpretations came to be known as the "New Divinity" or "New Haven Theology." This new religious ideology focused on, among other things, spiritual salvation through the suppression of vice and would ultimately provide religious justification for an enduring movement to suppress intemperance. But, initially, Dwight called for organized action to combat vice, broadly defined, and so his students began by organizing their fellow Yale undergraduates into voluntary associations against Sabbath breaking, dueling, profanity, fornication, and intemperance (Beecher, pub. 1866, vol. 1, pp. 26–33; Marsh, pub. 1866, pp. 10–12). These men would later carry the campaign against vice into their parishes and, in 1813, would begin to find some of the first voluntary "moral societies" or associations that one historian has described as "transitional organizations between churches and single-aim temperance associations" (Bernard, 1991, p. 344).[5]

A response by the challenged ministry was initiated by Dwight in the years immediately following the Jefferson victory in 1800. In his public oratory and theological writings, Dwight began to focus on a characterization of the new federal regime as comprised of dangerous "religious infidels" and the unsaved. In particular, he pointed to Jefferson's fascination with the French *philosophes* and the Republican's support of a strong political alliance with France as dangerously misguided. The case of the French republic offered concrete evidence of the anarchy and violence that would befall the republic that, under the influence of secular "infidel philosophies" of the Enlightenment, denied its religious obligations. France had "denied the existence of moral obligation, annihilated the distinction between virtue and vice, challenged and authorized the indulgence of every lust, strode down the barriers of truth, . . . and [thus] dared the thunder, of the Almighty" (Dwight, 1801, p. 534).

By demonizing the new secular authorities, Dwight had aligned religious leadership with the higher authority of God, who was now referred to as the "moral Governor." Perhaps more significant, he did so by appealing to a traditional religious characterization of the American nation drawn from covenant theology. This was a powerful imagery of the nascent republic as an "elected" or "chosen people"—a "new American Jerusalem"—which was bound to the deity by a national covenant or "heavenly contract" that specified its moral obligations. On the one hand, the newfound liberties and material abundance enjoyed by Americans following the Revolution was clear evidence of the republic's unique status as the "favorite land of heaven" (see Beecher, 1826, p. 3). On the other hand, the new republic was still engaged in a tenuous "experiment in civil liberties" that, under improper leadership, could yield results as disastrous as those of the French republic, fraught with anarchy and social disorder (Beecher, 1828). Unprecedented liberties and material abundance were evidence of Americans' holy "election" as a people, but also called upon a nation of Christians to exercise greater moral restraint in the face of increased temptation. In Dwight's (1778, p. 13) words, "Nothing obstructs the deliverance of America, but the crimes of its inhabitants." And as his protege, Lyman Beecher (pub. 1828, p. 48) warned collective indulgence in vices such as intemperance would inevitably bring the nation to destruction both economically and morally, thus leading to a failed republican experiment: "Communities which rise by the violation of the laws of humanity and equity, shall not prosper, and especially that wealth amassed by promoting intemperance, will bring upon the community intemperance, and poverty, and shame, as providential retribution." Thus, his sermons spun out vivid scenes of the "providential retribution" to surely follow if the republic were to betray its religious obligations under its national covenant with God: "Let loose from wholesome restraint, and taught sin by the example of the great, a scene most horrid to be conceived, but more dreadful to be experienced, will ensue. No people are more fitted for destruction, if they go to destruction, than we ourselves" (Beecher, pub. 1866, vol. 1, p. 193).

Reflected in these words is a type of religious apprehension that Max Weber (1922, 1930) referred to in his writings on Puritanism as "salvation anxiety." No longer able to enforce public adherence to strict colonial standards of moral conduct "from above," these religious leaders suffered from an acute preoccupation with the nation's potential for damnation and providential retribution—an anxiety that deepened as evidence of the uncontrollable immorality and vice of its people accumulated. As Beecher (pub. 1828, p. 4) bluntly put it, "A nation of drunkards would constitute a hell." Dwight and his followers believed themselves and their whole generation to be at a critical juncture with regard to the nation's spiritual progress and it's fulfillment of the terms of the national covenant: "All the great designs which God has to answer by planting our fathers here in this nation and world depend, as I believe, on the efforts of this generation to rescue their institutions from perversion" (Beecher, pub. 1866, vol. 2, p. 131).

Anxiety over the moral fate of the nation compelled these clergymen to instigate "vigorous, exterminating warfare" against what Dwight called the growing "sins of prosperity." Significantly, their appeal to the public hinged on a blend of two moral ideals: on the one hand, it was based on the Puritan imagery of a covenant between God and an "elect" people, and on the other hand, it was based on the republican vision of virtuous citizenship and independent nationhood. To Dwight and his followers, vice and moral misconduct imperiled the survival of a republican nation and its social order because they could corrupt the civic virtue and "self-government" of a citizenry from within. In particular, the vice of intemperance was a perditious "fiery flood" that could quickly consume the frail republic (Dwyer, 1977, p. 189). As Beecher warned,

> Republican institutions are guaranteed to the states, and the whole nation watches with sleepless vigilance the altar of liberty. But a mighty despot, whose army is legion, has invaded the land. . . . And now, ye venerable and honorable men, raised to seats of legislation in a nation which is the freest, and is destined to become the greatest, and may become the happiest upon earth—can you, will you behold unmoved the march of this mighty evil? . . . And deliberately dig the grave of our liberties—and entomb the last hope of enslaved nations—and nothing be done by the national government to stop the destroyer? (Beecher, pub. 1828, p. 100)

Defeat of this national foe, vice, would be achieved through domestic holy war—a "battle not man's but God's." Such an effort would require unification of the devout into an ecumenical "band of Christian heroes," forming a "phalanx of opposition" against encroaching immorality and vice (Beecher, pub. 1828, pp. 91–92). The war against vice would seek collective spiritual salvation. But it would also liberate those individuals enslaved by vice, such as the drunkard, who was a "shameless slave of appetite" (Kirkland, 1814, p. 12). Put simply, Dwight and his colleagues had proposed a moral crusade that would extend the republicans' War for Independence onto the spiritual plane.

The Theology of Temperance

The idea of a crusade against vice called for a new strategy by which to directly "regulate public sentiment"; in other words, some alternative to the colonial approach that had applied repressive laws to directly prohibit moral misconduct. As Lyman Beecher lamented, "Our fathers could enforce morality by law; but the times are changed; and unless we can regulate public sentiment, and secure morality in some other way, WE ARE UNDONE" (Beecher, pub. 1828, p. 33). This was achieved through the introduction of a new religious ideology that can be described as an original and deeply compromised Puritan theology. It was this new religious ideology that would ultimately provide a core of beliefs and rationale for temperance activism by Beecher's and subsequent generations.

In particular, this "New Divinity" bore strong consistencies with republicanism in its adoption of a more optimistic view of human empowerment in salvation, and in its more democratically inclusive vision of the Puritan "elect." In place of the traditional idea of election by God and the harsh belief that humans could do nothing to assure their salvation, Dwight suggested that humans had "freedom of choice" concerning sin, and therefore played an important role in their own salvation. By implication, this opened up the possibility of salvation to all who would "elect" themselves through the choice to abstain from moral misconduct; as Dwight's student Nathaniel Taylor put it, every soul had the ability to "choose aright" (McLoughlin, 1978; Mead, 1967). Thus, by 1830, Beecher (pub. 1866, vol. 2, p. 162) would observe that under the influence of these new ideas, "Thirty years ago, ten sermons were preached in New England, on *total depravity* and *election* to one that is preached on those subjects now" (italics in original).

The new emphasis on freedom of choice in salvation led to an alternative view of the conversion process, as one of rational decision-making and orderly spiritual preparation (Berk, 1974, p. 92). This was a view that was quite different from the traditional Puritan idea of human helplessness but also different from the internal focus and emotionalism that characterized conversion in revival religion. Distrusting the subjectivity and fleetingness of revival experiences, a "valid" conversion demanded self-control and would result from careful consideration and rational decision-making. This more subdued spirituality was recognizable by

> a mild, but constant and intense desire of heart for the awakening and conversion of sinners. When I say intense, I do not mean agitating, but strong and steady. A fullness and strength of desire, which does not ruffle the passions, and is compatible with the most cool and collected state of mind, both for planning and action. (Marsh, pub. 1866, p. 64)

Rational choice in salvation also implied a new role for the clergyman: he was to facilitate a rational and deliberate "turning" of the layperson from sinfulness using "moral education," a technique that prepared and moved the soul through the persuasive presentation of religious truths. Through "example and influence" the pastor taught moral restraint and "self-government" (Kirkland, 1814, p. 6); he was "God's agent and interpreter, who could tell one how to be saved, yet torment one with threats of damnation" (Cross, 1950, p. 28). Thus, Beecher (pub. 1866, vol. 2, pp. 75–76) described how persuasive argument and careful reasoning could be put to good use in moral education of the "infidel and skeptical class":

> They had the idea that ministers scorned them, and that ministers were this, that, and the other. But it was necessary to go over with them, and trip up their arguments; for until they were tripped up and crippled, logic was of little avail. So I put myself on the highest key with them, used the highest language and strongest arguments, and made them feel that somebody else knew something besides themselves; and then they came, meek as lambs, and were easily gained.

Finally, the idea of morally educating the public shifted the emphasis in religious practice away from traditional Puritan inward piety and onto politically focused moralism. Moral education taught the converted to take "VIGOROUS ACTION FOR GOD" (Beecher, pub. 1828) through efforts to reduce vice and moral misconduct in society at large, cultivating what Dwight called a "moral environment." Moral agents were to fight back against corruption and irreligion in secular government with the explicit goal of instituting a "moral government" modeled on divine institutions:

> Civil government is an ordinance of God, established for his glory, and for the good of men. Rulers stand in the place of God. . . . And in all acts of legislation they must be on the Lord's side—resisting all evil, protecting the people from evil doers, and sustaining the principles of God's moral government. (Marsh, pub. 1858, p. 15)

It is notable that this vision of a "moral government" was distinctively republican in its emphasis on individual freedom and the cultivation of civic virtue. Indeed, efforts to reform government would draw liberally on the strengths of a democracy, remodeling government "from below" through moral education of the electorate in correct voting choices. As Beecher (pub. 1828, p. 94) put it, "Republics must be prepared by moral sentiment for efficient legislation." It would be through the power of suffrage that a campaign against vice could ultimately reinstate a new regime of "godly magistrates" in the American republic:

> The suffrage of the community may be expected to put in requisition men of talents and integrity, who, sustained by their constituents, will not hesitate to frame the requisite laws, and to give to them their salutary power. Even now there may be an amount of suffrage, could it be concentrated and expressed, to sustain laws which might go to limit the evil [of vice and intemperance]; but it is scattered, it is dispersed, unorganized interest. (Beecher, pub. 1828, p. 94)

Organizing against Intemperance

It was in organizing the "scattered" and "dispersed" interests favoring anti-vice reform into voluntary moral societies, that the new religious ideology of Dwight and his followers was made readily available for mass consumption. In 1813, Beecher and other clergymen organized some of the first moral societies that quite soon thereafter began to focus specifically on suppressing the vice of intemperance. These organizations would prove significant in providing an infrastructure for the national temperance campaign, and in establishing within this infrastructure a core of ideas and symbolic practices informed by the unique religious ideology of its founders.[6] Thus, reflected in the temperance society's practice of signing the pledge to abstain from distilled spirits would be New Divinity theology's vision of conversion as a rational, deliberate choice, and "heavenly contract." Temperance oratory and written tracts would use moral education to inform the public of moral and medical "truths" regarding intoxicants (Keller, 1942). Temperance societies would agitate for government reform by organizing the suffrage toward moral reform, initially by amassing supporters at town meetings to vote down new liquor licenses and to encourage enforcement of colonial laws prohibiting vice. Later, a growing anti-vice constituency would take more daring political action, demanding new anti-alcohol legislation to increase prices, impose harsher sanctions on drunkenness as a civil offense, and, ultimately, institute prohibition on the local level (Dorchester, 1888; Krout, 1925).

Initially, the moral societies organized their assault on vice, broadly defined, seeking generally to rid society of "Sabbath-breakers, rumselling, tippling folk, infidels and ruff-scruff" (Beecher, pub. 1866, vol. 1, p. 251). However, in the practical context of implementing moral reform, the original emphasis of a crusade against vice in general appears to have quickly narrowed to a more specific focus on the vice of intemperance. It has been suggested that temperance became a central object of concern when it did because of a precipitous increase in rates of alcohol consumption and in alcohol-related social problems (Clark, 1976; Dorchester, 1886; Rorabaugh, 1979). However, attention to the unique religious ideology of the first moral societies suggests an alternative explanation. Under the influence of New Divinity theology's concept of conversion as a rational choice achieved through the discipline of moral education, abstinence from intoxicants became a necessary first step in what we might call a "triaged" approach to individual moral reform. In the practice of achieving a "turning" from immorality in converts through the methodical presentation of religious truths and careful guidance in rational decision-making, the disordering effects of drunkenness and the general "moral lethargy" it produced were an obvious initial barrier to success (Kirkland, 1814, p. 8). As one minister active in early temperance explained, within the mind under the influence of alcohol, "every moral and religious principle is dissipated" (Marsh, pub. 1859, p. 7). And Beecher (pub. 1828, pp. 35–36) corroborated that the drunkard suffered from "the extinction of all the finer feelings and amiable dispositions of the soul. . . . And as to religion, if he ever seemed to have any, all such affections declined as the emotions of artificial stimulants arose, until conscience has lost its power." This same viewpoint would be later reflected in the published minutes of the first meetings of the American Temperance Society as well:

> No sooner is a person brought under the power of intoxicating liquors, than he seems to be proof against the influence of all the means of reformation. If, at any time, the truth gains access to his mind, and impresses his heart, by a few draughts of this fatal poison, the impression is almost sure to be effaced. (American Temperance Society, 1835, p. 13)

Drunkenness also proved a significant obstacle to achieving the goal of moral reform at the collective level, which focused on the cultivation of a "moral environment" inhabited by a self-governed society compliant with a set of shared moral precepts. By disordering the mind of the individual, intoxicants fostered public disorder in a way that fornication, profanity, Sabbath-breaking, and other assorted vices did not. The disorder fostered by intemperance had no place in a democracy based on "self-government" and what Dwight called "rational liberty"; the drunkard [was] a menace to Dwight's ideal society because his intoxication deprive[d] him of 'reason' and 'self-control'" (Berk, 1974, p. 109).

On the specific cause of intemperance, however, the established churches generally proved to be "divided" and sometimes "apathetic" (Tyrrell, 1979, pp. 55–56), a fact that was apparently due largely to "wet" sentiment amidst the higher echelons of the church administrations.[7] For example, in approaching the 1812 Presbyterian General Assembly to appeal for organized church action on intemperance, Beecher found drinking to be "apparently universal" at official church functions, even to the point of "exhilaration" during ecclesiastical meetings (Beecher, pub. 1866, vol. 1, p. 179). According to Beecher's memoirs, after considering proposals for action on intemperance, church leadership concluded

> . . . that intemperance had been for some time increasing in a most alarming manner; but that, after the most faithful and prayerful inquiry, they were obliged to confess they did not perceive that anything could be done. The blood started through my heart when I heard this, and I rose instanter, and moved that a committee of three be appointed immediately, to report . . . [on] the ways and means of arresting the tide of intemperance. The committee was named and appointed. I was chairman, and on the following day brought in a report, the most important paper that ever I wrote. (Beecher, pub. 1866, vol. 1, p. 180)

It was in the abovementioned report that Beecher proposed the creation of independent "voluntary associations to aid the civil magistrate in the execution of the law" prohibiting intemperance.

The church hierarchy's disinterest in the temperance cause required moral activists to organize their campaign outside the auspices of the church. And in the long run, this would prove essential to the organizational growth and early success of the movement. As doctrinal controversy and resistance to change signaled a general decline in the churches' social influence, independent moral societies would offer interested clergymen a new kind of tool for promoting public morality, a democratic platform for influencing politics on moral issues and an alternative organizational base useful for attracting new converts and for saving souls. In contrast to the churches, temperance societies would evolve within a decentralized network of auxiliaries that could be rapidly proliferated, and which

could draw freely upon the prestige and skills of politically influential laymen in its highest ranks. As Beecher (pub. 1866, vol. 1, p. 190) explained, "That was a new thing in that day for the clergy and laymen to meet on the same level and co-operate. It was the first time there had ever been such a consultation between them in Connecticut in our day. The ministers had always managed things themselves, for in those days the ministers were all politicians."

Furthermore, independence from the church hierarchy would allow early temperance organizers to embrace the growing revival movement, or the "Second Great Awakening," as a rich source of spiritually readied moral agents. The conservative church hierarchy had staunchly resisted the revival movement as a heresy from its start in the first decade of the 19th century (Finney, pub. 1876; McLoughlin, 1959). Indeed, shortly after his ordination, Beecher himself had been appointed to spearhead a church committee to oust leading revivalist Charles Grandison Finney from the Presbyterian church. At the time, he had warned Finney that if the revivalist "streak of fire" entered his parish, he would meet Finney "at the State line, and call out the artillery-men, and fight every inch of the way" (Beecher, pub. 1866, vol. 2, p. 101). However, when Beecher later saw revivalism's powerful potential for "winning souls," he underwent his own "conversion" to revivalism—a gesture that years later would have him, too, tried for heresy by conservatives in the church. Ultimately, Beecher would personally invite Finney to conduct revival meetings in his own parish and would benefit directly from the awakening's potential to yield an abundant "harvest of souls" for the temperance cause (Beecher, pub. 1866, vol. 2, p. 90). In fact, revivals became so significant a resource for founding new temperance societies that Beecher came to view the awakening as "encouragement" from God (Beecher, pub. 1866, vol. 1, p. 182). Other clergymen described the success of revivals as a sign of divine endorsement for the temperance cause: "Now that God has so wonderfully revived religion in the nation, surely the temperance cause must follow in its wake, and soon witness blessed triumphs" (Marsh, pub. 1866, p. 81).

Indeed, Beecher and other early moral activists would not have to wait long to witness the "blessed triumphs" of a burgeoning movement to suppress intemperance. A short year after founding the first moral societies in Connecticut, they would see the proliferation of an additional 30 auxiliary societies in that state alone (Dorchester, 1888). By the 1830s, they would find themselves amidst the ranks of leadership for a temperance crusade of national scope, boasting a membership of over 1.5 million in over 8,000 local societies throughout the nation (Blocker, 1989).

Conclusion

This study has developed an alternative interpretation of the origins of American temperance, suggesting that the movement's beginnings are intrinsically linked to the response of clergymen in the early republic to a crisis of contested religious authority. At least initially, temperance was part of a larger effort by church leaders to secure a place for religious ideas in the public sphere and to guard collective salvation through the promotion of public obedience to religious prohibitions against vice. Historical change had brought about new practical problems for church leaders such as Dwight and Beecher, which included rising church disestablishment, the growing influence of secular authorities unsympathetic to the concerns of religious leadership, the challenge of ministering to an increasingly mobile and dispersed population, and doctrinal controversy. However, this study has emphasized that beneath these practical difficulties lay an even deeper crisis over the very meaning and relevance of the ministries' traditional religious ideas. Historical events and social change following the Revolution had brought about new challenges to the legitimacy of their core beliefs in human impotence in salvation, public obedience to religious authority and, most importantly, to their vision of the nation as a "holy commonwealth." For the first time, religious leaders faced a new and fully legitimate secular regime, one that with Jefferson offered a competing ideology of growing popular appeal. The new regime not only made a quite direct critique of revealed religion but also proposed a radically alternative vision for America emphasizing liberty, self-determination and political empowerment of the "common man."

I have suggested that, ultimately, the clergymen who went on to play leading roles in organizing temperance were willing to compromise on some of their traditional religious doctrine, if this allowed them to ensure public compliance with religious obligations to abstain from vice and immoral conduct. In the end, Dwight and his followers abandoned traditional Puritan dogma focused on human helplessness in salvation and inward piety. In place, they offered a new and more appealing religious ideology focused on individual freedom of choice in salvation and spiritual activism through democratic reform:

> Really bad ideas, such as original sin and divine complicity in evil were quietly set aside; others underwent drastic operations, and became no less harmless. . . . Damnation was postponed to the next world. Human depravity and regeneration by the Spirit of God were reconciled with "free moral agency," and moralized. . . . Such Calvinism was really not very objectionable, but it also was not Calvinism. It was the faith of the fathers ruined by the faith of their children. (Haroutunian, 1932, p. 281)

These modifications not only helped to restore the general appeal of religion, they also provided spiritual justification for instigating a public campaign against vice outside the auspices of the church, and therefore free from the constraints of tradition and sectarian controversy. Through moral education and persuasion of the public, clergymen could reassert the importance of religious prohibitions against vice on a mass basis. Moreover, by organizing the suffrage and voluntary moral activism of the masses, they could potentially cleanse corrupt government of "religious infidels" and fulfill their vision of a holy commonwealth in a radically new way: not through repressive measures enforced from above, but by creating a new, democratically elected "moral government" from below. Consequently, on the day of church disestablishment in his home state of Connecticut, Lyman Beecher could console himself with the thought that in voluntary efforts to campaign against vice and intemperance, clergymen had found a new means of preserving faith and morality in a changing nation: "They say ministers have lost their influence; the fact is, they have gained. By voluntary efforts, societies, missions, and revivals, they exert a deeper influence than ever . . ." (Beecher, pub. 1866, vol. 1, p. 253).

This study holds implications not only for interpreting the role of early temperance as a means for reasserting the authority of religious ideas but also suggests an alternative perspective on the meaning of the movement's unique ideology, and on how this new system of beliefs could operate independently to inspire and shape moral activism in America. I have argued that temperance activism in America arose out of a broader religious anxiety about the potential for rampant vice to bring social anarchy and heavenly retribution upon the new republic. The ultimate narrowing of the campaign against vice around the specific issue of intemperate drinking was a potential inherent in the particular system of religious ideas which early moral reformers had created. Their religious ideology emphasized rationality and inner-discipline in spiritual matters: religious awakening was a rational response to the careful consideration of religious truths conveyed through "moral education," while moral activism and other spiritual practices were carried out in a rational, detached manner—in "the most cool and collected state of mind, both for planning and action"

(Marsh, pub. 1866, p. 64). Consequently, drunkenness, more so than other vices such as fornication and profanity, was destined to become a central object of concern for moral reform. It fostered a mental disorderliness in the potential convert that proved a critical initial barrier to successful moral education. At the collective level, it fostered a social disorderliness completely incompatible with the ideals of a "moral environment" and self-governing society based on "rational liberty."

This study has also emphasized that the founding ideology of temperance blended moral ideals and imagery from both the Puritan and republican traditions. From this it follows that we should not be too quick to emphasize either its religious *or* political dimensions. Rather, we may best understand temperance ideology as a form of American "civil religion" (Bellah, 1970, 1975). This refers to the fact that, despite emphasis on religious pluralism and separation of church and state in America, a public religious dimension has persisted in our national political discourse. This is still with us today, for example, in the frequent use of biblical references during presidential inaugural addresses, including that of our current president who appealed for the public's commitment to a "new covenant." By drawing selectively on religious beliefs, symbols and rituals, American civil religion asserts political goals that obtain their inspiration and legitimacy from religious ones. It draws from the fund of religious ideas "powerful symbols of national solidarity . . . to mobilize deep levels of personal motivation for the attainment of national goals" (Bellah, 1970, p. 181).

As a type of civil religion, the founding ideology of American temperance was based on a masterful blend of Puritan and republican symbolism. Among adherents, these symbols deepened the significance of the movement's goals and justified the means of their attainment through "exterminating warfare" against public and government corruption. For example, rituals such as signing the temperance pledge not only "satisfied many patriotic longings" among participants, as Rorabaugh (1979, p. 194) has suggested, but also gave spiritual meaning and significance to participation by harking back to the Puritans' "heavenly contract" between God and the "elect." To be so "enlisted against intemperance" in "a band of Christian heroes" was made a duty of every Christian and true patriot (Beecher, pub. 1828, p. 4).

Temperance ideology drew one of its most powerful themes from missionary movements and episodes of religious crusading that have recurred throughout the history of Christianity (and for that matter, in other proselytizing religions as well, such as Islam). This was, of course, the idea of a holy war where the dramatic struggle between spiritual forces of good and evil would be played out in the world. Early reformers believed the American republic to be a "chosen people" blessed with new civil liberties and the revolutionary success, but still bound by the moral duties of its national covenant with God. The crusade against vice and intemperance, then, was powerfully conceived as a domestic holy war that would extend the War for Independence onto the spiritual plane. In voluntary societies, religious leaders would mobilize a "United Christian Army" to liberate the nascent republic from its enslavement to the internal tyrant, vice. This forceful idea, I am suggesting, could on its own compel vigorous moral activism because it held out two radically different outcomes for the American "experiment in civil liberties": national salvation achieved through the cultivation of a "rational liberty" that balanced republican freedoms with moral inhibitions, or "providential retribution," the inevitable result of unrestrained indulgence in vice and immorality. This was a powerful dualism that would sustain the enthusiasm of future generations of temperance activists, as historian J.A. Krout (1925, p. 124) observed: "Two pictures were constantly in their minds, one of a nation doomed to destruction because of the ravages of strong drink, the other of a nation happy and prosperous under a regimen of temperance." Through a careful alignment of the political and religious, temperance ideology had made inner-discipline, abstinence from vice and moral activism both spiritual requirements of the truly saved and civic duties of republican citizenship.

Acknowledgments

Source materials were obtained through the assistance of libraries at the Alcohol Research Group and Graduate Theological Union in Berkeley, CA, and through the Bancroft and Doe libraries of the University of California at Berkeley. This article has benefited from the comments of a number of people, but, in particular, from repeated and careful readings by Ron Roizen, Robin Room, Ann Swidler, and Jessica Warner. More broadly, my thoughts on Puritanism and temperance have been influenced by the ongoing discussions of the Study Group on Religion and Society at the Department of Sociology, University of California at Berkeley.

Notes

1. The observation that problems of contested authority experienced by political and religious elites can lead to the innovation of new ideologies is explored in the cultural histories of David

Zaret. For example, Zaret (1989) locates sources of liberal-democratic ideology in problems of contested authority arising for religious and political ideologues in the face of radical sectarian conflict during the English Revolution. A separate study drawing on similar arguments shows how pressures arising from the changing demands of laities led Puritan clergy in early modern England to introduce covenant theology and the notion of making a "heavenly contract" with God (Zaret, 1985).

2. Diaries and correspondence among temperance organizers, as well as their sermons and other public addresses, were often compiled and published by family members and temperance societies postmortem (or, at least, well after the actual recording of events) as tracts and edited volumes. In such cases, this is indicated next to the dates of reference citations in the text.

3. For fairly recent discussions of the Calvinist and Puritan political vision, and on its application in the colonies, see Miller (1961, 1967), Walzer (1972), and Zaret (1989).

4. Timothy Dwight (1752–1817) served as Yale College president from 1795 until he died. Lyman Beecher (1775–1863), served briefly as Congregational pastor in Long Island, was transferred to Litchfield, CT, where he stayed until 1826, at which point he was transferred again to a parish in Boston. Nathaniel Taylor (1786–1858) served as a pastor in Connecticut and ultimately took up Dwight's post at Yale in 1822.

5. It is worth noting that voluntary societies for the suppression of vice were not unique to the United States, and that Beecher, by reading international Christian publications, had been made well aware of similar organizations in England (Beecher, pub. 1866, vol. 1, p. 26). However, unlike the American case, English societies for "the reformation of manners" were sustained for only a brief period and did not evolve into a broader social movement (Curtis and Speck, 1976), a fact that, among other things, testifies to Tocqueville's observation that 19th-century Americans had a unique proclivity for voluntary participation.

6. Among the first societies was the Connecticut Society for the Reformation of Morals founded by Beecher, under Dwight's measured approval: "If my young friends think it best to proceed, God forbid that I should oppose or hinder them, or withhold my suffrage" (Beecher, pub. 1866, vol. 1, p. 180). The Massachusetts Society for the Suppression of Intemperance was also founded in this year by Presbyterian clergymen.

7. There was no clear biblical precedent for abstinence from intoxicants, especially with regard to wine, cider, and beer, which reformers ultimately defined as dangerous intoxicants. Moreover, unlike the Methodist and Quaker churches, those descended from Puritanism had no founding tradition of temperance (Cherrington, 1920; Warner et al., 1945). As a result, movement literature is replete with theological analyses and biblical justifications for temperance, as reformers quite narrowly came to define it (see, for example, Lees and Burns, 1894; Raymond, 1927).

References

American Temperance Society. Permanent Temperance Documents of the American Temperance Society, Vol. 1, Boston, MA: American Temperance Union, 1835 (reprint: Arno Press, New York, NY, 1972).

Banner, J.M. To the Hartford Convention: The Federalist Party and the Origins of Party Politics in Massachusetts, 1789–1815, New York: Alfred A. Knopf, Inc., 1970.

Beecher, L. A Reformation of Morals Practicable and Indispensable (sermon pamphlet), Andover, MA, 1814.

Beecher, L. The Memory of Our Fathers, Litchfield, Connecticut, 1826.

Beecher, L. Six Sermons on the Nature, Occasions, Signs, Evils and Remedy of Intemperance, Boston: T.R. Marvin, 1828.

Beecher, L. Autobiography, Correspondence, etc., of Lyman Beecher, Vols. 1 and 2, New York: Harper & Bros., 1866 (reprint: Harvard University Press, Cambridge, MA, 1961).

Bellah, R.N. Civil Religion in America. In: Bellah, R.N., Beyond Belief: Essays on Religion in a Post-Traditional World, New York: Harper & Row Publishers, Inc., 1970, pp. 168–189.

Bellah, R.N. The Broken Covenant: American Civil Religion in Time of Trial, 2nd Edition, Chicago, IL: University of Chicago Press, 1992.

Berk, S.E. Calvinism versus Democracy: Timothy Dwight and the Origins of American Evangelical Orthodoxy, Hamden, CT: Archon Books, 1974.

Bernard, J. From fasting to abstinence: The origins of the American temperance movement. In: Barrows, S. and Room R. (Eds.) Drinking: Behavior and Belief in Modern History, Berkeley, CA: Univ. of California Press, 1991, pp. 337–353.

Blocker, J.S. American Temperance Movements: Cycles of Reform, Boston, MA: Twayne Pubs., 1989.

Cherrington, E.H. The Evolution of Prohibition in the United States of America, Westerville, OH: American Issue Press, 1920 (reprint: Patterson Smith, Montclair, NJ, 1969).

Clark, N.H. Deliver Us from Evil: An Interpretation of American Prohibition, New York: W.W. Norton & Co., Inc., 1976.

Conroy, D.W. Puritans in taverns: Law and popular culture in Colonial Massachusetts, 1630–1720. In: Barrows, S. and Room, R. (Eds.) Drinking: Behavior and Belief in Modern History, Berkeley, CA: University of California Press, 1991, pp. 29–60.

Cross, W.R. The Burned-over District: The Social and Intellectual History of Enthusiastic Religion in Western New York, 1800–1850, Ithaca, NY: Cornell University Press, 1950.

Curtis, T.C. and Speck, W.A. The societies for the reformation of manners: A case study in the Theory and Practice of Moral Reform. Literat. Hist. **3**: 45–64, 1976.

Dorchester, D. The Inception of the Temperance Reformation. In: American Temperance Society. One Hundred Years of Temperance: A Memorial Volume of the Centennial Temperance Conference, New York: National Temperance Society and Publication House, 1886.

Dwight, T. A Sermon Preached at Stamford in Connecticut upon the General Thanksgiving, December 18, 1977, Hartford, CT, 1778.

Dwight, T. A discourse on some events of the last century. In: Smith, H.S., Handy, R.T. and Loetscher, L.A., American Christianity, Vol. 1, New York: Charles Scribner, 1801 (reprinted 1960).

Dwyer, E. The Rhetoric of Reform: A Study of Verbal Persuasion and Beliefs Systems in the Anti-Masonic and Temperance Movements, 1825–1860, PhD Dissertation, Yale University, 1977.

Gusfield, J.R. Symbolic Crusade: Status Politics and the American Temperance Movement, 2nd Edition, Champaign, IL: University of Illinois Press, 1986.

Haroutunian, J. Piety versus Moralism: The Passing of the New England Theology, New York: Henry Holt & Co., Inc., 1932.

Hatch, N.O. The Sacred Cause of Liberty: Republican Thought and the Millennium in Revolutionary New England, New Haven, CT: Yale University Press, 1977.

Heimert, A. Religion and the American Mind: From the Great Awakening to the Revolution, Cambridge, MA: Harvard University Press, 1966.

Jefferson, T. To Doctor Benjamin Waterhouse. In: American Christianity: An Historical Interpretation with Representative Documents, Vol. I, Smith, H.S., Handy, R.T. and Loetscher, L.A. New York: Charles Scribner's Sons, 1960, pp. 515–516.

Keller, C.R. The Second Great Awakening in Connecticut, New Haven, CT: Yale University Press, 1942.

Kirkland, J.T. Sermon Delivered Before the Massachusetts Society for Suppression of Intemperance, Boston: printed by John Eliot, 1814.

Krout, J.A. The Origins of Prohibition, New York: Alfred A. Knopf, Inc., 1925.

Lees, F.R. and Burns, D. The Temperance Bible-Commentary, London: National Temperance Publication Depot, 1894.

Lender, M. Drunkenness as an offense in early New England: A study of "Puritan" attitudes. Q. J. Stud Alcohol **34**: 353–366, 1973.

Lender, M.E. and Martin, J.K. Drinking in America: A History, New York: Free Press, 1982.

Levine, H.G. The Discovery of Addiction: Changing Conceptions of Habitual Drunkenness in America. J. Stud. Alcohol **39**: 143–174, 1978a.

Levine, H.G. Demon of the Middle Class: Self-Control, Liquor and the Ideology of Temperance in 19th-Century America, PhD Dissertation, University of California at Berkeley, 1978b.

Marsh, J. The Temperance Battle Not Man's but God's, New York: American Temperance Union, 1858.

Marsh, J. Putnam and the wolf; or: The monster destroyed. In: Select Temperance Tracts, New York: American Tract Society, 1859.

Marsh, J. Temperance Recollections: Labors, Defeats, Triumphs. An Autobiography, New York: C. Scribner's Sons, 1866.

McLoughlin, W.G. Modem Revivalism: Charles Grandison Finney to Billy Graham, New York: Ronald Press, 1959.

McLoughlin, W.G. Revivals, Awakenings, and Reform: An Essay on Religion and Social Change in America, 1607–1977, Chicago, IL: University. of Chicago Press, 1978.

Mead, S.E. Nathaniel William Taylor, 1786–1858: A Connecticut Liberal, Hamden, CT: Archon Books, 1967.

Miller, P. The New England Mind: The Seventeenth Century, Boston: Beacon Press, 1961.

Miller, P. Nature's Nation, Cambridge, MA: Harvard University Press, 1967.

Niebuhr, H.R. The Social Sources of Denominationalism, Hamden, CT: Shoe String Press, Inc., 1929.

Norwood, F.A. The Story of Methodism: A History of the United Methodists and Their Relations, Nashville, TN: Abingdon Press, 1974.

Nottingham, E.K. Methodism and the Frontier: Indiana Proving Ground, New York: Columbia University Press, 1944.

Raymond, I.W. The Teaching of the Early Church on the Use of Wine and Strong Drink, New York: Columbia University Press, 1927.

Rohrer, J.R. The Origins of the Temperance Movement: A Reinterpretation. J. Amer. Stud., 24: 228–235, 1990.

Rorabaugh, W.J. The Alcoholic Republic: An American Tradition, New York: Oxford University Press, Inc., 1979.

Smith, H.S., Handy, R.T. and Loetscher, L.A. American Christianity: An Historical Interpretation with Representative Documents, Vol. 1, New York: Charles Scribner's Sons, 1960.

Sweet, W.W. Religion on the American Frontier, Vol. 2: The Presbyterians, 1783–1840, New York: Harper & Row Publishers, Inc., 1936.

Tyrrell, I.R. Sobering Up: From Temperance to Prohibition to Antebellum America, 1800–1860, Westport, CT: Greenwood Publishing Group, Inc., 1979.

Walzer, M. The Revolution of the Saints: A Study in the Origins of Radical Politics, New York: Atheneum, 1972.

Warner, H.S., McPeek, F.W. and Jellinek, E.M. Philosophy of the temperance movement: A panel discussion. In: *Alcohol, Science and Society*, New Haven, CT: Journal of Studies on Alcohol, Inc., 1945, pp. 267–285.

Weber, M. Economy and Society: An Outline of Interpretive Sociology. Roth, G. and Wittich, C. (Eds.). Berkeley, CA: University of California Press, 1922 (reprinted 1978).

Youngs, J.W.T. The Congregationalists, Westport, CT: Greenwood Press, 1990.

Zaret, D. The Heavenly Contract: Ideology and Organization in Prerevolutionary Puritanism, Chicago, IL: University of Chicago Press, 1985.

Zaret, D. Religion and the rise of liberal-democratic ideology in 17th-century England. Amer. Social. Rev. 54: 163–179, 1989.

Laura A. Schmidt is a professor of Health Policy in the School of Medicine at the University of California at San Francisco. She holds a joint appointment in the Philip R. Lee Institute for Health Policy Studies and the Department of Anthropology, History and Social Medicine. Dr. Schmidt is also codirector of the Community Engagement and Health Policy Program for UCSF's Clinical and Translational Sciences Institute.

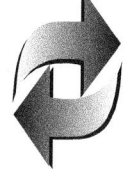

John J. Rumbarger

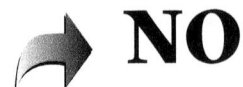

The Social and Ideological Origins of Drink Reform, 1800–1836

The roots of the temperance movement can be found in those social forces working to develop the expansionist tendencies of the American economy. Neither an abstract Puritan heritage nor paternalist conservatism can explain satisfactorily the dynamics that produced the movement to extirpate liquor drinking from America's culture. The earliest temperance societies, like that organized in Litchfield, Connecticut, in 1787, resulted from the efforts of wealthy farmers to curtail drinking among their laborers during harvest time. . . .

Nevertheless, these early societies defined the movement's strategic objective: the increase of productivity by the elimination of daily work breaks for alcoholic refreshment and its unpredictable consequences. These societies also illustrated a mutual desire on the part of property holders to obtain a uniform standard of labor, regardless of considerations that worked to set them in opposition to each other. These employers assumed that it was their prerogative to determine the social conditions that would lower the costs of production. In a market economy such considerations constituted sufficient reason to eliminate customary drinking, and the more so when labor scarcity deprived employers of a traditional instrument of capital accumulation, low wages.

Early concern about popular drinking was forcefully articulated by Benjamin Rush, whose writing on the subject became an ideological touchstone for the temperance movement. . . . His objective could best be obtained by employing "the force of severe manners" to curtail the social habits of drinking. . . .

Typical of the fruits of Rush's pioneering efforts was the temperance society formed by property owners in the Moreau-Northumberland region of Saratoga County, New York. At the beginning of the nineteenth century these agriculturally rich townships supported a diversified local economy of farming, lumbering, milling, and some rudimentary manufacturing. The political and social life of the area was dominated by a squirearchy, but, as elsewhere, it was difficult for them to engage in business enterprise without supplying workers with their customary alcoholic beverages. What distinguished Moreau-Northumberland's temperance pioneers was professional training among those who galvanized the squirearchy into action against liquor drinking.

Billy Clark had studied medicine; Esek Cowan had read law; Lebbius Armstrong was trained for the ministry. All three invested their surplus professional income in land and agricultural production. Clark, for example, owned several farms and had a large investment in a local paper mill. Cowan was a prosperous farm owner with a reputation for innovative husbandry. More important, however, for the purposes of temperance reform, was the common world view—quite like Rush's—the three shared. In one degree or another Moreau's temperance reformers believed society could improve with individual discipline and practical innovation, and that the criterion of improvement was business profits. William Hay, who subsequently headed the society, recalled that Clark was "convinced of the necessity of self-culture, and consequently acquired what are pertinently termed *business habits*." Hay admiringly described Clark as "pecuniarily successful as a physician and a businessman," and also wrote approvingly of Esek Cowan's various employments as a jurist, farmer, and classical scholar. For this kind of man "recreation was only change of employment," and employment was directed towards profit. . . .

These ideological conceptions nurtured temperance reform. But the reformers' stance towards other social classes was flexible: traditional rank or position was not an obstacle for association with like-minded men, provided the requisite social virtues of practical knowledge and disciplined effort could be demonstrated. Despite this apparent democratic appeal, the political ideology of a temperance "middle" class did not look to a reordering of society. Forged as it was in the crucible of business enterprise, it sought ultimately to redirect the energies and activities of capital and labor, but not to alter their social

---

Rumbarger, John J., "The Social and Ideological Origins of Drink Reform, 1800–1836," *Profits, Power, and Prohibition: Alcohol Reform and the Industrializing of America, 1800-1930*. Copyright ©1989 by State University of New York Press. Used with permission.

relationship. In the social context of Jeffersonian America, however, temperance ideology was radical in both theory and practice since it claimed to seek another reallocation of wealth and property according to utilitarian norms even as it sought an increase in social productivity. The assumption of the permanency of social stratification, to be dominated by a rationally selected elite, was but poorly masked by notions of individual worth taken to be demonstrated by the social virtues of innovation and discovery wedded to a discipline, including temperance, congenial to business. Because of this critical defect, temperance reformation, insofar as it envisioned a distinct "middle" class, was necessarily procapitalist.

The idea of a middle class proved especially valuable to the socialization process required by young America, which in the period 1820–50 could not compel people to alter their customary behavior sufficiently to modify the social order's value system. Indeed, the idea that personal characteristics and behavior were a form of capital may be seen as the *sine qua non* of American economic development in these years. Thus, all manner of ideologies, both secular and religious, that encouraged the development of internal modes of self-discipline as forms of "moral capital" were encouraged by the early advocates of liquor reform.

During the decades of the 1820s and 1830s temperance reform wherever it appeared became a political effort to create a social order universally congenial to entrepreneurial capitalism. It was during these years that the perceptions of men like Benjamin Rush and Billy Clark took root in business activity outside of agriculture, and attracted attention from such established institutions as the Protestant churches. But while local societies of employers who mutually agreed "that hereafter we will carry on our business without the use of distilled spirits as an article of refreshment, either for ourselves or those whom we may employ" remained on the reform scene, they proved insufficient to the task of extending temperance sentiment. To meet this need and to deal with the realities facing various enterprises, their politicization was required.

In Jeffersonian and Jacksonian America, maritime commerce ranked with agriculture in its importance to the economy. Here, too, liquor was customarily provided for laborers. . . .

In shipbuilding, workers enjoyed ceremonial provisions of strong drink in addition to their daily rations. At the completion of each major stage of construction they joined with shipowners and masters to toast their work's progress. Thus when the keel was put down, the ribs erected, the decking laid, and the masts raised and stepped there would be general celebrations fueled by large amounts of whiskey.

The earliest efforts at reform in these employment areas followed the boycott tactics that were being developed by agricultural temperance societies. In Medford, Massachusetts, for example, a local shipbuilder, Thacher Magoun, refused to permit rum or distilled spirits to be used in his shipyard. Magoun's 1817 no-rum edict was immediately interpreted by his laborers as "practically an increase in the working time, the employer thus saving the cost of time as well as the cost of the rum." Other Medford shipbuilders followed Magoun's lead, even to the point of raising wages. These boycotts could only be partially effective, however, because of the apprentice system and the grog shop, which furnished money and the means to smuggle the contraband refreshment into the yards.

By 1819, temperance advocates outside of agricultural societies had developed an analysis of the liquor problem that would eventually permit them to go beyond the limits of the boycott, and thus politicize the temperance movement. Thomas Hertell's *An Expose of the Causes of Intemperate Drinking and the Means by which It May Be Obviated* considered the entire social order to be the obstacle to temperance reform. Hertell implied that reform could only succeed if society in general were reformed with respect to drinking.

Hertell, who served for more than a dozen years on the bench of New York City's maritime court, asserted that his antiliquor convictions proceeded from the fact that "intemperate drinking is inimical to agricultural and mechanical, as well as moral improvement." He maintained that neither distillers nor the grog shop lay at the root of the problem; both were symptoms and consequences. The real cause of society's intemperate drinking was to be found in the "intemperate use of ardent liquor [which] originates in the fashions, habits, customs, and examples of what are called the upper or wealthy classes of the community." Because of the universal employment of such drinks by society's elites in both public and private, Hertell concluded that "inebriating drinks" had gained sanction as the "median universally adopted by society for manifesting friendship and good will, one to another."

Hertell believed that society's lower orders habitually emulated the upper, and so he argued that self-reformation by the wealthy must come before a general reform. Moreover, Hertell insisted that without a general temperance reform, nascent manufacturing enterprizes could not hope to succeed for "there is scarcely to be found among the laboring class, any who do not drink, and drink too much." Drinking customs were depriving manufacturers of quality manpower. "What single measure," he asked rhetorically, "would do more to further [manufacturing and agricultural development] than the destruction of the custom of giving ardent spirits to working people of every description."

Hertell's analysis of the liquor problem pulled together several strands in the developing temperance movement, and extended the focus of the reformers' concerns beyond agriculture and commerce to manufacturing. The reform impulse had derived from the pragmatic observation that customary drinking diminished productivity. Initially, reformers focused on the ordinary drinks—"ardent spirits"—of the working class as the principal source of abuse, and they continued to rely on the boycott as the means of curtailing and eliminating drinking.

On the other hand, Hertell insisted on the need of society's elites (including the churches) to exercise rigid self-restraint. Only when this class acted to end its sanction of drinking would "useful industry . . . become fashionable," and would "the already over-run and overrated learned professions" be abandoned for the "honorable calling" of the mechanical trades. Hertell looked to the formation of an antiliquor class consciousness that would act not only to protect its traditional base in agriculture and commerce, but also extend its concerns to American manufacturing. Of primary significance, however, is the fact that this attention to the responsibility of America's elite for the general well-being of society gave the temperance reform its peculiarly moralistic character, its ambivalence about the use of the state, and its connection with the Protestant churches.

During the years leading to the politicization of the temperance movement, American society underwent severe stress. Between 1800 and 1820, war and depression, accompanied by the introduction of the factory system, released latent hostilities that frequently expressed themselves in inchoate public drunkenness and disrespect towards religious and secular authority—or so it seemed to men like Lyman Beecher, the Congregationalist clergyman-reformer. Yet Beecher's consideration of social policy did not produce any effort to define the liquor problem in ways fundamentally different from those discussed. Indeed, during these years the established churches wedded themselves firmly to the emerging temperance movement in ways that sought to reinforce the movement's fundamental purposes. In 1812, for example, Beecher brought an ad hoc report before the General Association of Congregational and Presbyterian clergy wherein he asserted that intemperance was the mutual problem of the "Civil and Religious order," and recommended that employers cease providing liquor to their employees. Beecher also warned his colleagues that their efforts must remain within the boundaries of the "sanction of public sentiment," and thus echoed Benjamin Rush's plea for a regime of severe manners.

Ultimately the concerns of activist clergymen like Beecher were identical to those of men like Thomas Hertell and Mathew Carey, the Philadelphia publisher who helped establish the Philadelphia Society for the Promotion of National Industry. In 1820 Carey brought out Beecher's sermon, "The Means of National Prosperity," which encouraged the expansion of manufacturing, presupposing an abstemious social order, and outlined a role for the nation's churches in fostering this development. . . .

The larger vision of temperance reform articulated by Thomas Hertell and Lyman Beecher took firm root within the establishments of the Northeast during and immediately following the Napoleonic wars. Mercantile capital, the center of much early temperance concern, fueled the expansion of the nation's young manufacturing enterprises and brought to them the problems of absentee owners seeking to insure their investments in an unsure world. Made aware during these years of their own role in perpetuating the "drinking usages" of society, American capitalists organized to secure a dry working class. By 1834, Walter Channing, a pioneering member of the Massachusetts Society for the Suppression of Intemperance, recalled with some exaggerated pride that it was only when "men of great consideration . . . solemnly impressed with the ruinous progress of intemperance . . . came out as one man to make an open declaration of their convictions" that temperance reform began to progress.

The American Temperance Society (ATS), founded in January 1826 by Marcus Morton, a colleague of Channing, became the vehicle for the unified expression of class interest and coordinated action that Channing was to praise. Morton, who was "ahead of his time" in matters pertaining to labor reform, organized an umbrella society because of the deepening conviction that existing temperance societies were weak and ineffective. "Their object was," the ATS complained, "to regulate the use of ardent spirits, not to abolish it."

ATS envisioned a decentralized temperance apparatus, hierarchically organized from the local through the national level so that the smallest antiliquor organizations could "regulate their own movements and efforts according to their own views of necessity and expediency, and . . . their own wants and ability." The work of the ATS itself was to provide each and all with a common analysis of the liquor problem that corresponded to the class-conscious need for property owners to abstain totally from the use of distilled liquor, and to aid in the formation of state and local societies that adhered to this view of the problem. To oversee this work, Morton's group decided that a full-time paid secretary would be necessary and solicited contributions from "men of known and expansive benevolence, who are blessed with property," and who shared the view "that a system of general and powerful cooperation may be formed, and that a change may in a short time be effected, which will save an incalculable amount of property, and vast multitudes of valuable lives."

The man chosen to carry out the ATS reform was Justin Edwards of Andover Theological Seminary. In part Edwards's own previous skepticism about the efficacy of total abstinence from the use of distilled liquor became a major asset to the new organization. Prior to joining ATS as its secretary, Edwards had "thought [total abstinence] was going much too far . . . that the temperate use of ardent spirit was, for men who labor, in hot weather, necessary." What persuaded Edwards that the pledge of total abstinence by property owners was indeed efficacious was not theological conviction but an experiment conducted at one of the farms of a member of Morton's group in 1825. The result, Edwards testified, was that laborers "performed more labor with greater ease."

Equally and perhaps more important, in the eyes of ATS, total abstinence from hard liquor produced an apparent change in the attitude of laborers. According to Edwards the regime of enforced abstinence made the men "more respectful and uniform in their deportment . . . more contented with their living; more desirous of being present at morning and evening family devotion . . . more attentive at public worship on the Sabbath." Clearly this class-based reform effort saw a vital link between the docility of workers and their productivity on the one hand, and depriving them of liquor on the other.

The ATS, through the work of Edwards and secretaries of state societies affiliated with it, made repeated attempts to use the churches to advance the goal of abolition. Recognizing that distilleries were, for the most part, owned and operated by members of their own social class, ATS and its affiliates viewed the churches as the most appropriate vehicles available to them for the persuasion and coercion of their own. These efforts had profound and disruptive effects upon the churches and the movement itself, but what should not be lost sight of in the dogmatic hairsplitting over the extent to which abstinence was to be demanded is the intent of the reformers. "Ardent spirits" was the ordinary alcoholic beverage of workers. It had been the indifferent success of societies like the Massachusetts Society for the Suppression of Intemperance in seeking "to discontinue the too free use of ardent spirit" that had led to demands for total abolition. The ATS pledge committed affiliated societies to exclude all who "traffic" in ardent spirits and to "discountenance the use of them throughout the Community." It was thus that the churches became putative instruments of the reformers.

In their endeavor to persuade the churches to condemn both moderate drinking and the liquor traffic, ATS concentrated its efforts on the governing bodies of the various Protestant denominations. Such attempts met with indifferent success. The General Conference of the Methodist Episcopal Church, for example, condemned "the pestilential example of temperate drinking," but only inquired rhetorically if churches which tolerated manufacturers and sellers of whisky could be innocent of wrongdoing. The conference did not condemn the latter or move to excommunicate offending individuals. Thus, ATS had to rely upon the vague hopes of "some leading men" of the conference that by 1836 the church would be rid of the traffickers in drink.

The ATS also sought to bring pressure on the churches to expel liquor dealers through the efforts of such men as Wilbur Fisk, president of Wesleyan University, who castigated total abstinence church members for not insisting upon such expulsions and charged the churches with similar complicity. The ATS executive committee joined in this criticism: "From all parts of the country . . . the greatest difficulties in the way of Temperance Reformation . . . are those members of the church, who still sell ardent spirit."

Such pressures divided the established churches even though they produced condemnations of varying strength from national and state ecclesiastical organizations. The larger ones usually confined their expressions of opinion to vague generalities and left it to specific congregations to act. The Protestant clergy was also encouraged to advance the utilitarian purposes of the reformers. Thus, a Connecticut clergyman maintained that the cause would be well served "if farmers and mechanics would agree not to drink spirits themselves, and not provide them for their workmen."

By 1834 it was clear that the established churches had not made any deep inroads against either moderate drinking or the liquor traffic. In addition, their involvement in reform entailed a necessary hindrance to it since wine was of central importance to the Christian ritual as well as the ordinary drink of the wealthy. When, in the mid-1830s, ATS pushed for total abstinence from all alcoholic beverages and demanded state action against the liquor traffic, the difficulties posed by the churches appeared to outweigh their assets. As one clerical reformer acknowledged to the 1834 New York State Temperance Convention: "I have therefore been pained to see so many inclined to connect their religion with temperance. . . . And I know many individuals, who keep themselves aloof from the temperance society on this account, who would undoubtedly join the ranks, if the cause of temperance could be kept separate from everything else."

While the American Temperance Society concentrated its efforts on arousing the consciousness of property holders through the churches, state societies continued to recruit such people to the cause of temperance by stressing the utilitarian benefits of reform. In July 1833, the *Temperance Recorder,* the official organ of the New York State Temperance Society, reported that the consolidation of the Erie Canal's several towing firms into the Albany and Buffalo Towing Company had enabled the teamsters' employers to gain "control and government" over them, with the result that their intemperate drinking habits had been effectively checked. The same issue praised the society's forwarding of a circular letter to American consuls in Europe, warning émigrés that those who drank would find it difficult to obtain employment, and urging them to affiliate with a temperance society as an aid to finding work. The New York Society, which was dominated by mercantile and landed capitalists like Edward C. Delavan of Albany and Stephen Van Rensselaer of Saratoga, urged "the proprietors of our large, as well as our small manufacturing establishments . . . to take their subject into immediate consideration," since it was clear that intemperance was more dangerous to business prosperity than even foreign competition. The New Yorkers advised that temperance societies be organized within the factories themselves, and that proprietors and owners become the officers: "Unless proprietors or agents take the lead, nothing need be expected; but by their taking the course recommended . . . all under their control will be brought speedily into this 'ark of safety.'"

But the efforts of the New York Society and ATS to use the churches to arouse a class-conscious temperance sentiment in favor of overseas economic expansion ran afoul of the churches' difficulties and weakened the desired condemnation and divided the reformers. Many reformers recognized that the association of temperance with specific political and economic issues detracted from its class appeal. If the temperance movement were to gain the class support that its adherents believed was crucial, temperance morality would have to be divorced from specific secular and religious issues, and its moral appeal would have to come from an agency not associated with the churches.

In May 1833 ATS directors convened a national convention in Philadelphia to consider these questions and to chart the future course of reform. The four hundred delegates from twenty-four states represented the country's mercantile, manufacturing, and landed capital. Indicative of the range and scope of this class of men are Gerrit Smith and Stephen Van Rensselaer. Together with John Jacob Astor, Smith's father had acquired over one million acres of land in upstate New York, some 700,000 acres of which he passed on to his son in 1819. Van Rensselaer's holdings were equally vast. Both men were outstanding proponents of internal improvements and expanded trade with the West. Smith violently opposed a governmental role in expanding these markets, but Van Rensselaer was a strong advocate of such aid.

Other representatives of mercantile wealth included Edward C. Delavan, Roberts Vaux and his son, Richard, of Philadelphia, Samuel Ward of New York whose family's wealth had been invested in the banking firm of Prime, Ward, and King, Samuel Mifflin of Philadelphia, and John Tappan of Boston. Typical of emerging manufacturing representatives were Amasa Walker of Boston, Jonas Chickering, whose piano manufacturing concern of Stewart and Chickering developed the single casting iron frame for making grand pianos, and Matthew Newkirk, whose cotton goods business provided the funds for his railroad investments. Many of them, Delavan, Newkirk, and Smith, for example, had multiple investments in land, transportation, and manufacturing.

Also attending the first national temperance convention were luminaries from the first ranks of law, politics, religion, and science, many bearing some of the oldest family names in America. Reuben Hyde Walworth, chancellor of New York State, was named the convention's president. Joseph H. Lumpkin (whose brother Wilson was a Georgia planter and governor of the state), who would himself become a member of Georgia's Supreme Court, was named convention vice president. Timothy Pitkin, the author of the first major statistical account of American commerce, was a delegate from Connecticut. John McLean, who was to become president of the College of New Jersey, was a delegate. So also was Samuel L. Southard, Democratic senator from New Jersey. Amos Twitchell, a pioneer heart surgeon, represented New Hampshire. Jonas K. Converse of Burlington, Vermont, was a delegate, as were Philadelphia philanthropists John Sargent and Joseph B. Ingersoll; businessmen-publicists such as Mathew Carey, William Goodell, Thomas Bradford, Jr., and Sylvester Graham were typical delegates.

Other men of similar stature, like chemist Benjamin Silliman of Yale, or perhaps less well known, such as George Chambers, largest landowner in Franklin County, Pennsylvania and a reformer in education and agriculture, filled out the complement of delegates to the Philadelphia meeting. Their differences in economic interest, political affiliation, and religious persuasion were transcended by a fundamental class problem: the liquor question. . . .

In the end, this effort to rely solely upon the resources of property would fail because, as Gerrit Smith had already pointed out, America was a society where the demand for labor could not be met. Would-be employers would find the pledge inadequate and the law insufficient. But from the vantage point of 1834, the antiliquor movement had achieved astounding success. It had aroused the consciousness of virtually the entire propertied class, regardless of particular economic or political interest, to the importance of extirpating the use of distilled alcohol as a precondition of capitalist development. It had created a secular temperance morality that avoided the rigidities of various theologies while, at the same time, it had been able to enlist the churches in raising the consciousness of the "employing class." And it had developed its archetypal propaganda institution, the American Temperance Society, which was controlled by entrepreneurs of all sorts, and state and local temperance societies, which were to organize local property interests for the cause. Finally, the reform was being urged in the direction of a political attack on the liquor traffic itself.

When the United States Temperance Union and its affiliates met at Saratoga Springs in 1836, there appeared to remain but two mutually compatible tasks for the reform: first, spread the new gospel that "it has been proved a thousand times, that more labor can be accomplished in a month, or a year, under the influence of simple nourishing food and unstimulating drink than through the aid of alcohol"; second, organize and launch a political assault on the liquor traffic itself. To further these ends, the USTU named Reverend John Marsh and Edward C. Delavan to its principal offices. Both were fitting choices for the work. Marsh was related by marriage to the Tappan mercantile family of Boston and New York; his cousin Samuel would head the New York and Erie railroad. Delavan, on the other hand, was an active entrepreneur whose fortune had been made, ironically, as an importer of wine, and who came to the temperance reform after Nathaniel Prime, Lynde Catlin, and he had lost three hundred thousand dollars invested in the manufacture of steam engines and other heavy iron work because, they claimed, of "the unfortunate drinking habits [of the workers], which for best of motives, we ourselves encouraged."

JOHN J. RUMBARGER taught American political history at Rutgers University. A former editor of the *Prologue*, he later served as chief historian of the Federal Emergency Management Agency.

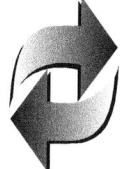

EXPLORING THE ISSUE

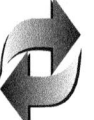

Was Antebellum Temperance Reform Driven by Theological Doctrine?

Critical Thinking and Reflection

1. What role did religion play in the efforts to reform the drinking habits of Americans in the first half of the nineteenth century? What role did industry play?
2. How did business interests affect the religious groups working toward temperance?
3. How did religious groups strategically align themselves with business interests?
4. What might have been a side effect of the interest convergence demonstrated between these two groups interested in temperance reform?

Is There Common Ground?

The temperance movement eventually led to the push for prohibition of alcohol and the passage of the 18th amendment in 1919. With the hindsight of the 21st amendment, we see that the efforts to legislate morality by both business and religious interests would eventually be for naught, and the ramifications of prohibition are myriad and include the rise of organized crime, a general contempt for the law and authority, and the relationship between the power and the judicial system. However, the legacy of the intermingling of these two interests would extend far beyond the reform era or even the early twentieth century when these two amendments were ratified.

Both Schmidt and Rumbarger are thinking in terms of social control as they construct arguments linking the need for either churches or businesses to operate more cohesively. Whether that meant adherence to the platform of the clergy or the demands of management, there is an element of overlap in their inherent views on the role of power and authority to shape behavior. Further, both articles articulate a prevailing view that drinking had become a problem in America at this time and begin to explore the limits of freedom in the Age of Jackson. Finally, both arguments hinge on the development of a grassroots campaign by interested laypersons who organized in groups supported by outside authorities. While neither perspective is particularly attentive to the sizable gender imbalance in these groups nor an exploration of what it might mean for women to collectively organize to address a pressing social issue, they are united in the contention that these organizations were characteristic of a developing republicanism in the adolescent nation.

Additional Resources

Barrows, S., & Room, R. (Eds.). (1991). *Drinking: Behavior and Belief in Modern History*. Berkeley, CA: University of California Press.

Fahey, D. M. (1996). *Temperance and Racism: John Bull, Johnny Reb, and the Good Templars*. Lexington, KY: The University Press of Kentucky.

Fletcher, H. B. (2007). *Gender and the American Temperance Movement of the Nineteenth Century*. New York: Routledge.

Gusfield, J. R. (1986). *Symbolic Crusade: Status Politics and the American Temperance Movement* (2nd ed.). Urbana, IL: University of Illinois Press.

Willis, L. (2011). *Southern Prohibition: Race, Reform, and Public Life in Middle Florida, 1821–1920*. Athens, GA: University of Georgia Press.

Internet References . . .

Roots of Prohibition (Companion site to Ken Burns' film *Prohibition*):

http://www.pbs.org/kenburns/prohibition/roots-of-prohibition/

Temperance Movement (Social Welfare History Project)

https://socialwelfare.library.vcu.edu/religious/the-temperance-movement/

Want a Drink, Anybody? (Lesson Plan from History Teaching Institute)

https://hti.osu.edu/opper/lesson-plans/want-drink-anybody-temperance

Women Led the Temperance Charge (Prohibition: An Interactive History)

http://prohibition.themobmuseum.org/the-history/the-road-to-prohibition/the-temperance-movement/

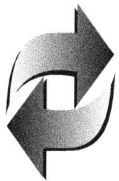

ISSUE

Selected, Edited, and with Issue Framing Material by:
Kevin R. Magill and Tony L. Talbert, *Baylor University*

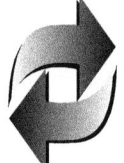

Was the Mexican War an Exercise in American Imperialism?

YES: **Ramón Eduardo Ruiz**, from "Manifest Destiny and the Mexican War," Dorsey Press (1988)

NO: **Norman A. Graebner**, from "The Mexican War: A Study in Causation," *Pacific Historical Review* (1980)

Learning Outcomes
After reading this issue, you will be able to: • Critically evaluate the causes of the Mexican War from the United States' and Mexican points of view. • Critically analyze the concepts of "manifest destiny" and "imperialism." • Critically analyze the strengths and weaknesses of the "American Empire." • Critically analyze the successes and failures of the Mexican War from the viewpoints of both the United States and Mexico. • Critically analyze the long-range effects of the Mexican War on both the United States and Mexico.

ISSUE SUMMARY

YES: Ramón Eduardo Ruiz believes that the Unites States demonstrated their imperialist tendencies by aggressively pursuing and waging war against Mexico in an effort to conquer and take her northern territories. Ruiz suggests that Mexico was never able to recover from this incursion.

NO: Norman A. Graebner suggests that the United States indeed adopted aggressive foreign policies designed to secure territory. However he argues that President Polk was not interested in war. Instead he suggests that the intention of his policies was to force Mexico to sell New Mexico and California to the United States and to recognize the legitimacy of the annexation of Texas.

The origins of the Mexican War began with the controversy over Texas, a Spanish possession for three centuries. In 1821, Texas became the northern-most province of the newly established country of Mexico. Sparsely populated with a mixture of Hispanics and Indians, the Mexican government encouraged immigration from the United States. By 1835, the Anglo population had swelled to 30,000 plus over 2,000 slaves, while the Mexican population was only 5,000. Fearful of losing control over Texas, the Mexican government prohibited further immigration from the United States in 1830, but it was too late. The Mexican government was divided and had changed hands several times. The centers of power were thousands of miles from Texas. In 1829, the Mexican government abolished slavery, an edict that was difficult to enforce. Finally, General Santa Anna attempted to abolish the federation and impose military rule over the entire country. Whether it was due to Mexican intransigence or the Anglos' assertiveness, the settlers rebelled in September 1835. The war was short-lived. Santa Anna was captured at the battled of San Jacinto in April 1836, and Texas was granted her independence.

For nine years, Texas remained an independent republic. Politicians were afraid that if Texas were annexed it would be carved into four or five states, thereby upsetting the balance of power between the evenly divided free states and slave states that had been created in 1819 by the Missouri Compromise. But the pro-slavery president John Tyler pushed through Congress a resolution annexing Texas in the final three days of his presidency in 1845.

The Mexican government was incensed and broke diplomatic relations with the United States. President James K. Polk sent John Slidell as the American emissary to Mexico to negotiate monetary claims of American citizens in Mexico, to purchase California, and to settle the southwestern boundary of Texas at the Rio Grande River and not farther north at the Nueces River, which Mexico recognized as the boundary. Upon Slidell's arrival, news leaked out about his proposals. The Mexican government rejected Slidell's offer. In March 1846, President Polk stationed General Zachary Taylor in the disputed territory along the Rio Grande with an army of 4,000 troops. On May 9, Slidell returned to Washington and informed Polk that he was rebuffed. Polk met with his cabinet to consider war. By chance that same evening, Polk received a dispatch from General Taylor informing him that on April 25 the Mexican army had crossed the Rio Grande and killed or wounded 16 of his men. On May 11, Polk submitted his war message claiming "American blood was shed on American soil." Congress voted overwhelmingly for war, 174 to 14 in the House and 40 to 2 in the Senate, despite the vocal minority of Whig protestors and intellectuals who opposed the war.

As David M. Pletcher points out in his balanced but critical book *The Diplomacy of Annexation: Texas, Oregon and the Mexican War* (University of Missouri Press, 1973), the long-range effects of the Mexican War on American foreign policy were immense. Between 1845 and 1848, the United States acquired more than 500,00 square miles of territory and increased its size by over a third of its present area. This included the annexation of Texas and the subsequent states of the southwest that stretched to the Pacific Coast, incorporating California and the Oregon Territory up to the 49th parallel. European efforts to gain a foothold in North America virtually ceased. By the 1850s, the British gradually abandoned their political aspirations in Central America, "content to compete for economic gains with the potent but unmilitary weapon of their factory system and their merchant marine." Meanwhile, the United States flexed its muscles at the end of the Civil War and used the Monroe Doctrine for the first time to force the French puppet ruler out of Mexico.

Walter Nugent's *Habits of Empire* (Knopf, 2008) is now the major synthesis of the political and military roots of American expansionism. Nugent bluntly argues that the United States was imperialistic from its very beginnings. American expansionism has gone through three phases: the first was the *continental* expansion across North America (exclusive of Canada) from 1783 to 1853, which resulted in the displacement of the Native Americans. Empire II was *overseas* expansion from 1867 to 1917, which resulted in the acquisition and rule over non-white populations in the Pacific and Central American regions. Since the end of World War II in 1945, the United States established the third *virtual-global* empire, which resulted in regime changes during the cold-war years against Russia and China as well as during the current war on terrorism.

Nugent spent most of his career writing about western American history. In this book he combines the expansion of the American people across the continent with the imperialist thrust of establishing an empire. The motivations are multi-causal—"spontaneous jingoism, national security demands, and visions of overseas markets for imperial goods." If there is one key factor, it is demographics. This is especially true for Empire I when the United States increased its population from one million in 1787 to thirty million on the eve of the Civil War. "During that period," said Stephen A. Douglas in deriding Lincoln's "House Divided" speech in a debate in 1858, "we have extended our territory from the Mississippi to the Pacific Ocean; we have acquired the Floridas and Texas, and other territory sufficient to double our geographical extent."

Nugent is also very critical of the United States' policy toward Mexico. He views Polk as a narrow-minded bigot whose one big idea was to acquire California and as much of the southwest as was possible either through negotiation or force. When the Mexican government, riddled with unstable governments, corrupt politicians, and incompetent generals, refused to negotiate, Polk maneuvered the Mexican government to attack American soldiers stationed in the disputed area between the Rio Grande and Nueces Rivers. This was not the only time, says Nugent, the chief executive maneuvered Congress into a fait accompli with regard to declaring war. "Madison came near to doing so in 1812. George H. W. Bush's troop buildup before the first Gulf War and George W. Bush's before Iraq were not novelties. There may be limits on presidential power, but there are no obvious ones on a president as commander-in-chief in sending troops and ships where he wants to." The two best historiographical essays on this topic are Jerald A. Combs, "Norman Graebner and the Realist View of American Diplomatic History," *Diplomatic History* (Summer 1987), and Dennis E. Berge, "Manifest Destiny and the Historians," in Michael P. Malone, ed., *Historians and the American West* (University of Nebraska Press, 1983).

The following selections reflect two opposing views on the nature of the United States' war with Mexico. In the first selection, Ramón Eduardo Ruiz argues that the United States waged a racist and aggressive war against Mexico for the purpose of conquering what became the American Southwest. In his view, Manifest Destiny was strictly an ideological rationale to provide noble motives for what were really acts of aggression against a neighboring country. Norman A. Graebner, the author of the second essay, was a very popular teacher with students at the University of Virginia and is considered one of the most prominent members of the "realist" school of diplomatic historians. His writings were influenced by the cold-war realists, political scientists, diplomats, and journalists of the 1950s who believed that American foreign policy oscillated between heedless isolationism and crusading wars without developing coherent policies that suited the national interests of the United States. According to Graebner, President James Polk assumed that Mexico was weak and that acquiring certain Mexican territories would satisfy "the long-range interests" of the United States. But when Mexico refused Polk's attempts to purchase New Mexico and California, he was left with three options: withdraw his demands, modify and soften his proposals, or aggressively pursue his original goals. According to Graebner, the president chose the third option.

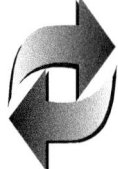

YES

Ramón Eduardo Ruiz

Manifest Destiny and the Mexican War

All nations have a sense of destiny. Spaniards braved the perils of unknown seas and the dangers of savage tribes to explore and conquer a New World for Catholicism. Napoleon's armies overran Europe on behalf of equality, liberty, and fraternity. Communism dictates the future of China and the Soviet Union. Arab expansionists speak of Islam. In the United States, Manifest Destiny in the 19th century was the equivalent of these ideologies or beliefs. Next-door neighbor Mexico felt the brunt of its impact first and suffered most from it.

What was Manifest Destiny? The term was coined in December 1845 by John L. O'Sullivan, then editor and cofounder of the *New York Morning News*. Superpatriot, expansionist, war hawk, and propagandist, O'Sullivan lived his doctrine of Manifest Destiny, for that slogan embodied what he believed. O'Sullivan spoke of America's special mission, frequently warned Europe to keep hands off the Western Hemisphere, later joined a filibustering expedition to Cuba, and had an honored place among the followers of President James K. Polk, Manifest Destiny's spokesman in the Mexican War.

Manifest Destiny voiced the expansionist sentiment that had gripped Americans almost from the day their forefathers had landed on the shores of the New World in the 17th century. Englishmen and their American offspring had looked westward since Jamestown and Plymouth, confident that time and fate would open to them the vast West that stretched out before them. Manifest Destiny, then, was first territorial expansion—American pretensions to lands held by Spain, France, and later Mexico; some even spoke of a United States with boundaries from pole to pole. But Manifest Destiny was greater than mere land hunger; much more was involved. Pervasive was a spirit of nationalism, the belief that what Americans upheld was right and good, that Providence had designated them the chosen people. In a political framework, Manifest Destiny stood for democracy as Americans conceived it; to spread democracy and freedom was the goal. Included also were ideals of regeneration, the conquest of virgin lands for the sake of their development, and concepts of Anglo-Saxon superiority. All these slogans and beliefs played a role in the Mexican question that culminated in hostilities in 1846.

Apostles of these slogans pointed out that Mexicans claimed lands from the Pacific to Texas but tilled only a fraction of them, and then inefficiently. "No nation has the right to hold soil, virgin and rich, yet unproducing," stressed one U.S. representative. "No race but our own can either cultivate or rule the western hemisphere," acknowledged the *United States Magazine and Democratic Review*. The Indian, almost always a poor farmer in North America, was the initial victim of this concept of soil use; expansionists later included nearly everyone in the New World, and in particular Mexicans. For, Caleb Cushing asked: "Is not the occupation of any portion of the earth by those competent to hold and till it, a providential law of national life?"

Oregon and Texas, and the Democratic Party platform of 1844, kindled the flames of territorial expansion in the roaring forties. Millions of Americans came to believe that God had willed them all of North America. Expansion symbolized the fulfillment of "America's providential mission or destiny"—a mission conceived in terms of the spread of democracy, which its exponents identified with freedom. Historian Albert K. Weinberg has written: "It was because of the association of expansion and freedom in a means-end relationship, that expansion now came to seem most manifestly a destiny."

Americans did not identify freedom with expansion until the forties. Then, fears of European designs on Texas, California, and Oregon, perhaps, prompted an identity of the two. Not only were strategic and economic interests at stake, but also democracy itself. The need to extend the area of freedom, therefore, rose partly from the necessity of keeping absolutistic European monarchs

---

"Manifest Destiny and the Mexican War" by Ramón Eduardo Ruiz from Main Problems in American History. Copyright ©1988 by Ramón Eduardo Ruiz. Reprinted by permission.

from limiting the area open to American democracy in the New World.

Other factors also impelled Americans to think expansion essential to their national life. Failure to expand imperiled the nation, for, as historian William E. Dodd stated, Westerners especially believed "that the Union gained in stability as the number of states multiplied." Meanwhile, Southerners declared the annexation of Texas essential to their prosperity and to the survival of slavery, and for a congressional balance of power between North and South. Others insisted that expansion helped the individual states to preserve their liberties, for their numerical strength curtailed the authority of the central government, the enemy of local autonomy and especially autonomy of the South. Moreover, for Southerners extension of the area of freedom meant, by implication, expansion of the limits of slavery. Few planters found the two ideas incompatible. Religious doctrines and natural principles, in their opinion, had ruled the Negro ineligible for political equality. That expansion favored the liberties of the individual, both North and South agreed.

In the forties, the pioneer spirit received recognition as a fundamental tenet of American life. Individualism and expansion, the mark of the pioneer, were joined together in the spirit of Manifest Destiny. Expansion guaranteed not just the political liberty of the person, but the opportunity to improve himself economically as well, an article of faith for the democracy of the age. Further, when antiexpansionists declared that the territorial limits of the United States in 1846 assured all Americans ample room for growth in the future, the expansionists-turned-ecologists replied that some 300 million Americans in 1946 would need more land, a prediction that overstated the case of the population-minded experts. And few Americans saw the extension of freedom in terms other than liberty for themselves—white, Anglo-Saxon, and Protestant. All these concepts, principles, and beliefs, then, entered into the expansionist creed of Manifest Destiny.

None of these was a part of the Mexican heritage, the legacy of three centuries of Spanish rule and countless years of pre-Columbian civilization. Mexico and the United States could not have been more dissimilar in 1846. A comparison of colonial backgrounds helps to bring into focus the reasons the two countries were destined to meet on the field of battle. One was weak and the other strong; Mexico had abolished slavery and the United States had not; Americans had their Manifest Destiny, but few Mexicans believed in themselves.

Daughter of a Spain whose colonial policy embraced the Indian, Mexico was a mestizo republic, a half-breed nation. Except for a small group of aristocrats, most Mexicans were descendants of both Spaniards and Indians. For Mexico had a colonial master eager and willing to assimilate pre-Columbian man. Since the days of the conqueror Hernán Cortés, Spaniards had mated with Indians, producing a Mexican both European and American in culture and race. Offspring of the Indian as well as the Spaniard, Mexican leaders, and even the society of the time, had come to accept the Indian, if not always as an equal, at least as a member of the republic. To have rejected him would have been tantamount to the Mexican's self-denial of himself. Doctrines of racial supremacy were, if not impossible, highly unlikely, for few Mexicans could claim racial purity. To be Mexican implied a mongrel status that ruled out European views of race.

Spain bequeathed Mexico not merely a racial attitude but laws, religious beliefs, and practices that banned most forms of segregation and discrimination. For example, reservations for Indians were never a part of the Spanish heritage. Early in the 16th century, the Spaniards had formulated the celebrated Laws of the Indies—legislation that clearly spelled out the place of the Indian in colonial society. Nothing was left to chance, since the Spanish master included every aspect of life—labor, the family, religion, and even the personal relations between Spaniard and Indian. The ultimate aim was full citizenship for the Indian and his descendants. In the meantime, the Church ruled that the Indian possessed a soul; given Christian teachings, he was the equal of his European conqueror. "All of the people of the world are men," the Dominican Bartolomé de las Casas had announced in his justly famous 1550 debate with the scholar Sepúlveda.

Clearly, church and state and the individual Spaniard who arrived in America had more than charity in mind. Dreams of national and personal glory and wealth dominated their outlook. Yet, despite the worldly goals of most secular and clerical conquerors, they built a colonial empire on the principle that men of all colors were equal on earth. Of course, Spain required the labor of the Indian and therefore had to protect him from the avarice of many a conquistador. Spaniards, the English were wont to say, were notorious for their disdain of manual labor of any type. But Spain went beyond merely offering the Indian protection in order to insure his labor. It incorporated him into Hispanic-American society. The modern Mexican is proof that the Indian survived: all Mexicans are Indian to some extent. That the Indian suffered economic exploitation and frequently even social isolation is undoubtedly true, but such was the lot of the poor in the Indies—Indian, half-breed, and even Spaniard.

Spain's empire, as well as the Mexican republic that followed, embraced not just the land but the people who had tilled it for centuries before the European's arrival. From northern California to Central America, the boundaries of colonial New Spain, and later Mexico, the Spaniard had embraced the Indian or allowed him to live out his life. It was this half-breed population that in 1846 confronted and fell victim to the doctrine of Manifest Destiny.

America's historical past could not have been more dissimilar. The English master had no room for the Indian in his scheme of things. Nearly all Englishmen—Puritans, Quakers, or Anglicans—visualized the conquest and settlement of the New World in terms of the exclusive possession of the soil. All new lands conquered were for the immediate benefit of the new arrivals. From the days of the founding of Jamestown and Plymouth, the English had pushed the Indian westward, relentlessly driving him from his homeland. In this activity, the clergy clasped hands with lay authorities; neither offered the red man a haven. Except for a few hardy souls, invariably condemned by their peers, Englishmen of church and state gave little thought to the Indian. Heaven, hell, and the teachings of Christ were the exclusive domain of the conquerors.

Society in the 13 colonies, and in the Union that followed, reflected English and European customs and ways of life. It was a transplanted society. Where the Indian survived, he found himself isolated from the currents of time. Unlike the Spaniards, whose ties with Africa and darker skinned peoples through .seven centuries of Moorish domination had left an indelible imprint on them, most Englishmen had experienced only sporadic contact with people of dissimilar races and customs. Having lived a sheltered and essentially isolated existence, the English developed a fear and distrust of those whose ways were foreign to them. The Americans who walked in their footsteps retained this attitude.

Many American historians will reject this interpretation. They will probably allege that American willingness to accept millions of destitute immigrants in the 19th century obviously contradicts the view that the Anglo-Saxon conqueror and settler distrusted what was strange in others. Some truth is present here, but the weight of the evidence lies on the other side. What must be kept firmly in mind is that immigration to the English colonies and later to the United States—in particular, the tidal wave of humanity that engulfed the United States in the post–Civil War era—was European in origin. Whether Italians, Jews, or Greeks from the Mediterranean, Swedes, Scots, or Germans from the North, what they had in common far outweighed conflicting traits and cultural and physical differences. All were European, offspring of one body of traditions and beliefs. Whether Catholics, Protestants, or Jews, they professed adherence to Western religious practices and beliefs. The so-called melting pot was scarcely a melting pot at all; the ingredients were European in origin. All spices that would have given the stew an entirely different flavor were carefully kept out—namely, the Negro and the Indian.

It was logical that Manifest Destiny, that American belief in a Providence of special design, should have racial overtones. Having meticulously kept out the infidel, Americans could rightly claim a racial doctrine of purity and supremacy in the world of 1846. Had not the nation of Polk's era developed free of those races not a part of the European heritage? Had the nation not progressed rapidly? Most assuredly, the answer was yes. When American development was compared to that of the former Spanish-American colonies, the reply was even more emphatically in the affirmative. After all, the Latin republics to the south had little to boast about. All were backward, illiterate, and badly governed states. Americans had just cause for satisfaction with what they had accomplished.

Unfortunately for Latin America, and especially Mexico, American pride had dire implications for the future. Convinced of the innate racial supremacy which the slogan of Manifest Destiny proclaimed throughout the world, many Americans came to believe that the New World was theirs to develop. Only their industry, their ingenuity, and their intelligence could cope fully with the continental challenge. Why should half-breed Mexico—backward, politically a waste-land, and hopelessly split by nature and man's failures—hold Texas, New Mexico, and California? In Mexico's possession, all these lands would lie virgin, offering a home to a few thousand savage Indians, and here and there a Mexican pueblo of people scarcely different from their heathen neighbors. Manifest Destiny simply proclaimed what most Americans had firmly believed—the right of Anglo-Saxons and others of similar racial origin to develop what Providence had promised them. Weak Mexico, prey of its own cupidity and mistakes, was the victim of this belief.

Manifest Destiny, writes Mexican historian Carlos Bosch García, also contradicts an old American view that means are as important as ends. He stresses that the key to the history of the United States, as the doctrine of Manifest Destiny illustrates, lies in the willingness of Americans to accept as good the ultimate result of whatever they have undertaken to do. That the red man was driven from his homeland is accepted as inevitable and thus justifiable. American scholars might condemn the maltreatment of the Indian, but few question the final verdict.

Equally ambivalent, says Bosch García, is the American interpretation of the Mexican War. Though some American scholars of the post–Civil War period severely censured the South for what they called its responsibility for the Mexican War, their views reflected a criticism of the slavocracy rather than a heartfelt conviction that Mexico had been wronged. Obviously, there were exceptions. Hubert H. Bancroft, a California scholar and book collector, emphatically denounced Polk and his cohorts in his voluminous *History of Mexico* (1883–88). Among the politicians of the era, Abraham Lincoln won notoriety—and probably lost his seat in the House of Representatives—for his condemnation of Polk's declaration of war against Mexico. There were others, mostly members of the Whig Party, which officially opposed the war; but the majority, to repeat, was more involved with the problem of the South than with the question of war guilt.

Most Americans, in fact, have discovered ways and means to justify Manifest Destiny's war on Mexico. That country's chronic political instability, its unwillingness to meet international obligations, its false pride in its military establishment—all those, say scholars, led Mexican leaders to plunge their people into a hopeless war. Had Mexico been willing to sell California, one historian declares, no conflict would have occurred. To paraphrase Samuel F. Bemis, distinguished Yale University diplomatic scholar, no American today would undo the results of Polk's war. Put differently, to fall back on Bosch García, American writers have justified the means because of the ends. Manifest Destiny has not only been explained but has been vindicated on the grounds of what has been accomplished in California and New Mexico since 1848. Or, to cite Hermann Eduard von Holst, a late 19th century German scholar whose writings on American history won him a professorship at the University of Chicago, the conflict between Mexico and the United States was bound to arise. A virile and ambitious people whose cause advanced that of world civilization could not avoid battle with a decadent, puerile people. Moral judgments that applied to individuals might find Americans guilty of aggression, but the standards by which nations survive and prosper upheld the cause of the United States. Might makes right? Walt Whitman, then editor of the *Brooklyn Daily Eagle*, put down his answer succinctly:

> We love to indulge in thoughts of the future extent and power of this Republic—because with its increase is the increase in human happiness and liberty. . . . What has miserable Mexico—with her superstition, her burlesque upon freedom, her actual tyranny by the few over the many—what has she to do with the great mission of peopling the New World with a noble race? Be it ours, to achieve that mission! Be it ours to roll down all of the up-start leaven of the old despotism, that comes our way.

The conflict with Mexico was an offensive war without moral pretensions, according to Texas scholar Otis A. Singletary. It was no lofty crusade, no noble battle to right the wrongs of the past or to free a subjugated people, but a war of conquest waged by one neighbor against another. President Polk and his allies had to pay conscience money to justify a "greedy land-grab from a neighbor too weak to defend herself." American indifference to the Mexican War, Professor Singletary concludes, "lies rooted in the guilt that we as a nation have come to feel about it."

American racial attitudes, the product of a unique colonial background in the New World, may also have dictated the scope of territorial conquest in 1848 and, ironically, saved Mexico from total annexation. Until the clash with Mexico, the American experience had been limited to the conquest, occupation, and annexation of empty or sparsely settled territories, or of those already colonized by citizens of the United States, as were Oregon and Texas. American pioneers had been reincorporated into the Union with the annexation of Oregon and Texas, and even with the purchase of Louisiana in 1803, for the alien population proved small and of little importance. White planters, farmers, and pioneers mastered the small Mexican population in Texas and easily disposed of the Indians and half-breeds in the Louisiana territory.

Expansionists and their foes had long considered both Indian and Negro unfit for regeneration; both were looked on as inferior and doomed races. On this point, most Americans were in agreement. While not entirely in keeping with this view, American opinions of Latin Americans, and of Mexicans in particular, were hardly flattering. Purchase and annexation of Louisiana and Florida, and of Texas and Oregon, had been debated and postponed partly out of fear of what many believed would be the detrimental effect on American democracy resulting from the amalgamation of the half-breed and mongrel peoples of these lands. Driven by a sense of national aggrandizement, the expansionists preferred to conquer lands free of alien populations. Manifest Destiny had no place for the assimilation of strange and exotic peoples. Freedom for Americans—this was the cry, regardless of what befell the conquered natives. The location of sparsely held territory had dictated the course of empire.

James K. Polk's hunger for California reflected national opinion on races as well as desire for land. Both that territory and New Mexico, nearly to the same extent, were almost barren of native populations. Of sparsely settled California, in 1845 the *Hartford Times* eloquently declared that Americans could "redeem from unhallowed hands a land, above all others of heaven, and hold it for the use of a people who know how to obey heaven's behests." Thus it was that the tide of conquest—the fruits of the conference table at Guadalupe Hidalgo—stopped on the border of Mexico's inhabited lands, where the villages of a people alien in race and culture confronted the invaders. American concepts of race, the belief in the regeneration of virgin lands—these logically ordered annexation of both California and New Mexico, but left Mexico's settled territory alone.

Many Americans, it is true, gave much thought to the conquest and regeneration of all Mexico, but the peace of 1848 came before a sufficiently large number of them had abandoned traditional thoughts on race and color to embrace the new gospel. Apparently, most Americans were not yet willing to accept dark-skinned people as the burden of the white man.

Manifest Destiny, that mid-19th-century slogan, is now merely a historical question for most Americans. Despite the spectacular plums garnered from the conference table, the war is forgotten by political orators, seldom discussed in classrooms, and only infrequently recalled by historians and scholars.

But Mexicans, whether scholars or not, have not forgotten the war; their country suffered most from Manifest Destiny's claims to California. The war of 1846–48 represents one of the supreme tragedies of their history. Mexicans are intimately involved with it, unlike their late adversaries who have forgotten it. Fundamental reasons explain this paradox. The victorious United States went to a post-Civil War success story unequaled in the annals of Western civilization. Mexico emerged from the peace of Guadalupe Hidalgo bereft of half of its territory, a beaten, discouraged, and divided country. Mexico never completely recovered from the debacle.

Mexicans had known tragedy and defeat before, but their conquest by Generals Zachary Taylor and Winfield Scott represented not only a territorial loss of immense proportions, but also a cataclysmic blow to their morale as a nation and as a people. From the Mexican point of view, their pride in what they believed they had mastered best—the science of warfare—was exposed as a myth. Mexicans could not even fight successfully, and they had little else to recall with pride, for their political development had enshrined bitter civil strife and callous betrayal of principle. Plagued by hordes of scheming politicians, hungry military men, and a backward and reactionary clergy, they had watched their economy stagnate. Guadalupe Hidalgo clearly outlined the scope of their defeat. There was no success story to write about, only tragedy. Mexicans of all classes are still engrossed in what might have been *if* General Antonio López de Santa Anna had repelled the invaders from the North.

Polk's war message to Congress and Lincoln's famous reply in the House cover some dimensions of the historical problem. Up for discussion are Polk's role in the affair, the responsibility of the United States and Mexico, and the question of war guilt—a question raised by the victorious Americans and their allies at Nuremberg after World War II. For if Polk felt "the blood of this war, like the blood of Abel, is crying to Heaven against him," as Lincoln charged, then not just the war but also Manifest Destiny stand condemned.

RAMÓN EDUARDO RUIZ (1921–2010) was professor emeritus of Latin American history at the University of California–San Diego. He is the author of fifteen books including *Triumphs and Tragedy: A History of the Mexican People* (W. W. Norton, 1972, 1993), *The Great Rebellion: Mexico, 1905–1924* (W. W. Norton, 1982), and *On the Rim of Mexico: Encounters of the Rich and Poor* (Basic Books, 1998).

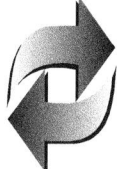

Norman A. Graebner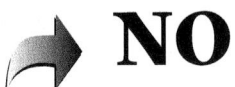

The Mexican War: A Study in Causation

On May 11, 1846, President James K. Polk presented his war message to Congress. After reviewing the skirmish between General Zachary Taylor's dragoons and a body of Mexican soldiers along the Rio Grande, the president asserted that Mexico "has passed the boundary of the United States, has invaded our territory and shed American blood upon the American soil.... War exists, and, notwithstanding all our efforts to avoid it, exists by act of Mexico." No country could have had a superior case for war. Democrats in large numbers (for it was largely a partisan matter) responded with the patriotic fervor which Polk expected of them. "Our government has permitted itself to be insulted long enough," wrote one Georgian. "The blood of her citizens has been spilt on her own soil. It appeals to us for vengeance." Still, some members of Congress, recalling more accurately than the president the circumstances of the conflict, soon rendered the Mexican War the most reviled in American history—at least until the Vietnam War of the 1960s. One outraged Whig termed the war "illegal, unrighteous, and damnable," and Whigs questioned both Polk's honesty and his sense of geography. Congressman Joshua R. Giddings of Ohio accused the president of "planting the standard of the United States on foreign soil, and using the military forces of the United States to violate every principle of international law and moral justice." To vote for the war, admitted Senator John C. Calhoun, was "to plunge a dagger into his own heart, and more so." Indeed, some critics in Congress openly wished the Mexicans well.

For over a century such profound differences in perception have pervaded American writings on the Mexican War. Even in the past decade, historians have reached conclusions on the question of war guilt as disparate as those which separated Polk from his wartime conservative and abolitionist critics....

In some measure the diversity of judgment on the Mexican War, as on other wars, is understandable. By basing their analyses on official rationalizations, historians often ignore the more universal causes of war which transcend individual conflicts and which can establish the bases for greater consensus. Neither the officials in Washington nor those in Mexico City ever acknowledged any alternatives to the actions which they took. But governments generally have more choices in any controversy than they are prepared to admit. Circumstances determine their extent. The more powerful a nation, the more remote its dangers, the greater its options between action and inaction. Often for the weak, unfortunately, the alternative is capitulation or war.... Polk and his advisers developed their Mexican policies on the dual assumption that Mexico was weak and that the acquisition of certain Mexican territories would satisfy admirably the long-range interests of the United States. Within that context, Polk's policies were direct, timely, and successful. But the president had choices. Mexico, whatever its internal condition, was no direct threat to the United States. Polk, had he so desired, could have avoided war; indeed, he could have ignored Mexico in 1845 with absolute impunity.

In explaining the Mexican War historians have dwelled on the causes of friction in American-Mexican relations. In part these lay in the disparate qualities of the two populations, in part in the vast discrepancies between the two countries in energy, efficiency, power, and national wealth. Through two decades of independence Mexico had experienced a continuous rise and fall of governments; by the 1840s survival had become the primary concern of every regime. Conscious of their weakness, the successive governments in Mexico City resented the superior power and effectiveness of the United States and feared American notions of destiny that anticipated the annexation of Mexico's northern provinces. Having failed to prevent the formation of the Texas Republic, Mexico reacted to Andrew Jackson's recognition of Texan independence in March 1837 with deep indignation. Thereafter the Mexican raids into Texas, such as the one on San Antonio in 1842, aggravated the bitterness of Texans toward Mexico, for such forays had no purpose beyond terrorizing the frontier settlements.

Such mutual animosities, extensive as they were, do not account for the Mexican War. Governments as divided and chaotic as the Mexican regimes of the 1840s usually have difficulty in maintaining positive and profitable relations with their neighbors; their behavior often produces annoyance, but seldom armed conflict. Belligerence toward other countries had flowed through U.S. history like a torrent without, in itself, setting off a war. Nations do not fight over cultural differences or verbal recriminations; they fight over perceived threats to their interests created by the ambitions or demands of others.

What increased the animosity between Mexico City and Washington was a series of specific issues over which the two countries perennially quarreled—claims, boundaries, and the future of Texas. Nations have made claims a pretext for intervention, but never a pretext for war. Every nineteenth-century effort to collect debts through force assumed the absence of effective resistance, for no debt was worth the price of war. To collect its debt from Mexico in 1838, for example, France blockaded Mexico's gulf ports and bombarded Vera Cruz. The U.S. claims against Mexico created special problems which discounted their seriousness as a rationale for war. True, the Mexican government failed to protect the possessions and the safety of Americans in Mexico from robbery, theft, and other illegal actions, but U.S. citizens were under no obligation to do business in Mexico and should have understood the risk of transporting goods and money in that country. Minister Waddy Thompson wrote from Mexico City in 1842 that it would be "with somewhat of bad grace that we should war upon a country because it could not pay its debts when so many of our own states are in the same situation." Even as the United States after 1842 attempted futilely to collect the $2 million awarded its citizens by a claims commission, it was far more deeply in debt to Britain over speculative losses. Minister Wilson Shannon reported in the summer of 1844 that the claims issue defied settlement in Mexico City and recommended that Washington take the needed action to compel Mexico to pay. If Polk would take up the challenge and sacrifice American human and material resources in a war against Mexico, he would do so for reasons other than the enforcement of claims. The president knew well that Mexico could not pay, yet as late as May 9, 1846, he was ready to ask Congress for a declaration of war on the question of unpaid claims alone.

Congress's joint resolution for Texas annexation in February 1845 raised the specter of war among editors and politicians alike. As early as 1843 the Mexican government had warned the American minister in Mexico City that annexation would render war inevitable; Mexican officials in Washington repeated that warning. To Mexico, therefore, the move to annex Texas was an unbearable affront. Within one month after Polk's inauguration on March 4, General Juan Almonte, the Mexican minister in Washington, boarded a packet in New York and sailed for Vera Cruz to sever his country's diplomatic relations with the United States. Even before the Texas Convention could meet on July 4 to vote annexation, rumors of a possible Mexican invasion of Texas prompted Polk to advance Taylor's forces from Fort Jesup in Louisiana down the Texas coast. Polk instructed Taylor to extend his protection to the Rio Grande but to avoid any areas to the north of that river occupied by Mexican troops. Simultaneously the president reinforced the American squadron in the Gulf of Mexico. "The threatened invasion of Texas by a large Mexican army," Polk informed Andrew J. Donelson, the American charge in Texas, on June 15, "is well calculated to excite great interest here and increases our solicitude concerning the final action by the Congress and the Convention of Texas." Polk assured Donelson that he intended to defend Texas to the limit of his constitutional power. Donelson resisted the pressure of those Texans who wanted Taylor to advance to the Rio Grande; instead, he placed the general at Corpus Christi on the Nueces River. Taylor agreed that the line from the mouth of the Nueces to San Antonio covered the Texas settlements and afforded a favorable base from which to defend the frontier.

Those who took the rumors of Mexican aggressiveness seriously lauded the president's action. With Texas virtually a part of the United States, argued the *Washington Union*, "We owe it to ourselves, to the proud and elevated character which America maintains among the nations of the earth, to guard our own territory from the invasion of the ruthless Mexicans." The *New York Morning News* observed that Polk's policy would, on the whole, "command a general concurrence of the public opinion of his country." Some Democratic leaders, fearful of a Mexican attack, urged the president to strengthen Taylor's forces and order them to take the offensive should Mexican soldiers cross the Rio Grande. Others believed the reports from Mexico exaggerated, for there was no apparent relationship between the country's expressions of belligerence and its capacity to act. Secretary of War William L. Marcy admitted that his information was no better than that of other commentators. "I have at no time," he wrote in July, "felt that war with Mexico was probable—and do not now believe it is, yet it is in the range of possible occurrences. I have officially acted on the hypothesis that our peace may be temporarily disturbed without however believing it will be." Still convinced that the administration had no grounds for alarm, Marcy wrote on August 12: "The presence of a considerable force in Texas will do no hurt and possibly may be of great use." In September William S. Parrott, Polk's special agent in Mexico, assured the president that there would be neither a Mexican declaration of war nor an invasion of Texas.

Polk insisted that the administration's show of force in Texas would prevent rather than provoke war. "I do not anticipate that Mexico will be mad enough to declare war," he wrote in July, but "I think she would have done so but for the appearance of a strong naval force in the Gulf and our army moving in the direction of her frontier on land." Polk restated this judgment on July 28 in a letter to General Robert Armstrong, the U.S. consul at Liverpool: "I think there need be but little apprehension of war with Mexico. If however she shall be mad enough to make war we are prepared to meet her." The president assured Senator William H. Haywood of North Carolina that the American forces in Texas would never aggress against Mexico; however, they would prevent any Mexican forces from crossing the Rio Grande. In conversation with Senator William S. Archer of Virginia on September 1, the president added confidently that "the appearance of our land and naval forces on the borders of Mexico & in the Gulf would probably deter and prevent Mexico from either declaring war or invading Texas." Polk's continuing conviction that Mexico would not attack suggests that his deployment of U.S. land and naval forces along Mexico's periphery was designed less to protect Texas than to support an aggressive diplomacy which might extract a satisfactory treaty from Mexico without war. For Anson Jones, the last president of the Texas Republic, Polk's deployments had precisely that purpose:

> Texas never actually needed the protection of the United States after I came into office.... There was no necessity for it after the 'preliminary Treaty,' as we were at peace with Mexico, and knew perfectly well that that Government, though she might bluster a little, had not the slightest idea of invading Texas either by land or water; and that nothing would provoke her to (active) hostilities, but the presence of troops in the immediate neighborhood of the Rio Grande, threatening her towns and settlements on the southwest side of that river.... But Donelson appeared so intent upon 'encumbering us with help,' that finally, to get rid of his annoyance, he was told he might give us as much protection as he pleased.... The protection asked for was only *prospective* and contingent; the *protection* he had in view was *immediate and aggressive*.

For Polk the exertion of military and diplomatic pressure on a disorganized Mexico was not a prelude to war. Whig critics of annexation had predicted war; this alone compelled the administration to avoid a conflict over Texas. In his memoirs Jones recalled that in 1845 Commodore Robert F. Stockton, with either the approval or the connivance of Polk, attempted to convince him that he should place Texas "in an attitude of active hostility toward Mexico, so that, when Texas was finally brought into the Union, *she might bring war with her*." If Stockton engaged in such an intrigue, he apparently did so on his own initiative, for no evidence exists to implicate the administration. Polk not only preferred to achieve his purposes by means other than war but also assumed that his military measures in Texas, limited as they were, would convince the Mexican government that it could not escape the necessity of coming to terms with the United States. Washington's policy toward Mexico during 1845 achieved the broad national purpose of Texas annexation. Beyond that it brought U.S. power to bear on Mexico in a manner calculated to further the processes of negotiation. Whether the burgeoning tension would lead to a negotiated boundary settlement or to war hinged on two factors: the nature of Polk's demands and Mexico's response to them. The president announced his objectives to Mexico's troubled officialdom through his instructions to John Slidell, his special emissary who departed for Mexico in November 1845 with the assurance that the government there was prepared to reestablish formal diplomatic relations with the United States and negotiate a territorial settlement....

Actually, Slidell's presence in Mexico inaugurated a diplomatic crisis not unlike those which precede most wars. Fundamentally the Polk administration, in dispatching Slidell, gave the Mexicans the same two choices that the dominant power in any confrontation gives to the weaker: the acceptance of a body of concrete diplomatic demands or eventual war. Slidell's instructions described U.S. territorial objectives with considerable clarity. If Mexico knew little of Polk's growing acquisitiveness toward California during the autumn of 1845, Slidell proclaimed the president's intentions with his proposals to purchase varying portions of California for as much as $25 million. Other countries such as England and Spain had consigned important areas of the New World through peaceful negotiations, but the United States, except in its Mexican relations, had never asked any country to part with a portion of its own territory. Yet Polk could not understand why Mexico should reveal any special reluctance to part with Texas, the Rio Grande, New Mexico, or California. What made the terms of Slidell's instructions appear fair to him was Mexico's military and financial helplessness. Polk's defenders noted that California was not a sine qua non of any settlement and that the president offered to settle the immediate controversy over the acquisition of the Rio Grande boundary alone in exchange for the cancellation of claims. Unfortunately, amid the passions of December 1845, such distinctions were lost. Furthermore, a settlement of the Texas boundary would not have resolved the California question at all.

Throughout the crisis months of 1845 and 1846, spokesmen of the Polk administration repeatedly warned the Mexican government that its choices were limited. In June 1845, Polk's mouthpiece, the *Washington Union*, had observed characteristically that, if Mexico resisted Washington's demands, "a corps of properly organized volunteers . . . would invade, overrun, and occupy Mexico. They would enable us not only to take California, but to keep it." American officials, in their contempt for Mexico, spoke privately of the need to chastize that country for its annoyances and insults. Parrott wrote to Secretary of State James Buchanan in October that he wished "to see this people well flogged by Uncle Sam's boys, ere we enter upon negotiations. . . . I know [the Mexicans] better, perhaps, than any other American citizen and I am fully persuaded, they can never love or respect us, as we should be loved and respected by them, until we shall have given them a positive proof of our superiority." Mexico's pretensions would continue, wrote Slidell in late December, "until the Mexican people shall be convinced by hostile demonstrations, that our differences must be settled promptly, either by negotiation or the sword." In January 1846 the *Union* publicly threatened Mexico with war if it rejected the just demands of the United States: "The result of such a course on her part may compel us to resort to more decisive measures . . . to obtain the settlement of our legitimate claims." As Slidell prepared to leave Mexico in March 1846, he again reminded the administration: "Depend upon it, we can never get along well with them, until we have given them a good drubbing." In Washington on May 8, Slidell advised the president "to take the redress of the wrongs and injuries which we had so long borne from Mexico into our own hands, and to act with promptness and energy."

Mexico responded to Polk's challenge with an outward display of belligerence and an inward dread of war. Mexicans feared above all that the United States intended to overrun their country and seize much of their territory. Polk and his advisers assumed that Mexico, to avoid an American invasion, would give up its provinces peacefully.

Obviously Mexico faced growing diplomatic and military pressures to negotiate away its territories; it faced no moral obligation to do so. Herrera and Paredes had the sovereign right to protect their regimes by avoiding any formal recognition of Slidell and by rejecting any of the boundary proposals embodied in his instructions, provided that in the process they did not endanger any legitimate interests of the American people. At least to some Mexicans, Slidell's terms demanded nothing less than Mexico's capitulation. By what standard was $2 million a proper payment for the Rio Grande boundary, or $25 million a fair price for California? No government would have accepted such terms. Having rejected negotiation in the face of superior force, Mexico would meet the challenge with a final gesture of defiance. In either case it was destined to lose, but historically nations have preferred to fight than to give away territory under diplomatic pressure alone. Gene M. Brack, in his long study of Mexico's deep-seated fear and resentment of the United States, explained Mexico's ultimate behavior in such terms:

> President Polk knew that Mexico could offer but feeble resistance militarily, and he knew that Mexico needed money. No proper American would exchange territory and the national honor for cash, but President Polk mistakenly believed that the application of military pressure would convince Mexicans to do so. They did not respond logically, but patriotically. Left with the choice of war or territorial concessions, the former course, however dim the prospects of success, could be the only one.

Mexico, in its resistance, gave Polk the three choices which every nation gives another in an uncompromising confrontation: to withdraw his demands and permit the issues to drift, unresolved; to reduce his goals in the interest of an immediate settlement; or to escalate the pressures in the hope of securing an eventual settlement on his own terms. Normally when the internal conditions of a country undermine its relations with others, a diplomatic corps simply removes itself from the hostile environment and awaits a better day. Mexico, despite its animosity, did not endanger the security interests of the United States; it had not invaded Texas and did not contemplate doing so. Mexico had refused to pay the claims, but those claims were not equal to the price of a one-week war. Whether Mexico negotiated a boundary for Texas in 1846 mattered little; the United States had lived with unsettled boundaries for decades without considering war. Settlers, in time, would have forced a decision, but in 1846 the region between the Nueces and the Rio Grande was a vast, generally unoccupied wilderness. Thus there was nothing, other than Polk's ambitions, to prevent the United States from withdrawing its diplomats from Mexico City and permitting its relations to drift. But Polk, whatever the language of his instructions, did not send Slidell to Mexico to normalize relations with that government. He expected Slidell to negotiate an immediate boundary settlement favorable to the United States, and nothing less.

Recognizing no need to reduce his demands on Mexico, Polk, without hesitation, took the third course which Mexico offered. Congress bound the president to the annexation of Texas; thereafter the Polk administration was free to formulate its own policies toward Mexico. With the Slidell mission Polk embarked upon a program of gradual coercion to achieve a settlement, preferably without war. That program led logically from his dispatching an army to Texas and his denunciation of Mexico in his annual message of December 1845 to his new instructions of January 1846, which ordered General Taylor to the Rio Grande. Colonel Atocha, spokesman for the deposed Mexican leader, Antonio López de Santa Anna, encouraged Polk to pursue his policy of escalation. The president recorded Atocha's advice:

> He said our army should be marched at once from Corpus Christi to the Del Norte, and a strong naval force assembled at Vera Cruz, that Mr. Slidell, the U.S. Minister, should withdraw from Jalappa, and go on board one of our ships of War at Vera Cruz, and in that position should demand the payment of [the] amount due our citizens; that it was well known the Mexican Government was unable to pay in money, and that when they saw a strong force ready to strike on their coasts and border, they would, he had no doubt, feel their danger and agree to the boundary suggested. He said that Paredes, Almonte, & Gen'l Santa Anna were all willing for such an arrangement, but that they dare not make it until it was made apparent to the Archbishop of Mexico & the people generally that it was necessary to save their country from a war with the U. States.

Thereafter Polk never questioned the efficacy of coercion. He asserted at a cabinet meeting on February 17 that "it would be necessary to take strong measures towards Mexico before our difficulties with that Government could be settled." Similarly on April 18 Polk told Calhoun that "our relations with Mexico had reached a point where we could not stand still but must treat all nations whether weak or strong alike, and that I saw no alternative but strong measures towards Mexico." A week later the president again brought the Mexican question before the cabinet. "I expressed my opinion," he noted in his diary, "that we must take redress for the injuries done us into our own hands, that we had attempted to conciliate Mexico in vain, and had forborne until forbearance was no longer either a virtue or patriotic." Convinced that Paredes needed money, Polk suggested to leading senators that Congress appropriate $1 million both to encourage Paredes to negotiate and to sustain him in power until the United States could ratify the treaty. The president failed to secure Calhoun's required support.

Polk's persistence led him and the country to war. Like all escalations in the exertion of force, his decision responded less to unwanted and unanticipated resistance than to the requirements of the clearly perceived and inflexible purposes which guided the administration. What perpetuated the president's escalation to the point of war was his determination to pursue goals to the end whose achievement lay outside the possibilities of successful negotiations. Senator Thomas Hart Benton of Missouri saw this situation when he wrote: "It is impossible to conceive of an administration less warlike, or more intriguing, than that of Mr. Polk. They were *men of peace, with objects to be accomplished by means of war;* so that war was a necessity and an indispensability to their purpose."

Polk understood fully the state of Mexican opinion. In placing General Taylor on the Rio Grande he revealed again his contempt for Mexico. Under no national obligation to expose the country's armed forces, he would not have advanced Taylor in the face of a superior military force. Mexico had been undiplomatic; its denunciations of the United States were insulting and provocative. But if Mexico's behavior antagonized Polk, it did not antagonize the Whigs, the abolitionists, or even much of the Democratic party. Such groups did not regard Mexico as a threat; they warned the administration repeatedly that Taylor's presence on the Rio Grande would provoke war. But in the balance against peace was the pressure of American expansionism. Much of the Democratic and expansionist press, having accepted without restraint both the purposes of the Polk administration and its charges of Mexican perfidy, urged the president on to more vigorous action. . . .

Confronted with the prospect of further decline which they could neither accept nor prevent, [the Mexicans] lashed out with the intention of protecting their self-esteem and compelling the United States, if it was determined to have the Rio Grande, New Mexico, and California, to pay for its prizes with something other than money. On April 23, Paredes issued a proclamation declaring a defensive war against the United States. Predictably, one day later the Mexicans fired on a detachment of U.S. dragoons. Taylor's report of the attack reached Polk on Saturday evening, May 9. On Sunday the president drafted his war message and delivered it to Congress on the following day. Had Polk avoided the crisis, he might have gained the time required to permit the emigrants of 1845 and 1846 to settle the California issue without war.

What clouds the issue of the Mexican War's justification was the acquisition of New Mexico and California, for contemporaries and historians could not logically condemn the war and laud the Polk administration for its territorial achievements. Perhaps it is true that time would have permitted American pioneers to transform California into another Texas. But even then California's acquisition by the United States would have emanated from the use of force, for the elimination of Mexican sovereignty, whether through revolution or war, demanded the successful use of power. If the power employed in revolution would have been less obtrusive than that exerted in war, its role would have been no less essential. There simply was no way that the United States could acquire California peacefully. If the distraught Mexico of 1845 would not sell the distant province, no regime thereafter would have done so. Without forceful destruction of Mexico's sovereign power, California would have entered the twentieth century as an increasingly important region of another country.

Thus the Mexican War poses the dilemma of all international relations. Nations whose geographic and political status fails to coincide with their ambition and power can balance the two sets of factors in only one manner: through the employment of force. They succeed or fail according to circumstances; and for the United States, the conditions for achieving its empire in the Southwest and its desired frontage on the Pacific were so ideal that later generations could refer to the process as the mere fulfillment of destiny. "The Mexican Republic," lamented a Mexican writer in 1848, ". . . had among other misfortunes of less account, the great one of being in the vicinity of a strong and energetic people." What the Mexican War revealed in equal measure is the simple fact that only those countries which have achieved their destiny, whatever that may be, can afford to extol the virtues of peaceful change.

NORMAN A. GRAEBNER (1915–2010) was the Randolph P. Compton Professor Emeritus of History at the University of Virginia. A renowned classroom teacher, he also wrote and edited numerous books, articles, and texts on American history, including *Foundations of American Foreign Policy: A Realist Appraisal from Franklin to McKinley* (Scholarly Resources, 1985) and *Empire on the Pacific: A Study in American Continental Expansion,* 2nd ed. (Regina Books, 1983).

EXPLORING THE ISSUE

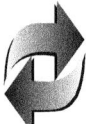

Was the Mexican War an Exercise in American Imperialism?

Critical Thinking and Reflection

1. Define imperialism by looking up the definition in a dictionary.
   a. Discuss whether or not the dictionary definition is too narrow.
   b. Does a nation need to control a country territorially to be imperialistic?
   c. Discuss whether or not the United States pursued an imperialistic policy toward Mexico in the 1840s.
2. Define Manifest Destiny.
   a. Where did the term originate?
   b. Did Manifest Destiny express the true feelings of the American people? Of American politicians? Or was it an exaggeration?
   c. Was Manifest Destiny merely a cover for American expansionist policies in Mexico?
   d. Was Manifest Destiny racist? Explain.
3. What evidence does Ramón Eduardo Ruiz provide to support his contention that the U.S.-Mexico War was motivated by racism and imperialism?
4. What is a "realist diplomatic historian"?
   a. Examine the influences of the cold war and influences of political scientists on Graebner's thinking.
   b. Analyze the following statement made by Graebner: "Nations do not fight over cultural differences or verbal recriminations; they fight over perceived threats to their interests created by the ambitions or demands of others."
5. Discuss the following three options which Polk could have taken after the Mexican government refused to back down in Texas or to sell New Mexico and California to the United States: (1) withdraw the demands; (2) scale down the demands; and (3) keep up the pressure until demands were met.
6. What other courses of action could President Polk have followed to achieve his objectives and to avoid a war?
7. Could California, like Texas, have become part of the United States through an internal revolution? Explain.
8. Has Mexico been hurt economically for the past 150 years because she lost control of Texas, New Mexico, and California?
9. Compare the cases of President Polk in 1846 with the two Presidents Bush in the ways in which they waged the Iraq Wars in 1991 and 2003.

Is There Common Ground?

Graebner disagrees with Walter Nugent over who started the Mexican War. He argues that Polk truly believed that President Paredes would back down and negotiate. Nugent, along with other writers such as Richard Kluger, in *Seizing Destiny: How America Grew from Sea to Shining Sea* (Knopf, 2007) maintains that Polk really wanted the war, especially after the Oregon boundary dispute with England was settled at the 49th parallel. Other historians support Graebner by putting the events into a broader focus. Walter A. McDougall, in *Promised Land, Crusader State: The American Encounter with the World since 1776*, states that aside from "sheer ambition" or "the fact that Americans inhabited an undeveloped continent devoid of serious rivals . . . expansion derived from the primordial exceptional American commitment to liberty." The four barriers to expansion, continued McDougall, included Indian tribes, British lords, Mexican juntas, and "U.S. federal authorities themselves telling farmers, trappers, ranchers, merchants and missionaries: No, you can't settle here, or do business there. Go back where you came from!" (p. 78). Finally, Robert Kagan, in *Dangerous Nation* (Knopf, 2006), emphasizes how the acquisition of California and the territories of New Mexico and Arizona could upset the balance of power between the equal number of free and slave states that had been created.

There are many issues that an instructor could discuss with students concerning the early foreign policy of the United States. First is the notion of American "exceptionalism." The policies of American isolationism, neutrality, and the Monroe Doctrine were premised on the rejection of the traditional European notion of balance-of-power politics. Manifest Destiny was a concept that extolled the spread of the unique American ideals of freedom, democracy, and capitalism across the North American continent (not including Canada). Europe, by contrast, was wedded to old-fashioned kingdoms that restrained economic development via mercantilist controls. American foreign policy was based on ideals; European diplomacy was based on cynical realism in which nations played games with one another to maintain a balance of power.

The issue of American "exceptionalism" raises several questions. Was Benjamin Franklin playing power politics when he violated the alliance with France and negotiated a separate peace treaty with England to gain American independence? Are there other examples in the pre–Civil War period in which American presidents negotiated realistic agreements with foreign countries? In his book *Unmanifest Destiny: Mayhem and Illusion in American Foreign Policy—From the Monroe Doctrine to Reagan's War in El Salvador* (Dial Press, 1984), journalist T. D. Allman asserts that American foreign policy has run amok, spreading its unmanifested destiny to Vietnam in the 1960s and early 1970s and to El Salvador and Nicaragua in the late 1980s. Was the American invasion of Grenada a violation of the Monroe Doctrine? Is American foreign policy imperialistic? Was Manifest Destiny merely a cover for American imperialism? Was Manifest Destiny also racist, as some Mexican historians contend? For a view that perceives empire as a way of life in the United States, consult the first chapter of Professor William Appleman Williams's classic *Tragedy of Diplomacy*, 2nd ed. (Delta, 1972). For the perspective of the Mexican side, see the collections on the Mexican War by Archie McDonald, ed., *The Mexican War: Crisis for American Democracy* (D. D. Heath, 1969) and Ramón Eduardo Ruiz, ed., *The Mexican War: Was It Manifest Destiny?* (Holt, Rinehart and Winston, 1969).

Additional Resources

Rodolfo Acuña, *Occupied America: A History of Chicanos*, 3rd ed. (Harper & Row, 1988)

Ernesto Chavez, *The U.S. War with Mexico: A Brief History with Documents* (Bedford/St. Martin's, 2008)

John S. D. Eisenhower, *So Far from God: The U. S. War with Mexico, 1846–1848* (Random House, 1989)

Amy S. Greenberg, *A Wicked War: Polk, Clay, Lincoln and the 1846 U.S. Invasion of Mexico* (Alfred A. Knopf, 2012)

Robert W. Merry, *A Country of Vast Designs: James K. Polk, the Mexican War and the Conquest of America* (Simon & Schuster, 2009)

Internet References . . .

A Continent Divided: The U.S.-Mexico War

library.uta.edu/usmexicowar/

A Guide to the Mexican War

www.loc.gov/rr/program/bib/mexicanwar/

Descendants of Mexican War Veterans

www.dmwv.org/

Mexican War Service Records

www.fold3.com/category_274/

Military Resources: Mexican War, 1846–1848

www.archives.gov/research/alic/reference/military/mexican-war.html

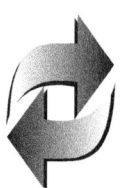

ISSUE

Selected, Edited, and with Issue Framing Material by:
Kevin R. Magill and Tony L. Talbert, *Baylor University*

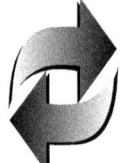

Was John Brown an Irrational Terrorist?

YES: **James N. Gilbert**, from "A Behavioral Analysis of John Brown: Martyr or Terrorist?" Ohio University Press (2005)

NO: **Scott John Hammond**, from "John Brown as Founder: America's Violent Confrontation with Its First Principles," Ohio University Press (2005)

Learning Outcomes

After reading this issue, you will be able to:

- Define "terrorism" and place this concept in a broad historical context that does not simply include the present.
- Determine whether John Brown's actions amount to terrorist tactics.
- Compare the abolitionists' goals for freedom for African American slaves with the political freedom sought by the founders of the American republic.
- Assess the legitimacy of employing violence to end the institution of slavery.

ISSUE SUMMARY

YES: James N. Gilbert believes that the actions of John Brown are a textbook definition of terrorism in modern society. Brown believed the United States was going to be incapable of the social reform needed to abolish slavery and therefore saw it as his responsibility to use violence to achieve that goal. Gilbert also discusses Brown's belief that adherence to a higher power was his justification for his acts of terror.

NO: Scott John Hammond instead believes that John Brown was committed to higher moral and political goals including the basic principals of human freedom, political equality, and legal egalitarianism. Therefore, he was not a terrorist, but a citizen committed to the ideals set forth by the founding fathers.

Opposition to slavery in the area that became the United States dates back to the seventeenth and eighteenth centuries, when Puritan leaders, such as Samuel Sewall, and Quakers, such as John Woolman and Anthony Benezet, published a number of pamphlets condemning the existence of the slave system. This religious link to antislavery sentiment is also evident in the writings of John Wesley as well as in the decision of the Society of Friends in 1688 to prohibit their members from owning bond servants. Slavery was said to be contrary to Christian principles. These attacks, however, did little to diminish the institution. Complaints that the English government had instituted a series of measures that "enslaved" the colonies in British North America raised thorny questions about the presence of *real* slavery in those colonies. How could American colonists demand their freedom from King George III, who was cast in the role of oppressive master, while denying freedom and liberty to African American slaves? Such a contradiction inspired a gradual emancipation movement in the North, which often was accompanied by compensation for the former slave owners.

In addition, antislavery societies sprang up throughout the nation to continue the crusade against bondage. Interestingly, the majority of these organizations were located in the South. Prior to the 1830s, the most prominent antislavery organization was the American

Colonization Society, which offered a twofold program: (1) gradual, compensated emancipation of slaves and (2) exportation of the newly freed to colonies outside the boundaries of the United States, mostly to Africa.

In the 1830s, antislavery activity underwent an important transformation. A new strain of antislavery sentiment expressed itself in the abolitionist movement. Drawing momentum both from the revivalism of the Second Great Awakening and the example set by England (which prohibited slavery in its imperial holdings in 1833), abolitionists called for the immediate end to slavery without compensation to masters for the loss of their property. Abolitionists viewed slavery not so much as a practical problem to be resolved, but rather as a moral offense incapable of resolution through traditional channels of political compromise. In January 1831, William Lloyd Garrison, who for many came to symbolize the abolitionist crusade, published the first issue of *The Liberator*, a newspaper dedicated to the immediate end to slavery. In his first editorial, Garrison expressed the self-righteous indignation of many in the abolitionist movement when he warned slaveholders and their supporters to "urge me not to use moderation in a cause like the present. I am in earnest—I will not equivocate—I will not excuse—I will not retreat a single inch—AND I WILL BE HEARD. . . ."

Unfortunately for Garrison, relatively few Americans were inclined to respond positively to his call. His newspaper generated little interest outside Boston, New York, Philadelphia, and other major urban centers of the North. This situation, however, changed within a matter of months. In August 1831, a slave preacher named Nat Turner led a rebellion of slaves in Southampton County, Virginia, that resulted in the death of 58 whites. Although the revolt was quickly suppressed and Turner and his supporters were executed, the incident spread fear throughout the South. Governor John B. Floyd of Virginia turned an accusatory finger toward the abolitionists when he concluded that the Turner uprising was "undoubtedly designed and matured by unrestrained fanatics in some of the neighboring states."

One of the weaknesses of most studies of abolitionism is that they generally are written from a monochromatic perspective. In other words, historians typically discuss whites within the abolitionist crusade and give little, if any, attention to the roles African Americans played in the movement. Whites are portrayed as the active agents of reform, while blacks are the passive recipients of humanitarian efforts to eliminate the scourge of slavery. Students should be aware that African Americans, slave and free, also rebelled against the institution of slavery both directly and indirectly, although very few rallied to the call of John Brown.

Benjamin Quarles in *Black Abolitionists* (Oxford University Press, 1969) describes a wide range of roles played by blacks in the abolitionist movement. The African American challenge to the slave system is also evident in the network known as the "underground railroad." Larry Gara, in *The Liberty Line: The Legend of the Underground Railroad* (University of Kentucky Press, 1961), concludes that the real heroes of the underground railroad were not white abolitionists but the slaves themselves who depended primarily upon their own resources or assistance they received from other African Americans, slave and free.

Other studies treating the role of black abolitionists in the antislavery movement include James M. McPherson, *The Struggle For Equality: Abolitionists and the Negro in the Civil War and Reconstruction* (Princeton University Press, 1964); Jane H. and William H. Pease, *They Who Would Be Free: Blacks' Search for Freedom, 1830–1861* (Atheneum, 1974); R. J. M. Blackett, *Building an Antislavery Wall: Black Americans in the Atlantic Abolitionist Movement, 1830–1860* (Louisiana State University Press, 1983) and *Beating Against the Barriers: The Lives of Six Nineteenth-Century Afro-Americans* (Louisiana State University Press, 1986); Ronald K. Burke, *Samuel Ringgold Ward: Christian Abolitionist* (Garland, 1995), Nell Irvin Painter, *Sojourner Truth: A Life, A Symbol* (W. W. Norton, 1997); and Catherine Clinton, *Harriet Tubman: The Road to Freedom* (2004). Frederick Douglass's contributions are evaluated in Benjamin Quarles, *Frederick Douglass* (Atheneum, 1968; originally published 1948), Nathan Irvin Huggins, *Slave and Citizen: The Life of Frederick Douglass* (Little, Brown, 1980), Waldo E. Martin, Jr., *The Mind of Frederick Douglass* (University of North Carolina Press, 1984), and William S. McFeely, *Frederick Douglass* (W. W. Norton, 1991).

The following essays focus on a white abolitionist who perhaps best fits the characterization of an "unrestrained fanatic" but who became a martyr in the antislavery pantheon when he was executed following his unsuccessful raid on the federal arsenal in Harpers Ferry, Virginia in 1859. James N. Gilbert argues that Brown's attack was comparable to recent acts of terrorism in the United States and that, despite the continuing tendency to portray his actions as those of a martyred hero, Brown clearly fits the modern definition of a domestic terrorist.

In the second selection, Scott John Hammond characterizes Brown in a more positive light. While recognizing flaws in Brown's personality and actions, Hammond nevertheless concludes that John Brown acted on the highest of principles to thwart evil by articulating an undiluted commitment to the basic principles of America's founding—individual liberty and political and legal equality.

YES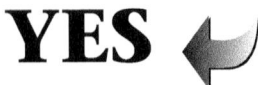

James N. Gilbert

A Behavioral Analysis of John Brown: Martyr or Terrorist?

The scholarly examination of the topic of terrorism has developed into a significant area of legal and criminological research. Academic and governmental studies pertaining to terrorist crimes and those who perpetrate them are now voluminous and continue to be actively pursued. Emerging as what appeared to be a new form of criminal deviance, the definition and cause of the "disease of the 70s" has challenged criminologists. While most contemporary documented incidents continue to occur outside the United States, the fear of domestic terrorism, as recent events have illustrated, remains a legitimate concern. The public and researchers alike have in the past commonly assumed that this country would continue to be spared from acts that conform to our contemporary definition of terrorist activity. Terrorism was associated with a foreign environment and viewed as exceptional in the history of American criminal violence.

But after February 26, 1993, when the New York World Trade Center was the target of a massive terrorist bombing, the attention of Americans became riveted upon the unique form of criminality that we have collectively termed terrorism. And of course this criminal act was followed by the far more deadly bombing in Oklahoma City and the attacks on the World Trade Center and the Pentagon on September 11, 2001. Although much of the media and public has treated these terrorist acts as precedent-setting domestic attacks, the history of terrorism in the United States actually dates to the founding of the nation. Of the many such violent episodes in our earlier history, John Brown's attack on Harpers Ferry in October 1859 is comparable to these more recent acts in terms of national terror and consequent social and political upheaval.

In late 1859 John Brown and twenty-one followers attempted to rally and arm large numbers of slaves by attacking and briefly holding the United States arsenal at Harpers Ferry, Virginia (presently West Virginia). Captured by federal military forces and local militia, Brown was hastily tried and executed. While the life and deeds of John Brown are immensely important for their impact on abolitionism and the American Civil War, this powerful historical figure is rarely defined as a terrorist. Instead, a vast collection of literature generally portrays Brown as either saint or madman. On one hand, there is the sympathetic traditional portrait of John Brown as an American hero of near mythical proportions. Such an image is certainly not viewed as criminally deviant, nor does it suggest the status of criminal folk hero. But while a minority historical judgment has questioned his sanity or the radical end-justification logic he appeared to employ, few even in this camp would declare his actions truly terrorist. Civil War and military historian John Hubbell reflects this multidimensional view. Stating that while John Brown was, "in fact, a combination of humility and arrogance, submission and aggression, murder and martyrdom," his true motivation may not have been calculated terroristic cause and effect, but "an unresolved resentment of his father; his hatred of slaveholders may have been the unconscious resolution of his anger."

Thus, one can only question how and why this imagery has persisted throughout the decades. Is the terrorist label lacking due to the singular rationale of his crimes: the massive evil of slavery? Alternatively, are we correct in excluding Brown from the definition of terrorist because his actions simply fail to conform to contemporary elements that constitute such a criminal? For example, a similar definitional confusion currently exists regarding various violent attacks on abortion clinics and their personnel by those who, like Brown, rationalize their violence by moral or religious conviction. Some would define convicted murderer Paul Hill as a domestic terrorist for his premeditated attack on an abortion doctor and an escort during the summer of 1994. Yet others would fail to define his actions as terroristic due to Hill's justification of his act as a "lesser evil."

In order to define Brown precisely as a terrorist rather than as a martyr, the meaning of terrorism must be explored. As with many singular, emotion-producing

---

Gilbert, James N. "A Behavioral Analysis of John Brown: Martyr or Terrorist?" from Russo, Peggy A. and Finkelman, Paul (eds) *Terrible Swift Sword: The Legacy of John Brown* (Ohio University Press, 2005), pp. 107–113, 114–116 (notes omitted). Copyright ©2005 by Ohio University Press. www.ohioswallow.com. Reprinted by permission.

labels of criminality, terrorism is easier to describe than define. The *Vice President's Task Force on Combating Terrorism* describes terrorism as a phenomenon involving "the unlawful use of threat of violence against persons or property to further political or social objectives." In a similar vein, the FBI's Terrorist Research and Analytical Center states that terroristic activity "is the unlawful use of force or violence against persons or property to intimidate or coerce a government, the civilian population, or any segment thereof, in furtherance of political or social objectives." Both definitions agree with views commonly provided by various governments. This traditional bureaucratic view stresses a triad in which both property and people are potential targets with the necessary presence of illegal actions and social or political motivations as the causative agent.

Additional attempts to conceptualize the terrorist often focus on the perpetrator's motive rather than legal definitions. To this economist Bill Anderson links the economic viewpoint, stressing that fundamental principles of economic theory are the real, often hidden, motives of such crimes. Anderson believes that after we "peel away the ideological skins and fig leaves that terrorists use to justify their violence, we come to the core reason for their actions: the terrorists' own desire for power and influence. In other words, the terrorists are seeking wealth transfers and/or power (all of which can be defined as economic or political rents) through violent means because they are not willing to pay the cost of participating in the political process."

Others prefer to explain away terrorism through an apologist approach, stressing the anger, hopelessness, and governmental violence brought against various victimized populations from which, inevitably, terrorists will be mobilized. Eqbal Ahmad, a research fellow at the Washington, D.C.–based Institute for Policy Studies, stresses this sympathetic theme when he links terrorism to government indifference to violence. He believes that individuals turn to terrorism to exercise "their need to be heard, the combination of anger and helplessness producing the impulse for retributive violence. The experience of violence by a stronger party has historically turned victims into terrorists." Thus, the apologist view firmly supports the recurring belief that terrorism is merely situational, constantly coming in and out of criminal focus according to prevailing political power or orientation. Sheikh Omar Abdel-Rahman clearly embraced the situational view when he claimed to be a victim rather than an alleged conspirator in the 1993 World Trade Center bombing. Angered over his conspiracy indictment and subsequent incarceration, he stated, "but what bothers me, and makes me feel bitter about the whole thing, is when a person who was called a freedom fighter then is now called, when the war is over, a terrorist."

A final view, particularly popular in fictional portrayals of terrorists, suggests individual psychopathology as the chief cause of terrorism. As detailed by political philosopher and professor of religion Moshe Amon, one form of terroristic crime may originate within the disturbed minds of some perpetrators, triggering myths and fantasies that can be categorized as messianic or apocalyptic. The messianic terrorist ideology streams from a conviction that one has special insight that produces an individual state of enlightenment. Terrorists are then convinced that "they are the only ones who see the real world, and the only ones who are not affected by its depravity. It is their mission, therefore, to liberate the blind people of this world from the rule of the unjust." Although this concept may be traced to early Hebrew origins, a more contemporary form is common among Latin American terrorists. Political scientist John Pottenger concludes, "The existence of social injustice and [the] individual's commitment to human liberation, demand that a radical change can turn the Christian into a revolutionary vanguard demonstrating that God not only intervenes in human history but He does so on the right side of the oppressed."

Other psychological theorists believe that the most common type of terrorist has a psychopathic or sociopathic personality. The classic traits of the psychopath—impulsiveness, lack of guilt, inability to experience emotional depth, and manipulation—are perceived as ideally suited to the commission of terrorism. The ability to kill often large numbers of strangers without compunction or to manipulate others to unwittingly further criminal ends convinces many that the psychopathic personality is a requirement for terroristic action.

With such definitions of terrorism in mind, how are we to view John Brown? After almost a century and a half, the actions of Brown have been preserved with stark clarity, yet his personality and related psychological motivations can only be surmised. John Brown was fifty-nine years old when he was executed by the state of Virginia for treason, conspiring with blacks to produce insurrection, and murder in the first degree. His criminal activities of record include embezzlement and assault with a deadly weapon against an Ohio sheriff in 1842. In 1856 a warrant was issued by a proslavery Kansas district court charging Brown with "organizing against slavery." A month later he and eight other men kidnapped and murdered five Kansans, including a constable and his two sons. The killings were particularly brutal: the victims were hacked to death by repeated sword blows. In December 1858 the state of Missouri and the federal government offered a reward for Brown's capture because he was the chief suspect in yet another criminal homicide. Finally, Brown's criminal activities culminated in the seizure of the federal armory at Harpers Ferry on October 16, 1859. A company of U.S. Marines captured him the following day, and history records his execution less than fifty days after his attack against the armory.

The question of whether John Brown was indeed a terrorist must be based on a definitional standard that defies emotional or mythical distortion. The linkage of Brown's cause to the horrors of slavery circumvents the true nature of the man and of his crimes. According to Albert Parry, author of a best-selling work on the history of terror and revolutionary violence, terrorists and those who study them offer innumerable explanations of their violence; yet their motivations can be compacted into three main concepts:

1. Society is sick and cannot be cured by half measures of reform.
2. The state is in itself violent and can be countered and overcome only by violence.
3. The truth of the terrorist cause justifies any action that supports it. While some terrorists recognize no moral law, others have their own "higher" morality.

Comparing John Brown's actions to these criteria produces an inescapable match. On many occasions Brown expressed his solid belief that society, particularly a society that would embrace slavery, was sick beyond its own cure. Brown had clearly given up on public policy reforms or legal remedies regarding slavery when he drafted his own constitution for the benefit of his followers. The document attempts to define his justifications for the upcoming attack at Harpers Ferry and utterly rejects the legal and moral foundation of the United States: "Therefore, we citizens of the United States and the Oppressed People, who by a Recent Decision of the Supreme Court are declared to have no rights which the white man is bound to respect; together with all other people regarded by the laws thereof, do for the time being, ordain and establish for ourselves the following provisional constitution and ordinances, the better to protect our persons, property, lives, and liberties: and to govern our actions."

As to the terroristic belief that violent government can only be overcome by violence, Brown's convictions were preserved for posterity by a note he handed to a jailer while being led to the gallows: "I John Brown am now quite *certain* that the crimes of this *guilty land: will* never be purged *away;* but with Blood. I had *as I now think: vainly* flattered myself that without *very much* bloodshed: it might be done."

With similar conformity, Brown's beliefs and actions demonstrated his rigid "higher" morality, which served to justify numerous crimes, including multiple homicides. As described by historian Stephen Oates, "Brown knew the Missourians would come after him ... yet he was not afraid of the consequences for God would keep and deliver him: God alone was his judge. Now that the work was done, he believed that he had been guided by a just and wrathful God."

Brown's deeds conform to contemporary definitions of terrorism, and his psychological predispositions are consistent with the terrorist model. As observed by David Hubbard, founder of the Aberrant Behavior Center and psychiatric consultant to the Federal Bureau of Prisons, the actions and personality of the terrorist are not "merely bizarre and willfully antisocial; but a reflection of deep-seated personal and cultural pathologies." Such behavioral pathology is commonly linked to the psychopathic personality or, less frequently, to some form of paranoia. Virtually unknown to mental health authorities during Brown's lifetime, the psychopathic personality is currently considered a relatively common criminal mental abnormality among violent offenders. Although psychopathic criminals account for a small percentage of overall lawbreakers, psychologist William McCord notes that they commit a disproportionate percentage of violent crime. While psychopaths may be encountered within any violent criminal typology, they appear to be particularly well represented in various crimes of serial violence, confidence fraud, and terrorism.

The concept of psychopathy focuses on the unsocialized criminal, who is devoid of conscience and consequently in repeated conflict with society; he or she fails to learn from prior experiences. As observed by Herbert Strean, professor of social work and psychotherapy researcher at Rutgers University, the psychopath is often arrogant, callous, and lacking in empathy and tends to offer plausible rationalizations for his or her reckless behavior. While John Brown demonstrated a guilt-free conscience on many occasions, his calculating leadership in the kidnapping and murder of five people in Kansas provided beyond question his capacity to free himself of normal emotion. On the night of May 26, 1856, Brown led a small party of followers to the various cabins of his political enemies, which included Constable James Doyle and his sons. During what would later be termed the Pottawatomie Massacre, the Brown party systematically dragged the five unarmed and terrified men from their homes and murdered them in a frenzy of brutal violence. "About a hundred yards down the road Salmon and Owen [Brown's sons] fell on the Doyles with broadswords. They put up a struggle, striking out, trying to shield themselves from the slashing blades as they staggered back down the road. But in a few moments the grisly work was done. Brown, who must have watched the executions in a kind of trance, now walked over and shot Doyle in the forehead with a revolver, to make certain work of it." When later questioned about his motives during the Kansas murders, Brown offered a classic messianic psychopathic rationalization. Without a trace of remorse, he stated that the victims all deserved to die as they "had committed murder in their hearts already, according to the Big Book . . . their killing had been decreed by Almighty God, ordained from eternity."

. . . John Brown does not stand alone in the annals of American-based terrorism. Yet he obviously remains a unique, paradoxical example of a terrorist whom history has often viewed through rose-colored lenses. As opposed to alarm or disgust, the deeds of John Brown have moved some to great literary inspiration, such as Stephen Vincent Benét's epic poem *John Brown's Body*. Ralph Waldo Emerson, writing shortly before Brown's execution, referred to Brown as "the Saint, whose fate yet hangs in suspense, but whose martyrdom, if it shall be perfected, will make the gallows glorious like the Cross." Other towering figures of the arts echo the purity of Brown while conveniently ignoring his murderous past. Henry David Thoreau wrote, "No man in America has ever stood up so persistently and effectively for the dignity of human nature, knowing himself for a man, and the equal of any and all governments. . . . He could not have been tried by a jury of his peers, because his peers did not exist." Other, more contemporary sources, including scores of textbooks, continue to echo such laudatory sentiments, informing generation after generation of young Americans that John Brown was a genuine hero. Typical of many such high school and middle school American history texts, one leading book praises Brown through Emerson's words as "a new saint," while another considers him "a martyr and hero, as he walked resolutely to the scaffold."

In a pragmatic sense, it is doubtful that the heroic legend of John Brown will ever include the terrorist truth of his crimes. As observed by guerrilla warfare essayist Walter Laqueur, "terrorism has long exercised a great fascination, especially at a safe distance . . . the fascination it exerts and the difficulty of interpreting it have the same roots: its unexpected, shocking and outrageous character." While many American terrorists exert a continuing fascination, none have occupied the unique position of John Brown. By contemporary definition, he was undoubtedly a terrorist to his core, demonstrating repeatedly the various axioms from which we shape this unique crime. Brown quite purposely waged war for political and social change while simultaneously committing the most heinous crimes. As political scientist Charles Hazelip would say when defining a terrorist, he had "crossed over the blurred line of demarcation between crime and war where political terrorism begins."

Yet John Brown's obsessive target, the focus of all his energy and murderous deeds, has by its nature absolved him from the cold label of *terrorist*. History and popular opinion have quite naturally found the greater criminality of slavery to far outweigh his illegal acts. The bold tactics at Harpers Ferry, coupled with his humanistic motives to free the Virginia slaves, compels us to forgive his disturbed personality and deadly past. The attack on a key government arsenal and armory, which in a contemporary context would horrify the nation, has been judged through the passage of time to be an inevitable, gallant first strike against the soon to be formed Southern Confederacy. When taken as a whole, and to the natural dismay of our justice system, Brown's actions quite convincingly demonstrate that if the weight of moral sentiment is on one's side, terroristic violence can be absorbed into a nation's historiography in a positive sense. [Christopher] Dobson and [Ronald] Payne conclude, "the main aim of terror is to make murderers into heroes." While many will continue to debate the magnitude of John Brown's terrorism, his heroic stature has been secured by the often paradoxical judgment of history.

JAMES N. GILBERT is a professor and former chair of the department of criminal justice at the University of Nebraska-Kearney, where he has taught since 1988. Specializing in criminal investigative theory, he is the author of *Criminal Investigation* (Pearson/Prentice Hall, 2009), now in its eighth edition, as well as numerous journal articles.

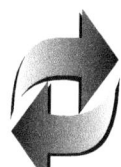

Scott John Hammond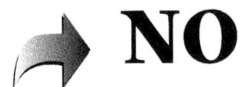

John Brown as Founder: America's Violent Confrontation with Its First Principles

John Brown moves at an angle through our history, a transfigured personage who is deemed a force of nature, an avenging angel wielding the scourge of God, a fearsome vessel of pure fanaticism that is seductive in the abstract as well as a terrifyingly demonic power in the flesh. Some would call him a tragic hero, flawed only in his insistence on purity in thought and action coupled with a mystical detachment from the political realities of his day; and some would see in him a prototerrorist, a criminal mind living on the lunatic fringe of history, condemned by rational people in both the North and South. Lincoln, in spite of his deep opposition to slavery, saw in Brown's raid the very archetype of lawless violence and was quick to distance both himself and his party from such obviously treasonous actions. For example, directing his remarks to Southern whites in a speech at the Cooper Union Institute on February 27, 1860, Lincoln declared: "You charge that we stir up insurrections among your slaves. We deny it; and what is your proof? Harper's [sic] Ferry! John Brown! John Brown is no Republican, and you have [yet] to implicate a single Republican in his Harper's [sic] Ferry enterprise." Conversely, Emerson praised Brown and remarked that Brown would elevate the gallows to a symbol of martyrdom on the same order and import as the Cross. It was, and perhaps still is, difficult for one to be objective or neutral about Osawatomie Brown: one was either with him or against him.

What we know of Brown's life fuels all these interpretations. As a lover of freedom steeled by a devotion to strict Calvinism, Brown appears to have been a practitioner of the Christian ethic framed by the imperative of universal love and compassion for others, especially those who suffer under the yoke of oppression and injustice. For in loving and caring for "the least" of his fellow human beings, he epitomized the purity of a love of human freedom that often comes from a sense of oneness with higher moral ends. Nonetheless, this is the same John Brown who, in the course of one night, assumed the visage of the Night Rider and personally directed and participated in the murder of five defenseless men. Since these men were supporters of slavery, and some of them had previously committed violence against Free State settlers, Brown's decision to kill them is perceived by some as part of his greater mission on behalf of even more defenseless slaves. Still, the manner in which Brown summarily executed these five resembles that of the vicious terrorist more than that of the righteous warrior, and the Pottawatomie Massacre chills the blood of even the most ardent foe of oppression.

These aspects of Brown's psyche reflect something about our own political soul—our "political psyche" writ large. If Brown embodies the essence of us all, then it might be conceded that Brown's more pathological qualities replicate a profound dissonance within our general political and social culture. We must consider the inevitable consequences inherent within a sociopolitical condition fractured by the collision between the ideals of democratic liberty and the appalling realities of slavery and racism. No American will impugn the principles of liberty and equality, for however they are construed or comprehended, the structuring principles of the American polity are derived from a noble vision and an aspiration for a free and dignified humanity. The presence of slavery in a country committed, at least in principle, to freedom is the worst possible incidence of ideational failure. Brown's fractured self is an embodiment of the tangled forces of light and darkness that grappled for the republic's soul; his character and actions demonstrate this, and in so doing, make him no different from the ruptured essence of our collective political self-consciousness. The Pottawatomie slaughter represents a symptom of the deeper malady, just as the abuse of any slave by an overseer represents the same

---

Hammond, Scott John. "John Brown as Founder: America's Violent Confrontation with Its First Principles," from Russo, Peggy A. and Finkelman, Paul (eds.) *Terrible Swift Sword: The Legacy of John Brown* (Ohio University Press, 2005), pp. 61–69, 70–71, 72–75 (excerpts; notes omitted). Copyright ©2005 by Ohio University Press. www.ohioswallow.com. Reprinted by permission.

type of symptomatic manifestation. In contrast to Brown's avenging violence in Kansas, the incident at Harpers Ferry was driven by a spirit imbued with the transfiguring fire of the idea of universal freedom, in the same manner as the Underground Railroad or the individual dissent of the most famous resident of Walden Pond. Both America and Brown reveal this self-negating duality.

That Brown could be so moved to action by the tragedy of his times further amplifies his character and conviction. Most citizens, absorbed in the daily process and considerations of private interest and obligation, ignore or suppress the maladies of the deeper social structure. The affairs of the state frequently demand too much concentration and emotional investment for the average citizen. Nevertheless, there will always be those among us who, like Brown, seriously regard the structuring principles of a political culture with unabashed sincerity and are thus impelled to hold our institutions and practices accountable to our own higher ideas and political ideals.

Brown judged society according to the laws of God, and he saw with a piercing clarity that neither the ruling political doctrine nor, more important, the commandments of Providence were being properly revered. Nothing could absolve us from the sin of slavery, and the distinctions between righteousness and evil were easily and sharply drawn. No ambiguity, no "gray in gray," no compromise or allowance would be tolerated; either one was with the warriors for freedom and divine righteousness or among the profane legions who served on behalf of sinful oppression. For Brown, unlike most of his fellow Americans, the only solution was an obvious one—brook no sympathy for or concession to the minions of evil, and unconditionally submit without hesitation or diffidence to the Higher Authority, never relenting until total emancipation was achieved or sublime retribution judiciously dispensed. This is what drove John Brown to act with such intensity of conviction, which magnified every hidden idiosyncrasy. Hence, Brown is at once liberator and fanatic, messiah and monster, the very incarnation of the conflicted American political soul.

This leads us to a more direct consideration of the notion of foundations and founding. The act of founding involves at least an abstract comprehension of those first principles that constitute a political soul and the resolve to forward those principles in an undiluted form. . . .

Upon examining those individuals who are noted for participating in an act of founding, we notice something unique that separates them from the ordinary politician, activist, or statesman. This is explained with considerable clarity by Machiavelli, who typically adds the ingredient of realpolitik to his observations of founding and reformative leadership. Given the fact that all founders and reformers will inevitably encounter resistance from those enemies who "profit from the old order," and assuming that a purely good leader will "bring about his own ruin among so many who are not good," Machiavelli notes that a lawgiver or prophet must go forth armed and prepared for struggle. Machiavelli's idea of a founder is consonant with the idea of virtue, or grandeur of soul—a character of extraordinary proportions, defined in terms of "ingenuity, skill, and excellence." Machiavelli seeks a type of transcending leadership, attaching a significant martial quality to his model founders. Even Moses, a religious founder, employs the might of God against Pharaoh in order to liberate the enslaved Israelites, something that those who follow the New Testament model of the suffering Christ would unequivocally reject.

Brown's actions are like those of a prophet-warrior. However, Machiavelli's armed prophet is also a conqueror; failure is associated with those who attempt to establish founding law without the enforcing power of arms. Brown does not seem to conform easily to the prophet-warrior model, for his arms were poor, his numbers few, and his plan thwarted by overextension and local hostility. Moses was at least able to extricate the Israelite slaves from their Egyptian oppressors. Moses conquered by overcoming the power of Egypt and then *founded* both a religion and a nation through the transmission of the Law of God. It is an understatement to say that Brown's achievement falls far short of this mark.

But if one considers the substance of Brown's commitment (the emancipation of the enslaved) and the method of Brown's action (confrontation with the sinful oppressor on behalf of the oppressed), Brown's character and actions do approximate the Machiavellian hero-founder. Furthermore, although he does not conquer in the physical or political sense, he does emerge triumphant. Brown was defeated but martyred, and in the end emancipation came for his people through the violence that he had prophesied. In a sobering moment of synchronicity, Lincoln's retrospective utterance in his second inaugural address, that "until every drop of blood drawn with the lash, shall be paid by another drawn with the sword," echoes Brown's last testimony. Two years earlier, Lincoln, at Gettysburg, had referred to a "new birth of freedom," and thus implicitly defined a new act of founding in the context and terms of the emancipation. From the blood and ashes of the war against slavery, the nation would be re-formed; Brown, who did not survive to witness the nation's second birth, nonetheless prophesied the act in his words. The nation was literally made anew but in a way that reaffirmed more completely the first principles of the republic. This represents an act of founding, and Brown's strike at Harpers Ferry was the prophetic prelude. Even though John Brown is distinct from Machiavelli's legendary types in a number of ways, he certainly shares in the role of founding/reforming visionary. Indeed, Lincoln, generally regarded as the heroic and tragic, even Christlike figure of the Civil War, resembles Brown in the end, only on a larger scale and from the comparatively more acceptable authority of his office. For Lincoln used violence to preserve the Union and purge the new nation of slavery. In his second inaugural address, he finally admits what he most likely knew from the beginning, that slavery was "somehow the cause of the war," and in so doing, for a brief moment toward the end of that war, the Great Emancipator shows himself akin to the Prophet of Osawatomie.

An alternative discussion of the founder-legislator is found in Rousseau's *Social Contract*. The Rousseauian founder is less applicable to the case of John Brown than the Machiavellian model. Rousseau's founder-legislator possesses a "superior intelligence" and is capable of "beholding all the passions of human beings without experiencing them." It is unlikely that Brown possessed a superior intelligence, and Brown's personality was far from the dispassionate character that Rousseau requires of his legislator. Furthermore, Rousseau's concept of the founder is identical to the concept of the first lawgiver and by no means resembles a prophet-warrior. Martial skill is not a requisite quality of Rousseau's founder, for Rousseau is always careful to mark an acute distinction between government based on consent and authority imposed by force. . . .

At another level, however, there is a similarity between Brown and Rousseau's founder. Rousseau's founder is an individual of superhuman qualities; indeed, Rousseau's description compares the creation of human first laws to the actions of gods. Rousseau's ideal founder is not afraid to act in a way that would challenge "human nature" itself. Brown seems to act against the natural order, but he does not intend to "change" human nature so much as to salvage it and even to save us from it. As a Calvinist, Brown undoubtedly believed that our nature is fixed by original sin; hence, he departed from Rousseau in yet another way. Brown fought against our sinful nature on behalf of redemption. Again, this seems to depart from Rousseau, but one must note that Rousseau's overall view of human nature was not much different from that of Calvin. Rousseau and Calvin both argued that humanity exists in a fallen condition, and although we cannot return to our original innocence, we can recover something of it through the affirmation of freedom and morality. For Calvin and John Brown, that higher state could be achieved through the Redeemer; for Rousseau, redemption is possible through the Social Contract. Both Rousseau and Brown sought a kind of recovery and affirmation of a better state of existence, and both insisted that in order to achieve such a goal, we must struggle mightily against our corrupted natures in order to reform and ennoble our humanity.

It should also be emphasized that the element of consent is vital to Rousseau. Brown's actions cannot admit of either direct or indirect consent of the governed for a number of reasons; most obvious of these is that Brown governed no one and possessed no legal or political authority, and that Brown was wholly dissociated from normal political channels. Even so, Brown acted in a way that relates indirectly to the notion of consensual governance. Brown sought neither the approval nor the consent of the populace, for the majority of the populace ignored, permitted, supported, or participated in the possession of human beings. More importantly, the law of God is not based on consent, but like Rousseau's general will, it is always right. Additionally, a minority of the population, both the enslaved victims and the various types of free dissenters and abolitionists, had been effectively deprived of their fundamental right to consent. The only rule that the slave knew was the rule of force, and the only rule that the abolitionist experienced was ultimately deemed immoral. The case of John Brown and his small group of followers and sympathizers exemplifies the latter, and it is compatible with Rousseau's theory of consent and resistance.

Even if Brown is not a founder-legislator in the strict Rousseauian sense, there are at least two arguments in the *Social Contract* that provide theoretical and moral support for Brown's extreme actions. First, Rousseau follows Locke in affirming that the notion of consent unequivocally requires unanimity. A political culture that either legitimizes or permits slavery violates this fundamental principle of universal consent. No one consents to be a slave; the enslaved population constitutes an excluded group that indicates a government based (partially) on force that is thus (wholly) illegitimate. Lincoln saw this as well and employed a similar argument in one of his many criticisms directed at the continued allowance of slavery. Even if one counters this argument by *incorrectly* objecting that Rousseau would not have included a slave population when considering the origins of the social contract, one would still have to take into account the abolitionists who, in acting against slavery from first principles, withdrew their consent to be governed by the current instrument. The unanimity that Rousseau demanded in theory never existed in practice under a regime that allowed slavery; thus, according to these standards, the Constitution, if it did indeed support or permit slavery (an issue that is in itself open to further analysis and argument within a different context) *was therefore not legitimate*. The founding act had occurred under an initial condition that was shaped by a great error.

This directs us back to our second point. Rousseau states without ambiguity that slavery is in every instance illegitimate and immoral. Freedom cannot be surrendered or usurped, for to "renounce liberty is to renounce being a man, to surrender the rights of humanity and even its duties." Thus, slavery can never be rendered legitimate or permitted by a government or any portion of its population. Rousseau makes this clear in the cases of both voluntary and involuntary submission. Slavery can be based neither on a voluntary arrangement nor on coercion or conquest. In the case of the former, one who agrees to be a slave is "out of one's mind," for it is madness to "renounce one's very humanity." Of course, American slavery was anything but voluntary, and for Rousseau, this form of slavery is equally inhumane. . . . As Rousseau powerfully states, "So, from whatever aspect we regard the question, the right of slavery is null and void, not only as being illegitimate, but also because it is absurd and meaningless. The words *slave* and *right* contradict each other, and are mutually exclusive. It will always be equally foolish for a man to say to a man or people: 'I make with you a convention wholly at your expense, and wholly to my advantage; I shall keep it as long as I like, and you will keep it as long as I like.'" Thus, not only is a social contract left unformed if it does not include the affirmation of *every* voice that is present within the polity, it is also morally incompatible given the presence of an enslaved group regardless of how the enslavement came about. In refusing to seek the consent of the majority, Brown chose to act on behalf of those who had been excluded from the founding act of consent and against a government that under Rousseau's definition can only be interpreted as illegitimate. Surely an analysis of Brown's actions from this perspective can better illuminate the questions that revolve around the accusation of his "lawlessness."

The notion of founding entails far more than establishment of institutions or governmental charters; it also, and above all, includes critical political and social reform in the pursuit of the higher principles of a given political culture. If we are to accept, along with such martyred luminaries as Lincoln and King, the proposition that the first principles of the American founding are to be understood as the guarantee of both individual liberty and the advance of political and legal equality, and if we add to this Rousseau's theoretical demolition of any claim to the alleged right to own human beings as property, then we can see in Brown's holy war against slavery an act that does indeed resonate with the spirit of the founding movement. . . .

Significantly, Brown made one major attempt to assume the mantle of legislator. The provisional constitution that was drafted and signed at the antislavery convention in Chatham, Ontario, was intended to provide the foundations for the new society that Brown envisioned establishing in the South after his successful liberation of the slaves and, as such, emulates the type of effort associated with a founder-legislator. In the Chatham document, Brown once again shares something in common with Lincoln in the latter's reaffirmation of the first principles established within the Declaration of Independence. Brown included in the Chatham document a statement that his provisional constitution was not meant to dissolve the federal constitution, but only to reaffirm the principles of the American Revolution through amendment and modification. The banner of the Spirit of '76 was to serve as the flag of the provisional government, thus echoing Lincoln's belief that the true founding of the nation began in the struggle for liberty and equality during the Revolution. In addition to the expression of higher political ideals, Brown also provided plans for framing a new government for the freed slaves and their allies, a proposed political system that, to many, was original and revolutionary. The Brown document departed dramatically from all previous constitutional examples because of such features as a supreme court that was to be elected by the widest possible popular vote; government officials who were "to serve without pay" and be removed and punished upon misconduct; extensive public reclamation of all property that was formerly acquired at the expense of the slaves; protection of female prisoners from violation; and plans for the "moral instruction" of the new citizens. Here again, Brown comes close to Rousseau's concept of the founder: a lawgiver who attempts to make human nature anew, one who is committed through law more than through force to the moral elevation of the human spirit. This is an example of Brown designing a more democratic government aimed toward human advancement and intended to restore the principles of the original American founding. . . . Brown's actions at Chatham are also similar to the steps taken at the convention of 1776, and once his supporters had signed the document, Brown felt prepared to enter the field of battle, knowing that his deeds were formally supported by written principles and political ideals as well as by his steadfast religious faith. At Chatham, Brown exchanged arms for pen and ink and, like Jefferson and Madison, attempted to establish a new order for humanity through law. . . .

In turning back to Harpers Ferry, we must also raise the following question: Why weren't more people of conscience moved to arms, as was John Brown? This can be partially explained by the close connection between abolition and nonviolent moral suasion, as in the case of William Lloyd Garrison and the Transcendentalists, but that connection notwithstanding, it is still remarkable that, after conceding the pacifism of most free opponents of slavery, we cannot remember another case that resembles or emulates the Harpers Ferry raid. This might be the best evidence on behalf of the case for Brown as founder, for his was an act consistent both with the tenets of scripture and with the political principles of the polity within which he lived. It was committed out of the purest motivations, it was directed to the achievement of the goal of purging the pathology responsible for the republic's social and cultural ills, and it anticipated the violent methods in which slavery was finally abolished. John Brown acted from high principles against evil, and while his methods were decidedly flawed, the moral necessity of his act of resistance remains evident. Although Brown's raid on Harpers Ferry was ultimately unsuccessful, he exemplifies the true spirit of just liberty; and while he contributed neither new law to support democracy nor any new concept to develop the idea of freedom, his deeds accelerated its progress. Thomas Jefferson proclaimed the egalitarian creed when he drafted the Declaration, but he was unable to renounce his own status as master or overcome his idiosyncratic ideas about racial difference. Abraham Lincoln sincerely and eloquently reaffirmed this creed on a higher and more authentically universal level at Gettysburg, but he was unable to act immediately and abolish the pernicious institution. John Brown, however, perhaps more than any founder since Thomas Paine, fully incorporated the creed into his actions and lived the idea of equality and racial friendship with unparalleled purity and ardor. John Brown compels us to think of him as a founder—one who, unlike Jefferson and Lincoln, appears to live and act on the fringes of society, but one who, on closer examination, springs from its very center.

Measuring the character and relevance of any historical figure is a task that lends itself to a certain degree of ambiguity. Figures such as Jefferson, Lincoln, and King have all been assessed differently by their champions and critics, and interpretations of their character and descriptions of their heroism as well as their lesser acts have all undergone continual redefinition. Yet they remain, for us, heroes all the same, for in spite of any inadequacies, they reflect the perpetual quest for the affirmation of higher political principle and remain among the great movers who helped shape the conscience and the development of the republic.

John Brown differs from these men because he shaped nothing tangible, at least nothing that we can point to today as the direct creation of his actions or product of his influence. However, he is similar to them because he represents the pursuit of high ideas consistent with action. In some aspects, John Brown is more relevant than they, for in his perpetually frustrated zeal for freedom and justice, he embodies the core of the American story; we see in the growth of the nation writ large the same constant buffeting between the idea of freedom and the reality of its interminable frustration that created a similar tension in the turbulent psyche of the Osawatomie Prophet. That tension was felt by the Sage of Monticello and was manifested in the visage of the Melancholy President, but it was *incarnate* in John Brown, and through that incarnation, the hope and dread of the American soul became flesh.

If some can embrace as a great hero the figure of Robert E. Lee, the defender of a commonwealth that included slavery as an accepted institution, then is it implausible to recognize heroism in the more astonishing figure of Brown? Lee never supported secession until the deed was committed, yet he chose to renounce his commission and past loyalties after years of distinction under arms only in order to side with his state. Other distinguished Southern warriors, such as David Farragut of Tennessee and Winfield Scott, Lee's fellow Virginian, went with the North, but Lee reluctantly followed the Old Dominion into the Confederacy. Is it fair to say that whereas Lee chose his homeland, Brown chose humanity? To his credit, Lee worried over the possibility of siding against his family and friends, thus exhibiting a tenderness for his communal roots and native land that is not as evident in Brown, so is it fair to argue that Lee chose to defend the hearth while Brown chose to fight for an abstraction? Whose abstraction is more meaningful: Lee's insistence on abiding with Virginia right or wrong or Brown's devotion to a people sealed in bondage? We must bear in mind that, in spite of his protestations, Lee owned slaves, and his wife owned even more than he did. Regardless of the answer to these questions, popular history has made its judgments, and Lee is known (by most) today as a gentleman warrior, acting from duty and on principle, while Brown is considered (by many) as the guerrilla fanatic, blinded by undignified zeal and without honor. But we must ask which of the two acted on the higher principle, which violated the greater law, which one carries more blood on his hands, and who between them is a more genuinely American hero? If it is madness to conduct a private, unruly, and suicidal war against an enemy that one perceives as the very cause of sinful oppression, then what state of mind could cause a man of principle to lead thousands into death out of questionable loyalty to a political system that acknowledges oppression as a venerable institution? Who acted on the real spirit of liberty as expressed in the motto Sic semper tyrannis? Without intending to detract from the achievement of either man, it is still instructive to compare the actions and motivations of these past contemporaries, one widely deemed a hero, the other, quite often, a villain. At Harpers Ferry, these two men of different principles fatally met, and it is primarily on principle that their legacies stand before us today.

If we are to judge heroes on the principles that they attempt to advance, then we must develop a more comprehensive sense of the value and purity of those ideals that stir one to action. By any measure, John Brown represents the more startling manifestation of the murky dynamics that course within the continual process of the unfolding and founding of America's first principles; thus, he represents an individual of heroic, if still frightening, proportions who speaks powerfully to us today as we continue to confront our higher purposes as a political culture and democratic nation. Perhaps for this reason he is the most typical founder of all: the most consistently idealistic, the most existentially frustrated, the most American.

Scott John Hammond is a professor of political science at James Madison University where he specializes in political philosophy. He is the author of *Political Theory: An Encyclopedia of Contemporary and Classic Terms* (Greenwood, 2008) and co-author of *Encyclopedia of Presidential Campaigns, Slogans, Issues, and Platforms* (Greenwood, 2008).

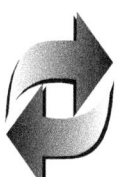

EXPLORING THE ISSUE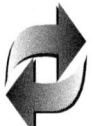

Was John Brown an Irrational Terrorist?

Critical Thinking and Reflection

1. Is it more appropriate to characterize John Brown as a domestic terrorist or a martyr? Explain.
2. What are the three main concepts that terrorists use to justify their actions? Did John Brown adhere to those concepts?
3. Is there a distinction to be drawn between Brown's antislavery activities in Kansas and his leadership of the raid on the federal arsenal at Harpers Ferry?
4. Is it legitimate to liken John Brown to Machiavelli's "prophet-warrior" and/or to Rousseau's "founder-legislator"?
5. Was Brown making "just war" on the institution of slavery?

Is There Common Ground?

Is John Brown representative of all abolitionists? While all of the abolitionists condemned the institution of slavery, few if any matched the behavior of John Brown. Some, like Garrison, used rhetorical or symbolic violence when speaking or writing of the immorality of the slave system in the United States. But burning copies of the Constitution of the United States was a far cry from executing proslavery settlers in Kansas or waging armed battle with local citizens and state troops in Virginia. But is such activity so different from American colonists waging war to free themselves from the bondage of an imperial power?

It is also important to remind ourselves that not all abolitionists agreed as to how best to attack the foundation of slavery in America. Some, like Garrison, took a moral suasionist approach that made no room for political action; others insisted that political involvement was essential in lobbying for the elimination of slavery. Most African American abolitionists, with the significant exception of Frederick Douglass who remained loyal to Garrison for a while longer, followed the political activists led by Theodore Dwight Weld and Arthur and Lewis Tappan. And as a group they tended to steer clear of John Brown. What does this suggest about the "radicalism" of abolitionists in general, whether black or white?

Additional Resources

Henry Mayer, *All on Fire: William Lloyd Garrison and the Abolition of Slavery* (St. Martin's, 1998)

Richard S. Newman, *The Transformation of American Abolitionism: Fighting Slavery in the Early Republic* (University of North Carolina Press, 2002)

Merrill D. Peterson, *John Brown: The Legend Revisited* (University of Virginia Press, 2002)

David S. Reynolds, *John Brown, Abolitionist: The Man Who Killed Slavery, Sparked the Civil War, and Seeded Civil Rights* (Alfred A. Knopf, 2005)

John Stauffer, *The Black Hearts of Men: Radical Abolitionists and the Transformation of Race* (Harvard University Press, 2002)

Internet References . . .

Abolitionist Movement

www.history.com/topics/abolitionist-movement

John Brown-Harpers Ferry

www.nps.gov/hafe/historyculture/john-brown.htm

John Brown's Holy War

www.pbs.org/wgbh/amex/brown

The African-American Mosaic

www.loc.gov/exhibits/african/afam005.html

The Trial of John Brown

http://law2.umkc.edu/faculty/projects/ftrials/johnbrown/brownhome.html

Unit 4

UNIT

Conflict and Resolution

The demand that the United States adhere to its principles of freedom and democracy and eradicate the evil of slavery finally erupted into violent conflict. Perhaps it was an inevitable step in the process of building a coherent nation from a number of distinct and diverse groups. The leaders, attitudes, and resources available to the North and the South were to determine the course of the war itself.

As part of the healing process (and lack thereof) that followed, most Americans concluded that the restoration of the Union superseded all local interests. Not all of the tensions generated by the war or by almost 300 years of political, economic, and social development had been resolved, but the framework had been established to secure a continuing commitment to the rights of citizenship in the American republic.

In 2015, author and activist Jim Wallis joined journalist and television commentator Roland Martin to discuss Wallis' book, *America's Original Sin: Racism, White Privilege and the Bridge to a New America*. While the transcripts from this interview could easily serve as the introduction to this unit's focus of topics for debate, it is essential that we not be lured into a singularity of topical focus that obscures the multiple antecedent (cause) and subsequent (effect) variables that should be considered as factors in the issues surrounding this tumultuous period in American history. As previously noted, each unit of this text offers examples of American history teetering on the head of pin sometimes tilting toward the ideals that point to our exceptional character as a nation of diverse people groups while at other times turning quickly toward dark realities of human behavior that undermines the legitimacy of the foundational value claims that make up the American narrative. Wallis is indeed correct that the historic issues of this era in U.S. history speak to a "deliberate dehumanizing and debasing of African-Americans" (J. Wallis, personal communication, January 28, 2016).

It is with this sentiment that we present to you the interdependent complexities of historic issues that do not shy away from acknowledging the realities that U.S. economic successes, past and present, and indeed U.S. political and social institutional failings are directly attributable to the enslavement of millions of African and African American women, children, and men prior to and during this period in history. Embedded in the topics for debate offered by Charles B. Dew, Gary W. Gallagher (slavery and warfare), Mark E. Neely, James M. McPherson (carnage and total war) are glimpses of the economic transitions that followed this period which established the conditions for a hybrid market economy where free market values are espoused as virtuous while simultaneously being violated in practice by monied and power interests who benefited from enslaved, indentured, and inequitably cast men, women, and children brought to and born on these American shores. As both northern and southern regions of the United States experienced a pre–Civil War agrarian and industrialization boom and the northern United States reaped the economic benefits of a post–Civil War southern confederacy collapse, a hybrid-ideology of economic, political, and social free-market capitalism and American Exceptionalism continued to thrive. It is important that the reader recognizes that Phillip Shaw Paludan's and Melvin E. Bradford's debate on the Abraham Lincoln's greatness or mediocrity is an extension of the conversation offered by Lisa J. McLeod and Adam Fairclough who examine the root causes of the failure of post–Civil War economic, political, and social reconstruction. For within these two topics of debate, like a Charlie Mingus quodlibet, the historic rhythmic counterpoint to the undeniably exceptional American narrative are the glaring exceptions to the American values of equity of opportunity for all people of the United States.

Whether we turn our ear to the tune of Reconstruction era promises of freedom and equality that were never realized due to the evolving definition of slavery as manifest in Jim Crow legislation and exploitation or listen to the equally resonate melody of the new waves of immigration that fed both the factory system and the nativist system of discrimination, the legacy of this historic musical score informs our contemporary political, economic, religious, social, intellectual, and area-focused ideological discussions and rhetorical reasoning. Lest we end the discussion of this unit of the text on a sour note, we offer to you a topic of debate that embodies the truly exceptional American experience as discussed by Albert J. Raboteau and John B. Boles who examine the resilient and defiant spirit of humanity as evidenced in African American slaves exercise of religious autonomy amidst relentless persecution.

Selected, Edited, and with Issue Framing Material by:
Kevin R. Magill and Tony L. Talbert, *Baylor University*

ISSUE

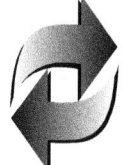

Was the Civil War Fought Over Slavery?

YES: **Charles B. Dew**, from "Apostles of Disunion: Southern Secession Commissioners and the Causes of the Civil War," University of Virginia Press (2001)

NO: **Gary W. Gallagher**, from "The Union War" Harvard University Press (2012)

Learning Outcomes
After reading this issue, you will be able to: • Describe the process used in the South to gain support for secession. • Understand that white southerners were not of one mind when it came to the decision to leave the Union. • Evaluate the major reason(s) why Union soldiers fought the Civil War. • Evaluate Union soldiers' attitudes toward the South, secession, and slavery. • Analyze the extent to which race and slavery were the keys to the sectional conflict leading to the American Civil War.

ISSUE SUMMARY

YES: Charles B. Dew presents documentation, which suggests that a number of white southerners attempted to gain support for secession in the southern states by arguing for the need to preserve slavery and white supremacy as social norms. Dew suggests that these appeals demonstrate the primary motive for secession.

NO: Gary W. Gallagher, analyzes the letters of white northern soldiers during the Civil War which suggest the common soldier cared little about slavery as an institution. Further, many of the letters were open hostility toward the idea that the union would African American troops. In other words, Gallagher believes the main motivation of these troops was saving the Union and not the abolition of slavery.

In April 1861, less than a month after his inauguration, President Abraham Lincoln attempted to send provisions to Fort Sumter in South Carolina, part of the newly formed Confederate States of America. Southern troops under the command of General P. G. T. Beauregard opened fire on the fort, forcing its surrender on April 1. The American Civil War had begun.

Numerous explanations have been offered for the cause of this "war between the states." Many contemporaries and some historians saw the conflict as the product of a conspiracy housed either in the North or South, depending upon one's regional perspective. For many in the northern states, the chief culprits were the planters and their political allies who were willing to defend southern institutions at all costs. South of the Mason-Dixon line, blame was laid at the feet of the fanatical abolitionists, like John Brown, and the free-soil architects of the Republican Party. Some viewed the secession and war as the consequence of a constitutional struggle between states' rights advocates and defenders of the U.S. federal government, whereas others focused upon the economic rivalries or the cultural differences between North and South. Embedded in each of these interpretations, however, is the powerful influence of the institution of slavery.

In the 85 years between the start of the American Revolution and the coming of the Civil War, Americans made the necessary political compromises on the slavery issue in order not to split the nation apart. The Northwest Ordinance of 1787 forbade slavery from spreading into those designated territories under its control, and the new Constitution written in the same year held out the possibility that the Atlantic slave trade would be prohibited after 1808.

There was some hope in the early nineteenth century that slavery might die from natural causes. The Revolutionary generation was well aware of the contradiction between the values of an egalitarian society and the practices of a slaveholding aristocracy. Philosophically, slavery was viewed as a necessary evil, not a positive good. The northern states were well on their way to abolishing slavery by 1800, and the erosion of the tobacco lands in Virginia and Maryland contributed to the lessening importance of a slave labor system.

Unfortunately, two factors—territorial expansion and the market economy—made slavery the key to the South's wealth in the 35 years before the Civil War. First, new slave states were created out of a population expanding into lands ceded to the United States as a result of the Treaty of Paris of 1783 and the Louisiana Purchase of 1803. Second, slaves were sold from the upper to the lower regions of the South because the invention of the cotton gin made it possible to harvest large quantities of cotton, ship it to the textile mills in New England and the British Isles, and turn it into cloth and finished clothing as part of the new, specialized market economy.

The slavery issue came to the forefront in 1820 when some northern congressmen proposed that slavery be banned from the states being carved out of the Louisiana Purchase. A heated debate ensued, but the Missouri Compromise drew a line that preserved the balance between free and slave states and that (with the exception of Missouri) prohibited slavery north of the 36° 30′ latitude.

The annexation of Texas in 1845 and the acquisition of New Mexico, Utah, and California, as a result of the Mexican-American War (see Issue 12), reopened the slavery question. Attempts at compromises in 1850 and 1854 only accelerated the conflict. The Kansas-Nebraska Act of 1854, which repealed the Missouri Compromise, allowed citizens in the new territories to decide whether or not they wanted slavery on the basis of the doctrine of popular sovereignty. As the second party system of Whigs and Democrats fell apart, the Republican Party, whose members hoped to confine slavery to existing slave states, mounted a successful challenge against the Democrats and in 1860 elected Abraham Lincoln as president of the United States, a result that 11 slaveholding states in the South refused to accept. In *America in 1857: A Nation on the Brink* (Oxford University Press, 1990), Kenneth M. Stampp argues that conflict became inevitable after the election of James Buchanan (not Lincoln) to the presidency, the continuing firestorm in Kansas, and the Supreme Court's decision in *Dred Scott*. Eric Foner, who has written extensively on the influence of the free soil ideology and its impact on the coming of the Civil War in such works as *Free Soil, Free Labor, Free Men: The Ideology of the Republican Party Before the Civil War* (Oxford University Press, 1970), also points out that the argument for states' rights as an explanation for the cause of the war is largely a product of the post–Civil War era and, hence, more or less an afterthought on the part of southerners who hoped to distance themselves from the institution of slavery that dominated their region in the antebellum period.

A challenge to the belief that slavery was the sole cause of the war can be found in the works of Joel Silbey. In "The Civil War Synthesis in American Political History," *Civil War History* (June 1964); *The Partisan Imperative: The Dynamics of American Politics Before the Civil War* (Oxford University Press, 1985); and *Party Over Section: The Rough and Ready Presidential Election of 1848* (University Press of Kansas, 2009), Silbey argues that historians, by positioning slavery as the major issue that divided the United States, have distorted "the reality of American political life between 1844 and 1861." Silbey is one of the "new political historians" who have applied the techniques of modern-day political scientists in analyzing the election returns and voting patterns of Americans' nineteenth- and early twentieth-century predecessors. These historians use computers and regression analysis of voting patterns, favor a quantitative analysis of past behavior, and reject the traditional sources of quotations from partisan newspapers and major politicians because these sources provide anecdotal and often misleading portraits of our past. Silbey and other new political historians maintain that all politics are local. Therefore, the primary issues for voters and their politicians in the 1860 election were ethnic and cultural, and party loyalty was more important than sectional considerations.

Another approach is presented by Michael F. Holt in *The Political Crisis of the 1850s* (John Wiley & Sons, 1978). Holt also is interested in analyzing the struggles for power at the state and local levels by the major political parties, but he is critical of the ethnocultural school represented by Silbey. In Holt's view, Silbey's emphasis on voter analysis does not explain why the Whig Party disappeared, nor why the Republican Party became the majority party in the northern and western states in the 1850s. Holt also rejects the more traditional view that the Civil War resulted from the "intensifying sectional disagreements over slavery." Instead, he promotes a more complicated picture of the events leading to the Civil War. Between 1845 and 1860, he maintains, three important things happened: (1) the breakdown of the Whig Party; (2) the realignment of voters; and (3) "a shift from a nationally balanced party system where both major parties competed on fairly even terms in all parts of the nation to a sectionalized polarized one with Republicans dominant in the North and Democrats in the South."

More recently, Gary W. Gallagher has challenged several of the interpretations of modern scholars of the era of the Civil War. His book *The Confederate War* (Harvard University Press, 1997), for example, attacked historians of the Confederacy for attributing the loss of the Civil War to class divisions between planters and non-planters or religious guilt over slave ownership. Gallagher reverts back to older interpretations which maintain that the North had the larger military forces and an industrial base which the South could not match. He marveled that southerners fought for national pride and kept the war going for four years.

In the following essays, Charles B. Dew makes a very powerful argument challenging the neo-Confederate insistence that the decision to secede was driven by the U.S. federal government's abuse of states' rights. Whose attitudes would provide a better window into the thinking of white southerners on the eve of the Civil War than those individuals commissioned to travel throughout the region to drum up support for secession?

Gary W. Gallagher takes issue with a number of scholars who grew up in the midst of the 1960s civil rights era for overemphasizing the slavery issue as the primary cause that the war was fought. At the same time, Gallagher accuses modern scholars of downplaying nationalism as the primary reason for fighting the war. Based on his examination of the letters of 350 Union soldiers, their patriotic envelopes, and the contemporary regimental histories, Gallagher sees soldiers expressing their patriotic feelings about democracy and the freedom to express one's opinions, as well as the more basic goal of earning enough money to live a comfortable life.

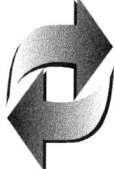

YES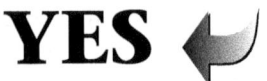

Charles B. Dew

Apostles of Disunion: Southern Secession Commissioners and the Causes of the Civil War

Slavery, States' Rights, and Secession Commissioners

"The Civil War was fought over what important issue?" So reads one of twenty questions on an exam administered by the Immigration and Naturalization Service to prospective American citizens. According to the INS, you are correct if you offer either one of the following answers: "Slavery or states rights."

It is reassuring to know that the INS has a flexible approach to one of the critical questions in American history, but one might ask how the single "issue" raised in the question can have an either/or answer in this instance—the only time such an option occurs on the test. Beyond that, some might want to know whether "slavery" or "states rights" is the more correct answer. But it is probably unfair to chide the test preparers at the INS for trying to fudge the issue. Their uncertainty reflects the deep division and profound ambivalence in contemporary American culture over the origins of the Civil War. One hundred and forty years after the beginning of that fratricidal conflict, neither the public nor the scholarly community has reached anything approaching a consensus as to what caused the bloodiest four years in this country's history....

There is, however, a remarkably clear window into the secessionist mind that has been largely ignored by students of this era. If we want to know what role slavery may or may not have played in the coming of the Civil War, there is no better place to look than in the speeches and letters of the men who served their states as secession commissioners on the eve of the conflict.

As sectional tension mounted in late 1860 and early 1861, five states of the lower South—Mississippi, Alabama, South Carolina, Georgia, and Louisiana—appointed commissioners to other slave states and instructed them to spread the secessionist message across the entire region. These commissioners often explained in detail why their states were exiting the Union, and they did everything in their power to persuade laggard slave states to join the secessionist cause. From December 1860 to April 1861, they carried the *gospel of disunion* to the far corners of the South.

The overwhelming majority of the commissioners came from the four Deep South states of Mississippi, Alabama, South Carolina, and Georgia. In Mississippi and Alabama the commissioners were appointed by the governor and thus took the field first. In South Carolina, Georgia, and Louisiana, the secession conventions chose the commissioners.

The number of men sent on this vital mission varied from state to state. Mississippi and Alabama named commissioners to every one of the fourteen other slave states. South Carolina, however, only appointed commissioners to those states which had announced they were calling secession conventions, so only nine representatives eventually went out from the cradle of the secession movement—to Alabama, Mississippi, Georgia, Florida, Louisiana, Texas, Arkansas, Virginia, and North Carolina. Georgia dispatched commissioners to six of these same states—Alabama, Louisiana, Texas, Arkansas, North Carolina, and Virginia—and added the border slave states of Maryland, Delaware, Kentucky, and Missouri to the list. The Louisiana Convention appointed a single commissioner, to neighboring Texas, and he did not arrive in Austin until well after the Texas Convention had passed its ordinance of secession.

In all, some fifty-two men served as secession commissioners in the critical weeks just before the Civil War. These individuals were not, by and large, the famous names of antebellum Southern politics. They were often relatively obscure figures—judges, lawyers, doctors,

---

Dew, Charles B., "Apostles of Disunion: Southern Secession Commissioners and the Causes of the Civil War," excerpts from pages 4, 18–21, 74–81. Copyright ©2001 by University of Virginia Press. Used with permission.

newspaper editors, planters, and farmers—who had had modest political careers but who possessed a reputation for oratory. Sometimes they were better known—ex-governors or state attorney generals or members of Congress. Often they had been born in the states to which they were sent; place of birth was clearly an important factor in the choice of a number of commissioners.

The commissioners appeared in a host of different venues. They addressed state legislatures, they spoke before state conventions called to consider the question of secession, they took the platform before crowds in meeting halls and in the streets, and they wrote letters to governors whose legislatures were not in session. To a man, what they had to say was, and remains, exceedingly instructive and highly illuminating.

Despite their enormous value, the commissioners' speeches and letters have been almost completely overlooked by historians and, as a consequence, by the public at large. This scholarly neglect is difficult to understand. Contemporaries in both North and South paid close attention to the commissioners' movements and what they had to say. Many of their speeches were reprinted in full in newspapers and official state publications, and several appeared in pamphlet form and apparently gained wide circulation. Accounts of the secession crisis published during and just after the war also devoted considerable space to their activities. In the late nineteenth century when editors at the War Department were assembling a documentary record of the Civil War, they included extensive coverage of the commissioners in the volume dealing with the onset of the conflict—a clear indication that they considered these men to be key players in the sequence of events leading up to the war.

Dwight Lowell Dumond highlighted the importance of the commissioners in his 1931 study of the secession movement, a book that remains the most detailed scholarly treatment of this subject. He described the commissioners' words as extraordinarily important and revealing. "From the speeches and writings of the commissioners, as nowhere else, one may realize the depth of feeling and the lack of sympathy between the two sections of the country," Dumond wrote. "Vividly denunciatory of a party pledged to the destruction of Southern institutions, almost tragic in their prophetic tone, and pleading for a unity of allied interests, they constitute one of the most interesting series of documents in American history," he went on to say.

Yet Professor Dumond's book provides little detailed coverage of what these men actually said, and that pattern has persisted in the torrent of literature on the Civil War that has appeared in subsequent decades. As Jon L. Wakelyn notes in his recent *Southern Pamphlets on Secession*, "No adequate study of the Lower South delegates sent to the Upper South exists," and that same observation could be made about the commissioners who addressed their remarks to fellow Southerners in the states of the Deep South as well. Indeed, Professor Wakelyn does not include the full text of a single commissioner's speech in his otherwise superb collection of pamphlet literature, even though, in my opinion, several of the addresses published in pamphlet form are among the most powerful and revealing expressions of the secessionist persuasion put to paper on the eve of the war.

I have managed to locate the full texts or detailed synopses of forty-one of the commissioners' speeches and public letters. It is, as Professor Dumond suggested, a truly remarkable set of documents. What is most striking about them is their amazing openness and frankness. The commissioners' words convey an unmistakable impression of candor, of white Southerners talking to fellow Southerners with no need to hold back out of deference to outside sensibilities. These men infused their speeches and letters with emotion, with passion, and with a powerful "Let's cut to the chase" analysis that reveals, better than any other sources I know, what was really driving the Deep South states toward disunion.

The explanations the commissioners offered and the arguments the commissioners made, in short, provide us with extraordinary insight into the secession of the lower South in 1860–61. And by helping us to understand the "why" of secession, these apostles of disunion have gone a long way toward answering that all-important question, "The Civil War was fought over what important issue?" . . .

John Smith Preston spent the war years in uniform. After serving in a number of different staff positions in the army, he found a home in the Confederate Bureau of Conscription. He took over that agency in 1863, was promoted to the rank of brigadier general in 1864, and headed the Conscript Bureau until the South went down to defeat. Preston lived for a time in England after the war, but in 1868 he went back to South Carolina. His reputation as an orator still intact, Preston was invited to return to his native state in 1868 to address the Washington and Jefferson Societies of the University of Virginia. On June 30 of that year, Preston spoke in Charlottesville to the young Virginians.

Much of his address was an eloquent tribute to the Founding Fathers and their principal handiwork—the Revolution, the state constitutions, and the Constitution of the United States. Through their efforts "your fathers achieved that liberty which comes of a free government, founded on justice, order and peace," Preston said. In order to preserve the principles and the constitutional forms established by the Revolutionary generation, "you, the immediate offspring of the founders, went forth to that death grapple which has prevailed against you," he continued. It was the North, "the victors," who rejected "the principles," destroyed "the forms," and defeated "the promised destiny of America," Preston charged. "The Constitution you fought for"—the Confederate Constitution—"embodied every principle of the Constitution of the United States, and guaranteed the free Constitution of Virginia. It did not omit one essential for liberty and the public welfare," he claimed. The Confederacy was in ashes, however, and so was true constitutional liberty. "That liberty was lost, and now the loud hosanna is shouted over land and sea—'Liberty may be dead, but the Union is preserved. Glory, glory, glory to Massachusetts and her Hessian and Milesian mercenaries,'" Preston declaimed. Yet all was not lost. Even though "cruel, bloody, remorseless tyrants may rule at Fort Sumter and at Richmond . . . they cannot crush that immortal hope, which rises from the blood soaked earth of Virginia," Preston believed. "I see the sacred image of regenerate Virginia, and cry aloud, in the hearing of a God of Right, and in the hearing of all the nations of the earth—ALL HAIL OUR MOTHER."

Passionate, unregenerate, unapologetic, unreconstructed—all these and more apply to Preston's remarks on this occasion. But so do words like "conveniently forgetful," "strongly revisionist," and "purposely misleading." Nowhere to be found are references to many of the arguments and descriptions he had used over and over again before the Virginia Convention in February 1861—things like "the subject race . . . rising and murdering their masters" or "the conflict between slavery and non-slavery is a conflict for life and death," or his insistence that "the South cannot exist without African slavery," or his portrait of the "fermenting millions" of the North as "canting, fanatics, festering in the licentiousness of abolition and amalgamation." All this was swept aside as Preston sought to paint the Civil War as a mighty struggle over differing concepts of constitutional liberty. Like Jefferson Davis and Alexander H. Stephens in their postwar writings, Preston was trying to reframe the causes of the conflict in terms that would be much more favorable to the South.

Preston was not the only former secession commissioner to launch such an effort after the war. Jabez L. M. Curry, who had served as Alabama's commissioner to Maryland in December 1860, became a leading figure in the drive to improve primary and secondary education in the postwar South. As agent for both the Peabody and Slater Funds and as supervising director of the Southern Education Board, Curry worked tirelessly to establish public schools and teacher training for both races in the states of the former Confederacy. Curry also worked diligently to justify the Lost Cause of the Confederacy. In his *Civil History of the Government of the Confederate States, with Some Personal Reminiscences,* published in Richmond in 1901, Curry offered an analysis of the coming of the war that closely paralleled the argument used by John S. Preston in 1868. "The object in quitting the Union was not to destroy, but to save the principles of the Constitution," Curry wrote. "The Southern States from the beginning of the government had striven to keep it within the orbit prescribed by the Constitution and failed." The Curry of 1901 would hardly have recognized the Curry of 1860, who told the governor of Maryland that secession meant "deliverance from Abolition domination," and who predicted that under Republican rule the South's slave-based social system would "be assaulted, humbled, dwarfed, degraded, and finally crushed out."

In 1860 and 1861 Preston, Curry, and the other commissioners had seen a horrific future facing their region within the confines of Abraham Lincoln's Union. When they used words like "submission" and "degradation," when they referred to "final subjugation" and "annihilation," they were not talking about constitutional differences or political arguments. They were talking about the dawning of an abominable new world in the South, a world created by the Republican destruction of the institution of slavery.

The secession commissioners knew what this new and hateful world would look like. Over and over again they called up three stark images that, taken together, constituted the white South's worst nightmare.

The first threat was the looming specter of racial equality. The commissioners insisted almost to a man that Republican ascendancy in Washington placed white supremacy in the South in mortal peril. Mississippi commissioner William L. Harris made this point clearly and unambiguously in his speech to the Georgia legislature in December 1860. "Our fathers made this a government for the white man," Harris told the Georgians, "rejecting the negro, as an ignorant, inferior, barbarian race, incapable of self-government, and not, therefore, entitled to be associated with the white man upon terms of civil, political, or social equality." But the Republicans intended "to overturn and strike down this great feature of our Union . . . and to substitute in its stead their new theory of the universal equality of the black and white races." Alabama's commissioners to North Carolina, Isham W. Garrott and Robert H. Smith, predicted that the white children of their state would "be compelled to flee from the land of their birth, and from the slaves their parents have toiled to acquire as an inheritance for them, or to submit to the degradation of being reduced to an equality with them, and all its attendant horrors." South Carolina's John McQueen warned the Texas Convention that Lincoln and the Republicans were bent upon "the abolition of slavery upon this continent and the elevation of our own slaves to an equality with ourselves and our children." And so it went, as commissioner after commissioner—Leonidas Spratt of South Carolina, David Clopton and Arthur F. Hopkins of Alabama, Henry L. Benning of Georgia—hammered home this same point.

The impending imposition of racial equality informed the speeches of other commissioners as well. Thomas J. Wharton, Mississippi's attorney general and that state's commissioner to Tennessee, said in Nashville on January 8, 1861, that the Republican Party would, "at no distant day, inaugurate the reign of equality of all races and colors, and the universality of the elective franchise." Commissioner Samuel L. Hall of Georgia told the North Carolina legislature on February 13, 1861, that only a people "dead to all sense of virtue and dignity" would embrace the Republican doctrine of "the social and political equality of the black and white races." Another Georgia commissioner, Luther J. Glenn of Atlanta, made the same point to the Missouri legislature on March 2, 1861. The Republican platform, press, and principal spokesmen had made their "purposes, objects, and motives" crystal clear, Glenn insisted: "hostility to the South, the extinction of slavery, and the ultimate elevation of the negro to civil, political and social equality with the white man." These reasons and these reasons alone had prompted his state "to dissolve her connexion with the General Government," Glenn insisted.

The second element in the commissioners' prophecy was the prospect of a race war. Mississippi commissioner Alexander H. Handy raised this threat in his Baltimore speech in December 1860—Republican agents infiltrating the South "to excite the slave to cut the throat of his master." Alabamians Garrott and Smith told their Raleigh audience that Republican policies would force the South either to abandon slavery "or be doomed to a servile war." William Cooper, Alabama's commissioner to Missouri, delivered a similar message in Jefferson City. "Under the policy of the Republican party, the time would arrive when the scenes of San Domingo and Hayti, with all their attendant horrors, would be enacted in the slaveholding States," he told the Missourians. David Clopton of Alabama wrote the governor of Delaware that Republican ascendancy "endangers instead of insuring domestic tranquility by the possession of channels through which to circulate insurrectionary documents and disseminate insurrectionary sentiments among a hitherto contented servile population." Wharton of Mississippi told the Tennessee legislature that Southerners "will not, cannot surrender our institutions," and that Republican attempts to subvert slavery "will drench the country in blood, and extirpate one or other of the races." In their speeches to the Virginia Convention, Fulton Anderson, Henry L. Benning, and John S. Preston all forecast a Republican-inspired race war that would, as Benning put it, "break out everywhere like hidden fire from the earth."

The third prospect in the commissioners' doomsday vision was, in many ways, the most dire: racial amalgamation. Judge Harris of Mississippi sounded this note in Georgia in December 1860 when he spoke of Republican insistence on "equality in the rights of matrimony." Other commissioners repeated this warning in the weeks that followed. In Virginia, Henry Benning insisted that under Republican-led abolition "our women" would suffer "horrors... we cannot contemplate in imagination." There was not an adult present who could not imagine exactly what Benning was talking about. Leroy Pope Walker, Alabama's commissioner to Tennessee and subsequently the first Confederate secretary of war, predicted that in the absence of secession all would be lost—first, "our property," and "then our liberties," and finally the South's greatest treasure, "the sacred purity of our daughters."

No commissioner articulated the racial fears of the secessionists better, or more graphically, than Alabama's Stephen F. Hale. When he wrote of a South facing "amalgamation or extermination," when he referred to "all the horrors of a San Domingo servile insurrection," when he described every white Southerner "degraded to a position of equality with free negroes," when he foresaw the "sons and daughters" of the South "associating with free negroes upon terms of political and social equality," when he spoke of the Lincoln administration consigning the citizens of the South "to assassinations and her wives and daughters to pollution and violation to gratify the lust of half-civilized Africans," he was giving voice to the night terrors of the secessionist South. States' rights, historic political abuses, territorial questions, economic differences, constitutional arguments—all these and more paled into insignificance when placed alongside this vision of the South's future under Republican domination.

The choice was absolutely clear. The slave states could secede and establish their independence, or they could submit to "Black Republican" rule with its inevitable consequences: Armageddon or amalgamation. Whites forced to endure racial equality, race war, a staining of the blood—who could tolerate such things?

The commissioners sent out to spread the secessionist gospel in late 1860 and early 1861 clearly believed that the racial fate of their region was hanging in the balance in the wake of Lincoln's election. Only through disunion could the South be saved from the disastrous effects of Republican principles and Republican malevolence. Hesitation, submission—any course other than immediate secession—would place both slavery and white supremacy on the road to certain extinction. The commissioners were arguing that disunion, even if it meant risking war, was the only way to save the white race.

Did these men really believe these things? Did they honestly think that secession was necessary in order to stay the frenzied hand of the Republican abolitionist, preserve racial purity and racial supremacy, and save their women and children from rape and slaughter at the hands of "half-civilized Africans"? They made these statements, and used the appropriate code words, too many times in too many places with too much fervor and raw emotion to leave much room for doubt. They knew these things in the marrow of their bones, and they destroyed a political union because of what they believed and what they foresaw.

But, we might ask, could they not see the illogicality, indeed the absurdity, of their insistence that Lincoln's election meant that the white South faced the sure prospect of either massive miscegenation or a race war to the finish? They seem to have been totally untroubled by logical inconsistencies of this sort. Indeed, the capacity for compartmentalization among this generation of white Southerners appears to have been practically boundless. How else can we explain Judge William L. Harris's comments before the Mississippi State Agricultural Society in November 1858? "It has been said by an eminent statesman," Harris observed on this occasion, " 'that nothing can advance the mass of society in prosperity and happiness, nothing can uphold the substantial interest and steadily improve the general condition and character of the whole, but this one thing—compensating rewards for labor.' " It apparently never occurred to Harris that this observation might apply to the hundreds of thousands of slaves working in Mississippi in 1858 as well as to the white farmers and mechanics of his adopted state. His mind could not even comprehend the possibility that slaves, too, were human beings who, if given the opportunity, might well respond to "compensating rewards" for their labor.

In setting out to explain secession to their fellow Southerners, the commissioners have explained a very great deal to us as well. By illuminating so clearly the racial content of the secession persuasion, the commissioners would seem to have laid to rest, once and for all, any notion that slavery had nothing to do with the coming of the Civil War. To put it quite simply, slavery and race were absolutely critical elements in the coming of the war. Neo-Confederate groups may have "a problem" with this interpretation, as the leader of the Virginia Heritage Preservation Association put it. But these defenders of the Lost Cause need only read the speeches and letters of the secession commissioners to learn what was really driving the Deep South to the brink of war in 1860–61.

CHARLES B. DEW is the Ephraim Williams Professor of American History at Williams College. Two of his books, *Apostles of Disunion and Ironmaker to the Confederacy: Joseph R. Anderson* and the *Tredegar Iron Works* (Yale University Press, 1966), received the Fletcher Pratt Award presented by the Civil War Round Table of New York for the best nonfiction book on the American Civil War. He is also the author of *Bond of Iron: Master and Slave at Buffalo Forge* (W. W. Norton, 1994), which received the Elliott Rudwick Prize from the Organization of American Historians.

Gary W. Gallagher

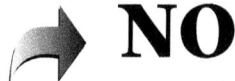 NO

The Union War

Introduction

The loyal American citizenry fought a war for Union that also killed slavery. In a conflict that stretched across four years and claimed more than 800,000 U.S. casualties, the nation experienced huge swings of civilian and military morale before crushing Confederate resistance. Union always remained the paramount goal, a fact clearly expressed by Abraham Lincoln in speeches and other statements designed to garner the widest popular support for the war effort. What Walt Whitman said of Lincoln and Union in the wake of the president's assassination applied equally to most loyal Americans. "UNIONISM, in its truest and amplest sense, form'd the hard-pan of his character," wrote the poet, who defined it as "a new virtue, unknown to other lands, and hardly yet really known here, but the foundation and tie of all, as the future will grandly develop." That hardpan of unionism held millions of Americans to the task of suppressing the slaveholders' rebellion, even as the human and material cost mushroomed. "By many has *this Union* been conserv'd and help'd," continued Whitman's tribute to Lincoln and Union, "but if one name, one man, must be pick'd out, he, most of all, is the Conservator of it, to the future. He was assassinated—but the Union is not assassinated—*ça ira!* One falls, and another falls. The soldier drops, sinks like a wave—but the ranks of the ocean eternally press on. Death does its work, obliterates a hundred, a thousand—President, general, captain, private—but the Nation is immortal."

Whitman celebrated a Union that carried great meaning for the mass of loyal citizens who joined him in equating it with "the Nation." It represented the cherished legacy of the founding generation, a democratic republic with a constitution that guaranteed political liberty and afforded individuals a chance to better themselves economically. From the perspective of loyal Americans, their republic stood as the only hope for democracy in a western world that had fallen more deeply into the stifling embrace of oligarchy since the failed European revolutions of the 1840s. Slaveholding aristocrats who established the Confederacy, believed untold unionists, posed a direct threat not only to the long-term success of the American republic but also to the broader future of democracy. Should armies of citizen-soldiers fail to restore the Union, forces of privilege on both sides of the Atlantic could pronounce ordinary people incapable of self-government and render irrelevant the military sacrifices and political genius of the Revolutionary fathers. Secretary of State William Henry Seward encapsulated much of this thinking in one sentence pertaining to the Republicans' agenda: "Their great work is the preservation of the Union and in that, the saving of popular government for the world."

Issues related to the institution of slavery precipitated secession and the outbreak of fighting, but the loyal citizenry initially gave little thought to emancipation in their quest to save the Union. By the early summer of 1862, long before black men donned blue uniforms in large numbers, victorious Union armies stood poised to win the war with slavery largely intact. Setbacks on battlefields in Virginia dictated that the bloodletting would continue, however, and as months went by, casualties mounted, and a shortage of manpower loomed, emancipation and African American military service assumed increasing importance. Eventually, most loyal citizens, though profoundly prejudiced by twenty-first-century standards and largely indifferent toward enslaved black people, embraced emancipation as a tool to punish slaveholders, weaken the Confederacy, and protect the Union from future internal strife. A minority of the white populace invoked moral grounds to attack slavery, though their arguments carried less weight than those presenting emancipation as a military measure necessary to defeat the Rebels and restore the Union. African American freedom still seemed problematic in the bloody summer of 1864, when Union armies bogged down in Georgia and Virginia and antiemancipation Democrats looked hopefully toward the November elections. Only striking victories at Atlanta and in the Shenandoah Valley in September and October retrieved the situation, setting up Lincoln's reelection and guaranteeing that slavery's extinction would be a nonnegotiable condition for peace.

THE UNION WAR by Gary W. Gallagher, Cambridge, Mass.: Harvard University Press, Copyright ©2011 by the President and Fellows of Harvard College. Used with permission.

Union armies composed of citizen-soldiers occupied a central position in the grand drama. Their hard and costly service salvaged the Union and, more than any other factor, made possible emancipation. They functioned as the most powerful national symbol and unifying institution, bringing together men from all over the country regardless of political affiliation. In a conflict marked by deep divisions within the loyal states, they represented self-sacrifice reminiscent of the Continental soldiers who had followed George Washington. They confirmed notions of American exceptionalism based on a long-standing antipathy toward professional soldiers and large standing armies. Observers who watched 150,000 veterans parade down Pennsylvania Avenue in the Grand Review at the end of the war gloried in the fact that the men soon would be on their way home—citizens who had performed their civic duty with the expectation of returning to civilian pursuits as soon as the Rebels capitulated. The wartime generation viewed surviving veterans and the Union dead—300,000 of the latter reinterred in national cemeteries established soon after Appomattox—as honored reminders of a free society's reliance on citizen-soldiers.

This book seeks to recover what Union meant to the generation that fought the war. That meaning has been almost completely effaced from popular understanding of the conflict; indeed, "Union" as defined in a political sense in the nineteenth century has disappeared from our vocabulary. Students and adults interested in the Civil War are reluctant to believe that anyone would risk life or fortune for something as abstract as "the Union." A war to end slavery seems more compelling, something powerfully reinforced by films such as *Glory*—easily the best of Hollywood's treatments of the conflict—and, *Gettysburg*. Although Lincoln remains a towering figure in the popular imagination, few Americans associate him with the widely held idea of the Union, as he put it in his second annual message to Congress in December 1862, as "the last best, hope of earth." Even within the specialized world of Civil War enthusiasts who purchase prints and other contemporary artworks, the Union and its military idols take a decidedly secondary position behind such Lost Cause icons as Robert E. Lee and "Stonewall" Jackson. Apart from Col. Joshua Lawrence Chamberlain and his 20th Maine Infantry, the Army of the Potomac's famous Irish Brigade, and various commanders and episodes at the battle of Gettysburg, the Union cause scarcely exists in that art. Were it not for Michael Shaara's Pulitzer Prize–winning novel *The Killer Angels,* Ken Burns's documentary *The Civil War,* and the director Ron Maxwell's film version of Shaara's book, even Chamberlain would be largely unknown.

Much Civil War scholarship over the past four decades has diminished the centrality of Union. Slavery, emancipation, and the actions of black people, unfairly marginalized for decades in writings about the conflict, have inspired a huge and rewarding literature since the mid-1960s. No longer can any serious reader fail to appreciate the degree to which African Americans figured in the political, social, and military history of the war. This has been one of the most heartening developments in the field since the great successes of the civil rights movement in the 1950s and 1960s. But the focus on emancipation and race sometimes suggests the war had scant meaning apart from these issues—and especially that the Union victory had little or no value without emancipation.

Historical context is crucial on this point. Anyone remotely conversant with nineteenth-century U.S. history knows that democracy as practiced in 1860 denied women, free and enslaved African Americans, and other groups basic liberties and freedoms most white northerners routinely attributed to their republic. Almost 99 percent of the residents in the free states were white (96.5 percent in the loyal states, which included slaveholding Missouri, Kentucky, Maryland, and Delaware), and their racial views offend our modern sensibilities. Yet a portrait of the nation that is dominated by racism, exclusion, and oppression obscures more than it reveals. Within the context of the mid-nineteenth-century western world, the United States offered the broadest political franchise and the most economic opportunity. Vast numbers of immigrants believed that however difficult the circumstances they might find, relocation in the United States promised a potentially brighter future. As one Irish-born Union soldier put it in early 1863, "this is my country as much as the man that was born on the soil and so it is with every man who comes to this country and becomes a citezen." If the Union lost the war, he added, "then the hopes of millions fall and. . . . the old cry will be sent forth from the aristocrats of europe that such is the common end of all republics." Without an appreciation of why the loyal citizenry went to great lengths to restore the Union, no accurate understanding of the era is possible.

The Union War focuses on one part of the population in the United States—citizens in the free states and four loyal slaveholding states who opposed secession and supported a war to restore the Union. This group encompassed Republicans as well as the portion of the Democratic Party that stridently opposed emancipation and other policies of the Lincoln administration but remained committed to a war against the rebellion. African American refugees who made their way to Union lines, soldiers in the United States Colored Troops (USCT), and antiwar Democrats or

Copperheads receive some attention but remain peripheral to my main line of inquiry. White unionists in the Confederacy fall outside my purview. Many U.S. soldiers, it is important to keep in mind, acted from motives unrelated to unionist or any other ideology, including an indeterminate number of poor men who enlisted primarily for financial reasons. Similarly, some of their fellow citizens on the home front exhibited minimal interest in the war's large issues, hoping for the least possible disruption in the usual rhythms of their daily lives.

By exploiting evidence relating to the substantial majority of the U.S. population that supported a war for Union, this book examines three fundamental questions. What did the war for Union mean in mid-nineteenth-century America? How and why did emancipation come to be part of the war for Union? How did armies of citizen-soldiers figure in conceptions of the war, the process of emancipation, and the shaping of national sentiment? Consideration of these questions proceeds from knowledge that pro-Union support could be grudging, especially as emancipation became more prominent and the central government took unprecedented steps to raise money and find manpower. The Lincoln administration dealt with political fissures, war weariness, apathy, and fluctuating levels of outright hostility to the war. Yet loyal citizens remained steadfast enough to push through to victory, despite far more casualties than in any previous American war and the absence of a direct physical threat from Rebel armies to their homes, farms, businesses, towns, and cities. They did so because they believed to do otherwise would betray the generation who established the Union as well as future Americans who would reap its political and economic benefits.

Although concerned with ideas about nation, this is not a study of the formation of American nationalism. I do not believe a new nation was born amid military upheaval in 1861–1865—though the service of more than 2 million men surely strengthened bonds of nationhood across the free states and to a lesser degree in the Border States except for Kentucky, which so loathed emancipation that it aligned with the defeated Confederacy after Appomattox. Nation building had been in progress for a long time, and an expansionist, democratic republic built on the blueprint of the Constitution and convinced of American exceptionalism had used diplomacy and violence to overspread the continent by mid-century.

Continuity marked loyal citizens' opinions and attitudes between 1860 and the early postwar decades. They routinely deployed "United States," "the Union," "the country" and "the nation" as synonyms. A Republican broadside from the 1864 presidential election perfectly captured this phenomenon, referring to Union, nation, and country in just a few sentences: "CITIZENS OF MICHIGAN! To-day is to be decided whether this Nation *lives, or dies* at the *hands of traitors!* . . . Be sure and vote for the Union, GOVERNMENT, AND COUNTRY. If the Union and government is not maintained, the nation is disgraced before the CIVILIZED WORLD." The citizens who labored to save the Union subscribed to a vision of their nation built on free labor, economic opportunity, and a broad political franchise they considered unique in the world. They believed victory over the slaveholders confirmed the nation, made it stronger in the absence of slavery's pernicious influence, set the stage for the country's continuing growth and vitality, and kept a democratic beacon shining in a world dominated by aristocrats and monarchs. It is this belief that led them into battle and ultimately to victory over the Confederacy. . . .

Although some have placed emancipation at the heart of the presidential election of 1864, soldiers' comments left no doubt that saving the nation, to use General Rosecrans's language, easily trumped killing slavery as a motivation to vote for the Union ticket of Lincoln and Andrew Johnson. Most states permitted their soldiers to vote in the field—though Delaware, Illinois, Indiana, New Jersey, and Oregon did not. Democrats complained vociferously, and perhaps with some merit, that Republicans conspired to suppress the anti-Lincoln military vote. Only twelve states counted soldiers' ballots separately. Those that can be identified favored Lincoln by a margin of 119,754 to 34,291—78 percent compared to 55 percent among the electorate as a whole. For soldiers, votes for Lincoln ensured that the war would be prosecuted vigorously until Rebels capitulated and the Union prevailed.

Three soldiers from New York, Maine, and Ohio recorded widely held opinions about the election. Edward King Wightman, a Democrat and noncommissioned officer in the 3rd New York Infantry, held "no very great respect" for Lincoln or McClellan and pronounced both parties' platforms "contemptible." He cast a ballot for Lincoln because the "main question seems to be whether we shall continue the war until the rebellion is subdued. "The integrity of the Union could "be restored only by force of arms and . . . such a course is necessary in order to vindicate the honor and establish the power of the Republic." Another noncommissioned officer, Abial Hall Edwards of the 29th Maine Infantry, believed the two parties in 1864 were "Unionists & Dis Unionists and I think as much of a war Democrat as I do of a Lincoln man." The Democratic platform called for a cessation of hostilities short of victory, which would "disgrace the memory of our fallin brothers[.]" Edwards craved peace but would vote for Lincoln, "remain here and if it need be lay down my life before we give up one iota of the victories we have gained to the Rebel hords." After Lincoln's victory, he explained to his future wife, "No Anna I do not desire the war to last 4 years longer. Neither do I want a peace that would disgrace us as a nation." John Marihugh of the 21st Ohio Infantry shared Edwards's sentiments. Deployed to Camp Butler near Springfield, Illinois, he summed up his ideas in one long sentence: "Wall a bout the election I think that Old Abe will be Electid with out mutch truble & if the Cop[perhead]s try too make truble down here we shall give them hell & that is whats the mater & I say three chears for Old Abe & the union."

Innumerable letters mirrored Marihugh's dislike of Copperheads and silence about emancipation as an issue in the election of 1864. Major Henry E. Richmond of the 4th New York Heavy Artillery touched on the nation, citizen-soldiers, and Copperheads in letters to his wife. He thought anyone who voted for McClellan would be "aiming a blow at & stabbing our National life to the heart." Pronouncing his military service "the noblest cause that a *loyal* citizen can do—the suppressing of the Rebellion against . . . our country & the best government that God ever vouchsafed to his children," Richmond insisted that "none but a copperhead or traitor" would support the Democrats or embrace peace short of Union victory. He considered any man who cast a ballot against Lincoln "no better than the enemy 100 yds in front, who fires his *bullets at us*." A second lieutenant in the 76th Ohio Infantry used fewer, though equally inflammatory, words to make the same point. "The peace sneaks of the north should know by this time," wrote Lyman U. Humphrey from near Chattanooga, "that their damnable cause must go down to nothingness and their names be forever damned to eternal infamy." The soldiers "burn indignantly at the doings of the traitors behind us." Asa M. Weston, another Ohioan serving in Georgia, hoped Lincoln would be reelected but worried that men in Kentucky units "will vote for McClellan . . . so much the more willingly I suppose because he suits [Copperhead politician Clement L.] Vallandigham."

Early Union regimentals contain excellent material on emancipation and its consequences—though just more than a third of the sixty-four examined here ignore the end of slavery as a noteworthy outcome of the war. The ideas, arguments, and descriptive narratives published in the conflict's immediate aftermath conform closely to wartime soldiers' testimony about war aims, black military service, and the ways in which racial attitudes affected behavior and political opinions. These opinions regarding emancipation should not obscure the very widely held belief among Union soldiers that slavery had caused the war.

Taken as a group, these regimentals underscore the degree to which emancipation figured in most soldiers' minds primarily as a means to achieve and uphold Union. Four examples from Ohio, New York, and Illinois illustrate this point. Chaplain Thomas M. Stevenson of the 78th Ohio Infantry observed that "to suppress the rebellion without interfering with slavery, is an absurdity which would be only taking the effect and leaving the cause." A restored Union could be safe only with emancipation. No other course would "make a loyal people in the South . . . As well make a mocking-bird out of a moccasin snake, or make the substance of opposite affinities unite." Lincoln understood this, and his proclamation "was the key that turned all our efforts into success, and opened the doors of victory and complete success to our arms." The wartime regimental of the 23rd New York Infantry reprinted a letter about Lincoln's proclamation, which, asserted its author, "does not seem to offend any one in this part of the army." The letter took Benjamin Butler's pronouncement about runaway slaves literally: "It is pretty well settled in these military circles that negroes during the continuance of this war are as clearly contraband as cannon, 'hard tack,' quinine, saltpeter, or mercurial ointment."

Wales Wood, adjutant of the 95th Illinois Infantry, flatly denied that emancipation had been the principal goal of the war. "It was claimed by some people, and there are probably those who still adhere to the opinion," he wrote in the autumn of 1865, "that the war against secession was carried on by the Government from the beginning with the prominent idea on the part of the Administration of abolishing slavery . . . , and that the incipient plan of emancipating the slaves was fully illustrated and carried into practice by the Proclamation of President Lincoln." That interpretation misconstrued the president's intent to offer the proclamation "only as a *war measure* to hurt traitors and kill rebellion." Although emancipation hurt the Rebel military effort, Wood believed the "negro question at all times during the progress of the war, was an annoying subject to military commanders, in endeavoring to carry out the policy of the Government." Wood also mentioned General Frémont's plan to seize slaves of Rebel owners in Missouri as a policy designed to help fight the war for Union, as did David Lathrop of the 59th Illinois Infantry. "General Fremont was far in advance of the nation's representatives, either in the field or cabinet," asserted Lathrop, "He realized that the only way to stop rebellion was to chastise rebels with the rod of justice."

Ovando J. Hollister of the 1st Colorado Volunteers detailed a lively discussion about emancipation among men in Company I of the 2nd U.S. Dragoons in September 1862. This group, who differed from the vast majority of Union men under arms because they were professional soldiers, "contained representatives of every shade of the idea, from the opposer of slavery on principle, to the tolerator of slavery on the ground of expediency, and the worshiper of slavery from long association and habit." Few Americans embraced fanatical devotion to any idea, mused Hollister, manifesting instead a very practical approach to life. Although motivation to fight the war against Rebels did not spring from a love of *"Liberty for all,"* true patriots "will rejoice that the destruction of chattel slavery in the United States, is an inseparable adjunct of the present upheaval of society." "Adjunct" was the crucial word for these men—though Hollister himself stood ardently against slavery on moral grounds—and set up the summary sentence. "We finally concluded," wrote Hollister with a swipe at slaveholders, "that because slavery is aggressive, if not because it is wrong, we muse necessarily war against it."

Chastising slaveholders through forced emancipation proved widely popular in the units covered by the regimentals. Lieutenant Bartholomew B. S. De Forest, quartermaster of the 81st New York Infantry, developed this theme. He hoped Rebel leaders would be punished severely in the aftermath of a war for "the preservation of our glorious Union." Black soldiers could help achieve that end, which would be complete only if slaveholders who "ruled with the iron hand of despotism" and "sought to perpetuate the institution of Slavery at the sacrifice of a Republican Government" had been utterly vanquished. Once Rebel armies had been dispersed and slavery abolished, "tyranny, that bitter foe of free institutions and humanity," would have been eradicated from American soil.

Regimental historians reached disparate conclusions about black military contributions. Very few perceived USCT regiments as decisive in any major battles, though several expressed admiration for black courage in smaller actions. Almost all welcomed the labor of African American soldiers because it freed white men from the kinds of noncombatant work they detested. A handful endorsed full citizenship for black soldiers based on their military service, though several drew a sharp line between the idea of equality within the wartime military sphere and in postwar society. Prejudice pervaded nearly all of the regimentals—often providing a jarring contrast to even the most appreciative accounts.

The chroniclers of the 117th and 115th New York Infantry acknowledged superior performances by USCT units at Petersburg and Olustee. Surgeon James A. Mowris of the 117th described the costly action outside Petersburg on June 15, 1864, where USCT men made their initial appearance on a big Virginia battlefield. The "brave fellows" had carried the outer line of Rebel works and then assaulted and captured a second line: "These black soldiers, were highly elated, even those who were severely wounded, greeted their white compatriots, with, 'Tell you boys, we made um get;' 'We druv em.'" The episode impressed white observers, noted Mowris with a touch of sarcasm: "Those who were politically the most conservative, suddenly experienced, an accession of respect for the chattel on this discovery of its 'equal' value in a possible emergency." Lieutenant James H. Clark of the 115th, a regiment that suffered heavy casualties at the battle of Olustee, described how one of the USCT regiments in that engagement "formed and maneuvered under fire, and suffered heavy losses." Although their colonel was killed, the black soldiers "preserved their line admirably and fought splendidly."

George W. Powers of the 38th Massachusetts Infantry typified those who found things to praise and criticize about black soldiers in combat. A veteran of operations in Louisiana and Virginia, he wrote in detail about two "native Louisiana regiments" in a skirmish on May 25, 1863, during the Port Hudson campaign. "A great deal of romance has been spoken and printed about this affair," Powers observed, "but, without wishing to detract in the least from the really valuable services rendered by the colored troops during the siege, especially in the engineer's department, it may be doubted if the exaggerated accounts of their bravery were of any real benefit to the 'colored boys in blue.'" Because it long had been fashionable "to decry the courage of the colored man, and deny him all the attributes of manhood, . . . when he proved himself something more than a beast of burden, public opinion went to the opposite extreme" and "asserted that this new freedman was the equal, if not the superior, of the Northern volunteer soldier." White soldiers even heard that General Banks said black soldiers "went where the white ones dared not go." Powers dismissed this as an improbable story that nonetheless "injured the general's popularity, and increased the prejudice already existing against the colored troops." On the night of May 26, Powers added in a short passage that twice damned African American comrades, a black regiment panicked and mistakenly fired a volley toward the 38th Massachusetts, but their aim was so bad "the bullets whistled harmlessly over head, and the panic soon subsided."

In his history of the 9th New Jersey Infantry, Hermann Everts ignored emancipation in the broader sense but inserted one comment critical of black soldiers. The 9th spent a good deal of time in proximity to USCT units, including in the trenches at Petersburg in the summer of

1864. Everts used a record of daily events in preparing the regimental, which included an entry for July 10, 1864, that suggested USCT soldiers lacked basic knowledge expected of veterans: "With the exception of the picket-firing, the night passed quietly. The picket-firing, so annoying, and so very unnecessary in most cases, was generally done by the negroes, as these troops need the sound of cannonballs around their heads and ears to keep their eyes open." Everts's observation accorded with other evidence from the first phase of the siege at Petersburg that suggested many white soldiers even doubted positive reports about the 54th Massachusetts in the assault at Fort Wagner—though some men changed their minds when they witnessed USCT troops overrun Rebel positions on June 15.

Black soldiers also emerged as less than exemplary in Col. W. W. H. Davis's narrative of the 104th Pennsylvania Infantry. Davis discussed the difficulty many white soldiers experienced with the idea of black enlistments, remarking that it took "some time to educate them up to this point." Deployed to South Carolina in early 1863, the 104th saw Col. Thomas Wentworth Higginson's 1st South Carolina Infantry (Union), the initial regiment of former slaves officially sanctioned by the War Department. "These African defenders of our national honor were lounging about camp and shore," recalled Davis with more than a hint of condescension, "clad in their blue dress coats and scarlet breeches. Our men gazed at them with strange interest, as it was the first time they had ever seen negroes equipped as soldiers. This sight carried me back to an earlier period in the history of the war, when arming the negroes to make soldiers of them dared not be talked about aloud." Davis also described how Brig. Gen. William Birney, son of the famous abolitionist James Gillespie Birney, detailed six men from the 104th to cook for a group of contraband laborers. This happened when two black regiments were posted near where the work was to be done and, insisted Davis, arose from Birney's wish "to degrade the white soldiers and insult the regiment . . . Is it then a cause of wonder that he was heartily despised by the white troops?"

The regimentals suggest that white soldiers reached no consensus about the postwar fate of USCT veterans and other freedpeople. Joseph Grecian, who wrote his history of the 83rd Indiana Infantry during the last part of the war, thought they should be educated "so as to be competent to take care and govern themselves. Meanwhile, they will be afforded means of accumulating a sufficient amount of wealth to take them to, and establish themselves in the Old World, from which they were brought, and thus they may become a 'polished shaft' in the hand of Providence to enlighten 'poor dark Africa.'" Lieutenant De Forest of the 81st New York printed a letter that affirmed USCT men "should be recognized as equal with the white soldier, when they are engaged in one common cause." Once a black soldier returned to civilian life, however, and "he lays off the blue jacket, he is a negro still, and should be treated as God designed he should be, as an inferior, with kindness and sympathy, but not as an equal, in a social point of view."

Henry T. Johns, a clerk in the 49th Massachusetts Infantry, presented deeply conflicting ideas about what the war would yield for African Americans. He presented his history in the form of letters to render the text "less didactic and stiff," signing his preface in early May 1864. Johns enthusiastically supported the Emancipation Proclamation and the enlistment of black soldiers, and in early 1863 predicted "Negro equality" but not "social equality" after the war. Talented black men would rise on their merits. Later in his text he envisioned a much bleaker future for freedpeople because they belonged to an inferior race. "Like the Indians," he prophesied, "they will disappear from before us"—perhaps returning to Africa. Yet at the end of the book he gave "all honor to our negro soldiers. They deserve citizenship. They will secure it." There would be much suffering in what he termed "the transition state," but a "nation is not born without pangs." . . .

GARY W. GALLAGHER is the John L. Nau III Professor of History of the American Civil War at the University of Virginia. He is the author of numerous scholarly studies of the Civil War, including *The Confederate War* (Harvard University Press, 1997), *Lee and His Generals in War and Memory* (Louisiana State University Press, 1998), and *Becoming Confederates: Paths to a New National Loyalty* (University of Georgia Press, 2013).

EXPLORING THE ISSUE

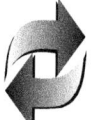

Was the Civil War Fought Over Slavery?

Critical Thinking and Reflection

1. What role did southern commissioners play in 1860 and 1861 in drumming up support for secession from the Union?
2. What arguments did southern commissioners make to justify secession?
3. Evaluate the continued support for the Union demonstrated by white southerners in several southern states right up to the time of secession.
4. Analyze the motivations of the Union soldiers for fighting the war.
5. Discuss the attitudes of northern soldiers toward the institution of slavery and the goal of preserving the Union.

Is There Common Ground?

Most historians of the Civil War era recognize the centrality of slavery in the sectional conflict that led ultimately to the secession of 11 southern states by 1861. The institution of slavery was so intricately wound into the fabric of southern society that even those who have insisted that the Civil War was a product of the propaganda of fanatics in either the North or South, blundering politicians, conflicting views of the Constitution of the United States, differences between the northern and southern economies, a conflict of cultures, or debates over majority rule and minority rights must realize how slavery imbedded itself into each of those factors. For those who insist that the debate was about states' rights, it is reasonably clear that the rights the southern states were seeking were the rights to keep the North and the federal government from meddling with the sanctity of the "peculiar institution." Similarly, scholars are hard-pressed to offer an economic explanation without recognizing that the most important economic institution in the South was slavery.

Charles B. Dew argues that the southern secessionist commissioners pushed the southern states into a Civil War in order to preserve the institution of slavery and the ideology of white supremacy. This interpretation is challenged in David Goldfield's recent book *America Aflame: How the Civil War Created a Nation* (Bloomsbury, 2011) which gives a more sympathetic portrait of the white slave owner who was proud of his ancestral heritage and felt himself losing political clout via attacks from abolitionists and northern evangelicals. At the same time, northerners were participating in slavery through their participation in the purchase of cotton goods for their factory.

Another comparison can be made regarding the motivations of the soldiers. Were they fighting to preserve the union and a democratic system that extended political and economic freedoms to its citizens? James McPherson's *For Cause and Comrade: Why Men Fought the Civil War* (Oxford, 1997) provides a variety of viewpoints on the grass-roots soldiers. Gary W. Gallagher finds sentiments toward African American soldiers that would be considered racist by modern standards. Most white soldiers believed that African Americans would make good support troops, serving as ditch diggers, supply officers, cooks, and laundrymen. Gallagher's critics say that the 350 soldiers' letters may not be a representative sample of attitudes. Is it possible that slavery and nationalism became fused together during the war? One may also argue that military necessity rather than human kindness was the main reason for Lincoln's Emancipation Proclamation in January 1863. Nevertheless, the president used all of his political leverage to attain the Thirteenth Amendment in March 1865, which freed the slaves and which passed the House of Representatives by only three votes. This is certainly the conclusion presented to viewers of Stephen Spielberg's recent movie *Lincoln*.

Additional Resources

Edward L. Ayers, *What Caused the Civil War? Reflections on the South and Southern History* (W. W. Norton, 2005)

Steven A. Canning, *Crisis of Fear: Secession in South Carolina* (Simon & Schuster, 1970)

James Oakes, *Freedom National: The Destruction of Slavery in the United States, 1861–1865* (W. W. Norton, 2012)

Michael Perman, ed., *The Coming of the American Civil War*, 3rd ed. (D. C. Heath, 1993)

David Potter, *The Impending Crisis, 1848–1861* (Harper & Row, 1976)

Internet References . . .

History Detectives: Causes of the Civil War

www.pbs.org/opb/historydetectives/feature/causes-of-the-civil-war

The American Civil War Center: The Causes of the Civil War

www.tredegar.org/caused-civil-war.aspxhttp://

The Causes of the Civil War

www.historynet.com/causes-of-the-civil-war

The Civil War Home Page

www.civil-war.net/pages/troops_furnished_losses.html

ISSUE

Selected, Edited, and with Issue Framing Material by:
Kevin R. Magill and Tony L. Talbert, *Baylor University*

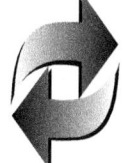

Are Historians Wrong to Consider the War Between the States a "Total War"?

YES: Mark E. Neely, Jr., from "Was the Civil War a Total War?" *Civil War History* (2004)

NO: James M. McPherson, from "From Limited to Total War, Missouri and the Nation, 1861–1865," *Magazine of the Missouri Historical Society* (1992)

Learning Outcomes
After reading this issue, you will be able to: • Define "total war." • Distinguish "total war," "unconditional surrender," and "modern war" from earlier types of warfare. • List arguments for and against the Civil War as a total war and critically analyze the validity of these arguments.

ISSUE SUMMARY

YES: Mark E. Neely convincingly asserts that the U.S. Civil War was not a "total war" based upon three factors. First, President Lincoln's continued insistence that Union generals made a distinction between combatants and non-combatants in the exercise of the war (though Grant and Sherman openly disagreed). Second, Lincoln's continued willingness to negotiate relatively lenient terms of peace that instead of demanding unconditional surrender offered Confederate leaders the opportunity of enter into discussions as long as they accepted the full restoration of the Union and the abandonment of slavery. And third, Neely contents that the U.S. Civil War did in fact have limitations and codes of conduct, which means it was not in fact a total war. He even cites the work of Brian Bond who argues that a true total war is unattainable.

NO: In stark contrast, Jame M. McPherson asserts that whether the notion of "total war" was the official policy Lincoln and his generals it was exactly that which was accomplished through the destruction of the southern states' economies, the dismantling of the symbiotic state-based Confederacy, and the complete abolition of a system of slavery that served as both the philosophical and cultural zeitgeist of the Confederacy. Simply put, McPherson argues that "total war" was indeed the outcome with the extensive destruction of Southern civilian populations and the south's economy as a whole.

The confusion around the issue of whether the Civil War was a total war centers around the terms which historians use to describe the conflict. Are the terms "unconditional surrender" and "modern war" synonymous with total war? Was the policy of unconditional surrender that the Americans applied against Germany and Japan to end World War II also used by Lincoln against the Confederacy? Apparently Jefferson Davis thought so when Lincoln's negotiators at the Hampton Roads Peace Conference in early 1865 demanded "no cessation of hostilities short of an end of the war and the disbanding of all forces hostile to the government."

Yet even though Lincoln was determined to free the slaves, he stopped short of unconditional surrender when he drafted a bill after the Hampton Roads conference which would have compensated the former slave owners $400 per slave if they ended the war before April 1865. Professor Neely also points out that if Lincoln really believed in unconditional surrender, he could have demanded "the exclusion of Confederate political leaders from future public office, disenfranchisement of Confederate soldiers, enfranchisement of freed blacks, legal protection for the Republican Party in former Confederate states, recognition of West Virginia's statehood, the partition of other Southern states, no reprisals against ex-slaves who served in Union armies, and so on."

Many historians consider the Civil War the most modern war because of the enormous number of casualties suffered—over 600,000 lives, 400,000 on the Union side and 200,000 on the Confederate. There is some question as to whether the weapons used, such as the development of the rifle musket, gave an advantage to the defense in repelling frontal assaults engaged by the infamous Pickett's charge at Gettysburg, which caused so many deaths. Professor Grady McWhiney and Perry D. Jamieson argue in *Attack and Die: Civil War Military Tactics and the Southern Heritage* (University of Alabama Press, 1982) that the "celtic heritage" caused Southerners to engage in these frontal attacks. But Professors Herman Hattaway and Archer Jones in *How the North Won: A Military History of the Civil War* (University of Illinois Press, 1983) downplay the importance of specific battles and actions taken by individuals and believe that the North was victorious because the Union was more effective than the Confederacy in marshaling its resources.

Professor Mark Neely challenges the conventional wisdom of the time when he denies that the Civil War was a total war. According to Neely, not until after World War II when improved technology with its aerial bombing raids rendered the distinction between combatants and noncombatants meaningless that true "total war" was a reality. In his assessment of Sherman, Neely believes his rhetoric was more ferocious than his actions. Sherman did not make war against noncombatants. Whatever atrocities that were suffered in the war were mostly by soldiers against other soldiers on both sides. Whenever possible, Sherman tried to restrain his men from destroying the lives of civilians and their personal property. (South Carolina was the exception because it started the war.) If one seeks the earliest application of total war, Neely says it can be found in the speeches of President Jefferson Davis.

Neely also argues that the Lincoln administration did not mobilize its economy or its scientific community very well. There was no Manhattan Project that developed America's first atomic bomb. Nor were key industries mobilized under the rubric of state planning. Neely's argument on this point is partially substantiated by Stanley L. Engerman and J. Matthew Galman, "The Civil War Economy: A Modern View" in Steg Forster, et al., *The American Civil War and the German Wars of Unification, 1861–1871* (Cambridge University Press, 1997), who argue that it was the South and not the North that had to levy taxes, draft white Southerners, and engage in economic planning because its economic base was primarily agricultural.

Professor McPherson makes a strong case that the Civil War was a total war. Statistically, the war was devastating: 620,000 soldiers lost their lives, a number that equals almost all the number of soldiers killed in all the other American wars combined. One quarter of white men of military age lost their lives. Altogether, about 4 percent of southern people, black and white, were killed. Most were not killed in combat, but were victims of malnutrition and disease. It has been estimated that the war destroyed two-thirds of the region's wealth including the market value of slaves. In short, McPherson believes the Union war effort was "total" in its objectives because it destroyed the Confederate government and ended slavery.

McPherson argues familiarly that Lincoln shifted the objective of the war from restoring the Union with or without slavery intact to the destruction of both the Confederacy and slavery. His case for a shift from partial to total war is supported in his essay on "Union Generalship, Political Leadership and Total War" in the Forster collection cited above. Professor Edward Hagerman agrees with McPherson by saying that when Lincoln fired McClellan, he shifted his objective from a limited to a total war.

Did the North wage a total war against the South? In the YES selection, Professor Mark E. Neely, Jr., denies that the Civil War was a total war because the Union leaders respected the distinction between combatants and noncombatants and did not fully mobilize the country's economic resources. In the NO selection, Professor James M. McPherson says that Lincoln shifted the policy from limited to total war in the fall of 1862 and accomplished his objectives of abolishing slavery and destroying the Confederate government.

YES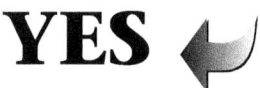

Mark E. Neely, Jr.

Was the Civil War a Total War?

... The idea of total war was first applied to the Civil War in an article about William T. Sherman published in the *Journal of Southern History* in 1948: John B. Walters's "General William T. Sherman and Total War."[1] After this initial use of the term, it was quickly adopted by T. Harry Williams, whose influential book *Lincoln and His Generals*, published in 1952, began with this memorable sentence: "The Civil War was the first of the modern total wars, and the American democracy was almost totally unready to fight it." Among the more popular Civil War writers, the idea also fared well. Bruce Catton, for example, wrote in a 1964 essay on "The Generalship of Ulysses S. Grant" that "He was fighting . . . a total war, and in a total war the enemy's economy is to be undermined in any way possible." Scholarly writers continued to use the term as well. In his masterful *Battle Cry of Freedom: The Civil War Era*, Princeton University's James M. McPherson writes, "By 1863, Lincoln's remarkable abilities gave him a wide edge over Davis as a war leader, while in Grant and Sherman the North acquired commanders with a concept of total war and the necessary determination to make it succeed." Professor McPherson's book forms part of the prestigious Oxford History of the United States. In another landmark volume, "*A People's Contest": The Union and the Civil War* (Harper & Row's New American Nation series), historian Phillip Shaw Paludan writes, "Grant's war making has come to stand for the American way of war. For one thing, that image is one of total war demanding unconditional surrender."[2]

Surely any idea about the military conduct of the Civil War that has been championed by Williams, Catton, McPherson, and Paludan, that is embodied in the Oxford History of the United States and in the New American Nation series, can fairly be called accepted wisdom on the subject. Most writers on the military history of the war, if forced to articulate a brief general description of the nature of that conflict, would now say, as McPherson has, that the Civil War began in 1861 with a purpose in the North "to suppress this insurrection and restore loyal Unionists to control of the southern states. The conflict was therefore a limited war . . . with the limited goal of restoring the status quo ante bellum, not an unlimited war to destroy an enemy nation and reshape its society." Gradually, or as McPherson puts it, "willy-nilly," the war became "a total war rather than a limited one." Eventually, "Union generals William Tecumseh Sherman and Philip Sheridan saw more clearly than anyone else the nature of modern, total war, a war between peoples rather than simply between armies, a war in which the fighting left nothing untouched or unchanged." President Lincoln came to realize the nature of the military contest and "sanctioned this policy of 'being terrible' on the enemy." Finally, "when the Civil War became a total war, the invading army intentionally destroyed the economic capacity of the South to wage war." Northern victory resulted from this gradual realization and the subsequent application of new and harsh doctrines in the war's later phase. . . .

Northerner and Southerner alike have come to agree on the use of this term, total war, but what does it mean exactly? It was never used in the Civil War itself. Where does it come from? . . .

Unfortunately, like many parts of everyday vocabulary, total war is a loose term with several meanings. Since World War II, it has come to mean, in part, a war requiring the full economic mobilization of a society. From the start, it meant the obverse of the idea as well: making war on the economic resources of the enemy rather than directly on its armed forces alone. Yet there was nothing really new about attacking an enemy's economic resources; that was the very essence of naval blockades and they long predated the Civil War. The crucial and terrible new aspect of the notion of total war was embodied in the following idea, part of a definition of the term cited in the *Oxford English Dictionary*: "Every citizen is in a sense a combatant and also the object of attack." Every systematic definition of the term embodies the concept of destroying the ages-old distinction between civilians and soldiers, whatever other ideas may be present. Another citation in the *OED*, for example, terms it "a war to which all resources and the whole population are committed; loosely, a war conducted without any scruple or limitations." *Webster's . . . Unabridged* dictionary describes total war as "warfare that uses all possible means of attack, military, scientific, and psychological, against both enemy troops and civilians." And James Turner Johnson, in his study of *Just War Tradition and the Restraint of War,* asserts that in total war "there must be disregard of restraints imposed by custom, law, and morality on the prosecution of the war. Especially, . . . total war bears hardest on noncombatants, whose traditional protection from harm according to the traditions of just and limited warfare appears to evaporate here."

Close application of this twentieth-century term (the product of the age of strategic bombing and blitzkrieg and powerful totalitarian governments capable of mobilizing science and psychology) to the Civil War seems fraught with difficulty. Surely no one believes, for example, that the Civil War was fought "without any scruple or limitations." From the ten thousand plus pages of documents in the eight full volumes of the *Official Records* dealing with prisoners of war, to the many copies of General Orders No. 100, a brief code of the laws of war distributed throughout the Union army in 1863, evidence abounds that this war knew careful limitation and conscientious scruple. Even World War II followed the rules bearing on prisoners of war. Any assessment of the Civil War's nearness to being a total war can be no more than that: an assertion that it *approached* total war in some ways. By no definition of the term can it be said to *be* a total war.

Occasionally, the term total war approximates the meaning of modernity. T. Harry Williams used the terms interchangeably, as in this passage from a later work in which he hedged a bit on calling the Civil War a total war: "Trite it may be to say that the Civil War was the first of the modern wars, but this is a truth that needs to be repeated. If the Civil War was not quite total, it missed totality by only a narrow margin."

Modernity is not a very useful concept in military history. Surely every war is thought to be modern by its participants—save possibly those fought by Japan in the strange era when firearms were consciously rejected. As a historian's term, modern when applied to warfare has a widely accepted meaning different from total. Modern warfare generally connotes wars fought after the French Revolution by large citizen armies equipped with the products of the Industrial Revolution and motivated more by ideology than the lash or strictly mercenary considerations. The Civil War certainly was a modern war in that sense, but it was not a total war in the sense that civilians were commonly thought of as legitimate military targets.

Perhaps no one who maintains the Civil War was a total war means it so literally. Historian Brian Bond provides a useful idea when he writes, "strictly speaking, total war is just as much a myth as total victory or total peace. What is true, however, is that the fragile barriers separating war from peace and soldiers from civilians—already eroded in the First World War—virtually disappeared between 1939 and 1945." Seeing how often that fragile barrier broke in the Civil War will tell how nearly it approached being a total war. All such matters of degree contain dangers for the historian trying to answer the question; the risk of sinking under a mass of piecemeal objections raised afterward by critics is very high. Even the most conservative of Civil War generals occasionally stepped over the boundaries of customarily accepted behavior in nineteenth-century warfare. General George B. McClellan, for example, did so in the Peninsula campaign, after only about a year's fighting. On May 4, 1862, he informed Secretary of War Edwin M. Stanton: "The rebels have been guilty of the most murderous & barbarous conduct in placing torpedoes [land mines] *within* the abandoned works, near wells & springs, near flag staffs, magazines, telegraph offices, in carpet bags, barrels of flour etc. Fortunately we have not lost many men in this manner—some 4 or 5 killed & perhaps a dozen wounded. I shall make the prisoners remove them at their own peril." . . .

John B. Walters cited General Sherman's use of prisoners to clear mines as an example of his total war practices, but Sherman's reaction was in fact exactly like McClellan's. When Sherman saw a "handsome young officer" with all the flesh blown off one of his legs by a Confederate mine in Georgia in December 1864, he grew "very angry," because "this was not war, but murder." Sherman then retaliated by using Confederate prisoners to clear the mines. What at first may seem an incident suggesting the degeneration of warfare, in fact proves the belief of the protagonists in rules and codes of civilized behavior that have in the twentieth century long since vanished from the world's battlefields. The real point is that Union and Confederate authorities were in substantial agreement about the laws of war, and they usually tried to stay within them.

Leaving aside similar isolated instances caused by temporary rage, can a historian seeking to describe the war's direction toward or away from total war examine larger aspects of the war where the "fragile barriers" between soldiers and civilians may have broken down? Since the conscious application of a new doctrine in warfare forms part of the total war interpretation, can a historian focus on certain figures in high command who held such doctrines and applied them to the enemy in the Civil

War? Throughout, can the historian keep an eye on the dictionary definition of total war to measure the proximity of the Civil War to it? Surely this can be done, and short of a study of the Civil War day by day, there can hardly be any other test. . . .

Sherman is the Civil War soldier most often quoted on the subject of total war. An article about him gave rise to this interpretation of the Civil War, and indeed it is now widely held that, as historian John E. Marszalek has expressed it, William T. Sherman was the "Inventor of Total Warfare." "We are not only fighting hostile armies, but a hostile people, and must make old and young, rich and poor, feel the hard hand of war, as well as their organized armies," Sherman told Gen. Hency W. Halleck on Christmas Eve 1864. As early as October 1862 he said, "We cannot change the hearts of these people of the South, but we can make war so terrible . . . [and] make them so sick of war that generations would pass away before they would again appeal to it."[3]

The gift of sounding like a twentieth-century man was peculiarly Sherman's. Nearly every other Civil War general sounds ancient by comparison, but many historians may have allowed themselves to be fooled by his style while ignoring the substance of his campaigns.

Historians, moreover, quote Sherman selectively. In fact, he said many things and when gathered together they do not add up to any coherent "total-war philosophy," as one historian describes it. Sherman was not a philosopher; he was a general and a garrulous one at that. "He talked incessantly and more rapidly than any man I ever saw," Maj. John Chipman Gray reported. "It would be easier to say what he did not talk about than what he did." Chauncey Depew said Sherman was "the readiest and most original talker in the United States." And what Sherman said during the war was often provoked by exasperating, momentary circumstance. Therefore, he occasionally uttered frightening statements. "To secure the safety of the navigation of the Mississippi River I would slay millions," Sherman told Gen. John A. Logan on December 21,1863. "On that point I am not only insane, but mad . . . For every bullet shot at a steam-boat, I would shoot a thousand 30-pounder Parrotts into even helpless towns on Red, Oachita, Yazoo, or wherever a boat can float or soldier march." This statement was all the more striking, coming from a man widely reputed by newspaper critics to be insane. On another occasion, Sherman said, "To the petulant and persistent secessionists, why, death is mercy, and the quicker he or *she is* disposed of the better" (italics added).[4]

In other moods and in different circumstances, Sherman could sound as mild as Robert E. Lee. "War," the alleged inventor of total war wrote on April 19, 1863, "at best is barbarism, but to involve all—children, women, old and helpless—is more than can be justified." And he went on to caution against seizing so many stores that family necessities were endangered. Later, in the summer of 1863 when General Sherman sent a cavalry expedition toward Memphis from Mississippi, General Grant instructed him to "impress upon the men the importance of going through the State in an orderly manner, abstaining from taking anything not absolutely necessary for their subsistence while travelling. They should try to create as favorable an impression as possible upon the people." These may seem hopeless orders to give General Sherman, but his enthusiastic reply was this: "It will give me excessive pleasure to instruct the Cavalry as you direct, for the Policy you point out meets every wish of my heart."[5]

Scholars who pay less heed to the seductively modern sound of Sherman's harsher statements and look closely instead at what he actually did on his celebrated campaigns in Georgia and the Carolinas, find a nineteenth-century soldier at work—certainly not a man who made war on noncombatants. Joseph T. Glatthaar's study of Sherman's campaigns confirmed that, for the most part, Sherman's men did not physically abuse civilians who kept to themselves: atrocities were suffered mostly by soldiers on *both* sides; in Georgia and the Carolinas, Sherman's army recovered the bodies of at least 172 Union soldiers hanged, shot in the head at close range, with their throats slit, or "actually butchered." And only in South Carolina, the state blamed for starting the war, did Sherman fail to restrain his men in their destruction of private property. Before the idea of total war came to Civil War studies, shrewd students of the conflict had noted the essentially nineteenth-century nature of Sherman's campaigns. Gamaliel Bradford's *Union Portraits,* for example, written during World War I, observed: "Events . . . have made the vandalism of Sherman seem like discipline and order. The injury done by him seldom directly affected anything but property. There was no systematic cruelty in the treatment of noncombatants, and to the eternal glory of American soldiers be it recorded that insult and abuse toward women were practically unknown during the Civil War."[6]

Though not a systematic military thinker, General Sherman did compose a letter addressing the problem of noncombatants in the Civil War, and it described his actual policies better than his frequently quoted statements of a more sensational nature. He sent the letter to Maj. R. M. Sawyer, whom Sherman left behind to manage Huntsville, Alabama, when he departed for Meridian, Mississippi, early in 1864. Sherman also sent a copy to his brother, Republican Senator John Sherman, with an eye to possible publication:

> In my former letters I have answered all your questions save one, and that relates to the treatment of inhabitants known or suspected to be hostile or "Secesh." This is in truth the most difficult business of our army as it advances and occupies the Southern country. It is almost impossible to lay down rules, and I invariably leave the whole subject to the local commanders, but am willing to give them the benefit of my acquired knowledge and experience. In Europe, whence we derive our principles of war, wars are between kings or rulers through hired armies, and not between peoples. These remain, as it were, neutral, and sell their produce to whatever army is in possession.
>
> Napoleon when at war with Prussia, Austria, and Russia bought forage and provisions of the inhabitants and consequently had an interest to protect the farms and factories which ministered to his wants. In like manner the allied Armies in France could buy of the French inhabitants whatever they needed, the produce of the soil or manufactures of the country. Therefore, the general rule was and is that war is confined to the armies engaged, and should not visit the houses of families or private interests. But in other examples a different rule obtained the sanction of historical authority. I will only instance one, where in the siege of William and Mary the English army occupied Ireland, then in a state of revolt. The inhabitants were actually driven into foreign lands, and were dispossessed of their property and a new population introduced.
>
> ... The question then arises, Should we treat as absolute enemies all in the South who differ from us in opinion or prejudice, kill or banish them, or should we give them time to think and gradually change their conduct so as to conform to the new order of things which is slowly and gradually creeping into their country?
>
> When men take up arms to resist a rightful authority, we are compelled to use like force. ... When the provisions, forage, horses, mules, wagons, etc., are used by our enemy, it is clearly our duty and right to take them also, because otherwise they might be used against us. In like manner all houses left vacant by an inimical people are clearly our right, and as such are needed as storehouses, hospitals, and quarters. But the question arises as to dwellings used by women, children and non-combatants. So long as non-combatants remain in their houses and keep to their accustomed peaceful business, their opinions and prejudices can in no wise influence the war, and therefore should not be noticed; but if any one comes out into the public streets and creates disorder, he or she should be punished, restrained, or banished. ... If the people, or any of them, keep up a correspondence with parties in hostility, they are spies, and can be punished according to law with death or minor punishment. These are well-established principles of war, and the people of the South having appealed to war, are barred from appealing for protection to our constitution, which they have practically and publicly defied. They have appealed to war, and must abide its rules and laws.

Excepting incidents of retaliation, Sherman by and large lived by these "principles of war."[7]

Leaving "the whole subject" to local commanders nevertheless permitted considerable latitude for pillage or destruction and was in itself an important principle. Moreover, Sherman, who was a critic of universal suffrage and loathed the free press, thought a volunteer army, the product of America's ultra-individualistic society, would inevitably loot and burn private property. His conservative social views thus led to a career-long fatalism about pillage.[8]

Sherman's purposes in the Georgia and Carolinas campaigns, usually pointed to as the epitome of total war in the Civil War, are obscured by two months of the general's letters to other generals describing his desire to cut loose from Atlanta and his long, thin line of supply to march to the sea. From mid-September to mid-November 1864, Sherman worried the idea, and his superiors, explaining it in several ways. At first he argued from his knowledge of the political disputes between Jefferson Davis and Georgia governor Joseph E. Brown that the march would sever the state from the Confederacy. "They may stand the fall of Richmond," Sherman told Grant on September 20, "but not of all Georgia." At the same time he belittled the effects of mere destruction: "the more I study the game the more I am convinced that it would be wrong for me to penetrate much farther into Georgia without an objective beyond. It would not be productive of much good. I can start east and make a circuit south and back, *doing vast damage to the State,* but resulting in no permanent good" (italics added).[9]

Less than three weeks later, Sherman gave a rather different explanation to Grant: "Until we can repopulate Georgia, it is useless to occupy it, but the utter destruction of its roads, houses, and people will cripple their military resources. By attempting to hold the roads we will lose 1,000 men monthly, and will gain no result. I can make the march, and make Georgia howl."

Ten days after that, he more or less combined his different arguments in a letter to General Halleck. "This movement is not purely military or strategic," he now said, "but it will illustrate the vulnerability of the South." Only when Sherman's armies arrived and "fences and corn and hogs and sheep" vanished would "the rich planters of the Oconee and Savannah" know "what war means." He spoke more tersely to his subordinates. "I want to prepare for my big raid," he explained on October 19 to a colonel in charge of supply, and with that Sherman arranged to send his impedimenta to the rear.

With plans more or less set, Sherman explained to Gen. George Thomas, who would be left to deal with Confederate Gen. John Bell Hood's army, "I propose to demonstrate the vulnerability of the South, and make its inhabitants feel that war and individual ruin are synonymous terms." Delays ensued and Sherman decided to remain in place until after election day. On the twelfth he cut his telegraph lines, and the confusing explanations of the campaign ceased pouring out of Georgia.

Sherman did not attempt the "utter destruction" of Georgia's "people." He did not really attack noncombatants directly or make any serious attempt to destroy "the economic capacity of the south to wage war," as one historian has described his purpose. After capturing Atlanta, for example, Sherman moved to capture Savannah and then attacked the symbolic capital of secession, South Carolina. He did not attack Augusta, Georgia, which he knew to contain "the only powder mills and factories remaining in the South." Though he did systematically destroy railroad lines, Sherman otherwise had little conception of eliminating essential industries. Indeed, there were few to eliminate, for the South, in comparison with the North, was a premodern, underdeveloped, agrarian region where determined men with rifles were the real problem—not the ability of the area's industries to manufacture high-technology weapons. Despite scorching a sixty-mile-wide swath through the Confederacy, Sherman was never going to starve this agrarian economy into submission, either. He had remarked in the past on how well fed and even shod the Confederate armies were despite their backward economy.

What Sherman was doing embodied traditional geopolitical objectives in a civil war: convincing the enemy's people and the world that the Confederate government and upper classes were too weak to maintain nationhood. He did this with a "big raid." "If we can march a well-appointed army right through his [Jefferson Davis's] territory," Sherman told Grant on November 6, 1864, "it is a demonstration to the world, foreign and domestic, that we have a power which Davis cannot resist." In *Battle Cry of Freedom* this statement is followed by ellipsis marks and the statement, "I can make the march, and make Georgia howl!" But that appears to be a misquotation. In fact, Sherman went on to say something much less vivid and scorching:

> This may not be war, but rather statesmanship, nevertheless it is overwhelming to my mind that there are thousands of people abroad and in the South who will reason thus: If the North can march an army right through the south, it is proof positive that the North can prevail in this contest, leaving only open the question of its willingness to use that power.
>
> Now, Mr. Lincoln's election, which is assured, coupled with the conclusion just reached, makes a complete, logical whole.

And Mr. Lincoln himself endorsed the view. In his letter congratulating Sherman on his Christmas capture of Savannah, the president counted the campaign "a great success" not only in affording "the obvious and immediate military advantages" but also "in showing to the world that your army could be divided, putting the stronger part to an important new service, and yet leaving enough to vanquish the old opposing force of the whole—Hood's army." This, Lincoln said, "brings those who sat in darkness, to see a great light." Neither Sherman nor Lincoln put the emphasis on the role of sheer destructiveness or economic deprivation. . . .

In fact, no Northerner at any time in the nineteenth century embraced as his own the cold-blooded ideas now associated with total war. If one seeks the earliest application of the idea (rather than the actual term) to the Civil War, it lies perhaps in the following document, written in the midst of the Civil War itself:

> [T]hey [the U.S.] have repudiated the foolish conceit that the inhabitants of this confederacy are still citizens of the United States, for they are waging an indiscriminate war upon them all, with a savage ferocity unknown to modern civilization. In this war, rapine is the rule: private residences, in peaceful rural retreats, are bombarded and burnt: Grain crops in the field are consumed by the torch and when the torch is not convenient, careful labor is bestowed to render complete the destruction of every article of use or ornament remaining in private dwellings, after their inhabitants have fled from the outrages of a brutal soldiery.
>
> Mankind will shudder to hear of the tales of outrages committed on defenceless females

by soldiers of the United States now invading our homes: yet these outrages are prompted by inflamed passions and madness of intoxication.

The source of the idea was, of course, Confederate, and it was a high Confederate source indeed: Jefferson Davis.

It may sound as though Davis was describing Sherman's march through Georgia or perhaps Sheridan in the Shenandoah Valley—most probably in a late speech, in 1864 or 1865. In fact, President Davis made the statement in 1861, in his Message to Congress of July 20. Davis not only described total war three years before Sherman entered Georgia; he described total war before the First Battle of Bull Run had been fought. It was fought the day *after* Davis delivered his message to Congress.

The first application of the *idea* to the Civil War came, then, in Confederate propaganda. Though it may not be a sectional interpretation now, it was an entirely sectional idea in the beginning. Its origins give perhaps the best clue to the usefulness of the idea in describing the Civil War. Total war may describe certain isolated and uncharacteristic aspects of the Civil War but is at most a partial view.

The point is not merely semantic. The use of the idea of total war prevents historians from understanding the era properly. . . .

Likewise, the economic aspect of total war is misleading when used to describe characteristics of the Civil War reputedly more forward looking than naval blockades. The ideas of economic planning and control from World War II cannot be applied to the Civil War. Hardly anyone then thought in such macroeconomic terms. Abraham Lincoln did calculate the total daily cost of the war, but he did not do so to aid long-range economic planning for the Union war effort. Instead he used the figure to show how relatively inexpensive it would be for the U.S. government to purchase the freedom of all the slaves in the border states through compensated emancipation. At $400 a head, the $2 million daily war expenditure would buy every slave in Delaware at "less than one half-day's cost," and "less than eighty seven days cost of this war would, at the same price, pay for all in Delaware, Maryland, District of Columbia, Kentucky, and Missouri."

From the Confederate perspective, the economic insight seems ironically somewhat more appropriate. The blockade induced scarcities on which almost all Confederate civilian diarists commented—coffee, shoe leather, and needles were sorely missed. The Confederate government's attempts to supply scarce war necessities led some historians to call the resulting system "state socialism" or a "revolutionary experience." Yet these were the outcome less of deliberate Northern military strategy (the blockade aside) than of the circumstance that the South was agrarian and the North more industrialized.

For its part, the North did little to mobilize its resources—little, that is, that would resemble the centralized planning and state intervention typical of twentieth-century economies in war. There was no rationing, North or South, and the Yankees' society knew only the sacrifice of men, not of materials. As Phillip Paludan has shown, agriculture thrived, and other parts of Northern society suffered only modestly; college enrollments fell, except at the University of Michigan, but young men still continued to go to college in substantial numbers. Inflation and a graduated income tax did little to trouble the claims made by most Republicans of surprising prosperity in the midst of war. The Republican president stated in his annual message to the United States Congress in December 1864:

> It is of noteworthy interest that the steady expansion of population, improvement and governmental institutions over the new and unoccupied portions of our country have scarcely been checked, much less impeded or destroyed, by our great civil war, which at first glance would seem to have absorbed almost the entire energies of the nation.
> . . . It is not material to inquire *how* the increase has been produced, or to show that it would have been *greater* but for the war. . . . The important fact remains demonstrated, that we have *more* men *now* than we had when the war *began*. . . . This as to men. Material resources are now more complete and abundant than ever.
> The national resources, then, are unexhausted, and, as we believe, inexhaustible.

Democrats generally conceded prosperity by their silence and focused instead on race and civil liberties as campaign issues.

The essential aspect of any definition of total war asserts that it breaks down the distinction between soldiers and civilians, combatants and non-combatants, and this no one in the Civil War did systematically, including William T. Sherman. He and his fellow generals waged war the same way most Victorian gentlemen did, and other Victorian gentlemen in the world knew it. That is one reason why British, French, and Prussian observers failed to comment on any startling developments seen in the American war: there was little new to report. The conservative monarchies of the old world surely would have seized with delight on any evidence that warfare in the New World was degenerating to the level of starving and killing civilians. Their observers encountered no such spectacle. It required airplanes and tanks and heartless twentieth-century ideas born in the hopeless trenches of World War I to break down distinctions adhered to in practice by almost all Civil War generals. Their war did little to usher in the shock of the new in the twentieth century.

Notes

1. John B. Walters, "General William T. Sherman and Total War," *Journal of Southern History* 14 (November 1948): 447–80. See also John B. Walters, *Merchant of Terror: General Sherman and Total War* (Indianapolis, Ind.: Bobbs-Merrill, 1973). Phillip Paludan mistakes the origins of Walters's ideas as being a product of the Vietnam War era, ignoring the anti-Yankee roots of the idea apparent in the earlier article. See Philip Paludan, *"A People's Contest": The Union and the Civil War* (New York: Harper & Row, 1988), 456. Other books on Sherman embracing the total war thesis include: John G. Barrett, *Sherman's March through the Carolinas* (Chapel Hill: Univ. of North Carolina Press, 1956); Burke Davis, *Sherman's March* (New York: Random House, 1980); and James M. Reston Jr., *Sherman's March and Viet Nam* (New York: Macmillan, 1984).

2. T. Harry Williams, *Lincoln and His Generals* (New York: Alfred A. Knopf, 1952), 3; Bruce Catton, "The Generalship of Ulysses S. Grant," in *Grant, Lee, Lincoln and the Radicals: Essays on Civil War Leadership,* ed. Grady McWhiney (New York: Harper Colophon, 1966), 8; James M. McPherson, *Battle Cry of Freedom: The Civil War Era* (New York: Oxford Univ. Press, 1988), 857; Paludan, *"A People's Contest,"* 296.

3. OR 44:798; OR 17, 2:261.

4. McPherson, *Battle Cry of Freedom,* 809; John Chipman Gray and John Codman Ropes, *War Letters 1862–1865* (Boston: Houghton, Mifflin, 1927), 425, 427; Edmund Wilson, *Patriotic Gore: Studies in the Literature of the American Civil War* (New York: Oxford Univ. Press, 1962), 205; OR 31, 3:459; OR 32, 2:281.

5. OR 24, 2:209; John Y. Simon, ed., *The Papers of Ulysses S. Grant,* 16 vols. to date (Carbondale: Southern Illinois Univ. Press, 1967–), 9:155, 156n.

6. Joseph T. Glatthaar, *The March to the Sea and Beyond: Sherman's Troops in the Savannah and Carolinas Campaigns* (New York: New York Univ. Press, 1985), 72–73, 127–28; Gamaliel Bradford, *Union Portraits* (Boston: Houghton, Mifflin, 1916), 154n–155n, Paludan, though he says Sherman "helped announce the coming of total war," also states that "Sherman's idea of war was more description than doctrine." Paludan, *"A People's Contest."* 291, 302.

7. Rachel Sherman Thorndike, ed., *The Sherman Letters: Correspondence between General and Senator Sherman from 1837 to 1891* (New York: Charles Scribner's Sons, 1894), 228–30.

8. Ibid. 175–76, 181–82, 185; M. A. DeWolfe Howe, ed., *Home Letters of General Sherman* (New York: Charles Scribner's Sons, 1909), 209.

9. OR 39, 2:412.

MARK E. NEELY is currently the McCabe Greer Professor of Civil War History at Penn State University. A specialist on Abraham Lincoln and the American Civil War, he is the author of *The Fate of Liberty: Abraham Lincoln and Civil Liberties* (Oxford University Press, 1991), which won the Pulitzer and Bell I. Wiley prizes; *The Last Best Hope of Earth: Abraham Lincoln and the Promise of America* (Harvard University Press, 1993); *The Civil War and the Limits of Destruction* (Harvard University Press, 2007); and, most recently, *Lincoln and the Triumph of the Nation: Constitutional Conflict in the American Civil War* (University of North Carolina Press, 2011). From 1972 to 1992, he served as director of The Lincoln Museum in Ft. Wayne, Indiana.

James M. McPherson

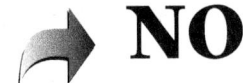

From Limited War to Total War, 1861–1865

A few years after the Civil War, Mark Twain described that great conflict as having "uprooted institutions that were centuries old, changed the politics of a people, transformed the social life of half the country, and wrought so profoundly upon the entire national character that the influence cannot be measured short of two or three generations." This profound transformation was achieved at enormous cost in lives and property. Fully one-quarter of the white men of military age in the Confederacy lost their lives. And that terrible toll does not include an unknown number of civilian deaths in the South. Altogether nearly 4 percent of the Southern people, black and white, civilians and soldiers, died as a consequence of the war. This percentage exceeded the human cost of any country in World War I and was outstripped only by the region between the Rhine and the Volga in World War II. The amount of property and resources destroyed in the Confederate States is almost incalculable. It has been estimated at two-thirds of all assessed wealth, including the market value of slaves.

This is the negative side of that radical transformation described by Mark Twain. The positive side included preservation of the United States as a unified nation, the liberation of four million slaves, and the abolition by constitutional amendment of the institution of bondage that had plagued the nation since the beginning, inhibited its progress, and made a mockery of the libertarian values on which it was founded. No other society in history freed so many slaves in so short a time—but also at such a cost in violence.

The Civil War mobilized human resources on a scale unmatched by any other event in American history except, perhaps, World War II. For actual combat duty the Civil War mustered a considerably larger proportion of American manpower than did World War II. And, in another comparison with that global conflict, the victorious power in the Civil War did all it could to devastate the enemy's economic resources as well as the morale of its home-front population, which was considered almost as important as enemy armies in the war effort. In World War II this was done by strategic bombing; in the Civil War it was done by cavalry and infantry penetrating deep into the Confederate heartland.

It is these factors—the devastation wrought by the war, the radical changes it accomplished, and the mobilization of the whole society to sustain the war effort that have caused many historians to label the Civil War a "total war." Recently, however, some analysts have questioned this terminology. They maintain that true total war—or in the words of Carl von Clausewitz, "absolute war"—makes no distinction between combatants and noncombatants, no discrimination between taking the lives of enemy soldiers and those of enemy civilians; it is war "without any scruple or limitations," war in which combatants give no quarter and take no prisoners.

Some wars have approached this totality—for example, World War II, in which Germany deliberately murdered millions of civilians in eastern Europe, Allied strategic bombing killed hundreds of thousands of German and Japanese civilians, and both sides sometimes refused to take prisoners and shot those who tried to surrender. In that sense of totality, the Civil War was not a total war. Although suffering and disease mortality were high among prisoners of war, and Confederates occasionally murdered captured black soldiers, there was no systematic effort to kill prisoners. And while soldiers on both sides in the Civil War pillaged and looted civilian property, and several Union commanders systematized this destruction into a policy, they did not deliberately kill civilians. Mark Neely, the chief critic of the notion of the Civil War as a total war, maintains that "the *essential* aspect of any definition of total war asserts that it breaks down the distinction between soldiers and civilians, combatants and noncombatants, and this no one in the Civil War did systematically."

Even William T. Sherman, widely regarded as the progenitor of total war, was more bark than bite according to Neely. Sherman wrote and spoke in a nervous, rapid-fire, sometimes offhand manner; he said extreme things about

---

McPherson, James M., "From Limited War to Total War, 1861–1865," Gateway Heritage; Magazine of the Missouri Historical Society 12. Copyright ©1992 Missouri History Museum. Used with permission.

"slaying millions" and "repopulating Georgia" if necessary to win the war. But this was rhetorical exaggeration. One of Sherman's most widely quoted statements—"We are not only fighting hostile armies, but a hostile people, and must make old and young, rich and poor, feel the hard hand of war"—did not really erase the distinction between combatants and noncombatants, for Sherman did not mean it to justify killing civilians.

To note the difference between rhetoric and substance in the Civil War is to make a valid point. The rhetoric not only of Sherman but also of many other people on both sides was far more ferocious than anything that actually happened. Northerners had no monopoly on such rhetoric. A Savannah newspaper proclaimed in 1863: "Let Yankee cities burn and their fields be laid waste," while a Richmond editor echoed: "It surely must be made plain at last that this is to be a war of extermination." A month after the firing on Fort Sumter, a Nashville woman prayed that "God may be with us to give us strength to conquer them, to exterminate them, to lay waste every Northern city, town and village, to destroy them utterly." Yankees used similar language. In the first month of the war a Milwaukee judge said that Northern armies should "restore New Orleans to its native marshes, then march across the country, burn Montgomery to ashes, and serve Charleston in the same way. . . . We must starve, drown, burn, shoot the traitors." In St. Louis the uneasy truce between Union and Confederate factions that had followed the riots and fighting in May 1861 broke down a month later when the Union commander Nathaniel Lyon rejected a compromise with pro-Confederate elements, which included the governor, with these words: "Rather than concede to the State of Missouri for one single instant the right to dictate to my Government in any matter . . . I would see you . . . and every man, woman, and child in the State, dead and buried."

These statements certainly sound like total war, war without limits or restraints. But of course none of the scenarios sketched out in these quotations literally came true—not even in Missouri, where reality came closer to rhetoric than anywhere else. Therefore, those who insist that the Civil War was not a total war appear to have won their case, at least semantically. Recognizing this, a few historians have sought different adjectives to describe the kind of conflict the Civil War became: One uses the phrase "destructive war"; another prefers "hard war."

But these phrases, though accurate, do not convey the true dimensions of devastation in the Civil War. All wars are hard and destructive in some degree; what made the Civil War distinctive in the American experience? It *was* that overwhelming involvement of the whole population, the shocking loss of life, the wholesale devastation and radical social and political transformations that it wrought. In the experience of Americans, especially Southerners, this approached totality; it *seemed* total. Thus the concept, and label, of total war remains a useful one. It is what the sociologist Max Weber called an "ideal type"—a theoretical model used to measure a reality that never fully conforms to the model, but that nevertheless remains a useful tool for analyzing the reality.

That is the sense in which this essay will analyze the evolution of the Civil War from a limited to a total war. Despite that fierce rhetoric of destruction quoted earlier, the official war aims of both sides in 1861 were quite limited. In his first message to the Confederate Congress after the firing on Fort Sumter by his troops had provoked war, Jefferson Davis declared that "we seek no conquest, no aggrandizement, no concession of any kind from the States with which we were lately confederated; all we ask is to be let alone." As for the Union government, its initial conception of the war was one of a domestic insurrection, an uprising against national authority by certain lawless hotheads who had gained temporary sway over the otherwise law-abiding citizens of a few Southern states—or as Lincoln put it in his proclamation calling out seventy-five thousand state militia to put down the uprising, "combinations too powerful to be suppressed by the ordinary course of judicial proceedings." This was a strategy of limited war—indeed, so limited that it was scarcely seen as a war at all, but rather as a police action to quell a large riot. It was a strategy founded on an assumption of residual loyalty among the silent majority of Southerners. Once the national government demonstrated its firmness by regaining control of its forts and by blockading Southern ports, those presumed legions of Unionists would come to the fore and bring their states back into the Union. To cultivate this loyalty, and to temper firmness with restraint, Lincoln promised that the federalized ninety-day militia would avoid "any devastation, any destruction of, or interference with, property, or any disturbance of peaceful citizens."

None other than William Tecumseh Sherman echoed these sentiments in the summer of 1861. Commander of a brigade that fought at Bull Run, Sherman deplored the marauding tendencies of his poorly disciplined soldiers. "No curse could be greater than invasion by a volunteer army," he wrote. "No Goths or Vandals ever had less respect for the lives and properties of friends and foes, and henceforth we should never hope for any friends in Virginia. . . . My only hope now is that a common sense of decency may be infused into this soldiery to respect life and property."

The most important and vulnerable form of Southern property was slaves. The Lincoln administration went out of its way to reassure Southerners in 1861 that it had no designs on slavery. Congress followed suit, passing by an overwhelming majority in July 1861 a resolution affirming that Union war aims included no intention "of overthrowing or interfering with the rights or established institutions of the States"—in plain words, slavery—but intended only "to defend and maintain the supremacy of the Constitution and to preserve the Union with all the dignity, equality, and rights of the several States unimpaired."

There were, to be sure, murmurings in the North against this soft-war approach, this "kid-glove policy." Abolitionists and radical Republicans insisted that a rebellion sustained *by* slavery in defense *of* slavery could be crushed only by striking *against* slavery. As Frederick Douglass put it: "To fight against Slaveholders, without fighting against slavery, is but a half-hearted business, and paralyzes the hands engaged in it.... Fire must be met with water. War for the destruction of liberty must be met with war for the destruction of slavery." Several Union soldiers and their officers, some with no previous antislavery convictions, also began to grumble about protecting the property of traitors in arms against the United States.

The first practical manifestation of such sentiments came in Missouri. Thus began a pattern whereby events in that state set the pace for the transformation from a limited to a total war, radiating eastward and southward from Missouri. The commander of the Western Department of the Union army in the summer of 1861, with headquarters at St. Louis, was John C. Frémont, famed explorer of the West, first Republican presidential candidate (in 1856), and now ambitious for military glory. Handicapped by his own administrative incompetence, bedeviled by a Confederate invasion of southwest Missouri that defeated and killed Nathaniel Lyon at Wilson's Creek on August 10 and then marched northward to the Missouri River, and driven to distraction by Confederate guerrilla bands that sprang up almost everywhere, Frémont on August 30 took a bold step toward total war. He placed the whole state of Missouri under martial law, announced the death penalty for guerrillas captured behind Union lines, and confiscated the property and emancipated the slaves of Confederate activists.

Northern radicals applauded, but conservatives shuddered and border-state Unionists expressed outrage. Still pursuing a strategy of trying to cultivate Southern Unionists as the best way to restore the Union, Lincoln feared that the emancipation provision of Frémont's edict would alarm our Southern Union friends, and turn them against us—perhaps ruin our rather fair prospect for Kentucky.... To lose Kentucky is nearly the same as to lose the whole game. Kentucky gone, we can not hold Missouri, nor, as I think, Maryland. These all against us, and the job on our hands is too large for us. We would as well consent to separation at once, including the surrender of this capitol.

Lincoln thus revoked the confiscation and emancipation provisions of Frémont's decree. He also ordered the general to execute no guerrillas without specific presidential approval. Lincoln feared that such a policy would only provoke reprisals whereby guerrillas would shoot captured Union soldiers "man for man, indefinitely." His apprehensions were well founded. One guerrilla leader in southeast Missouri had already issued a counterproclamation declaring that for every man executed under Frémont's order, he would "HANG, DRAW, and QUARTER a minion of said Abraham Lincoln."

Lincoln probably had the Missouri situation in mind when he told Congress in his annual message of December 1861 that "in considering the policy to be adopted for suppressing the insurrection, I have been anxious and careful that the inevitable conflict for this purpose shall not degenerate into a violent and remorseless revolutionary struggle." But that was already happening. The momentum of a war that had already mobilized nearly a million men on both sides was becoming remorseless even as Lincoln spoke, and it would soon become revolutionary.

Nowhere was this more true than in Missouri. There occurred the tragedy of a civil war within the Civil War, of neighbor against neighbor and sometimes literally brother against brother, of an armed conflict along the Kansas border that went back to 1854 and had never really stopped, of ugly, vicious, no-holds-barred bushwhacking that constituted pretty much a total war in fact as well as in theory. Bands of Confederate guerrillas led by the notorious William Clarke Quantrill, Bloody Bill Anderson, and other pathological killers, and containing such famous desperadoes as the James and Younger brothers, ambushed, murdered, and burned out Missouri Unionists and tied down thousands of Union troops by hit-and-run raids. Union militia and Kansas Jayhawkers retaliated in kind. In contrapuntal disharmony guerrillas and Jayhawkers plundered and pillaged their way across the state, taking no prisoners, killing in cold blood, terrorizing the civilian population, leaving large parts of Missouri a scorched earth.

In 1863 Quantrill's band rode into Kansas to the hated Yankee settlement of Lawrence and murdered almost every adult male they found there, more than 150 in all. A year later Bloody Bill Anderson's gang took twenty-four unarmed Union soldiers from a train, shot them in the head, then turned on a posse of pursuing militia and slaughtered 127 of them including the wounded and captured. In April 1864 the Missourian John S. Marmaduke, a Confederate general (and later governor of Missouri), led an attack on Union supply wagons at Poison Springs, Arkansas, killing in cold blood almost as many black soldiers as Nathan Bedford Forrest's troops did at almost the same time in the more famous Fort Pillow massacre in Tennessee.

Confederate guerrillas had no monopoly on atrocities and scorched-earth practices in Missouri. The Seventh Kansas Cavalry—"Jennison's Jayhawkers"—containing many abolitionists including a son of John Brown, seemed determined to exterminate rebellion and slaveholders in the most literal manner. The Union commander in western Missouri where guerrilla activity was most rife, Thomas Ewing, issued his notorious Order No. 11 after Quantrill's raid to Lawrence. Order No. 11 forcibly removed thousands of families from four Missouri counties along the Kansas border and burned their farms to deny the guerrillas the sanctuary they had enjoyed in this region. Interestingly, Ewing was William T. Sherman's brother-in-law. In fact, most of the Union commanders who subsequently became famous as practitioners of total war spent part of their early Civil War careers in Missouri—including Grant, Sherman, and Sheridan. This was more than coincidence. What they saw and experienced in that state helped to predispose them toward a conviction that, in Sherman's words, "we are not only fighting hostile armies, but a hostile people" and must make them "feel the hard hand of war."

That conviction took root and began to grow among the Northern people and their leaders in the summer of 1862. Before then, for several months in the winter and spring, Union forces had seemed on the verge of winning the war without resorting to such measures. The capture of Forts Henry and Donelson, the victories at Mill Springs in Kentucky, Pea Ridge in Arkansas, Shiloh in Tennessee, Roanoke Island and New Bern in North Carolina, the capture of Nashville, New Orleans, and Memphis, the expulsion of organized Confederate armies from Missouri, Kentucky, and West Virginia, the Union occupation of much of the lower Mississippi Valley and a large part of the state of Tennessee, and the advance of the splendidly equipped Army of the Potomac to within five miles of Richmond in May 1862 seemed to herald the Confederacy's doom. But then came counteroffensives by Stonewall Jackson and Robert E. Lee in Virginia and by Braxton Bragg and Kirby Smith in Tennessee, which took Confederate armies almost to the Ohio River and across the Potomac River by September 1862.

Those deceptively easy Union advances and victories in early 1862 had apparently confirmed the validity of a limited-war strategy. Grant's capture of Forts Henry and Donelson, for example, had convinced him that the Confederacy was a hollow shell about to collapse. But when the rebels regrouped and counterpunched so hard at Shiloh that they nearly whipped him, Grant changed his mind. He now "gave up all idea," he later wrote, "of saving the Union except by complete conquest." Complete conquest meant not merely the occupation of territory, but also the crippling or destruction of Confederate armies. For if these armies remained intact they could reconquer territory, as they did in the summer of 1862. Grant's new conception of the war also included the seizure or destruction of any property or other resources used to sustain the Confederate war effort. Before those Southern counteroffensives, Grant said that he had been careful "to protect the property of the citizens whose territory was invaded"; afterwards his policy became to "consume everything that could be used to support or supply armies."

"Everything" included slaves, whose labor was one of the principal resources used to support and supply Confederate armies. If the Confederacy "cannot be whipped in any other way than through a war against slavery," wrote Grant, "let it come to that." Union armies in the field as well as Republican leaders in Congress had been edging toward an emancipation policy ever since May 1861 when General Benjamin Butler had admitted three escaped slaves to his lines at Fort Monroe, labeled them contraband of war, and put them to work for wages to help support and supply *Union* forces. By the summer of 1862, tens of thousands of these contrabands had come within Union lines. Congress had forbidden army officers to return them. Legislation passed in July 1862 declared free all of those belonging to masters who supported the Confederacy. Frémont in Missouri turned out to have been not wrong, but a year ahead of his time.

By the summer of 1862 Lincoln too had come to the position enunciated a year earlier by Frederick Douglass: "To fight against slaveholders, without fighting against slavery, is but a half-hearted business." Acting in his capacity as commander in chief with power to seize property used to wage war against the United States, Lincoln decided to issue a proclamation freeing all slaves in those states engaged in rebellion. Emancipation, he told his cabinet in July 1862, had become "a military necessity, absolutely essential to the preservation of the Union. . . . We must free the slaves or be ourselves subdued. The slaves [are] undeniably an element of strength to those who [have] their service, and we must decide whether that element should be with us or against us. . . . Decisive and extensive measures must be adopted. . . . We [want] the army to strike more vigorous blows. The Administration must set an example, and strike at the heart of the rebellion." After a wait of two months for a victory to give the proclamation credibility, Lincoln announced it on September 22, 1862, to go into effect on January 1, 1863.

With this action Lincoln embraced the idea of the Civil War as a revolutionary conflict. Things had changed a great deal since he had promised to avoid "any devastation, or destruction of, or interference with, property." The Emancipation Proclamation was just what the *Springfield Republican* pronounced it: "the greatest social and political revolution of the age." No less an authority on revolutions than Karl Marx exulted: *"Never* has such a gigantic transformation taken place so rapidly." General Henry W. Halleck, who had been called from his headquarters in St. Louis (where he was commander of the Western Department) to Washington to become general in chief, made clear the practical import of the Emancipation Proclamation in a dispatch to Grant at Memphis in January 1863. "The character of the war has very much changed within the last year," he wrote. "There is now no possible hope of reconciliation with the rebels. . . . We must conquer the rebels or be conquered by them. . . . Every slave withdrawn from the enemy is the equivalent of a white man put *hors de combat*." One of Grant's field commanders explained that the new "policy is to be terrible on the enemy. I am using negroes all the time for my work as teamsters, and have 1,000 employed."

The program of "being terrible on the enemy" soon went beyond emancipating slaves and using them as teamsters. In early 1863 the Lincoln administration committed itself to a policy that had first emerged, like other total-war practices, in the trans-Mississippi theater. The First Kansas Colored Volunteers, composed mostly of contrabands from Missouri, were the earliest black soldiers to see combat, in 1862, and along with the Louisiana Native Guards the first to take shape as organized units. Arms in the hands of slaves constituted the South's ultimate revolutionary nightmare. After initial hesitation, Lincoln embraced this revolution as well. In March 1863 he wrote to Andrew Johnson, military governor of occupied Tennessee: "The bare sight of fifty thousand armed, and drilled black soldiers on the banks of the Mississippi, would end the rebellion at once. And who doubts that we can present that sight, if we but take hold in earnest?" By August 1863 Lincoln could declare in a public letter that "the emancipation policy, and the use of colored troops, constitute the heaviest blow yet dealt to the rebellion."

Well before then the conflict had become remorseless as well as revolutionary, with Lincoln's approval. Two of the generals he brought to Washington from the West in the summer of 1862, John Pope and Henry W. Halleck, helped to define and enunciate the remorselessness. Both had spent the previous winter and spring in Missouri, where experience with guerrillas had shaped their hard-war approach. One of Pope's first actions upon becoming commander of the Army of Virginia was a series of orders authorizing his officers to seize Confederate property without compensation, to execute captured guerrillas who had fired on Union troops, and to expel from occupied territory any civilians who sheltered guerrillas or who refused to take an oath of allegiance to the United States. From Halleck's office as general in chief in August 1862 went orders to Grant, now commander of Union forces in western Tennessee and Mississippi. "Take up all active [rebel] sympathizers," wrote Halleck, "and either hold them as prisoners or put them beyond our lines. Handle that class without gloves, and take their property for public use. . . . It is time that they should begin to feel the presence of the war."

With or without such orders, Union soldiers in the South were erasing the distinction between military and civilian property belonging to the enemy. A soldier from St. Louis with his regiment in west Tennessee wrote home that "this thing of guarding rebels' property has about 'played out.'" "The iron gauntlet," wrote another officer in the Mississippi Valley, "must be used more than the silken glove to crush this serpent."

Inevitably, bitter protests against this harshness reached Lincoln from purported Southern Unionists. A few months earlier the president would have rebuked the harshness, as he had rebuked Frémont, for alienating potential Unionist friends in the South. But in July 1862 Lincoln rebuked the protesters instead. He asked one of them sarcastically if they expected him to fight the war "with elder-stalk squirts, charged with rose water?" Did they think he would "surrender the government to save them from losing all"? Lincoln had lost faith in those professed Unionists:

> The paralysis—the dead palsy—of the government in this whole struggle is, that this class of men will do nothing for the government . . . except [demand] that the government shall not strike its open enemies, lest they be struck by accident! . . . This government cannot much longer play a game in which it stakes all, and its enemies stake nothing. Those enemies must understand that they cannot experiment for ten years trying to destroy the government, and if they fail still come back into the Union unhurt.

Using one of his favorite metaphors, Lincoln warned Southern whites that "broken eggs cannot be mended." The rebels had already cracked the egg of slavery by their own rash behavior; the sooner they gave up and ceased the insurrection, "the smaller will be the amount of [eggs] which will be past mending."

William Tecumseh Sherman eventually became the foremost military spokesman for remorseless war and the most effective general in carrying it out. Sherman too had spent part of the winter of 1861–1862 in Missouri where he stored up impressions of guerrilla ferocity. Nonetheless, even as late as July 1862, as commander of Union occupation forces around Memphis, he complained of some Northern troops who took several mules and horses from farmers. Such "petty thieving and pillaging," he wrote, "does us infinite harm." This scarcely sounds like the Sherman that Southerners love to hate. But his command problems in western Tennessee soon taught him what his brother-in-law Thomas Ewing was also learning about guerrillas and the civilian population that sheltered them across the river in Arkansas and Missouri. Nearly every white man, woman, and child in Sherman's district seemed to hate the Yankees and to abet the bushwhackers who fired into Union supply boats on the river, burned railroad bridges and ripped up the tracks, attacked Union picket outposts, ambushed Northern soldiers unless they moved in large groups, and generally raised hell behind Union lines. Some of the cavalry troopers who rode with Nathan Bedford Forrest and John Hunt Morgan on devastating raids behind Union lines also functioned in the manner of guerrillas, fading away to their homes and melting into the civilian population after a raid.

These operations convinced Sherman to take off the gloves. The distinction between enemy civilians and soldiers grew blurred. After fair warning, Sherman burned houses and sometimes whole villages in western Tennessee that he suspected of harboring snipers and guerrillas. The Union army, he now said, must act "on the proper rule that all in the South *are* enemies of all in the North. . . . The whole country is full of guerrilla bands. . . . The entire South, man, woman, and child, is against us, armed and determined." This conviction governed Sherman's subsequent operations which left smoldering ruins in his track from Vicksburg to Meridian, from Atlanta to the sea, and from the sea to Goldsboro, North Carolina.

When Mississippians protested, Sherman told them that they were lucky to get off so lightly: A commander

> may take your house, your fields, your everything, and turn you all out, helpless, to starve. It may be wrong, but that don't alter the case. In war you can't help yourselves, and the only possible remedy is to stop the war. . . . Our duty is not to build up; it is rather to destroy both the rebel army and whatever of wealth or property it has founded its boasted strength upon.

When Confederate General John Bell Hood charged him with barbarism for expelling the civilian population from Atlanta, Sherman gave Hood a tongue-lashing. Accusations of barbarity, he said, came with a fine irony from "you who, in the midst of peace and prosperity, have plunged a nation into war . . . who dared and badgered us to battle, insulted our flag . . . turned loose your privateers to plunder unarmed ships, expelled Union families by the thousands [and] burned their houses. . . . Talk thus to the marines, but not to me, who have seen these things." Sherman vowed to "make Georgia howl" in his march from Atlanta to Savannah, and afterwards expressed satisfaction with having done so. He estimated the damage to Confederate resources "at $100,000,000; at least $20,000,000 of which has inured to our advantage, and the remainder is simple waste and destruction." And this turned out to be mere child's play compared with what awaited South Carolina.

Sherman was convinced that not only the economic resources but also the will of Southern civilians sustained the Confederate war effort. His campaigns of devastation were intended to break that will as much as to destroy the resources. This is certainly a feature of modern total war; Sherman was a pioneer in the concept of psychological warfare as part of a total war against the whole enemy population. Sherman was well aware of the fear that his soldiers inspired among Southern whites. This terror "was a power," he wrote, "and I intended to utilize it . . . to humble their pride, to follow them to their inmost recesses, and to make them fear and dread us. . . . We cannot change the hearts and minds of those people of the South, but we can make war so terrible . . . [and] make them so sick of war that generations would pass away before they would again appeal to it."

This strategy seemed to work; Sherman's destruction not only deprived Confederate armies of desperately needed supplies; it also crippled morale both on the home front and in the army. Numerous soldiers deserted from Confederate armies in response to letters of despair from home in the wake of Sherman's juggernaut. One Southern soldier wrote after the march through Georgia: "I hev concludud that the dam fulishness uv tryin to lick shurmin Had better be stoped, we have gettin nuthin but hell & lots uv it ever since we saw the dam yankys & I am tirde uv it . . . thair thicker than lise on a hen and a dam site ornraier." After the march through South Carolina, a civilian in that state wrote: "All is gloom, despondency, and inactivity. Our army is demoralized and the people panic stricken. To fight longer seems to be madness."

Philip Sheridan carried out a similar policy of scorched earth in the Shenandoah Valley. Interestingly, Sheridan too had spent most of the war's first year in Missouri. There as well as subsequently in Tennessee and Virginia he saw the ravages of Confederate guerrillas, and responded as Sherman did. If guerrilla operations and Union counterinsurgency activities in Virginia during 1864 were slightly less vicious than in Missouri, it was perhaps only because the proximity of Washington and Richmond and of large field armies imposed some restraint. Nevertheless, plenty of atrocities piled up in John Singleton Mosby's Confederacy just east of the Blue Ridge and in the Shenandoah Valley to the west. In retaliation, and with a purpose similar to Sherman's to destroy the Valley's resources which helped supply Lee's army, Sheridan carried out a campaign of devastation that left nothing to sustain Confederate armies or even to enable the Valley's inhabitants to get through the winter. In little more than a week, wrote Sheridan in one of his reports, his army had "destroyed over 2,000 barns filled with wheat, hay, and farming implements; over seventy mills filled with flour and wheat; have driven in front of the army over 4,000 head of stock, and have killed and issued to the troops not less than 3,000 sheep." That was just the beginning, Sheridan promised. By the time he was through, "the Valley, from Winchester up to Staunton, ninety-two miles, will have little in it for man or beast."

Several years later, while serving as an American observer at German headquarters during the Franco-Prussian War, Sheridan lectured his hosts on the correct way to wage war. The "proper strategy," said Sheridan, consisted first of "inflicting as telling blows as possible on the enemy's army, and then in causing the inhabitants so much suffering that they must long for peace, and force the government to demand it. The people must be left nothing but their eyes to weep with over the war."

Abraham Lincoln is famed for his compassion; he issued many pardons and commuted many sentences of execution; the concluding passage of his second inaugural address, beginning "With malice toward none; with charity for all," is one of his most familiar utterances. Lincoln regretted the devastation and suffering caused by the army's scorched-earth policy in the South. Yet he had warned Southerners in 1862 that the longer they fought, the more eggs would be broken. He would have agreed with Sherman's words to a Southerner: "You brought all this on yourselves." In 1864, after the march to the sea, Lincoln officially conveyed to Sherman's army the "grateful acknowledgments" of the nation; to Sheridan he offered the "thanks of the nation, and my own personal admiration, for [your] operations in the Shenandoah Valley." And while the words in the second inaugural about malice toward none and charity for all promised a generous peace, the victory that must precede that peace could be achieved only by hard war—indeed, by total war. Consider *these* words from the second inaugural:

> Fondly do we hope—fervently do we pray—that this mighty scourge of war may speedily pass away. Yet if God wills that it continue, until all the wealth piled by the bond-man's two hundred and fifty years of unrequited toil shall be sunk, and until every drop of blood drawn with the lash, shall be paid by another drawn with the sword, as was said three thousand years ago, so still it must be said "the judgments of the Lord, are true and righteous altogether."

The kind of conflict the Civil War had become merits the label of total war. To be sure, Union soldiers did not set out to kill Southern civilians. Sherman's bummers destroyed property; Allied bombers in World War II destroyed hundreds of thousands of lives as well. But the strategic purpose of both was the same: to eliminate the resources and break the will of the people to sustain war. White people in large parts of the Confederacy were indeed left with "nothing but their eyes to weep with." This was not pretty; it was not glorious; it did not conform to the image of war held by most Americans in 1861 of flags waving, bands playing, and people cheering on a spring afternoon. But as Sherman himself put it, in a speech to young men of a new generation fifteen years after the Civil War, the notion that war is glorious was nothing but moonshine. "When . . . you come down to the practical realities, boys," said Sherman, "war is all hell."

JAMES M. MCPHERSON is the George Henry Davis '86 Professor Emeritus of United States History at Princeton University. The author of 17 books, his major works include *The Struggle for Equality: Abolitionists and the Negro in the Civil War and Reconstruction* (Princeton University Press, 1964); *The Negro's Civil War: How American Negroes Felt and Acted During the War for the Union* (Pantheon Books, 1965); *Ordeal by Fire: The Civil War and Reconstruction* (3rd ed., McGraw-Hill, 2001); and *Battle Cry for Freedom: The Civil War Era* (Oxford University Press, 1988), for which he won the Pulitzer Prize.

EXPLORING THE ISSUE

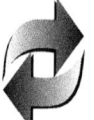

Are Historians Wrong to Consider the War Between the States a "Total War"?

Critical Thinking and Reflection

1. (a) Define total war.
   (b) Given your definition, compare the arguments of Professors Neely and McPherson for their respective positions.
   (c) For example, do you agree with McPherson that the distinction between combatants and noncombatants refers to the twentieth-century world wars and that it is possible to have a total war without such a distinction? Critically evaluate the arguments of both authors.
2. Critically evaluate the different arguments of Neely and McPherson about the rhetoric and actions of General William T. Sherman. Did Sherman wage a total war? How similar and how different were Sherman's actions compared to those of the Allied Commanders in World War II?
3. Professor Neely argues that neither Lincoln, Grant, nor Sherman had a total war philosophy. Critically analyze what he means by this. How does Professor McPherson counter this argument?
4. Professor Neely argues elsewhere that President Lincoln's surrender terms—end hostilities, abolish the Confederacy, and emancipate the slaves—were lenient surrender terms. McPherson disagrees. Critically discuss.
5. Was it politically possible for Lincoln to have been tougher when Lee surrendered and have demanded the following?
   - Exclude all Confederate political leaders from public office.
   - Disenfranchise all Confederate soldiers.
   - Give free blacks the right to vote.
   - Give legal protection to the Republic party in former Confederate states.
   - Recognize the statehood of West Virginia.
   - Partition the Southern states.
   - Protect the ex-slaves who fought in the Union from reprisals.
   Critically discuss.

Is There Common Ground?

The "total war" issue raises a side question. Was the North's victory inevitable because of its superior leadership, nationalist ideology, and its overwhelming numbers in terms of population and natural resources? Most historians argue yes, but Professor James M. McPherson disagrees with the conventional wisdom. In a Gettysburg symposium, edited by Gabor S. Boritt, on *Why the Confederacy Lost* (Oxford University Press, 1992), McPherson dismisses all the external and internal explanations for the South's defeat listed above. In his critique, McPherson applies the theory of *reversibility*. Briefly stated, the hindsight provided by knowing the outcome of the war allows the writer to attribute causes that explain the northern victory. But what if the South had won the Civil War? Could the same external explanations that are attributed to the Union victory also be used to explain a Confederate win? Would Jefferson Davis's leadership emerge as superior to Abraham Lincoln's? Would the great military leaders be Robert E. Lee, Thomas "Stonewall" Jackson, and Braxton Bragg instead of Grant, Sherman, and Sheridan? Would one Confederate soldier be considered equal to four Union soldiers? Would a triumvirate of yeoman farmers, slaveholding planters, and small industrialists have proven the superiority of agrarian values over industrial ones?

In addition to the theory of reversibility, McPherson advances the theory of *contingency* as an explanation for the Union victory. During the war, four turning points that altered the course of the war could have gone either way. First, during the summer of 1862 the southern victories prolonged the war. Second, at the Battle of Antietam in the fall of 1862, the southern advance into the North stalled. Third, the battle of Gettysburg in July 1863 turned the tide of war in favor of the Union. Fourth, the Atlanta and western campaigns in the fall of 1864 enabled Lincoln to win the presidential election and eventually led the northern forces to defeat the Confederacy and abolish slavery. These arguments merit serious consideration by students and scholars seeking to characterize the nature of the American Civil War.

Additional Resources

Edward Ayers, *Valley of the Shadow: Two Communities in the American Civil War* (W. W. Norton, 2000)

Stig Forster and Jorg Nagler, eds., *On the Road to Total War: The American Civil War and the German Wars of Unification, 1861–1871* (Cambridge University Press, 1997)

James M. McPherson, *Battle Cry of Freedom: The Civil War Era* (Oxford University Press, 1998)

James M. McPherson and William J. Cooper, Jr., eds., *Writing the Civil War: The Quest to Understand* (University of South Carolina Press, 1998)

Robert Toplin, ed., *Ken Burns' The Civil War: The Historians Respond* (Oxford University Press, 1996)

Internet References . . .

AmericanCivilWar.com

http://americancivilwar.com/index.html

Images of Battle—The American Civil War

www.lib.unc.edu/mss/exhibits/civilwar/index.html

The Valley of the Shadow Project

http://valley.vcdh.virginia.edu/

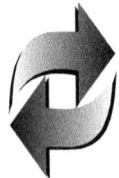

ISSUE

Selected, Edited, and with Issue Framing Material by:
Kevin R. Magill and Tony L. Talbert, *Baylor University*

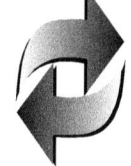

Did African American Slaves Exercise Religious Autonomy?

YES: Albert J. Raboteau, from "Slave Autonomy and Religion," *Journal of Religious Thought* (1982)

NO: John B. Boles, from "Masters & Slaves in the House of the Lord: Race and Religion in the American South, 1740–1870," University Press of Kentucky (1988)

Learning Outcomes

After reading this issue, you will be able to:

- Explain how slave owners could employ religion to control their slaves.
- Understand ways in which slaves used religious activities to gain personal autonomy.
- Discuss the importance of African American preachers in the antebellum period.
- Evaluate the biracial religious culture of the antebellum South.
- Assess the extent to which Christianity pacified slaves or caused them to resist their enslavement.

ISSUE SUMMARY

YES: Albert J. Raboteau asserts that the exercise of religion among African American slaves in the 19th century United States allowed for the development of a cohesive organization founded within a common lived experience. Through the development of an autonomous religious culture African American slaves formed a philosophical and pragmatic bond of interests that resulted in the pursuit of freedom from oppression.

NO: John B. Boles counters the notion of the segregated congregational religious experience among Anglos and African American slaves in the southern region of the United States during the 19th century. While Boles acknowledges the importance of religious customs and organizational structures within the enslaved African American population he asserts that Anglos and African Americans shared a common religious experience both in philosophy (interpretation of Christian text) and practice (attendance in worship services).

Since the mid-1950s, few issues in American history have generated more interest among scholars than the institution of slavery. Books and articles analyzing the treatment of slaves, comparative slave systems, the profitability of slavery, slave rebelliousness (or lack thereof), urban slavery, the slave family, and slave religion have abounded. This proliferation of scholarship, stimulated in part by the civil rights movement, contrasts sharply with slavery historiography between the two world wars, which was monopolized by a single book—Ulrich B. Phillips's apologetic and blatantly racist *American Negro Slavery* (D. Appleton, 1918). Phillips, a native Georgian who taught for most of his career at Yale, based his sweeping view of the southern slave system upon plantation records left by some of the wealthiest slave owners. He concluded that American slavery was a benign institution controlled by paternalistic masters. These owners, Phillips insisted, rarely treated their bondservants cruelly but, instead, paternalistically provided food, clothing, housing, and other necessities of life to their slaves, who he characterized as childlike, acquiescent human property.

Although African American historians such as George Washington Williams, W. E. B. Du Bois, Carter G. Woodson, and John Hope Franklin produced scholarly works emphasizing the brutal impact of slavery, their views received almost no consideration from the wider academic community. Consequently, recognition of a "revisionist" interpretation of slavery was delayed until the post–World War II era when, in the wake of the *Brown* desegregation case, Kenneth Stampp, a white northern historian, published *The Peculiar Institution: Slavery in the Ante-Bellum South* (Alfred A. Knopf, 1956). Stampp also focused primarily upon antebellum plantation records, but his conclusions were literally a point-by-point rebuttal of the Phillips thesis. The institution of slavery, he said, was a harsh, oppressive system in which slave owners controlled their servants through fear of the lash. Further, in contrast to the image of the passive, happy-go-lucky "Sambo" described by Phillips, Stampp argued that slaves were "a troublesome property" who resisted their enslavement in subtle as well as overt ways.

Three years later, Stanley Elkins synthesized these seemingly contradictory interpretations in his controversial study *Slavery: A Problem in American Institutional and Intellectual Life* (University of Chicago Press, 1959). Elkins clearly accepted Stampp's emphasis on the harshness of the slave system by hypothesizing that slavery was a "closed" system in which masters dominated their slaves in the same way that Nazi concentration camp guards in World War II had controlled the lives of their prisoners. Such an environment, he insisted, generated severe psychological dysfunctions which produced the personality traits of Phillips's "Sambo" character type.

As the debate over the nature of slavery moved into the 1960s and 1970s, several scholars, seeking to provide a history of the institution "from the bottom up," began to focus upon the slaves themselves as a contributing force in the slave system. Interviews with ex-slaves had been conducted in the 1920s and 1930s under the auspices of Southern University in Louisiana, Fisk University in Tennessee, and the Federal Writers Project of the Works Progress Administration. Drawing upon these interviews and previously ignored slave autobiographies, sociologist George Rawick's *From Sundown to Sunup: The Making of the Black Community* (Greenwood, 1972) and historians John Blassingame's *The Slave Community: Plantation Life in the Antebellum South* (Oxford University Press 1972) and Eugene D. Genovese's *Roll, Jordan, Roll: The World the Slaves Made* (Pantheon, 1974), among others, portrayed a multifaceted community life over which slaves held a significant degree of influence. This community, operating beyond the view of the "Big House," was, in Genovese's phrase, "the world the slaves made."

Religion was an integral part of that community life among slaves by the antebellum period and has received attention in virtually every scholarly treatment of the institution of slavery. In the colonial period, however, whites made little more than sporadic attempts to proselytize among newly arrived Africans who brought with them their traditional religious belief systems. More attention began to be directed toward the religious lives of enslaved peoples during the evangelical Protestant revivals from the mid-eighteenth century to the early decades of the 1800s, as masters offered religious instruction to their chattel property, various Christian denominations directed missionary activities toward slaves, and as African American bondservants began to adapt the white man's religion to their own spiritual needs. Genovese's *Roll, Jordan, Roll* (cited above) places religious practice at the heart of the slave community. Slaves, says Genovese, were able to create a syncretized African-Christianity that served them in multiple ways: as an instrument of accommodation or resistance, emotional fervor, and spiritual comfort and relief from their daily labors and troubles. They took from their master's religion what was useful to them, particularly the themes of faith, love, and deliverance, and gave less thought to doctrine or denominational structure. Lawrence W. Levine, in *Black Culture and Black Consciousness: Afro-American Folk Thought from Slavery to Freedom* (Oxford University Press, 1977), studies slave songs, spirituals, and folk tales to conclude that slaves practiced their religion in a world that they shared with one another apart from their masters. Albert Raboteau's *Slave Religion: The "Invisible Institution" in the Antebellum South* (Oxford University Press, 1978) insists that this separate religious life enabled slaves to develop a strong sense of community and to develop leaders within that community. Sterling Stuckey offers a slightly different conclusion in *Slave Culture: Nationalist Theory and the Foundations of Black America* (Oxford University Press, 1987) by pointing out that many slaves lacked access to regular religious services or embraced Sunday as a day off and, hence, were scarcely touched by Christianity. In contrast to the interpretations presented in the preceding works, Orville Burton's *In My Father's House Are Many Mansions: Family and Community in Edgefield, South Carolina* (University of North Carolina Press, 1985) suggests that Christianity functioned as a means of social control over slaves to maintain docility and obedience.

Some of these contrasting interpretive currents are reflected in the following essays on the nature of slave religion. In the first selection, Albert Raboteau describes the ways in which the acceptance of Christianity produced numerous opportunities for slaves to assume control over their own religious activities. Slave preachers assumed positions of leadership in the black community that could not be limited by whites, and slaves realized greater autonomy in black-controlled churches or in secret religious gatherings. This religious autonomy, according to Raboteau, permitted slaves to resist some of the dehumanizing elements of the slave system.

John Boles admits that slaves in the antebellum South worshiped in a variety of ways (in independent black churches, plantation chapels, or informal, secret gatherings), but he concludes that the typical site for slave religious activities was the church of their masters. Although potentially restrictive, such a setting vitalized the slave community by offering bondservants from different plantations an opportunity to mingle freely with one another. Moreover, says Boles, nowhere else in southern society were blacks treated so nearly as equals to whites than in these biracial churches, where they were admitted to membership, addressed by whites as "brother" or "sister" (the same terms used for fellow white members), and allowed to participate with limited equality in church discipline.

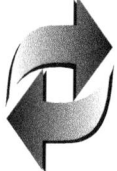

YES ← Albert J. Raboteau

Slave Autonomy and Religion

One of the perennial questions in the historical study of American slavery is the question of the relationship between Christianity and the response of slaves to enslavement. Did the Christian religion serve as a tool in the hands of slaveholders to make slaves docile or did it serve in the hands of slaves as a weapon of resistance and even outright rebellion against the system of slavery? Let us acknowledge from the outset that the role of religion in human motivation and action is very complex; let us recognize also that Christianity played an ambiguous role in the stances which slaves took toward slavery, sometimes supporting resistance, sometimes accommodation. That much admitted, much more remains to be said. Specifically, we need to trace the convoluted ways in which the egalitarian impulse within Christianity overflowed the boundaries of the master-slave hierarchy, creating unexpected channels of slave autonomy on institutional as well as personal levels. To briefly sketch out some of the directions which religious autonomy took among slaves in the antebellum South is the purpose of this essay.

Institutional Autonomy

From the beginning of the Atlantic slave trade in the fifteenth century. European Christians claimed that the conversion of slaves to Christianity justified the enslavement of Africans. For more than four centuries Christian apologists for slavery would repeat this religious rationalization for one of history's greatest atrocities. Despite the justification of slavery as a method of spreading the gospel, the conversion of slaves was not a top priority for colonial planters. One of the principal reasons for the refusal of British colonists to allow their slaves religious instruction was the fear that baptism would require the manumission of their slaves, since it was illegal to hold a fellow Christian in bondage. This dilemma was solved quickly by colonial legislation stating that baptism did not alter slave status. However, the most serious obstacle to religious instruction of the slaves could not be legislated away. It was the slaveholder's deep-seated uneasiness at the prospect of a slave laying claim to Christian fellowship with his master. The concept of equality, though only spiritual, between master and slave threatened the stability of the system of slave control. Christianity, complained the masters, would ruin slaves by allowing them to think themselves equal to white Christians. Far worse was the fear, supported by the behavior of some Christian slaves, that religion would make them rebellious. In order to allay this fear, would-be missionaries to the slaves had to prove that Christianity would make better slaves. By arguing that Christian slaves would become obedient to their masters out of duty to God and by stressing the distinction between spiritual equality and worldly equality, the proponents of slave conversion in effect built a religious foundation to support slavery. Wary slaveholders were assured by missionaries that "scripture, far from making an Alteration in civil Rights, expressly directs, *that every Man abide in the Condition wherein he is called, with great indifference of Mind* concerning outward circumstances."

In spite of missionary efforts to convince them that Christianity was no threat to the slave system, slaveowners from the colonial period on down to the Civil War remained suspicious of slave religion as a two-edged sword. Clerical assurances aside, the masters' concern was valid. Religious Instruction for slaves had more than spiritual implications. No event would reveal these implications as clearly as the series of religious revivals called the Great Awakenings which preceded and followed the Revolution. The impact of revival fervor would demonstrate how difficult it was to control the egalitarian impulse of Christianity within safe channels.

The first Great Awakening of the 1740s swept the colonies with the tumultuous preaching and emotional conversions of revivalistic, evangelical Protestantism. Accounts by Whitefield, Tennent, Edwards, and other revivalists made special mention of the fact that blacks were flocking to hear the message of salvation in hitherto unseen numbers. Not only were free blacks and slaves attending revivals in significant numbers, they were

Raboteau, Albert J. "Slave Autonomy and Religion," Journal of Religious Thought, 1982. Copyright ©1982 by Howard University. Used with permission.

taking active part in the services as exhorters and preachers. The same pattern of black activism was repeated in the rural camp meetings of the second Great Awakening of the early nineteenth century.

The increase in slave conversions which accompanied the awakenings was due to several factors. The evangelical religion spread by the revivalists initiated a religious renaissance in the South where the majority of slaves lived. The revival became a means of church extension, especially for Methodists and Baptists. The mobility of the Methodist circuit rider and the local independence of the Baptist preacher were suited to the needs of the rural South. Among the Southerners swelling the ranks of these denominations, were black as well as white converts.

Moreover, the ethos of the revival meeting, with its strong emphasis upon emotional preaching and congregational response, not only permitted ecstatic religious behavior but encouraged it. Religious exercises, as they were termed, including fainting, jerking, barking, and laughing a "holy laugh," were a common, if spectacular, feature of revivals. In this heated atmosphere slaves found sanction for an outward expression of religious emotion consonant with their tradition of danced religion from Africa. While converting to belief in a "new" God, slaves were able to worship in ways hauntingly similar to those of old.

Extremely important for the development of black participation in revival religion was the intense concentration upon individual inward conversion which fostered an inclusiveness that could become egalitarianism. Evangelicals did not hesitate to preach to racially mixed congregations and had no doubt about the capacity of slaves to share the experience of conversion to Christ. Stressing plain doctrine and emotional preaching, emphasizing the conversion experience instead of religious instruction, made Christianity accessible to illiterate slave and slaveholder alike. The criterion for preachers was not seminary training but evidence of a converted heart and gifted tongue. Therefore, when an awakened slave showed talent for preaching, he preached, and not only to black congregations. The tendency of evangelical Protestantism to level the souls of all men before God reached its logical conclusion when blacks preached to and converted whites.

By the last quarter of the eighteenth century a cadre of black preachers had begun to emerge. Some of these pioneer black ministers were licensed, some not; some were slaves, others free. During the 1780s a black man named Lewis preached to crowds as large as four hundred in Westmoreland County, Virginia. Harry Hosier traveled with Methodist leaders, Asbury, Coke, Garretson, and Whatcoat and was reportedly such an eloquent preacher that he served as a "drawing card" to attract larger crowds of potential converts, white and black. In 1792 the mixed congregation of the Portsmouth, Virginia Baptist Church selected a slave, Josiah Bishop, as pastor, after purchasing his freedom and also his family's. Another black preacher, William Lemon, pastored a white Baptist church in Gloucester County, Virginia, for a time at the turn of the century.

In 1798, Joseph Willis, a freeman, duly licensed as a Baptist preacher, began his ministry in southwest Mississippi and Louisiana. He formed Louisiana's first Baptist church at Bayou Chicot in 1812 and served as its pastor. After developing several other churches in the area, he became the first moderator of the Louisiana Baptist Association in 1818. Uncle Jack, an African-born slave, joined the Baptist church and in 1792 began to preach in Nottoway County, Virginia. White church members purchased his freedom and he continued to preach for over forty years. Henry Evans, a free black licensed as a local preacher by the Methodists, was the first to bring Methodist preaching to Fayetteville, North Carolina. Initially preaching to black people only, he attracted the attention of several prominent whites and eventually the white membership of his congregation increased until the blacks were crowded out of their seats. Evans was eventually replaced by a white minister, but continued to serve as an assistant in the church he had founded until his death.

That black preachers should exhort, convert, and even pastor white Christians in the slave South was certainly antithetical to the premise of slave control. Though such occasions were rare, they were the ineluctable result of the impulse unleashed by revivalistic religion. Of greater importance for the development of autonomy in the religious life of slave was the fact that black preachers, despite threats of punishment, continued to preach to slaves and in some few cases even founded churches. An early historian of the Baptists applauded the anonymous but effective ministry of these black preachers:

> Among the African Baptists in the Southern states there are a multitude of preachers and exhorters whose names do not appear on the minutes of the associations. They preach principally on the plantations to those of their own color, and their preaching though broken and Illiterate, is in many cases highly useful.

Several "African" Baptist churches sprang up before 1800. Some of these black congregations were independent to the extent that they called their own pastors and officers, joined local associations with white Baptist churches, and sent their own delegates to associational meetings. Though the separate black church was primarily an urban phenomenon, it drew upon surrounding rural areas for its membership, which consisted of both free blacks and slaves, Sometimes these black churches were founded amidst persecution. Such was the case with the African Baptist Church of Williamsburg, Virginia, whose history was chronicled in 1810:

> This church is composed almost, if not altogether of people of colour. Moses, a black man, first preached among them, and was often taken up and whipped, for holding meetings. Afterwards Gowan Pamphlet . . . became popular among the blacks, and began to baptize, as well as to preach. It seems, the association had advised that no person of colour should be allowed to preach, on the pain of excommunication; against this regulation, many of the blacks were rebellious, and continued still to hold meetings. Some were excluded and among this number was Gowan. . . . Continuing still to preach and many professing faith under his ministry, not being in connexion with any church himself, he formed a kind of church out of some who had been baptized, who, sitting with him, received such as offered themselves; Gowan baptized them, and was moreover appointed their pastor; some of them knowing how to write, a churchbook was kept; they increased to a large number; so that in the year 1791, the Dover association, stat[ed] their number to be about five hundred. The association received them, so far, as to appoint persons to visit them and set things in order. These making a favourable report, they were received, and have associated ever since.

Several features of this narrative deserve emphasis as significant examples of black religious autonomy. Ignoring the threat of excommunication, not to mention physical punishment, blacks rebelled against white religious control and insisted on holding their own meetings, led by their own ministers. They gathered their own church, apparently according to the norms of Baptist polity, accepted their own members, kept their own minutes, and finally succeeded in joining the local association, all the while growing to a membership of five hundred by 1791!

In Savannah, Georgia, a slave named Andrew Bryan established an African Baptist Church, against white objection and persecution. In 1790, Bryan's church included two hundred and twenty-five full communicants and approximately three hundred and fifty converts, many of whom did not have their masters' permission to be baptized. In 1803, a Second African Church of Savannah was organized from the first, and a few years later a third came into being. Both of the new churches were led by black pastors. After Bryan's death, his nephew, Andrew Marshall, became pastor of the First African Church and by 1830 his congregation had increased in size to two thousand, four hundred and seventeen members.

The labors of these early black preachers and their successors were crucial in the formation of slave religion. In order to adequately understand the development of Christianity among the slaves, we must realize that slaves learned Christianity not only from whites but from other slaves as well. Slave preachers, exhorters, and church-appointed watchmen instructed their fellow slaves, nurtured their religious development, and brought them to conversion in some cases without the active involvement of white missionaries or masters at all. The early independence of black preachers and churches was curtailed as the antebellum period wore on, particularly in periods of reaction to slave conspiracies, when all gatherings of blacks for whatever purpose were viewed with alarm. For slaves to participate in the organization, leadership, and governance of church structures was perceived as dangerous. Surely it was inconsistent, argued the guardians of the system, to allow blacks such authority. As the prominent South Carolinian planter, Charles Cotesworth Pinkney, declared before the Charleston Agricultural Society in 1829, the exercise of religious prerogatives left slaves too free from white control. "We look upon the habit of Negro preaching as a widespreading evil; not because a black man cannot be a good one, but . . . because they acquire an influence independent of the owner, and not subject to his control. . . . when they have possessed this power, they have been known to make an improper use of it." No doubt, Pinkney and his audience had in mind the African Methodist Church of Charleston which had served as a seedbed of rebellion for the Denmark Vesey conspiracy of 1822. (Following discovery of the plot, whites razed the church to the ground.)

Regardless of periodic harassment by civil and ecclesiastical authorities, black preachers continued to preach and separate black churches continued to be organized. Just as Pinkney and others warned, in preaching and in church life some blacks found channels for self-expression and self-governance. To be sure, the exercise of such autonomy was frequently modified by white supervision, but it was nonetheless real. In various sections of the antebellum South, black churches kept gathering members, over the years swelling in size to hundreds and in a few instances thousands of members. Certainly, the vast majority of slaves attended churches under white control. However, even in racially mixed churches some black Christians found opportunities to exercise their spiritual gifts and a measure of control over their religious life. This was so especially in Baptist churches because Baptist polity required that each congregation govern itself. In some churches committees of black members were constituted to oversee their own conduct. These committees listened to black applicants related their religious experience and heard the replies of members charged with moral laxity. Meeting once a month, committees of "brethren in black" conducted business, reported their recommendations to the general meeting and gave to black church members experience in church governance. This experience laid a foundation upon which freedmen would rapidly build their own independent churches after emancipation.

Hampered though it was, the exercise of religious autonomy among slaves was a fact of antebellum life. It was due to the nature of the revival fervor of the Great Awakenings of the eighteenth and early nineteenth centuries which first brought the slaves to conversion in large numbers and also created a situation in which it became possible for black freemen and slaves to preach and even pastor. (By way of contrast, these avenues to spiritual authority would not open for blacks in either the Church of England or the Roman Catholic Church for a long time to come.) To the extent possible, then, black Christians proved not at all reluctant about deciding their own religious affairs and managing their own religious institutions. For the vast majority of slaves, however, institutional religious autonomy was not possible. This did not stop them from seeking religious independence from whites in more secretive ways.

Personal Autonomy

Like their colonial predecessors, antebellum missionaries to the slaves had to face objections from whites that religion for slaves was dangerous. Beginning in the 1820s, a movement led by prominent clerics and laymen attempted to mold southern opinion in support of missions to the slaves. Plantation missionaries created an ideal image of the Christian plantation, built upon the mutual observance of duties by masters and by slaves. One leader of the plantation mission stated the movement's basic premise when he predicted that "religious instruction of the Negroes will *promote our own morality and religion*." For, when "one class rises, so will the other; the two are so associated they are apt to rise or fall together. Therefore, servants do well by your masters and masters do well by your servants." In this premise lay a serious fallacy: for while the interests of master and slave occasionally coincided, they could never cohere. No matter how devoted master was to the ideal of a Christian plantation, no matter how pious he might be, the slave knew that the master's religion did not countenance the slaves' freedom in this world.

Precisely because the interests of master and slave extended only so far and no further, there was a dimension of the slaves religious life that was secret. The disparity between the master's ideal of religion on the plantation and that of the slaves led the slaves to gather secretly in the quarters or in brush arbors (aptly named hush harbors) where they could pray, preach, and sing, free from white control. Risking severe punishment, slaves disobeyed their masters and stole off under cover of secrecy to worship as they saw fit. Here it was that Christianity was fitted to their own peculiar experience.

It was the slaveholding gospel preached to them by master's preacher which drove many slaves to seek true Christian preaching at their own meetings. "Church was what they called it," recalled former slave Charlie Van Dyke, "but all that preacher talked about was for us slaves to obey our masters and not to lie and steal." To attend secret meetings was in itself an act of resistance against the will of the master and was punished as such. In the face of the absolute authority of the Divine Master, the authority of the human master shrank. Slaves persisted in their hush harbor meetings because there they found consolation and communal support, tangible relief from the exhaustion and brutality of work stretching from "day clean" to after dark, day in and day out. "Us niggers," remarked Richard Carruthers, describing a scene still vivid in his memory many years later, "used to have a prayin' ground down in the hollow and sometimes we come out of the field . . . scorchin' and burnin' up with nothin' to eat, and we wants to ask the good Lawd to have mercy. . . . We takes a pine torch . . . and goes down in the hollow to pray. Some gits so joyous they starts to holler loud and we has to stop up they mouth. I see niggers git so full of the Lawd and so happy they draps unconscious."

In the hush harbor slaves sought not only substantive preaching and spiritual consolation they also talked about and prayed for an end to their physical bondage. "I've heard them pray for freedom," declared one former slave. "I thought it was foolishness then, but the old time folks always felt they was to be free. It must have been something 'vealed unto 'em." Though some might be skeptical, those slaves who were confident that freedom would come, since God had revealed it, were able to cast their lives in a different light. Hope for a brighter future irradiated the darkness of the present. Their desire for freedom in this world was reaffirmed in the songs, prayers, and sermons of the hush harbor. This was just what the master—those who didn't believe in prayer, as well as those who did—tried to prevent. The external hush harbor symbolized an internal resistance, a private place at the core of the slaves' religious life which they claimed as their own and which, in the midst of bondage, could not be controlled.

For evangelical Christians, black or white, full admission into membership in the church required that the candidate give credible testimony about the inner workings of the Spirit upon his or her heart. The conversion experience, as described by ex-slaves, was typically a visionary one, inaugurated by feelings of sadness and inner turmoil. Frequently the individual "convicted of sin" envisioned Hell and realized that he was destined for damnation. Suddenly, the sinner was rescued from this danger and led to a vision of Heaven by an emissary from God. Ushered into God's presence, the person learned that he was not damned but saved. Awakening, the convert realized that he was now one of the elect and overwhelmed with the joyful feeling of being "made new" shouted out his happiness. For years afterwards, this "peak" experience remained a fixed point of identity and value in the convert's life. He knew that he was saved, and be knew it not just theoretically but experientially. Confident of their election and their value in the eyes of God, slaves who underwent conversion, gained in this radical experience a deeply rooted identity which formed the basis for a sense of purpose and an affirmation of self-worth—valuable psychic barriers to the demeaning and dehumanizing attacks of slavery.

Conversion, as an experience common to white and black Christians, occasionally led to moments of genuine emotional contact, in which the etiquette of racial relationships was forgotten. A dramatic instance of one such occasion was recounted by a former slave named Morte:

> One day while in the field plowing I heard a voice . . . I looked but saw no one . . . Every thing got dark, and I was unable to stand any longer . . . With this I began to cry, Mercy! Mercy! Mercy! As I prayed an angel came and touched me, and I looked new . . . and there came a soft voice saying, "My little one, I have loved you with an everlasting love. You are this day made alive and freed from hell. You are a chosen vessel unto the Lord." . . . I must have been in this trance more than an hour. I went on to the barn and found my master waiting for me. . . . I began to tell him of my experiences . . . My master sat watching and listening to me, and then he began to cry. He turned from me and said in a broken voice, "Morte I believe you are a preacher. From now on you can preach to the people here on my place . . . But tomorrow morning. Sunday. I want you to preach to my family and my neighbors." . . . The next morning at the time appointed I stood up on two planks in front of the porch of the big house and, without a Bible or anything. I began to preach to my master and the people. My thoughts came so fast that I could hardly speak fast enough. My soul caught on fire, and soon I had them all in tears . . . I told them that they must be born again and that their souls must be freed from the shackles of hell.

The spectacle of a slave reducing his master to tears by preaching to him of his enslavement to sin certainly suggests that religion could bend human relationships into interesting shapes despite the iron rule of slavery. Morte's power over his master was spiritual and (as far as we know) it was temporary. It was also effective.

While commonality of religious belief might lead to moments of religious reciprocity between blacks and whites, by far the more common relationship, from the slaves' side, was one of alienation from the hypocrisy of slaveholding Christians. As Frederick Douglass put it, "Slaves knew enough of the orthodox theology of the time to consign all bad slaveholders to hell." On the same point, Charles Ball commented that in his experience slaves thought that heaven would not be heaven unless slaves could be avenged on their enemies. "A fortunate and kind master or mistress, may now and then be admitted into heaven, but this rather as a matter of favour, to the intercession of some slave, than as a matter of strict justice to the whites, who will, by no means, be of an equal rank with those who shall be raised from the depths of misery in this world." Ball concluded that "The idea of a revolution in the conditions of the whites and blacks, is the cornerstone of the religion of the latter. . . ."

Slaves had no difficulty distinguishing the gospel of Christianity from the religion of their masters. Ex-slave Douglas Dorsey reported that after the minister on his plantation admonished the slaves to honor their masters whom they could see as they would God whom they could not see, the driver's wife who could read and write a little would say that the minister's sermon "was all lies." Charles Colcock Jones, plantation missionary, found that his slave congregation did not hesitate to reject the doctrine preached in a sermon he gave in 1833:

> I was preaching to a large congregation on the *Epistle of Philemon:* and when I insisted upon fidelity and obedience as Christian virtues in servants and upon the authority of Paul, condemned the practice of *running away*, one half of my audience deliberately rose up and walked off with themselves, and those that remained looked any

thing but satisfied, either with the preacher or his doctrine. After dismission, there was no small stir among them: some solemnly declared "that there was no such an Epistle in the Bible:" others, "that I preached to please the masters:" others, "that it was not the Gospel:" others, "that they did not care if they ever heard me preach again!" . . . There were some too, who had strong objections against me as a preacher because I was a *master* and said, "his people have to work as well as we."

The slaves' rejection of white man's religion was clearly revealed in their attitudes toward morality. While white preachers repeated the command, "Do not steal," slaves simply denied that this precept applied to them since they themselves were stolen property. Josephine Howard put the argument this way: "Dey allus done tell us it am wrong to lie and steal, but why did de white folks steal my mammy and her mammy . . . Dat de sinfulles' stealin' dey is." Rachel Fairley demanded, "How could they help but steal when they didn't have nothin'? You didn't eat if you didn't steal." Henry Bibb declared that under slavery "I had a just right to what I look, because it was the labor of my hands." Other slaves concluded that it was not morally possible for one piece of property to steal another since both belonged to the same owner: it was merely a case of taking something out of one tub and putting it in another. This view of stealing referred only to master's goods, however, for a slave to steal from another slave was seriously wrong. As the saying went, "a slave that will steal from a slave is called *mean as master*." Or as one ex-slave remarked, "This is the lowest comparison slaves know how to use: just as mean as white folks." . . .

Not all slaves, however, were able to distinguish master's religion from authentic Christianity, and were led to reject this religion totally. In 1839, Daniel Alexander Payne explained how this could happen:

> The slaves are sensible of the oppression exercised by their masters: and they see these masters on the Lord's day worshipping in his holy Sanctuary. They hear their masters professing Christianity; they see their masters preaching the gospel; they hear these masters praying in their families and they know that oppression and slavery are inconsistent with the Christian religion; therefore they scoff at religion itself—mock their masters, and distrust both the goodness and justice of God.

Frederick Douglass too remembered being shaken by "doubts arising . . . from the sham religion which everywhere prevailed" under slavery, doubts which "awakened in my mind a distrust of all religion and the conviction that prayers were unavailing and delusive." Unable to account for the evil of slavery in a world ruled by a just God, some slaves abandoned belief. "I pretended to profess religion one time," recalled one former slave, "I don't hardly know what to think about religion. They say God killed the just and unjust; I don't understand that part of it. It looks hard to think that if you ain't done nothing in the world you be punished just like the wicked. Plenty folks went crazy trying to get that straightened out." There is no way of estimating how many slaves felt these doubts, but they indicate how keenly aware slaves were of the disparity between the gospel of Christ and what they termed "white man's religion."

At the opposite extreme from the agnostic slave was the slave who developed a life of exemplary Christian virtue which placed him in a position of moral superiority over his master. William Grimes, for example, was possessed of a sense of righteousness which led him to take a surprising attitude toward his master when punished for something he had not done:

> It grieved me very much to be blamed when I was innocent. I knew I had been faithful to him, perfectly so. At this time I was quite serious, and used constantly to pray to my God. I would not lie nor steal. . . . When I considered him accusing me of stealing, when I was so innocent, and had endeavored to make him satisfied by every means in my power, that I was so, but he still persisted in disbelieving me, I then said to myself if this thing is done in a green tree what must be done in a dry? I forgave my master in my own heart for all this, and prayed to God to forgive him and turn his heart.

Grimes is of course alluding to the sacrifice of Christ and identifying himself with the innocent suffering servant who spoke the words concerning green and dry wood on his way to death on Calvary. From this vantage point Grimes is able forgive his master. Note however the element of threat implied in the question, "if this thing is done in a green tree (to the innocent) what must be done in a dry (to the guilty)?" Those who are guilty of persecuting the innocent, like Grimes's master, will be judged and punished. (The full context of the biblical allusion includes a terrifying prediction of the destruction of Jerusalem.) What did it mean to Grimes's self-image to be able to have moral leverage by which he might elevate his own dignity. A similar impulse lay behind the comment of Mary Younger, a fugitive slave in Canada, "if those slaveholders were to come here, I would treat them well, just to shame them by showing that I had humanity." To assert one's humanity in the face of slavery's power to dehumanize, perhaps explained Grimes's careful adherence to righteousness, a righteousness which might at first glance seem merely servile.

Conclusion

In the slave society of the antebellum South, as in most societies, the Christian religion both supported and undermined the status quo. On the one hand, Nat Turner claimed that God's will moved him to slaughter whites, on the other, "good" slaves protected their masters out of a sense of duty. Slave religion, however was more complex than these alternatives suggest. Institutionally, the egalitarian impulse of evangelical Protestantism, leveling all men before God and lifting some up to declare his word with power and authority, gave slaves and free blacks the opportunity to exercise leadership. Usually this leadership was not revolutionary and from the perspective of political strategy it was overwhelmingly conservative. Yet political action is not the only measure of resistance to oppression. Despite political impotence, the black preacher was still a figure of power as an unmistakable symbol of the talent and ability of black men, a fact which contradicted the doctrine of inherent black inferiority. As white slaveholders occasionally recognized, black preachers were anomalous, if not dangerous, persons under the system of slave control precisely because their authority could not be effectively limited by whites.

Nor were slave owners able to control the spirit of religious independence once it had been imbibed by their slaves. Continually this spirit sought to break out of the strictures confining slave life. When possible, it sought expression in separate institutions controlled by blacks. When that proved impossible, it found expression in secret religious gatherings "out from under the eye of the master." In both cases, the internal autonomy of the slave's own moral will proved impossible to destroy. Throughout the history of Christianity, earthly rulers (civil and religious) have been troubled by the claim that individuals owed obedience to a higher authority than their own. Antebellum slaveholders and missionaries faced the same problem. When slaves disobeyed their masters in order to obey God, a long tradition of Christian heroism validated their assertion of human freedom

The emotional ecstasy of slave religion has been criticized as compensatory and otherworldly, a distraction from the evils of this world. And so it was. But it was much more. Individually, slaves found not only solace in their religion but, particularly in the conversion experience, a source of personal identity and value. Collectively, slaves found in the archetypical symbol of biblical Israel their identity as a community, a new chosen people bound for Divine deliverance from bondage. From this communal identity mutual support, meaning, and hope derived. In the ecstasy of religious performance individual and communal identity and values were dramatically reaffirmed time and time again. In the hand-clapping, footstomping, headshaking fervor of the plantation praise house, the slaves, in prayer, sermon, and song, fit Christianity to their own peculiar experience and in the process resisted, even transcended the dehumanizing bonds of slavery.

ALBERT J. RABOTEAU earned his PhD in religious studies at Yale University and has taught at Princeton University since 1982, where he currently serves as the Henry W. Putnam Professor of Religion. He is the author of numerous works on the topic of African American religion, including *A Fire in the Bones: Reflections on African-American Religious History* (Beacon Press, 1995) and *Canaan Land: A Religious History of African Americans* (Oxford University Press, 1999).

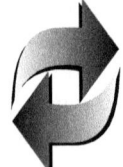

John B. Boles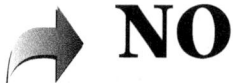

Masters & Slaves in the House of the Lord: Race and Religion in the American South, 1740–1870

Race and religion have probably always been controversial topics in the South, as elsewhere, particularly when their intersection has called into question widely accepted folkways about the place of blacks in southern society. Different interpreters have suggested that the South has been haunted by God and preoccupied with race, so perhaps we should not expect a scholarly consensus on how the two intertwined in the decades from the Great Awakening to Reconstruction. The last generation of our own times has witnessed a remarkable burst of scholarship on blacks and race relations in the region and similar if not quite as prolific discovery of southern religious history. . . .

Most laypersons today seem completely unaware that a century and a half ago many churches in the Old South had significant numbers of black members: black and white co-worshipers heard the same sermons, were baptized and took communion together, and upon death were buried in the same cemeteries. Such practices seem inconceivable today, when the old cliché that Sunday morning at 11:00 A.M. is the most segregated hour in America still rings true. When I was a boy in the rural South thirty years ago, we all supported the Lottie Moon Christmas offering to send missionaries to convert the "heathen" in Africa and elsewhere, but the church deacons and the congregation would have been scandalized had one of the black converts traveled from Africa expecting to worship with us. Yet a century earlier biracial attendance at Baptist churches like ours was the norm in the rural South.

Blacks worshiped in a variety of ways, and some did not participate in any Christian worship, for, especially in the colonial period, a smattering of blacks practiced Islam and others clung tenaciously to traditional African religions. All non-Christian religious activity was discouraged by most slaveowners, who were as ethnocentric as they were concerned about the potential for unrest and rebellion they sensed in their slaves' participation in what to whites were strange and exotic rites. In addition, many slaveowners in the seventeenth and eighteenth centuries were hesitant to attempt to convert their bondspeople to Christianity—if they themselves were Christians—out of fear that conversion might loosen the ties of their bondage. The English knew of slavery long before they had any New World settlements and had considered it a backward institution that might be promoted by Catholic Spain but not by the England of Elizabeth. Even so, the English believed that certain persons might be held in bondage—convicted felons, war prisoners, in some cases heathens, that is, nonbelievers in Christianity. It took several generations before Englishmen in the North American mainland colonies came to accept the practicality of African slavery, then argue the necessity of it, and finally surpass their Spanish rivals in its applications. To the extent that they needed any noneconomic justification, they assumed that the Africans not being Christians made it morally acceptable to enslave them. But if Africans' "heathenism" justified making them slaves, would not their conversion at the very least call into question the rightness of keeping them in bondage? On at least several occasions in the seventeenth century blacks had won their freedom in court by proving they had been baptized. Hence any moral uneasiness that might have existed among less-than-devout slaveowners for nor sharing the gospel with their slaves was entirely overcome by their uneasiness about the stability of their work force should they do so. To clarify this ambiguity obliging laws were passed in the late seventeenth century specifying that a person's "civil state" would not be affected by his conversion to Christianity. . . .

Yet despite the difficulties inherent in converting the slave—the whites' hesitancy to have their slaves hear Christian doctrines and no doubt a hesitancy on the part

---

Boles, John B. "Masters and Slaves in the House of the Lord: Race and Religion in the American South 1740–1870," *Masters and Slaves in the House of the Lord*, 1988. Copyright © 1988 by University Press of Kentucky. Used with permission.

of some slaves to give up traditional beliefs, even if those beliefs had been attenuated by a long presence in the New World—in the middle decades of the eighteenth century increasing numbers of bondspeople became members of Christian churches. A dramatic shift was occurring in the history of black Americans, most of whom before 1750 had been outside the Christian church, for within a century the majority of slaves were worshiping in one fashion or another as Christians. After emancipation, freedpersons continued to find in their churches solace from the cares of the world and joy and a purpose for living in a society that continued to oppress black people. Everyone acknowledges the significance of the church in the black community after freedom; less understood is black worship during the antebellum era and earlier. Yet the half-century following 1740 was the critical period during which some whites broke down their fears and inhibitions about sharing their religion with the slaves in their midst, and some blacks—only a few at first—came to find in Christianity a system of ideas and symbols that was genuinely attractive. . . .

Several aspects of African traditional religion bore close enough parallels to Christianity that bondspeople who were initially disinterested in the white man's religion could—once they glimpsed another side to it—see sufficient common ground between the whites' Christianity and their own folk religions to merit closer examination. That willingness, that openness, on the part of blacks to the claims of Christianity was all the entée white Christian evangelicals needed. Most West African religions assumed a tripartite hierarchy of deities—nature gods, ancestral gods, and an omnipotent creator god who was more remote though more powerful than the others. This conception was roughly transferable to the Christian idea of the trinity. West Africans understood that spirit possession was a sure sign of contact with the divine, an experience not totally dissimilar from the emotional fervor of evangelistic services. Before the mid-eighteenth century slaves had not come into contact with white evangelicals, who were also largely of the lower social order, who worshiped with emotional abandon, and who spoke movingly of being possessed by the Holy Spirit and knowing Jesus as their personal savior. But such evangelical Christians came increasingly to minister to slaves, and they would bridge the chasm between the races and introduce large and growing numbers of slaves to evangelical Christianity.

During the second quarter of the eighteenth century, Evangelicalism and Pietism swept across England and Europe, and the quickening of heartfelt religion soon leapfrogged to the New World in the person of George Whitefield. The resulting Great Awakening occurred primarily north of Maryland, but Whitefield's preaching and the example of his life gained disciples in South Carolina and Georgia. None of Whitefield's followers were more devout than members of the prominent Bryan family in Georgia, and . . . the two Bryan brothers sincerely believed Jesus' call for repentance was addressed to all persons, black and white, bond and free. Consequently, they undertook to promote Christianity among their own and neighboring slaves, but they did so in such a way as to support the institution of slavery. From today's perspective, their paternalistic efforts toward the blacks under their control seem a truncated version of Christianity, but they did present the faith to the slaves in a way that was acceptable to the larger society. A subtle shift in rationales had occurred that would have a far-reaching influence on whites and blacks. At first it had been deemed appropriate to enslave Africans because they were considered heathens; by the mid-eighteenth century some Anglican clergy had begun to argue that it was appropriate to enslave Africans because they might thereby be converted to Christianity. In that sense this development foreshadowed an important tradition of elite white evangelism to blacks, and through such efforts then and in the future thousands of slaves came to know Christianity and, in various ways, to appropriate its message for their own ends.

Another development of the mid-eighteenth century was to be even more important for the growth of Christianity among the slaves than the limited Anglican awakening in the aftermath of Whitefield. In the quarter of a century following 1745 three evangelical Protestant groups planted their seeds in the colonial South—first the Presbyterians, then the Separate Baptists (later the term Separate was dropped as this species came almost completely to swallow all competing versions of believers in adult baptism), and finally the Methodists (first only a subset of the Church of England but after 1784 an independent denomination). These three churches grew at different rates and had different constituencies. The Presbyterians never experienced the extensive growth among rural southerners that the other two did but found increasing support from among those on the upper rungs of society, supplanting the erstwhile Anglican (the postrevolutionary Episcopal) church in influence among the elite. Presbyterian church members, disproportionately wealthy, of course owned disproportionate numbers of slaves, and continuing the elite paternalism pioneered by the Anglican Bryans in colonial Georgia, they tended to minister to blacks by providing them special ministers and separate accommodations. A form of religious noblesse oblige motivated some of them to devise ways to bring the gospel message to their blacks, especially after abolitionists charged that southern whites neglected the spiritual well-being of their slaves. Moreover, the developing argument that slavery was a progressive institution designed by God to effect the Christianization of Africans gave slaveholders a moral obligation to consider the religious needs of their bondspeople. This sentiment, especially strong among Presbyterians and Episcopalians, produced the significant "mission to the slaves" movement of the late antebellum period. . . .

Although the Presbyterian church was to remain relatively small but influential beyond its numbers, the Baptists and Methodists experienced remarkable growth, especially after the Great Revival at the beginning of the nineteenth century. It would be inappropriate in this brief overview to rehearse the reasons for the success these two evangelical denominations had in the rural South; to an extraordinary degree they became the folk churches of the region. Certainly in their youthful decades, the 1750s through 1790s, when their appeal was even more emphatically to those whites who lived at the margins of society—poor, isolated, largely nonslaveholding—the Baptists and Methodists maintained a fairly consistent antislavery stance. Especially south of Maryland, both denominations recognized the political explosiveness of such beliefs if preached incautiously. They tended to criticize slavery in the abstract, delineate its evils both to the slaves and even more to the whites, emphasize that slaves were persons with souls precious in the sight of God, and suggest that slavery be ended "insofar as practicable"—or words to that effect. This is not to argue that they were insincere or hypocritical. Rather, they understood the realities of the economic and social-control imperatives of the institution and occasionally stated explicitly that if they boldly attacked slavery, they would not be allowed to preach to the blacks, thereby—by their lights—causing the unfortunate bondspeople not to hear the gospel. It is easy from today's perspective, and probably incorrect, to see as self-serving such remarks as Methodist Francis Asbury's summation of his position in 1809: "Would not an *amelioration* in the condition and treatment of slaves have produced more practical good to the poor Africans, than any attempt at their *emancipation*? The state of society, unhappily, does not admit of this: besides, the blacks are deprived of the means of instruction; who will take the pains to lead them into the way of salvation, and watch over them that they may not stray, but the Methodists? . . . What is the personal liberty of the African which he may abuse, to the salvation of his soul; how may it be compared?"

The point is not the limited emancipationist impulse in the evangelical denominations and how it was thwarted over time by political and racial pressures. More appropriate here is the way the lower-class structure of the early Baptist and Methodist churches, most of whose members did not own slaves and felt estranged from the wealthier whites who did, enabled them to see blacks as potential fellow believers in a way that white worshipers in more elite churches seldom could. From the moment of their organization, typical Baptist or Methodist churches included black members, who often signed (or put their "X") on the founding documents of incorporation. Black membership in these two popular denominations was substantial from the last quarter of the eighteenth century through the Civil War. Without claiming too much or failing to recognize the multitude of ways slaves were not accorded genuine equality in these biracial churches it is still fair to say that nowhere else in southern society were they treated so nearly as equals.

Because church membership statistics for the antebellum period are incomplete, and because churches varied in their definitions of membership, a quantitatively precise portrait of the extent to which blacks and whites worshiped together is impossible to obtain. Historian John Blassingame has written that "an overwhelming majority of the slaves throughout the antebellum period attended church with their masters. Then, after the regular services ended, the ministers held special services for the slaves." Such special services were more typical of Episcopal and Presbyterian churches; Methodist and Baptist preachers would usually, sometimes toward the end of the service, call for something like "a special word for our black brothers and sisters" and then turn to them in the back pews or in the balcony and address them with a didactic sermon that often stressed obedience to their earthly masters. Sarah Fitzpatrick, a ninety-year-old former slave interviewed in 1938, recalled that "us 'Niggers' had our meetin' in de white fo'ks Baptist Church in de town o' Tuskegee. Dere's a place up in de loft dere now dat dey built fer de 'Nigger' slaves to 'tend church wid de white fo'ks. White preacher he preach to de white fo'ks an' when he git thu' wid dem he preach some to de 'Niggers.' Tell 'em to mind dere Marster an' b'have deyself an' dey'll go to Hebben when dey die."

Slaves saw through these words and felt contempt for the self-serving attention they received. More important to them was the remainder of the service that they heard and participated in with the rest of the congregation. Here the slaves heard a more complete version of the gospel, and despite whatever social-control uses some ministers tried to put religion to in a portion of the Sunday service, most slaves found grounds for hope and a degree of spiritual liberation through their participation in these biracial churches. As Blassingame concluded, "Generally the ministers tried to expose the slaves to the major tenets of Christianity. . . . [And] only 15 percent of the Georgia slaves who had heard antebellum whites preach recalled admonitions to obedience."

Slaves worshiped apart from whites on some occasions, often with the knowledge of their owners and often without the white supervision the law called for. Some black churches were adjuncts to white churches, and completely independent and autonomous black churches existed in southern cities. Blacks worshiped privately and often secretly in their cabins and in the fields. Sometimes, and especially when their owner was irreligious, slaves had to slip away to hidden "brush arbors" deep in the woods to preach, shout, sing, and worship. But such practices should not lead us to forget that the normative worship experience of blacks in the antebellum South was in a biracial church. "Including black Sunday School scholars and catechumens," Blassingame writes, "there were probably 1,000,000 slaves under the regular tutelage of Southern churches in 1860." When David T. Bailey examined some 40 autobiographies of blacks and 637 interviews of slaves on the subject of religion, he discovered that 32 percent of the autobiographers who mentioned religion reported that they had gone to white churches, 14 percent said their master led the services for them, and another 14 percent attended worship services at special plantation chapels, whereas 36 percent mentioned that they had attended black prayer meetings. Of the former slaves interviewed, 43.5 percent mentioned attending white churches, 6.5 percent reported master-led services, 6.5 percent described plantation chapels, and only 24 percent discussed attendance at black prayer meetings.

Such substantial black participation in churches normally considered white indicates that white evangelicals, even in the late antebellum period, when they had moved up the social scale, joined the establishment, and come to support the institution of slavery, still felt a Christian responsibility to include slaves in the outreach of the church. Their idea of mission assumed that slaves were persons with souls precious in God's sight. In fact, many white evangelicals came to believe that part of their responsibility to God involved Christianizing the slave work force. It was to that end, they reasoned, that God had sanctioned slavery. . . . [A]bolitionist charges that the southern church ignored the slaves infuriated southern clergymen and caused them to redouble their efforts to bring slaves into the church. During the Civil War clergy feared that God was chastising the region for not sufficiently supporting the mission effort to the blacks, and religiously inspired attempts to amend slavery by correcting the worst abuses, teaching bondspeople to read (so the Scriptures would be accessible to them), and providing missionaries for them . . . almost reformed slavery out of existence in Confederate Georgia.

Devout white clergy often took seriously their responsibilities toward the blacks in their midst, and their paternalistic and racist assumptions should not blind us to their convictions that slaves too were God's children and that white slaveowners stood under God's judgment for the way they treated their bondspeople. It is difficult to understand today how devout whites could define blacks legally as chattel and yet show real concern for the state of their souls. Could genuine Christians so compartmentalize their charity? Apparently so, given their assumptions that blacks were a race of permanent children. A misguided sense of Christian responsibility led well-meaning, decent whites to justify slavery as the white man's duty to Africans, for it was, they argued, through the order and discipline bondage provided that slaves learned—sampled?—Christianity and Western civilization. Almost like whistling in the dark to drive away one's fears, white churchmen sometimes were particularly anxious to Christianize their slaves as though only thus could the institution be justified and their guilt be lessened.

Blacks too must have derived a substantial reward from their participation in the institutional churches or they would not have been involved with them to such an extent for so long. The manuscript records of hundreds of local Baptist churches across the South allow us to see a seldom-studied aspect of white-black interaction that helps explain the attraction biracial churches held for slaves. First, . . . blacks were accorded a semblance of equality when they joined antebellum Baptist churches. White members often addressed them as brother or sister, just as they did fellow white members. This equality in the terms of address may seem insignificant today, but in an age when only whites were accorded the titles of Mr. and Mrs., and it was taboo for a white to so address a black, any form of address that smacked of equality was notable. Behind it lay the familial idea, accepted by whites in principle if not always in practice, that in the sight of God all were equal and were members of His spiritual family. Incoming or outgoing members of Baptist churches were accepted or dismissed with "letters" attesting to their good standing, and slaves asking to join Baptist churches were expected to "bring their letter" just as prospective white members were. Churches seem to have routinely supplied such letters to their members of both races who moved to other locations. New members, black and white, were usually given the "right hand of fellowship" after their letters were accepted or after they came to the altar following the minister's sermon-ending call for conversion to "confess their sins and accept Christ's mercy." Individual churches often varied in this practice, as in much else in the South, where strict uniformity in anything was the exception.

Blacks usually sat in a separate section of the church, perhaps a balcony or a lean-to. There is evidence, however, that slaves sat scattered throughout Anglican churches in colonial Virginia and that sometimes they sat with or next to the pew of their master. Today, such segregated seating would seem to contradict the idea of spiritual equality, but the contradiction probably did not seem so stark to slaves, who were excluded from most other white-dominated functions. The white women often sat apart from the white men, too; in that age segregation by gender was almost as common as that by race, and the familiarity of such separation might well have lessened the negative connotation although it accentuated each subgroup's sense of separate identity. That is, the sense of both a separate women's culture and a separate black culture might have been inadvertently strengthened by the prevalent mode of segregated seating under a common roof. In fact, for some blacks who were isolated on farms and small plantations with no or only a few fellow slaves, the gathering together on Sunday at the church house with slaves from other farms may have been the primary occasion for experiencing a sense of black community. For such slaves the forced segregation in seating may have seemed both natural and desirable because they hungered for close interaction with persons of their own kind. That interaction may have been a stronger attraction than the worship itself. No doubt many bondspeople found their marriage partners through such social involvement at church—certainly much white courtship began there. Perhaps, then, for slaves dispersed on farms outside the plantation district, the slave community was largely created and vitalized in the one arena in which slaves belonging to different owners could freely mingle—the biracial church service.

As with church membership practices, there was an important but limited degree of equality in slaves' participation in antebellum church discipline.... [C]ertainly no one would want to argue that whites completely forgot or transcended the racial mores of a slave society in the confines of the church building, but it is significant that slaves were allowed to give testimony—sometimes even conflicting with white testimony—and that on occasion their witness overruled the charges of whites. This occurred in a society that did not allow blacks to testify against whites in civil courts. Moreover, blacks were not disciplined out of proportion to their numbers; on the whole, they were charged with infractions similar to those of whites; and they were held to the same moral expectations as whites with regard to profanity, drunkenness, lying, adultery, failure to attend church, and fighting. There surely were charges against blacks that had no parallel for whites—for example, blacks alone were charged with running away. But nowhere else in southern society were slaves and whites brought together in an arena where both were held responsible to a code of behavior sanctioned by a source outside the society—the Bible. The Scriptures were interpreted in culturally sanctioned ways, but whites as well as blacks were occasionally found wanting.

Blacks discovered in the church and in church discipline a unique sphere wherein to nurture (and be recognized by whites to have) moral responsibility and what Timothy L. Smith has called "moral earnestness." Through the church slaves found a meaning for their lives that could give a touch of moral grandeur to the tragic dimension of their bondage. Images of the children of Israel and the suffering servant provided ways to accept their life predicament without feelings of self-worthlessness. The church offered a spark of joy in the midst of pain, a promise of life-affirming forgiveness to soften the hopelessness of unremitting bondage, an ultimate reward in heaven for unrewarded service in this world. Participation in the biracial churches was one of the ways slaves found the moral and psychological strength to survive their bondage.

It is important to remember that social interaction does not necessarily imply social equality, in a variety of contexts outside the churches slaves and masters mingled closely without narrowing the gap between freedom and bondage. In many ways such interaction could even magnify the sense of enslavement. Yet it would be a mistake so to emphasize the belittling possibilities of white-black interaction that we fail to see the alternative possibilities inherent in the biracial churches. Slaves apparently had their image of being creatures of God strengthened by the sermons they heard—even when that was not the intention of the ministers—and the discipline they accepted. Their evident pleasure in occasionally hearing black preachers speak to biracial congregations no doubt augmented their sense of racial pride. Taking communion together with whites, serving as deacons or Sunday school teachers, being baptized or confirmed in the same ceremonies, even contributing their mite to the temporal upkeep of the church, could surely have been seen as symbolic ways of emphasizing their self-respect and equality before God. Slaves certainly were not dependent on white-controlled institutions to nurture their sense of self-worth, but neither were they adverse to seizing opportunities wherever they found them and using them for that purpose. In a society that offered few opportunities for blacks to practice organizational and leadership skills or hear themselves addressed and see themselves evaluated morally on an equal basis with whites, small matters could have large meanings. Blacks did not discover in the biracial churches an equality of treatment that spiritually transported them out of bondage, but they found in them a theology of hope and a recognition of self-worth that fared them well in their struggle to endure slavery.

As Robert L. Hall documents in his analysis of religion in antebellum Florida, blacks worshiped in a variety of ways in the antebellum South besides in biracial Protestant churches. In most southern cities and large towns there were completely independent black churches, with black ministers, black deacons or elders, and a panoply of self-help associations connected to and supported by the church. Usually such churches, like the St. James African Episcopal Church in Baltimore, were under the control of free blacks, although many if not most of the members were slaves. Although the surrounding white-dominated churches tended to ignore societal ills, emphasize conversion, and minister primarily to individuals, the black churches tended to minister to all the social and religious needs of their parishioners. There was a communal and social thrust in the independent black churches that was notably absent from the mainstream white churches of the South. (That difference even today sets many black churches apart from white.) Often the black churches had very large memberships, and sometimes their meeting places had the largest seating capacity in the city.

Blacks also worshiped in black churches that were adjunct to white churches. Such situations typically arose after the biracial church built a new sanctuary and, with the black members perhaps outnumbering the white, the blacks were allowed ("allowed" seems more accurate than "forced") to conduct separate services in the old structure. The motivation of the whites here is not clear; they often indicated that the blacks preferred their own services, but to what extent whites desired segregated white churches for essentially racist reasons is impossible to determine. In most cases when blacks were split off into separate "African" churches, as they were known, a committee of whites was assigned to oversee their services. The supervision seems to have been honored more in the breach, however. In a variety of other ways black church members were often given some autonomy in regulating portions of their worship life, again apparently more because the blacks desired such separation than because whites required it. These small islands of black autonomy within the biracial church were perhaps the beginning of the complete racial separation that would come after the Civil War.

Not all the organized churches in the South were Protestant, although Protestantism was far more dominant in the South than elsewhere in the nation. There were pockets of Catholic strength in Maryland, Kentucky, and Missouri, and in south Louisiana Catholicism was preponderant. Most southern cities had at least one Catholic church, usually attended primarily by immigrant workers. Louisiana and Maryland had rural Catholic churches as well, with numbers of black Catholic parishioners. Catholic masters sometimes required that their slaves worship as Catholics, though their bondspeople may have preferred the neighboring Baptist or Methodist churches either as a subtle form of rebellion against their masters or because of the appeal of the demonstrative emotionalism of the evangelical churches. In various ways the Catholic church ministered to bondspeople; separate black orders and sisterhoods were established and the sacraments extended. Because it was a minority church in a rabidly Protestant region and was concerned not to attract notoriety, the Catholic church never questioned the morality of slavery. An occasional Catholic institution or order might own slaves, as did the Jesuits in Maryland, though this property in humans was divested for reasons of ethics and economics. . . .

In addition to the various kinds of formal churches—biracial, adjunct, and independent black churches and plantation chapels—to which slaves had access, black worshipers also gathered in more informal, often secret settings. The evidence for this is to be found in black memoirs and slave narratives, although even these sources suggest that most blacks worshiped in one or another of the formal churches. There are many reasons why slaves would choose to worship in a manner less subject to white supervision or control. Some masters sought to prevent slaves from worshiping at all, which forced slaves to develop an underground religion and to meet secretly either in their cabins at night or in the brush arbors. Slaves who were allowed (or required) to attend a biracial church (or any formal service carefully monitored by whites) in which the minister placed too much emphasis on the "slaves-obey-your-master" homily and thereby neglected to preach the gospel in its fullness often sought an alternative worship experience. There must have been other times when slaves felt inhibited in the presence of whites and simply desired a time and a place to preach, sing, and shout without having to suffer the condescending glances of less emotionally involved white churchgoers. Although slaves worshiping apart and secretively may have developed a distinctly black Christianity significantly different from that which they heard in the more formal institutions, there is no unambiguous evidence that they did so. More probably the services in the brush arbors were simply a longer, more emotionally demonstrative version of those in the biracial churches, with more congregational participation. No precise record exists of the theology implicit in such brush arbor meetings or of special emphases that might have developed, but the similarity in worship practice and ecclesiology of the autonomous black churches that emerged after the Civil War to the earlier biracial churches argues against the evolution of any fundamentally different system in the brush arbors.

A momentous change in the nature of church practice in the South took place at the beginning of Reconstruction. Blacks in significant numbers—eventually all of them—began to move out of the biracial churches and join a variety of independent black denominations. As Katharine Dvorak notes in her insightful essay, the blacks left on their own volition; they were not forced out. At first many white churchmen tried to persuade them to stay, but within several decades the degenerating racial climate of the region led these same churchmen on occasion to applaud the new segregated patterns of worship, so different from the common practice before the Civil War.

Of course, that freedpersons wanted to leave the biracial churches is a commentary on the less-than-complete equality they had enjoyed in them. Blacks had a strong sense of racial identity, reinforced by their having been slaves and, within the confines of the churches, by their segregated seating. The complete sermons they had heard for years, not just the self-serving words the white ministers directed specifically at them, had engendered in blacks a sense of their moral worth and equality in the sight of God. The biracial churches simultaneously nurtured this sense of moral equality and thwarted it by their conformity to the demands of the slave society. Black participation in the biracial churches—as preachers, deacons, stewards, and Sunday school teachers—had given them practical leadership and administrative experience, as had their islands of autonomy within the demographically biracial churches. Theologically and experientially blacks were ready to seize the moment offered by emancipation to withdraw from their old allegiances and create autonomous denominations. No better evidence of the freedom slaves had not enjoyed in the biracial churches exists than the rapidity with which blacks sought to establish separate denominations after the Civil War. And no better evidence exists of the extent to which slaves in the biracial churches accepted evangelical Christianity as their preferred expression of religious faith and molded their lives to its demands than the denominations they created after emancipation.

The worship services and institutional arrangements in the new black churches bore a very close resemblance to the biracial churches from which the blacks withdrew. In fact, black Baptist and Methodist services were closer to the early nineteenth-century post–Great Revival services of the evangelical churches than those of the postbellum all-white churches. Blacks had assimilated the theology and order of service in the biracial churches. Rejecting the modernizing tendencies of the white churches toward less emotion, shorter sermons, an emphasis on choir singing rather than congregational singing, and seminary-trained ministers, they more truly carried on the pioneer evangelical traditions. It should not have been surprising to anyone that when born-again Baptist presidential candidate Jimmy Carter wanted to appeal to blacks in 1976, he spoke to them in their churches. Despite the differences—black services are longer, the music is more expressive, emotions are more freely expressed, there is greater congregational participation—the kinship between the white and black Baptist churches of today is readily apparent, and it points back to a time more than a century ago when the religious culture of the South was fundamentally biracial.

JOHN B. BOLES earned his PhD from the University of Virginia and currently teaches at Rice University, where he is the William P. Hobby Professor of History. A specialist in the American South and southern religion, Boles served for thirty years as the editor of the prestigious *Journal of Southern History*. He also is the author of numerous books, including *The Great Revival, 1787–1805: The Origins of the Southern Evangelical Mind* (University Press of Kentucky, 1972), *Black Southerners, 1619–1869* (University Press of Kentucky, 1983), and *The Irony of Southern Religion* (Peter Lang, 1994).

EXPLORING THE ISSUE

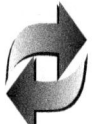

Did African American Slaves Exercise Religious Autonomy?

Critical Thinking and Reflection

1. According to Raboteau, how did American slaves develop both institutional and personal autonomy in the antebellum South?
2. What impact did Christianity have on the racial status quo in the antebellum South?
3. How could religion be used as a form of resistance to the institution of slavery?
4. What factors contributed to the growth of Christianity among enslaved persons?
5. Discuss in detail the influence of the biracial church on the lives of slaves in the antebellum South.

Is There Common Ground?

Both Albert Raboteau and John Boles recognize that the religious practices of African American slaves in the antebellum South included both formal participation in biracial church congregations and more informal efforts by the slaves to carve out some degree of autonomy free from the supervision of their masters. Both are equally aware that the message of Christianity was subject to different interpretations or understandings depending on whether masters or slaves were in charge of delivering that message. Antebellum white southerners for the most part crafted the Gospel to legitimize slavery and developed a multi-pronged justification to satisfy themselves that slavery and Christianity were not at odds with one another. African American preachers and exhorters, however, were far more inclined to focus upon the liberationist nature of the Exodus and the egalitarian character of the New Testament. The real point of debate, therefore, is which of these religious experiences was most prominent in the lives of American slaves.

One of the most intriguing issues for students of American slavery is the relationship between religion and resistance. Specifically, did slaves find in Christianity a palliative that conditioned them to seek salvation only in God's heavenly kingdom or did it steel their resolve to seek deliverance from their bondage in the earthly realm? Actually, there was a certain dualism evident in the slaves' religious life. Some obviously were pacified by a fatalistic attitude that slavery was their permanent status, yet hopeful that salvation would be achieved in the heavenly afterlife. Slave owners, of course, attempted to ensure their bondservants' loyalty and passivity. For their own part, slaves much preferred to hear Bible readings related to Moses's deliverance of the Israelites from Egypt, and it should be remembered that Gabriel Prosser, Denmark Vesey, and Nat Turner all employed religious symbolism and apocalyptic language to foster their revolutionary conspiracies in the antebellum South.

Additional Resources

Carol V. R. George, *Segregated Sabbaths: Richard Allen and the Rise of Independent Black Churches, 1760–1840* (Oxford University Press, 1973)

Vincent Harding, "Religion and Resistance Among Antebellum Negroes, 1800–1860," in August Meier and Elliott Rudwick, eds., *The Making of Black America*, 2 vols. (Atheneum, 1969); vol. 1, pp. 179–197

Charles Joyner, *Down by the Riverside: A South Carolina Slave Community* (University of Illinois Press, 1984)

Orlando Patterson, *Slavery and Social Death: A Comparative Study* (Harvard University Press, 1982)

Mechal Sobel, *Trabelin' On: The Slave Journey to an Afro-Baptist Faith* (Princeton University Press, 1979)

Internet References . . .

African American Christianity

http://nationalhumanitiescenter.org/tserve/nineteen/nkeyinfo/aareligion.htm

Facts About the Slave Trade and Slavery

https://www.gilderlehrman.org/history-by-era/slavery-and-anti-slavery/resources/facts-about-slave-trade-and-slavery

Slavery and the Making of America

www.pbs.org/wnet/slavery/timeline/

Slavery in America

www.uen.org/themepark/liberty/slavery.shtml

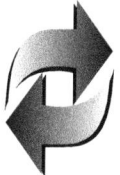

ISSUE

Selected, Edited, and with Issue Framing Material by:
Kevin R. Magill and Tony L. Talbert, *Baylor University*

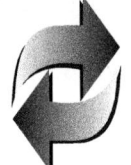

Was Abraham Lincoln America's Greatest President?

YES: Phillip Shaw Paludan, from "The Presidency of Abraham Lincoln," University Press of Kansas (1994)

NO: Melvin E. Bradford, from "Remembering Who We Are: Observations of a Southern Conservative," University of Georgia Press (1985)

Learning Outcomes

After reading this issue, you will be able to:

- Evaluate the criteria historians use to assess presidential performance.
- Analyze Lincoln's leadership from the perspective of the concept of the "imperial presidency."
- Identify and assess Lincoln's policies as a wartime president.
- Summarize the major points of criticism of Lincoln's presidency.

ISSUE SUMMARY

YES: Phillip Shaw Paluden offers a portrait of greatness in his description of Abraham Lincoln who was first and foremost deeply committed to the process of the American "political-constitutional system." Paluden primary thesis asserting Lincoln's status as America's greatest President is rooted in the notion that "Lincoln was not either a constitutionalist or an egalitarian" in his commitment to preserving the Union and ending slavery. Instead, Lincoln's ideological devotion to the notion that "Constitutional government" and full equality were not simply complementary but codependent. Therefore, Lincoln's greatness lied in his commitment to the "process" and fully expected that both equality and the union would survive.

NO: In contrast Melvin E. Bradford seeks to challenge what he calls the "myth of the American Messiah." Bradford contends that indeed Lincoln was at the heart of many of the changes that were brought about during the era and simply put would never have come to pass if not for Lincoln pushing them forward (e.g., emancipation of African American enslaved peoples, increased powers of federalism, eventual ratification of Reconstruction Amendments after Lincoln's death, etc.). While many would consider this a sign of Lincoln's greatness Bradford argues that it is an example of "Lincoln's dishonesty and obfuscation" of the nation's constitutional principles as established by the Founding Father's commitment to republican principles. Moreover, Bradford argues that Lincoln's failure as a U.S. President is evidenced by his overstep of authority as granted by Article II of the U.S. Constitution and his setting in motion the rise of the "imperial Presidency" which is what the Founding Fathers intended to prevent.

The American Civil War (1861–1865) produced what Arthur Schlesinger, Jr. has called "our greatest national trauma." To be sure, the War Between the States was a searing event that etched itself on the collective memory of the American people and inspired an interest that has made it the most thoroughly studied episode in American history. During the last century and a quarter, scholars have identified a variety of factors (including slavery, economic sectionalism, cultural distinctions between North and South, the doctrine of states' rights, and the irresponsibility of abolitionists and proslavery advocates) that contributed to sectional tensions and that ultimately led to war. Although often presented as "sole causes," these factors are complicated, interconnected, and controversial. Consequently, historians must consider as many of them as possible in their evaluations of the war, even if they choose to spotlight one or another as the main explanation (see Issue 14).

Most historians, however, agree that the war would not have occurred had 11 southern states not seceded from the Union to form the Confederate States of America following Abraham Lincoln's election to the presidency in 1860. Why was Lincoln viewed as a threat to the South? A southerner by birth, Lincoln's career in national politics (as a congressman representing his adopted state of Illinois) apparently had been short-circuited by his unpopular opposition to the Mexican War. His attempt to emerge from political obscurity a decade later failed when he was defeated by Stephen Douglas in a bid for a Senate seat from Illinois. This campaign, however, gained for Lincoln a reputation as a powerful orator, and in 1860 Republican Party managers passed over some of their more well-known leaders, such as William Henry Seward, and nominated the moderate Mr. Lincoln for the presidency. His victory was guaranteed by factionalism within Democratic ranks, but the election results revealed that the new president received only 39 percent of the popular vote. This fact, however, provided little solace for Southerners, who mistook the new president's opposition to the extension of slavery into the territories as evidence that he supported the abolitionist wing of the Republican Party. Despite assurances during the campaign that he would not tamper with slavery where it already existed, Lincoln could not prevent the splintering of the Union.

Given such an inauspicious beginning, few observers at the time could have predicted that future generations would view Lincoln as our nation's greatest president. What factors have contributed to this assessment? The answer would appear to lie in his role as commander-in-chief during the Civil War. Is this reputation deserved?

Lincoln's assassination at the hands of John Wilkes Booth shortly following the end of the Civil War pretty much guaranteed for the fallen leader a martyrdom that had the potential to cloud balanced appraisals of his leadership. Biographer Stephen B. Oates, in *Abraham Lincoln: The Man Behind the Myths* (Harper & Row, 1984), accurately reminds us that Lincoln, at the time of his assassination, was perhaps the most hated president in history. But since Arthur Schlesinger, Jr. first polled experts on the subject in 1948, historians consistently have rated Lincoln the nation's best chief executive. George Washington, Thomas Jefferson, Theodore and Franklin Roosevelt, and Woodrow Wilson have done well in presidential polls conducted by Gary Maranell (1970), Steve Neal (1982), and Robert K. Murray (1983), but none so well as Abraham Lincoln. Another president, Harry Truman, himself ranked Lincoln in the category of "great" chief executives. Truman wrote of Lincoln: "He was a strong executive who saved the government, saved the United States. He was a President who understood people, and, when it came time to make decisions, he was willing to take the responsibility and make those decisions, no matter how difficult they were. He knew how to treat people and how to make a decision stick, and that's why his is regarded as such a great Administration."

Some of the most insightful writing on various aspects of Lincoln's life appeared almost 50 years ago but still offer incisive interpretations of many aspects of Lincoln's political career and philosophy. See, for example, David Donald, *Lincoln Reconsidered: Essays on the Civil War Era* (Knopf, 1956) and Richard Current, *The Lincoln Nobody Knows* (McGraw-Hill, 1958). Lincoln's responsibility for the precipitating event of the war is explored in Richard N. Current, *Lincoln and the First Shot* (Lippincott, 1963). Doris Kearns Goodwin, *Team of Rivals: The Political Genius of Abraham Lincoln* (Simon & Schuster, 2005) is a beautifully written more recent appraisal of Lincoln's approach to leadership. Goodwin, in particular, notes that in the selection of cabinet members, Lincoln chose individuals representing many different factions but who overcame their contentiousness to handle competently the burdens of wartime governing.

The best studies of Lincoln's attitudes toward race and slavery are by the generally sympathetic Benjamin Quarles, *Lincoln and the Negro* (Oxford University Press, 1962), and by LaWanda Cox, *Lincoln and Black Freedom: A Study in Presidential Leadership* (University of South Carolina Press, 1981). Lerone Bennett, *Forced Into Glory: Abraham Lincoln's White Dream* (Johnson Publishing, 2000) characterizes Lincoln as a white supremacist and argues that African American slaves themselves were far more effective agents of emancipation than was the "Great Emancipator."

The selections that follow assess Lincoln's presidency from dramatically different perspectives. Phillip Shaw Paludan sees unparalleled greatness in the leadership of the United States' 16th chief executive. Lincoln's greatness, Paludan concludes, derived from his ability to mobilize public opinion in the North behind his goal of saving the Union and freeing the slaves. Significantly, Paludan does not separate these accomplishments. Rather, he argues that they were inextricably connected; one could not be realized without the other.

Melvin Bradford offers a sharp critique of the conclusions reached by Paludan. By pursuing an anti-southern strategy, Bradford argues, President Lincoln perverted the republican goals advanced by the Founding Fathers and destroyed the Democratic majority that was essential to the preservation of the Union. Furthermore, Bradford asserts, Lincoln abused his executive authority by cynically expanding the scope of presidential powers to an unhealthy extent. Finally, Bradford charges that Lincoln was uncommitted to the cause of black Americans.

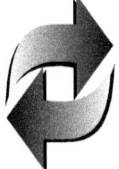

YES ← Phillip Shaw Paludan

The Presidency of Abraham Lincoln

The oath is a simple one, made all the more austere because there is no coronation, no anointing by priest or predecessor. The office has passed from one person to another months before, first by popular election and then by a ritualistic casting of votes by presidential electors, whose names are forgotten if anyone knew them in the first place. The only requirement on the day the president takes office is an oath or affirmation: "I do solemnly swear that I will faithfully execute the Office of President of the United States, and will to the best of my ability, preserve, protect and defend the Constitution of the United States."

Each president in the history of the nation has tried to protect and defend the Constitution—some with more dedication than others. Each responded to the challenges and the opportunity that his time gave him. No president had larger challenges than Abraham Lincoln, and the testimony to his greatness rests in his keeping of that oath, which led him to be responsible for two enormous accomplishments that are part of folk legend as well as fact. He saved the Union and he freed the slaves.

He preserved the unity of the nation both in size and in structure. There were still thirty-six states at the end of his presidency; there might have been twenty-five. The population of the nation when he died was 30 million; it might have been 20 million. The constitutional instrument for changing governments was still in 1865 what it had been in 1861—win a free election and gain the majority of the electoral votes. Another option might have existed—secede from the country and make war if necessary after losing the election. A divided nation might have been more easily divided again—perhaps when angry westerners felt exploited by eastern capitalists, perhaps when urban minorities felt oppressed by powerful majorities. And there were lasting international consequences from Lincoln's achievement: Foreign oppressors of the twentieth century were not allowed to run free, disregarding the two or perhaps three or four countries that might have existed between Canada and Mexico.

Because of Lincoln, 4 million black Americans gained options beyond a life of slavery for themselves and their children. Men, women, and children were no longer bought and sold, denied their humanity—because of Lincoln, but certainly not because of Lincoln alone. Perhaps 2 million Union soldiers fought to achieve these goals. Women behind the lines and near the battlefields did jobs that men would not or could not do. Workers on farms and in factories supplied the huge army and the society that sustained it. Managers and entrepreneurs organized the resources that helped gain the victory. But Lincoln's was the voice that inspired and explained and guided soldiers and civilians to continue the fight.

Black soldiers, too, preserved the Union and freed slaves. And these black soldiers were in the army because Lincoln wanted them there, accepted the demands of black and white abolitionists and growing numbers of soldiers and sailors that they be there. Hundreds of thousands, perhaps millions, of slaves, given the chance, walked away from slavery and thus "stole" from their masters the labor needed to sustain the Confederacy and the ability of those masters to enslave them. No one would ever again sell their children, their husbands, their wives; no one would rape and murder and mutilate them, control their work and much of their leisure.

Lincoln kept his oath by leading the nation, guiding it, insisting that it keep on with the task of saving the Union and freeing the slaves.

Too often historians and the general populace (which cares very much, and may define itself in vital ways by what Lincoln did and means) have divided his two great achievements. They have made saving the Union, at least for the first half of his presidency, a different task from freeing the slaves. They have noted that Lincoln explained to Horace Greeley that he could not answer Greeley's "Prayer of Twenty Million" and simply free the slaves. His prime goal, he told Greeley, was to save the Union, and he would free none, some, or all the slaves to save that Union. But before Lincoln wrote those words he had already decided that to save the Union he would have to free the slaves.

. . . Freeing the slaves and saving the Union were linked as one goal, not two optional goals. The Union that Lincoln wanted to save was not a union where slavery was safe. He wanted to outlaw slavery in the territories and thus begin a process that would end it in the states. Slave states understood this; that is why they seceded and why the Union needed saving.

Freeing the slaves, more precisely ending slavery, was the indispensable means to saving the Union. In an immediate practical sense, those 180,000 black soldiers were an essential part of the Union army in the last two years of the war. They made up almost 12 percent of the total Union land forces by 1865, adding not only to Union numbers but subtracting from the Confederate labor force. Moreover, those black soldiers liberated even where they did not march. Their example was noted throughout the South so that slaves far from Union occupation knew that blacks could be soldiers, not just property, and they began to march toward freedom.

Ending slavery also meant saving the Union in a larger sense. Slavery had endangered the Union, hurting black people but also hurting white people, and not only by allowing them to be brutes, as Jefferson had lamented. Slavery had divided the nation, threatening the processes of government by making debate over the most crucial issue of the age intolerable in the South and, for decades, dangerous in the Congress of the United States. To protect slavery the Confederate States of America would challenge the peaceful, lawful, orderly means of changing governments in the United States, even by resorting to war. Lincoln led the successful effort to stop them and thus simultaneously saved the Union and freed the slaves.

Why does it matter that Lincoln linked saving the Union and the emancipation of the nation from slavery? First, it is necessary to get the historical record straight. It matters also because in understanding our history Americans gain access to the kind of faith that Lincoln held that our means, our legal processes, our political-constitutional system work to achieve our best ideals. Too many people, among them the first black justice of the United States Supreme Court, Thurgood Marshall, have doubted that respect for the law and the Constitution can lead to greater equality. "The system" too often has been the villain, "institutional racism" the disease that obstructs the struggle for equality. The underlying premise of this book is that the political-constitutional system, conceived of and operated at its best, inescapably leads to equality. Lincoln operated on that premise and through his presidency tried to achieve that goal.

But how did he do that? One of his accomplishments, the one that took most of his time, was fighting and winning a war. He chose the generals, gathered the armies, set the overall strategy; he restrained the dissenters and the opponents of the war; he helped to gather the resources that would maintain the Union economy and that would enable the Union military to remain strong and unrelenting. He kept himself and his party in office, the only party that was dedicated to saving the Union and ending slavery. And he kept an eye on foreign affairs, seeing to it that Great Britain remained willing to negotiate and to watch the conflict rather than joining or trying to stop it. . . .

I am particularly interested in what Lincoln said, for the most important power of a president, as Richard Neustadt has argued, is the power to persuade. Thus it is vital for a president to inform and to inspire, to warn and to empower the polity, to bring out the "better angels of our nature"—better in the sense of allowing the nation to achieve its best aspirations. "Events have controlled me," Lincoln said, but what he did most effectively was to define those events and to shape the public opinion that, he noted, was "everything in this country." In the 1840s a Whig newspaper came close to the mark I am admiring in assessing Lincoln:

> Put the case that the same multitude were addressed by two orators, and on the same question and occasion; that the first of these orators considered in his mind that the people he addressed were to be controlled by several passions . . . the orator may be fairly said to have no faith in the people; he rather believes that they are creatures of passion, and subject to none but base and selfish impulses. But now a second orator arises, a Chatham, a Webster, a Pericles, a Clay; his generous spirit expands itself through the vast auditory, and he believes that he is addressing a company of high spirited men, citizens. . . . When he says "fellow citizens," they believe him, and at once, from a tumultuous herd they are converted into men . . . their thoughts and feeling rise to an heroical heights, beyond that of common men or common times. The second orator "had faith in the people"; he addressed the better part of each man's nature, supposing it to be in him—and it *was* in him.

At their best American presidents recognize that their duty as the chief opinion maker is to shape a public understanding that opens options and tells the truth about what the people can be and what their problems are. Appealing to the fears we have, manipulating them to win office or pass a law or achieve another goal, does not so much *reflect* who we are as it in fact *creates* who we are. It affirms us as legitimately fearful—afraid of something that our leaders confirm to be frightening—and as being citizens whose fears properly define us.

Appealing to better angels is more complicated—it requires calling on history for original aspirations—reminding Americans for example that the basic ideal of the nation is that "all men are created equal." Equally vital, such an appeal also requires reminding Americans that they have in fact established institutions that work to that end—not only reminding them of their aspirations but also reassuring them that their history, their lived experience, reveals legitimate paths to achieving those goals. History thus acts to recall the nation's best dreams, but it also restores faith that the means to approach the dream live, abide in the institutions as well as in the values that shape the nation.

I believe that a history of the presidency of Abraham Lincoln can show how Lincoln managed to shape a public understanding, how at times he failed, but how he usually succeeded. Thus he set a standard that makes it legitimate that we, when the better angels of our nature prevail, define ourselves in important ways by who Lincoln was, by what he did, and by what he said.

The Lincoln presidency did not end through the operation of the political-constitutional system. There was no joyous ritual, no abiding process that had gone on for generations. It was the first assassination of a president in history. A single bullet erased the decision by the people of the Union that Abraham Lincoln should be their president. It was stunning, an awful repudiation of the system that helped define them as a people, that they had been fighting for over the last four years, that had cost them such blood and treasure.

Yet the process endured. Reacting to the murder of the president newspapers throughout the country spoke of the need to "let law and order resume their sway," as the *San Francisco Chronicle* noted. "The law must reign supreme," the *Philadelphia Evening Bulletin* declared, "or in this great crisis chaos will overwhelm us, and our own maddening feeling bring upon us national wreck and ruin which traitor arms have failed to accomplish." More specifically there was admiration and recognition for a system that could overcome even assassination. "When Andrew Johnson was sworn in as President," the Reverend Joseph Thompson told a New York audience, "the Statue of Liberty that surmounts the dome of the Capitol and was put there by Lincoln, looked down on the city and on the nation and said 'Our Government is unchanged—it has merely passed from the hands of one man into those of another.'"

The words reflected part of a larger legacy. The Union was saved, and thus the political-constitutional process endured—the nation would change governments, settle controversies, and debate alternatives at the polls, in legislative halls, and in courtrooms, not on bloody battlefields. It would be a nation whose size and diversity gave it wealth and opportunities for its citizens and huge potential influence in the world. Future autocrats would have reason to fear that influence, just as future immigrants would be drawn to it. Its power would not always be used well. Native Americans who "obstructed" national mission, foreign governments deemed "un-American" had reason to fear and to protest against invasions of their rights and the destruction of their people. But within the nation itself, because of what it stood for and fought for and preserved, there remained a conscience that could be appealed to in the name of the ideals it symbolized and had demonstrated in its greatest war. Saving the Union had meant killing slavery.

Slavery was dead. Its power to divide the Union, to erode and destroy constitutional and political debate was over. No longer was the highest court in the land able to rule that under the Constitution black people had no rights that white people had to respect and that no political party legally could say otherwise. No longer could men, women, and children be bought and sold: treated as things without ties to each other, without the capacity to fulfill their own dreams. The Thirteenth Amendment, ending slavery throughout the nation and moving through the states toward ratification, ensured that. And in the vain of that amendment came protection for civil rights and suffrage. Blacks were promised that they would enter the political arena and the constitutional system—this time as participants, not as objects.

This more perfect Union was achieved chiefly through an extraordinary outreach of national authority. Certainly Lincoln extended presidential power beyond any limits seen before his time—the war demanded that; Congress agreed, the Supreme Court acquiesced, and the people sustained his power. If one compares Lincoln's use of power with executive actions before 1861, popular and even scholarly use of a word such as "dictatorship" makes limited sense. Lincoln had produced, as Edwin S. Corwin observes, "a complete transformation in the President's role as Commander in Chief." Yet war was about the expansion of power, and Congress also stepped forward, expanding national power, extending its authority. Even state governments reached further than precedent admitted, increasing expenditures, strengthening their police powers over health, morals, and safety, and establishing new regulatory agencies to shape the economy.

After the war public pressures demanded a return to peacetime boundaries. Executive authority in most areas, once the fight between Johnson and Congress was settled, rapidly contracted. A few outbursts of presidential influence showed that the White House was still occupied. Grant fought senators bitterly over the Santo Domingo Treaty and presided over an effective Treaty of Washington, which resolved claims against the British for building rebel raiders. Hayes sent federal troops to settle labor protests and worked for civil service reforms. Garfield, Arthur, and Harrison also kept busy; Cleveland's vetoes showed signs of vigor. Generally, however, the presidency declined in power. With the exception of Grant a series of one-term presidents did little to inspire demands that they stay in office. For the rest of the century no president came within miles of Lincoln's power or even close to Polk or Jackson, for that matter. By 1886 Woodrow Wilson was able to write that national government in the United States was "congressional government." M. Ostrogorsky, telling foreign audiences about America, described a lawmaking environment in which "after the [civil] war the eclipse of the executive was complete and definitive"; Lord Bryce told British and American audiences in 1894 that "the domestic authority of the President is in time of peace small." These late-nineteenth-century images may have inspired Theodore Lowi to assert in 1992 that "by 1875 you would not know there had been a war or a Lincoln."

But Lord Bryce had added a caveat about the president's domestic authority: In time of war, "especially in a civil war, it expands with portentous speed." Clearly it had been thus with Lincoln. Despite calls to retreat from the vast domains of Civil War there is a sense in which Lincoln's legacy of power in the presidency survived the retreat. Certainly presidential authority, like the national authority with which it was connected, diminished when the war was over. But national power was still available after Appomattox and for the fundamental purpose that had called it forth originally: to destroy slavery and its vestiges. The fight between Congress and Lincoln's successor has obscured the fact that congressional Republicans were acting in the same cause for which Lincoln had acted. They were not recapturing power lost to the president; they were claiming power that they had shared increasingly with Lincoln.

Before Lincoln died many of the more radical Republicans had been attacking him for moving too slowly toward emancipation and then for yielding too much to military necessity and Southern loyalists. After early statements of satisfaction with Johnson they quickly came to their senses as Johnson proved not only to be slower than Lincoln to march to their goals but also to be a bitter racist obstructionist. Thus they fought against Johnson and for goals that Lincoln had espoused and had used his power to try to achieve: civil rights, education, suffrage for the freedmen. The army, which had been the major instrument of Lincoln's expanding egalitarianism and which looked to its commander in chief for direction, shifted its allegiance to Congress. Soldiers such as Grant, whom Lincoln had charged with leading the army to save the Union, did not think it incongruous to support Congress in its battle to preserve the gains of war. And when legislators moved to weaken executive power over the army with the Tenure of Office and the Command of the Army acts, they were trying to save Lincoln's legacy by weakening Johnson.

Although President Grant retreated on other issues, he tried to protect former slaves from white Southerners' efforts to restore as much of the prewar South as they could. Grant sent troops into Louisiana, Mississippi, North Carolina, and South Carolina to effect the Force Acts and to destroy the Ku Klux Klan. A vocal element in the Republican party continued to push for federal intervention in the South in the form of national civil rights and suffrage-enforcement laws well into the 1890s. Despite retreating from the broadest definitions of federal power when it interpreted the Civil War amendments, the Supreme Court struck down laws that kept blacks off juries, and that denied Chinese Americans equal chances to work, and it upheld federal power to protect blacks from political violence. The Justice Department prosecuted thousands of election officers under this power. Local juries usually acquitted their white neighbors, but the national prohibition remained. Because of the Lincoln presidency the constitutional system carried promises of equality, and the processes to bring those promises to life endured. One hundred years after Lincoln had been awakened by the Kansas Nebraska Act to the dangers of slavery to the constitutional system, blacks and whites would see the United States Supreme Court strike down inequality in that system (that case would, interestingly enough, also involve Kansas).

Not every element, even in that reformed constitutional system, promised equal justice. The Union that Lincoln and his forces had saved remained a Union of states. Lincoln's respect for those states, demonstrated in his commitment to reconstruct them rather than to allow Congress to govern territories and in his insistence that only a constitutional amendment, ratified by states, would secure slavery's death, strengthened later arguments that states should control the fate of their citizens, old and new. Lincoln's abiding insistence that the Constitution guided his actions meant that black equality could be hindered or denied by constitutional claims of states' rights and local self-government. Brutal racism could find shelter in such legal arguments.

Yet the triumph and the irony of his administration resided in Lincoln's commitment to the Constitution; without that there would have been no promises to keep to 4 million black Americans. Because so many Americans cherished the Union that the Constitution forged, they made war on slave masters and their friends, on a government that Alexander Stephens claimed rested "on the great truth that the negro is not the equal of the white man; that slavery . . . is his natural and normal condition."

Without the president's devotion to and mastery of the political-constitutional institutions of his time, in all probability the Union would have lacked the capacity to focus its will and its resources on defeating that Confederacy. Without Lincoln's unmatched ability to integrate egalitarian ends and constitutional means he could not have enlisted the range of supporters and soldiers necessary for victory. His great accomplishment was to energize and mobilize the nation by affirming its better angels, by showing the nation at its best: engaged in the imperative, life-preserving conversation between structure and purpose, ideal and institution, means and ends.

PHILLIP SHAW PALUDAN (1938–2007) was a professor of history at the University of Kansas for over 30 years before accepting the distinguished chair in Lincoln studies at the University of Illinois, Springfield. In addition to his study of Lincoln's presidency, which won the Lincoln Prize, he is the author of *Victims: A True Story of the Civil War* (University of Tennessee Press, 1981) and *A People's Contest: The Union and Civil War, 1861–1865* (Harper & Row, 1988).

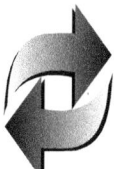

Melvin E. Bradford

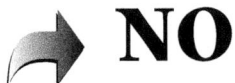

Remembering Who We Are: Observations of a Southern Conservative

The Lincoln Legacy: A Long View

With the time and manner of his death Abraham Lincoln, as leader of a Puritan people who had just won a great victory over "the forces of evil," was placed beyond the reach of ordinary historical inquiry and assessment. Through Booth's bullet he became the one who had "died to make men free," who had perished that his country's "new birth" might occur: a "second founder" who, in Ford's theater, had been transformed into an American version of the "dying god." Our common life, according to this construction, owes its continuation to the shedding of the sacred blood. Now after over a century of devotion to the myth of the "political messiah," it is still impossible for most Americans to see through and beyond the magical events of April 1865. However, Lincoln's daily purchase upon the ongoing business of the nation requires that we devise a way of setting aside the martyrdom to look behind it at Lincoln's place in the total context of American history and discover in him a major source of our present confusion, our distance from the republicanism of the Fathers, the models of political conduct which we profess most to admire. . . .

Of course, nothing that we can identify as part of Lincoln's legacy belongs to him alone. In some respects the Emancipator was carried along with the tides. Yet a measure of his importance is that he was at the heart of the major political events of his era. Therefore what signifies in a final evaluation of this melancholy man is that many of these changes in the country would never have come to pass had Lincoln not pushed them forward. Or at least not come so quickly, or with such dreadful violence. I will emphasize only the events that he most certainly shaped according to his relentless will, alterations in the character of our country for which he was clearly responsible. For related developments touched by Lincoln's wand, I can have only a passing word. The major charges advanced here, if proved, are sufficient to impeach the most famous and respected of public men. More would only overdo.

The first and most obvious item in my bill of particulars for indictment concerns Lincoln's dishonesty and obfuscation with respect to the nation's future obligations to the Negro, slave and free. It was of course an essential ingredient of Lincoln's position that he make a success at being anti-Southern or antislavery without at the same time appearing to be significantly impious about the beginnings of the Republic (which was neither anti-Southern nor antislavery)—or significantly pro-Negro. He was the first Northern politician of any rank to combine these attitudes into a viable platform persona, the first to make his moral position on slavery in the South into a part of his national politics. It was a posture that enabled him to unite elements of the Northern electorate not ordinarily willing to cooperate in any political undertaking. And thus enabled him to destroy the old Democratic majority—a coalition necessary to preserving the union of the states. Then came the explosion. But this calculated posturing has had more durable consequences than secession and the Federal confiscation of property in slaves. . . .

In the nation as a whole what moves toward fruition is a train of events set in motion by the duplicitous rhetoric concerning the Negro that helped make Abraham Lincoln into our first "sectional" president. Central to this appeal is a claim to a kind of moral superiority that costs absolutely nothing in the way of conduct. Lincoln, in insisting that the Negro was included in the promise of the Declaration of Independence and that the Declaration bound his countrymen to fulfill a pledge hidden in that document, seemed clearly to point toward a radical transformation of American society. Carried within his rejection of Negro slavery as a continuing feature of the American regime, his assertion that the equality clause of the Declaration of Independence was "the father of all moral principle among us," were certain muted corollaries. By promising that the peculiar institution would be made to disappear if candidates for national office adopted the proper "moral attitude" on that subject, Lincoln recited as a litany the

---

Bradford, Melvin E. "Remembering Who We Are: Observations of a Southern Conservative," *Modern Age*, Spring 1982. Copyright ©1982 by Intercollegiate Studies Institute. Used with permission.

general terms of his regard for universal human rights. But at the same time he added certain modifications to this high doctrine: modifications required by those of his countrymen to whom he hoped to appeal, by the rigid racism of the Northern electorate, and by "what his own feelings would admit." The most important of these reservations was that none of his doctrine should apply significantly to the Negro in the North. Or, after freedom, to what he could expect in the South. It was a very broad, very general, and very abstract principle to which he made reference. By it he could divide the sheep from the goats, the wheat from the chaff, the patriot from the conspirator. But for the Negro it provided nothing more than a technical freedom, best to be enjoyed far away. Or the valuable opportunity to "root, hog, or die." For the sake of such vapid distinctions he urged his countrymen to wade through seas of blood.

To be sure, this position does not push the "feelings" of that moralist who was our sixteenth president too far from what was comfortable for him. And it goes without saying that a commitment to "natural rights" which will not challenge the Black Codes of Illinois, which promises something like them for the freedman in the South, or else offers him as alternative the proverbial "one-way-ticket to nowhere" is a commitment of empty words. It is only an accident of political history that the final Reconstruction settlement provided a bit more for the former slave—principally, the chance to vote Republican; and even that "right" didn't last, once a better deal was made available to his erstwhile protectors. But the point is that Lincoln's commitment was precisely of the sort that the North was ready to make—while passing legislation to restrict the flow of Negroes into its own territories, elaborating its own system of segregation by race, and exploiting black labor through its representatives in a conquered South. Lincoln's double talk left his part of the country with a durable heritage of pious self-congratulation. . . .

The second heading in this "case against Lincoln" involves no complicated pleading. Neither will it confuse any reader who examines his record with care. For it has to do with Lincoln's political economy, his management of the commercial and business life of the part of the Republic under his authority. This material is obvious, even though it is not always connected with the presidency of Abraham Lincoln. Nevertheless, it must be developed at this point. For it leads directly into the more serious charges upon which this argument depends. It is customary to deplore the Gilded Age, the era of the Great Barbecue. It is true that many of the corruptions of the Republican Era came to a head after Lincoln lay at rest in Springfield. But it is a matter of fact that they began either under his direction or with his sponsorship. Military necessity, the "War for the Union," provided an excuse, an umbrella of sanction, under which the essential nature of the changes being made in the relation of government to commerce could be concealed. Of his total policy the Northern historian Robert Sharkey has written, "Human ingenuity would have had difficulty in contriving a more perfect engine for class and sectional exploration, creditors finally obtaining the upper hand as opposed to debtors, and the developed East holding the whip over the underdeveloped West and South." Until the South left the Union, until a High Whig sat in the White House, none of this return to the "energetic government" of Hamilton's design was possible. Indeed, even in the heyday of the Federalists it had never been so simple a matter to translate power into wealth. Now Lincoln could try again the internal improvements of the early days in Illinois. The difference was that this time the funding would not be restrained by political reversal or a failure of credit. For if anything fell short, Mr. Salmon P. Chase, "the foreman" of his "green printing office," could be instructed "to give his paper mill another turn." And the inflationary policy of rewarding the friends of the government sustained. The euphemism of our time calls this "income redistribution." But it was theft in 1864, and is theft today.

A great increase in the tariff and the formation of a national banking network were, of course, the cornerstones of this great alteration in the posture of the Federal government toward the sponsorship of business. From the beginning of the Republican Party Lincoln warned his associates not to talk about their views on these subjects. Their alliance, he knew, was a negative thing: a league against the Slave Power and its Northern friends. But in private he made it clear that the hidden agenda of the Republicans would have its turn, once the stick was in their hand. In this he promised well. Between 1861 and 1865, the tariff rose from 18.84 percent to 47.56 percent. And it stayed above 40 percent in all but two years of the period concluded with the election of Woodrow Wilson. Writes the Virginia historian Ludwell H. Johnson, it would "facilitate a massive transfer of wealth, satisfying the dreariest predictions of John C. Calhoun." The new Republican system of banking (for which we should note Lincoln was directly accountable) was part of the same large design of "refounding." The National Banking Acts of 1863 and 1864, with the earlier Legal Tender Act, flooded the country with $480 million of fiat money that was soon depreciated by about two-thirds in relation to specie. Then all notes but the greenback dollar were taxed out of existence, excepting only United States Treasury bonds that all banks were required to purchase if they were to have a share in the war boom. The support for these special bonds was thus the debt itself—Hamilton's old standby. Specie disappeared. Moreover, the bank laws controlled the money supply, credit, and the balance of power. New banks and credit for farms, small businesses, or small town operations were discouraged. And the Federalist model, after four score and seven years, finally achieved.

As chief executive, Lincoln naturally supported heavy taxes. Plus a scheme of tax graduation. The war was a legitimate explanation for these measures. Lincoln's participation in huge subsidies or bounties for railroads and in other legislation granting economic favors is not so readily linked to "saving the Union." All of his life Lincoln was a friend of the big corporations. He had no moral problem in signing a bill which gifted the Union Pacific Railway with a huge strip of land running across the West and an almost unsecured loan of $16,000 to $48,000 per mile of track. The final result of this bill was the Credit Mobilier scandal. With other laws favoring land speculation it helped to negate the seemingly noble promise of the Homestead Act of 1862—under which less than 19 percent of the open lands settled between 1860 and 1900 went to legitimate homesteaders. The Northern policy of importing immigrants with the promise of this land, only to force them into the ranks of General Grant's meatgrinder or into near slavery in the cities of the East, requires little comment. Nor need we belabor the rotten army contracts given to politically faithful crooks. Nor the massive thefts by law performed during the war in the South. More significant is Lincoln's openly disgraceful policy of allowing special cronies and favorites of his friends to trade in Southern cotton—even with "the enemy" across the line—and his calculated use of the patronage and the pork barrel. Between 1860 and 1880, the Republicans spent almost $10 million breathing life into state and local Republican organizations. Lincoln pointed them down that road. There can be no doubt of his responsibility for the depressing spectacle of greed and peculation concerning which so many loyal Northern men of the day spoke with sorrow, disappointment, and outrage....

A large part of the complaint against Lincoln as a political precedent for later declensions from the example of the Fathers has to do with his expansion of the powers of the presidency and his alteration of the basis for the Federal Union. With reference to his role in changing the office of chief magistrate from what it had been under his predecessors, it is important to remember that he defined himself through the war powers that belonged to his post. In this way Lincoln could profess allegiance to the Whig ideal of the modest, self-effacing leader, the antitype of Andrew Jackson, and, in his capacity as Commander-in-Chief, do whatever he wished. That is, if he could do it in the name of preserving the Union. As Clinton Rossiter has stated, Lincoln believed there were "no limits" to his powers if he exercised them in that "holy cause." Gottfried Dietze compares Lincoln in this role to the Committee of Public Safety as it operated in the French Revolution. Except for the absence of mass executions, the results were similar. War is of course the occasion for concentration of power and the limitation of liberties within any nation. But an internal war, a war between states in a union of states, is not like a war to repel invasion or to acquire territory. For it is an extension into violence of a domestic political difference. And it is thus subject to extraordinary abuses of authority—confusions or conflations of purpose which convert the effort to win the war into an effort to effect even larger, essentially political changes in the structure of government. War, in these terms, is not only an engine for preserving the Union; it is also an instrument for transforming its nature. But without overdeveloping this structure of theory, let us shore it up with specific instances of presidential misconduct by Lincoln: abuses that mark him as our first imperial president. Lincoln began his tenure as a dictator when between April 12 and July 4 of 1861, without interference from Congress, he summoned militia, spent millions, suspended law, authorized recruiting, decreed a blockade, defied the Supreme Court, and pledged the nation's credit. In the following months and years he created units of government not known to the Constitution and officers to rule over them in "conquered" sections of the South, seized property throughout both sections, arrested upwards of twenty thousand of his political enemies and confined them without trial in a Northern "Gulag," closed over three hundred newspapers critical of his policy, imported an army of foreign mercenaries (of perhaps five hundred thousand men), interrupted the assembly of duly elected legislatures and employed the Federal hosts to secure his own reelection—in a contest where about thirty-eight thousand votes, if shifted, might have produced an armistice and a negotiated peace under a President McClellan. To the same end he created a state in West Virginia, arguing of this blatant violation of the explicit provisions of the Constitution that it was "expedient." But the worst of this bold and ruthless dealing (and I have given but a very selective list of Lincoln's "high crimes") has to do with his role as military leader per se: as the commander and selector of Northern generals, chief commissary of the Federal forces, and head of government in dealing with the leaders of an opposing power. In this role the image of Lincoln grows to be very dark—indeed, almost sinister.

The worst that we may say of Lincoln is that he led the North in war so as to put the domestic political priorities of his political machine ahead of the lives and the well-being of his soldiers in the field. The appointment of the venal Simon Cameron of Pennsylvania as his secretary of war, and of lesser hacks and rascals to direct the victualing of Federal armies, was part of this malfeasance. By breaking up their bodies, the locust hoard of contractors even found a profit in the Union dead. And better money still in the living. They made of Lincoln (who winked at their activities) an accessory to lost horses, rotten meat, and worthless guns. But all such mendacity was nothing in comparison to the price in blood paid for Lincoln's attempts to give the nation a genuine Republican hero. He had a problem with this project throughout the entire course of the war. That is, until Grant and Sherman "converted" to radicalism. Prior to their emergence all of Lincoln's "loyal" generals disapproved of either his politics or of his character. These, as with McClellan, he could use and discharge at will. Or demote to minor tasks. One thinks immediately of George G. Meade—who defeated Lee at Gettysburg, and yet made the mistake of defining himself as the defender of a separate Northern nation from whose soil he would drive a foreign Southern "invader." Or of Fitz John Porter, William B. Franklin, and Don Carlos Buell—all scapegoats thrown by Lincoln to the radical wolves. In place of these heterodox professionals, Lincoln assigned such champions of the "new freedom" as Nathaniel P. ("Commissary") Banks, Benjamin F. ("Beast") Butler, John C. Fremont, and John A. McClernand. Speaking in summary despair of these appointments (and adding to my list, Franz Sigel and Lew Wallace), General Henry Halleck, Lincoln's chief-of-staff, declared that they were "little better than murder." Yet in the East, with the Army of the Potomac, Lincoln made promotions even more difficult to defend, placing not special projects, divisions, and brigades but entire commands under the authority of such "right thinking" incompetents as John Pope (son of an old crony in Illinois) and "Fighting Joe" Hooker. Or with that "tame" Democrat and late favorite of the radicals, Ambrose E. Burnside. Thousands of Northern boys lost their lives in order that the Republican Party might experience rejuvenation, to serve its partisan goals. And those were "party supremacy within a Northern dominated Union." A Democratic "man-on-horseback" could not serve those ends, however faithful to "the Constitution as it is, and the Union as it was" (the motto of the Democrats) they might be. For neither of these commitments promised a Republican hegemony. To provide for his faction both security and continuity in office, Lincoln sounded out his commanders in correspondence (much of which still survives), suborned their military integrity, and employed their focus in purely political operation. Writes Johnson:

> Although extreme measures were most common in the border states, they were often used elsewhere too. By extreme measures is meant the arrest of anti-Republican candidates and voters, driving anti-Republican voters from the polls or forcing them to vote the Republican ticket, preventing opposition parties from holding meetings, removing names from ballots, and so forth. These methods were employed in national, state and local elections. Not only did the army interfere by force, it was used to supply votes. Soldiers whose states did not allow absentee voting were sent home by order of the President to swell the Republican totals. When voting in the field was used, Democratic commissioners carrying ballots to soldiers from their state were . . . unceremoniously thrown into prison, while Republican agents were offered every assistance. Votes of Democratic soldiers were sometimes discarded as defective, replaced by Republican ballots, or simply not counted.

All Lincoln asked of the ordinary Billy Yank was that he be prepared to give himself up to no real purpose—at least until Father Abraham found a general with the proper moral and political credentials to lead him on to Richmond. How this part of Lincoln's career can be reconciled to the myth of the "suffering savior" I cannot imagine.

We might dwell for some time on what injury Lincoln did to the dignity of his office through the methods he employed in prosecuting the war. It was no small thing to disavow the ancient Christian code of "limited war," as did his minions, acting in his name. However, it is enough in this connection to remember his policy of denying medicines to the South, even for the sake of Northern prisoners held behind the lines. We can imagine what a modern "war crimes" tribunal would do with that decision. There may have been practicality in such inhumane decisions. *Practicality* indeed! As Charles Francis Adams, Lincoln's ambassador to the Court of St. James and the scion of the most notable family in the North, wrote in his diary of his leader, the "President and his chief advisers are not without the spirit of the serpent mixed in with their wisdom." And he knew whereof he spoke. For practical politics, the necessities of the campaign of 1864, had led Lincoln and Seward to a decision far more serious than unethical practices against prisoners and civilians in the South. I speak of the rejection by the Lincoln administration of peace feelers authorized by the Confederate government in Richmond: feelers that met Lincoln's announced terms for an end to the Federal invasion of the South. The emissary in this negotiation was sponsored by Charles Francis Adams. He was a Tennessean living in France, one Thomas Yeatman. After arriving in the United States, he was swiftly deported by direct order of the government before he could properly explore the possibility of an armistice on the conditions of reunion and an end to slavery. Lincoln sought these goals, but only on his terms. And in his own time. He wanted total victory. And he needed a still-resisting, impenitent Confederacy to justify his re-election. We can only speculate as to why President Davis allowed the Yeatman mission. We know that he expected little of such peace feelers. (There were many in the last stages of the conflict.) He knew his enemy too well to expect anything but subjection, however benign the rhetoric used to disguise its rigor. Adams's peace plan was perhaps impossible, even if his superiors in Washington had behaved in good faith. The point is that none of the peace moves of 1864 was given any chance of success. Over one hundred thousand Americans may have died because of the Rail-Splitter's rejection of an inexpedient peace. Yet we have still not touched upon the most serious of Lincoln's violations of the Presidential responsibility. I speak, finally, of his role in bringing on the War Between the States.

There is, we should recall, a great body of scholarly argument concerning Lincoln's intentions in 1860 and early 1861. A respectable portion of this work comes to the conclusion that the first Republican president expected a "tug," a "crisis," to follow his election. And then, once secession had occurred, also expected to put it down swiftly with a combination of persuasion, force, and Southern loyalty to the Union. The last of these, it is agreed, he completely overestimated. In a similar fashion he exaggerated the force of Southern "realism," the region's capacity to act in its own pecuniary interest. The authority on Lincoln's political economy has remarked that the Illinois lawyer-politician and old line Whig always made the mistake of explaining in simple economic terms the South's hostile reaction to anti-slavery proposals. To that blunder he added the related mistake of attempting to end the "rebellion" with the same sort of simplistic appeals to the prospect of riches. Or with fear of a servile insurrection brought on by his greatest "war measure," the emancipation of slaves behind Southern lines, beyond his control. A full-scale Southern revolution, a revolution of all classes of men against the way he and some of his supporters thought, was beyond his imagination. There was no "policy" in such extravagant behavior, no human nature as he perceived it. Therefore, on the basis of my understanding of his overall career, I am compelled to agree with Charles W. Ramsdell concerning Lincoln and his war. Though he was no sadist and no warmonger, and though he got for his pains much more of a conflict than he had in mind, Lincoln hoped for an "insurrection" of some sort—an "uprising" he could use.

The "rational" transformation of our form of government which he had first predicted in the "Springfield Lyceum Speech" required some kind of passionate disorder to justify the enforcement of a new Federalism. And needed also for the voting representatives of the South to be out of their seats in the Congress. It is out of keeping with his total performance as a public man and in contradiction of his campaigning after 1854 not to believe that Lincoln hoped for a Southern attack on Fort Sumter. As he told his old friend Senator Orville H. Browning of Illinois: "The plan succeeded. They attacked Sumter—it fell, and thus did more service than it otherwise could." And to others he wrote or spoke to the same effect. If the Confederacy's offer of money for Federal property were made known in the North and business relations of the sections remained unaffected, if the Mississippi remained open to Northern shipping, there would be no support for "restoring" the Union on a basis of force. Americans were in the habit of thinking of the unity of the nation as a reflex of their agreement in the Constitution, of law as limit on government and on the authority of temporary majorities, and of revisions in law as the product of the ordinary course of push and pull within a pluralistic society, not as a response to the extralegal authority of some admirable abstraction like equality. In other words, they thought of the country as being defined by the way in which we conducted our political business, not by where we were trying to go in a body. Though once a disciple of Henry Clay, Lincoln changed the basis of our common bond away from the doctrine of his mentor, away from the patterns of compromise and dialectic of interests and values under a limited, Federal sovereignty with which we as a people began our adventure with the Great Compromise of 1787–1788. The nature of the Union left to us by Lincoln is thus always at stake in every major election, in every refinement in our civil theology; the Constitution is still to be defined by the latest wave of big ideas, the most recent mass emotion. Writes Dietze:

> Concentrations of power in the national and executive branches of government, brought about by Lincoln in the name of the people, were processes that conceivably complemented each other to the detriment of free government. Lincoln's

administration thus opened the way for the development of an omnipotent national executive who as a spokesman for the people might consider himself entitled to do whatever he felt was good for the Nation, irrespective of the interests and rights of states, Congress, the judiciary, and the individual....

But in my opinion the capstone of this case against Lincoln . . . is what he has done to the language of American political discourse that makes it so difficult for us to reverse the ill effects of trends he set in motion with his executive fiat. When I say that Lincoln was our first Puritan president, I am chiefly referring to a distinction of style, to his habit of wrapping up his policy in the idiom of Holy Scripture, concealing within the Trojan horse of his gasconade and moral superiority an agenda that would never have been approved if presented in any other form. It is this rhetoric in particular, a rhetoric confirmed in its authority by his martyrdom, that is enshrined in the iconography of the Lincoln myth preserved against examination by monuments such as the Lincoln Memorial, where his oversized likeness is elevated above us like that of a deified Roman emperor....

MELVIN E. BRADFORD (1934–1993) was a professor of literature at the University of Dallas from 1967 until his death. His publications include *Against the Barbarians and Other Reflections on Familiar Themes* (University of Missouri Press, 1992) and *Original Intentions: On the Making and Ratification of the United States Constitution* (University of Georgia Press, 1993).

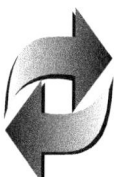

EXPLORING THE ISSUE

Was Abraham Lincoln America's Greatest President?

Critical Thinking and Reflection

1. What were the major issues Abraham Lincoln faced as president of the United States, and how effective was he in addressing these matters?
2. What were Lincoln's major goals in the Civil War?
3. How did Lincoln respond to his opponents during the war?
4. Based on your understanding of his leadership during the Civil War, was Abraham Lincoln an effective commander-in-chief?
5. What approach did President Lincoln take with respect to the institution of slavery?

Is There Common Ground?

Historians consistently rank Abraham Lincoln in the highest echelon of American presidents even when they do not place him in the top spot. Over the years, Lincoln has had competition from George Washington, mainly for being the first president and providing a sterling role model for those who followed, and Franklin D. Roosevelt, for his leadership during the Great Depression and most of World War II. Nevertheless, Lincoln more often than not ends up on the top of the heap. Melvin Bradford's assessment, therefore, is extreme in its departure from tradition. At the same time, however, most Lincoln scholars, without embracing many of Bradford's specific conclusions, would agree that during the Civil War, Lincoln plumbed the well of executive powers and found it almost limitless. Lincoln himself told Senator Chandler in 1864, "I conceive that I may in this emergency do things on military grounds which cannot be done constitutionally even by Congress." To this end, he suspended the writ of habeas corpus, suppressed hostile newspapers, declared a blockade of southern ports before war was declared, raised a national army without an enabling act, and prepared for the reconstruction of the Union without seeking anyone's advice on how best to proceed. Clearly, however, most historians view these steps as necessary in prosecuting the war against the recalcitrant Southerners who formed the Confederacy.

Additional Resources

Gabor S. Boritt, ed., *The Historian's Lincoln: Pseudohistory, Psychohistory, and History* (University of Illinois Press, 1988)

David Donald, *Lincoln* (Simon & Schuster, 1996)

Allen C. Guelzo, *Lincoln's Emancipation Proclamation: The End of Slavery in America* (Simon & Schuster, 2004)

Mark E. Neely, Jr., *The Fate of Liberty: Abraham Lincoln and Civil Liberties* (Oxford University Press, 1991)

Stephen B. Oates, *With Malice Toward None: The Life of Abraham Lincoln* (Harper & Row, 1977)

Internet References . . .

Abraham Lincoln Historical Digitization Project

lincoln.lib.niu.edu/

Abraham Lincoln Institute

www.abrahamlincoln.org/

Abraham Lincoln Online

www.abrahamlincolnonline.org/

American President—Abraham Lincoln (1809–1865)

millercenter.org/president/lincoln

Two Hundred Years of Abraham Lincoln

www.smithsonianmag.com/history-archaeology/life-of-lincoln.html

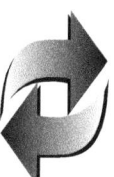

ISSUE

Selected, Edited, and with Issue Framing Material by:
Kevin R. Magill and Tony L. Talbert, *Baylor University*

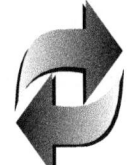

Did Reconstruction Fail as a Result of Racism?

YES: Lisa J. McLeod, from "Transubstantiation of Andrew Johnson: White Epistemic Failure in Du Bois' Black Reconstruction," *Phylon* (2014)

NO: Adam Fairclough, from "Was the Grant of Black Suffrage a Political Error? Reconsidering the Views of John W. Burgess, William A. Dunning, and Eric Foner on Congressional Reconstruction," *Journal of the Historical Society* (2012)

Learning Outcomes

After reading this issue, you will be able to:

- Explain the major tenets of whiteness studies and the concept of "racial bribery."
- Explain President Andrew Johnson's hopes for Reconstruction.
- Understand the basic arguments of Burgess, Dunning, and Foner regarding Reconstruction.
- Identify the benefits and issues surrounding black suffrage.
- Explain the arguments for Congress' enactment of black suffrage as being a failure.

ISSUE SUMMARY

YES: Lisa J. McLeod discusses W. E. B. Du Bois's *Black Reconstruction* to highlight white people's epistemic and moral failure in the Post–Civil War era. President Johnson went from poor white farmer to champion of the plantation owner. McLeod suggests that the failed legacy of Reconstruction continues to affect social institutions and white consciousness today.

NO: Adam Fairclough believes that policy regarding the integration of African Americans into the political process ensured Reconstruction would be unsuccessful. He suggests that more radical policy and a political revolution would have been required for an effective Reconstruction.

Issue Framing with Justin Kruger

Given the complexities of the post–civil war years, it is unsurprising that Reconstruction (1865–1877) is a controversial historical time period in the United States. For the better part of a century following the war, historians typically characterized Reconstruction as a total failure that had proved detrimental to all Americans—Northerners and Southerners, whites and blacks. Prior to 1960s, this was the thinking of many historians who wrote about this era from two basic assumptions: first, that the South was capable of solving its own problems without federal government interference and second, the former slaves were intellectually inferior to whites and incapable of running a democratic government. From this interpretation, a vengeful Congress, dominated by radical Republicans, imposed military rule upon the southern states. Carpetbaggers from the North, along with traitorous white scalawags and their black accomplices in the South, established coalition governments that rewrote state constitutions, raised taxes, looted state treasuries, and disenfranchised former Confederates while extending the ballot to the freedmen. This era finally ended in 1877 when courageous southern White Democrats successfully "redeemed" their region from "Negro rule" by toppling the Republican state governments.

There can be little doubt that racism played a major role in this interpretation, and historians, potentially, failed to recognize the complex nuances of this period. Many academics such as W. E. B. Du Bois challenged this traditional historical thinking but received little notice in mainstream American scholarship. However, after the 1960s, we began to see historians revisit this period with new questions and increased attention to Du Bois's scholarship. One such question being, why were the Radical Republicans unable to complete their vision for fully integrating Freedmen into society? Another asking how might their vision otherwise have come to fruition? Several historians suggest that the Fourteenth and Fifteenth Amendments could have only been adopted under the conditions of a *more* radical reconstruction. Certain historians also suggest that this never could have been the case because of the nation's commitment to free labor was an ideology barrier to postwar assistance and relational progress. Perhaps too it is fair to say that the alienating wage slavery and poor wages we see for people today is the neoliberal evolution of the Southern legacy of slavery and the oppressive, but better working conditions in the industrial North.

Nuancing these newer arguments, some have noted positives have also come from Reconstruction. Some scholars argue that state constitutions written in the South were some of the most democratic documents up to that time—a time when Freedman *took* their voting and economic rights. Eric Foner claims that Reconstruction, while perhaps not all that radical, offered African Americans at least a temporary vision of a free society, and that Freedmen were better treated than freed slaves in other societies. He claims that although Freedmen had been stripped of their rights the majority of Southern states by 1900, during Reconstruction they had cultivated a legacy of freedom that would inspire future generations of African Americans. Perhaps then the questions should not be about the failure of Reconstruction but about how ideology allowed the promise of the Radical Republicans die. Conversely, C. Vann Woodward claims, in "Reconstruction: A Counterfactual Playback," an essay in *The Future of the Past* (Oxford University Press, 1988), that Foner's conclusions are erroneous by offering evidence that former slaves were in fact as poorly treated in the United States as they were in other countries. He also maintains that confiscating former plantations and redistributing land to former slaves would have failed in the same way that the Homestead Act of 1862 failed to generate equal distribution of government lands to poor white settlers. From this perspective, many debate if redistribution would have led to a more peaceful and egalitarian society.

The following articles offer us an interesting discussion of race and politics during Reconstruction. Lisa McLeod draws on W. E. B. Du Bois' *Black Reconstruction in America: 1860–1888* to argue that the white supremacy directed society post–Civil War and should be considered front and center in the failure of Reconstruction. To her, the overarching ideology of whiteness and its supremacy was present in all aspects of society during Reconstruction. Du Bois wrote *Black Reconstruction* in 1935 as a rebuttal to the other histories of the day, many of which are now referred to as white supremacist histories. His argument suggests Reconstruction was considered a disaster, primarily because of its effects on whites. McLeod offers that racism, while rampant prior and during the Civil War, was not inevitable. She contends that poor white workers could have found common ground along economic and class lines with newly freed blacks. Instead, she argues, a racial commitment to whiteness became as central to Reconstruction as did overt racism. Poor whites allying with rich whites allowed for race to supersede class.

McLeod then lays out the foundation for President Andrew Johnson's vision of Reconstruction and his vision for white society. She highlights his political decision and norms, which led to white ignorance, oppression, and white supremacy. McLeod further asserts that Johnson did not consider blacks to be fully human and did not think of them when imagining the post–Civil War U.S. South. Accordingly, this thinking guided President Johnson's actions and are present in the stereotypes he drew on when describing African Americans, in limiting reparations and social supports, and limiting black voting rights (which he thought would start a race war and be unfair to whites). Even in meetings, Johnson showed racism in describing interactions with black academics, clergy, and troops.

President Johnson also fundamentally believed that blacks were no worse off than poor whites. During Reconstruction, blacks believed the "American Assumption" that hard work would equal wealth. McLeod argues that Johnson's "white ignorance" led him to completely ignore the lack of opportunities available to blacks and the constant threats of physical violence during Reconstruction. McLeod provides examples where Johnson, time and again, fell to racist understandings that positioned blacks as more than livestock, but less than human. They were "humanoid entities" to him—entitled to some rights but less than those afforded whites.

In the second article, Fairclough examines the works of three prominent white Reconstruction historians: John W. Burgess (early 1900s), William A. Dunning (up to the 1930s), and Eric Foner (contemporary). He asserts that history is constantly rewritten to address the needs and desires of a time, a place, and a people. Therefore, the early views of Reconstruction via historians like Dunning and Burgess need to be reconsidered, as did Foner's 1988 classic, *Reconstruction: America's Unfinished Revolution, 1863–1877*. Dunning and Burgess argue that Reconstruction was bad for whites and see Reconstruction as a major political blunder that could have been avoided. To Fairclough, the unfortunate assertions of racism (i.e., black inferiority) espoused by both Burgess and Dunning does not automatically invalidate their other claims about the reasons for the failure of Reconstruction (i.e., constitutional, legal, economic, and political issues). Specifically, Fairclough agrees that Dunning's assertion that black suffrage was a political error and a major failure of Reconstruction. With Burgess, Fairclough also agrees that Johnson's implementation of black codes and the vetoing of the Freedmen's Bureau and civil rights bills were massive mistakes.

Fairclough also highlights the thinking of Dunning and Burgess noting that the mistake of Black suffrage is not that it was attempted, but that it was not properly protected and enacted by Congress. To them, the national government did not go far enough to produce a law-abiding South protecting African American from the violence levied by angry white southerners. In their estimation, Southern states were let back into the United States much too quickly because Northern Republicans believed black suffrage "would facilitate a swift termination of military rule and constitute a guarantee of loyalty on the part of readmitted states." Viewed as a cheap alternative to prolonged military occupation of the South, the passage of black suffrage offered no protections to blacks against the physical violence or against state governments who used "fraud, intimidation, violence, and legislation" to limit/erase newly minted black voting rights in the South. Foner conversely argues that the passage and promise of black suffrage was a success because it included freedom even despite of its poor enactment. To Fairclough, though, the failure of the federal government to sustain protections for African Americans in the South is a major reason Reconstruction failed. He suggests the extent of racial opposition and violence toward blacks was underestimated. The article offers a new look at Dunning and Burgess, who for many had been cast aside because of their white supremacist sympathies in Reconstruction. While Fairclough notes the abhorrent racial attitudes of their writings, he also acknowledges that some of their arguments are valid (i.e., black suffrage was a failure because Congress did not use enough federal power to ensure its success, rather they abdicated responsibility to state governments who almost immediately limited it).

Many academics now discussing the idea of reparations as a way to make up for the failure of Reconstruction to adequately create a new society. Modern society was built on the backs of slaves. African Americans have largely been unable to share in the economic, social, or existential material bounty of their struggle. Clear and targeted historical disenfranchisement of Africa Americans still pervades almost every aspect of social life in both the North and South. Educational, judicial, relational, political, and economic, disenfranchisement, and the racist legacy of Reconstruction are due to U.S. societies' unwillingness to enforce basic human rights.

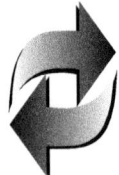

YES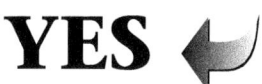

Lisa J. McLeod

Transubstantiation of Andrew Johnson: White Epistemic Failure in Du Bois' Black Reconstruction

Introduction

The depth and breadth of Du Bois' vision cannot be ignored; his work can and should be recognized as giving meaning to several areas of study. In this chapter, I advance that Du Bois was specifically a pioneer in the systematic and critical study of whiteness in the United States, as well as a global phenomenon. Whiteness, I argue, was a central concern for Du Bois from his earliest published work to the end of his life nearly 60 years later; while I am not the first to make such a claim (see, e.g., Hancock; Owen; Rabaka; Shuford; Sullivan), my focus here is upon his 1935 masterpiece, Black Reconstruction in America: 1860–1888. Black Reconstruction is perhaps most known for its groundbreaking revision of white supremacist histories describing the "disastrous" aftermath of the Civil War (718), including Du Bois' demonstration of the devastating role that race consciousness played in the American labor movement: the well-known "psychological wages of whiteness" that prevented white workers from aligning themselves with black workers against the white moneyed class (700; see also Roediger, passim). However, Black Reconstruction also suggests that white supremacy drove many of the legal, political, and economic developments that emerged post-Reconstruction and continued well into the 20th century. Du Bois holds that the white South's campaign to exploit and brutalize the black population did not end in 1865, but began a steady march of triumph, with few stumbles to the end of the 19th century. With the final withdrawal of the federal government from the South, the end of Reconstruction left black southerners, Du Bois tells us, "near naked to their enemies" (670).

Black Reconstruction is, of course, an epic work—more than 700 pages divided into 17 chapters and is a rich source of documentation and analysis along several themes. Regarding the growth of white supremacy and its postwar role, the book offers an extensive and detailed analysis that has yet to be fully appreciated. In this paper, my primary focus is on chapter VIII, "The Transubstantiation of a Poor White." Du Bois demonstrates in this, the longest chapter, that the infamous "choice" presented to poor white southerners to ally with wealthy whites or poor blacks was first made just a few short weeks after his elevation to the presidency by Andrew Johnson, "the most pitiful figure of American history" (22). By describing with great sensitivity Johnson's limitations at this pivotal moment, Du Bois provides an incisive portrait of "whiteness"—one installment in his ongoing discursive engagement with that phenomenon. His identification of whiteness' ontological myths and epistemic shortcomings anticipates much of the work done by philosophers of race at the end of the 20th century.

The Tragedy of Reconstruction: An Overview

While it will come as no surprise that racial justice did not spring into being, fully formed, after the Treaty of Appomattox, many Americans do not understand the extent to which white supremacy explicitly undermined the potential for racial equality in the decades following the Civil War. In Black Reconstruction, Du Bois demonstrates that this outcome was not, in some deep sense, inevitable. The defeat of the Confederacy and end of American institutional slavery might have motivated the majority of white American workers to find common cause with the formerly enslaved black Americans to negotiate with the monied interests against which both groups were arrayed. According to Du Bois, "the white laborers realized that Negroes were part of a group of millions of workers who were slaves by law, and whose competition kept white labor out of the work of the South and threatened its wages and stability in the North" (p. 19). That they identified instead with wealthy white and expended valuable energy to demean not only black labor but black Americans across social circumstances is a key moment in the development of white supremacy. Crucially, Andrew Johnson not only reflects this racial moment but acts to encourage white racial loyalty at every juncture.

For Du Bois, Johnson's ascent to the presidency made him "the real emancipator of four millions of black slaves, . . . [w]hat more splendid opportunity could the champion of labor and the exploited have had to start a nation towards freedom?" (p. 252). This comment, I think, Is not merely Du Boisian sarcasm, for not only might Johnson have seen the economic interests linking white and black labor against the plantocracy and Northern industry, but his own personal sense of worth as a hard-working common man should have (and certainly had in the past) driven his policy choices. Instead, Johnson's racial commitments—both conscious and perhaps less so—set the stage for the "Redemption" of the South, a wave of brutal violence that by 1900 saw the disfranchisement of African Americans in every Southern state. The Supreme Court's legal validation of Jim Crow affirmed white supremacy three decades *after* the end of the Civil War (*Plessy v. Ferguson*, 163 U.S. 537, 1896).

Du Bois tells us that if no black Americans had survived the Civil War, "peace would have been difficult because of hatred, loss, and bitter grief. *But its logical path would have been straight*" (238, emphasis added). That is, the reconciliation of North and South would have involved negotiations over the points of contention at stake in the war, with the North entitled to the privileges of the victor—presumably the subjugation of the South, including the confiscation of Southern land and great influence in its subsequent political restructuring. Instead, Du Bois argues, the white leaders of the North and South faced each other in light of a shared goal that overrode any motive the North may have had to subjugate the South: the continued depression of wages (and prices of raw materials) achieved through the availability of unpaid black labor. The black man, he writes, "loom[ed] like a dark ghost on the horizon. He was the child of force and greed, and the father of wealth and war" (238).

As mentioned above, in simple economic terms, white labor *should* have allied themselves with those who were newly freed from slavery and thus shared their interest in just compensation; that they did not require explanation. Du Bois claims that the threat of previously enslaved African Americans gaining "civil and political rights, education and land" prompted white labor to overcome their former alienation from the plantocracy. "The Poor White South," for Du Bois, "deserted its economic class and itself" choosing instead "racial bribery" (p. 239). Indeed, he writes, white workers were seduced by what he calls the "American idea" according to their envisioning themselves as "future exploiters" (17). For the majority of whites, then, maintaining the basic economic conditions of the Antebellum South—especially the tremendous social and economic gap between black labor and white—had great appeal.

This objective might appear to us inimical to the triumphal narrative of "the war that freed the slaves," but this tension only demonstrates the complexity of the material and ideological motivations that emerged and evolved during the Civil War. For example, the abolition—democrats, a coalition of progressive members of Congress and black activists that Du Bois christened thusly, did conceive of the Union victory as an opportunity to enact the conviction that "the reduction of a human being to real estate was a crime against humanity" (20). According to Du Bois, they openly challenged the social and political elevation of whites with proposed legislation designed to mandate racial equality:

> Only one forward step President Lincoln insisted upon and that was the real continued freedom of the emancipated slave; but the abolition-democracy went beyond this because it was convinced that here was no logical stopping place; and it looked forward to civil and political rights, education and land, as the only complete guarantee of freedom, in the face of a dominant South which hoped from the first, to abolish slavery only in name (239).

That the vision of the abolition democrats eventually gave way to a resurrected South, for Du Bois, is prefigured in the person of Andrew Johnson.

White Ignorance and White Supremacy in Theory

"Whiteness studies" emerged in the 1990s as a relatively late offshoot of critical race theory (Delgado and Stefancic, 1997). For my purposes, its relevant insights can be formulated as follows: (1) "white" is a racial identity, and whites have a race; (2) whether or not all white people can be said to be racists, all white people do benefit from structural racism, which might better be termed "white supremacy," and (3) white people tend to be ignorant of (1) and (2), assuming that their experiences are race-neutral, and free from racial entanglements unless and until they interact with people of color. While Du Bois is not often cited as a key theorist of whiteness, his analysis of Andrew Johnson presents a rich and compelling illustration of the sort of white racial myopia central to the insights of whiteness studies.

Black Reconstruction is, of course, recognized for its explanation of the role of whiteness in American class conflicts (e.g., Roediger). Du Bois' discussion of Johnson's particular affliction is less often noted, but tremendously significant in illustrating how the maintenance of white identity—and white supremacy—required that whites not only deny their material interests but also compromise their ability to accurately perceive the world around them. In this regard, Du Bois anticipates the work of philosopher Charles Mills and others on the phenomenon of "white ignorance" (Mills et al., in Sullivan and Tuana). In this paper, I focus on two elements of Mills' critique that resonate with Du Bois' examination of Andrew Johnson: first, the often *explicit* conviction that black Americans are "subhuman"; and second, that white epistemic tendencies discourage many (mostly White) people from accurately perceiving the abundant evidence *against* the lesser humanity of African-descended people. Mills calls the predictable confluence of these fundamentally flawed epistemic norms "white ignorance" (24–25).

Due to such cognitive biases, many (but not all or only) white Americans fail to question or seek explanation for quite obvious and predictable differences in life chances that (on average) separate along race lines. Whether or not they are aware of it, those afflicted with white ignorance assume that such inequalities are explicable in terms of the failings of people of color—the *sub-humanity* of those who are not white, regardless of centuries of evidence to the contrary. Consequently, such cognitive weaknesses result in "incorrect judgments about the rights and wrongs of moral situations" (22). As an example, we might consider the present failure of (white) moral outrage in response to long-standing evidence that current social conditions in the United States quite literally deprive African Americans of *years* of life. From infant mortality to life expectancy, white Americans benefit, on average, from these same systems (Centers for Disease Control, 2012; 2013). During the summer of 2012, there was widespread outrage over the persistence of high rates of unemployment, which stood at approximately 8.2 percent (Bureau of Labor Statistics, 2012). This outrage helped to elide the fact that the rate for African Americans (14.4 percent) was just less than *double* that of white Americans (7.4 percent) for the same period. Little attention is paid to the fact that the "American" unemployment rate has been significantly lower, on average, than that in the black community for as long as such records have been kept (Censky). In a racially just country, one not in the thrall of white supremacy and white ignorance, this disparity would be intolerable.

White Americans are primed to presume "normal Americans" as white, and white people free of racial bias, in part due to the general construction of the United States as a "white" country (Lopez; Painter). For Mills, white supremacy determines not only the perceived racial identity but also the dominant "epistemic ground and product" in the United States ("White Ignorance" 17). The "white" view of the world is shared by those who are *reasonable*, and viewpoints that challenge this worldview are marginalized or seen as biased. By virtue of this condition, often called "white privilege," white people generally tend to lack the skills that would enable us to explore racially linked inequities in community across racial boundaries (Hoagland 110). Moreover, even when such investigations do take place, whites' ability to do critique is framed by a history of white supremacy in power relations, myths, and ideologies. Our habits of communication themselves often go unquestioned (Taylor 146).

In short, whites have constructed ourselves as the objective, disinterested observers in matters of race, and insisted that our perspectives are the proper perspectives from which to make knowledge claims. Our ignorance about white supremacy has underwritten the "reality" that white supremacy does not function in an oppressive fashion in the United States regardless of the testimony that may be offered by racial "Others." Du Bois' analysis of Reconstruction in general, and Johnson in particular, reveals the extent to which such epistemic shortcomings (and related moral failures) contributed to the ultimate failure of Reconstruction, and the postwar reinscription of white supremacy in the United States.

Johnson's Whiteness in *Black Reconstruction*

> When [Johnson] asked that plantations be divided in the South and lands opened in the West, he had in mind white men, who would thus become rich or at least richer. But for Negroes, he had nothing of the sort in mind, except the bare possibility that, if given freedom, they might continue to exist and not die out.
>
> –W.E.B. Du Bois, *Black Reconstruction*, pp. 243–244

White Ignorance and Black Subhumanity

With a dry sarcasm reminiscent of Mark Twain, Du Bois writes in *Black Reconstruction* that "[Johnson] was a thick-and-thin advocate of universal suffrage in the hands of the laborer and the common man, until he realized that some people actually thought that Negroes were men" (281). Du Bois, I think, did not intend this quip as mere hyperbole. The speed and extent of Johnson's "transubstantiation" indicates that the political salience of these formerly enslaved people escaped his notice until he came face to face with abolition-democrats in Congress (242). Because Johnson's political vision failed to include freed black people, he found himself confronted with a choice he had not anticipated: between the unsavory "increased political power of a restored Southern oligarchy" and (the apparently even more unsavory) "votes for Negroes" (237). Ironically, of course, Johnson's rehabilitation of the Southern aristocracy also denied the spoils of war to poor and working-class Southern whites, of whom he had always counted himself as one. His willingness to ally himself with those former Confederate landowners rather than his fellow "poor whites" is, for Du Bois, eloquent testimony to the abhorrence with which he viewed civil rights for Black people.

Du Bois' account of Johnson's "transubstantiation" from an enemy of the rich to an ally of the former Confederacy depends heavily on his "inability to see Negroes as men" (322). This is no mere rhetorical flourish on Du Bois' part, but the identification of an epistemic shortcoming among white Americans that persists today. Johnson's failure to recognize the full humanity of black Americans is echoed in Charles Mills' contention that "white ignorance" involves, in part, the perception of black people as "subpersons." For Mills, "subpersons are humanoid entities who, because of racial phenotype/genealogy, culture, are not fully human and therefore have a different and inferior schedule of rights and liberties applying to them" (*Racial Contract* 56). On his view, the United States presents a political system in which racialized hierarchy is central; the lack of genuine concern for this ongoing situation depends, in part, on the perception of people of color as less than human.

Because Johnson was himself a slave owner, his inability to foresee the "problem" of freed Black Americans may seem odd; on the conception of white ignorance advanced by Mills, however, the inability of white Americans to "see" black people is not surprising. Mills posits that human perception "is also in part *conception*, the viewing of the world through a particular conceptual grid" ("White Ignorance," 23–24). Johnson's conceptual grid of relevant political actors in the postwar situation would not obviously include black Americans because it *never had*. To be clear, Johnson's mistake was not a mere oversight; rather, it was part and parcel of an overall metaphysics according to which black Americans were fundamentally morally different from—and inferior to—whites. Du Bois makes clear that Johnson viewed black people as, at best, a *resource* (chattel or cheap labor).

If Johnson's prewar conception of African Americans' humanity was morally lacking, his postwar conception was morally and politically disastrous at a crucial point in U.S. history. Du Bois recounts representative instances in which Johnson's inability to perceive black Americans as fully human (e.g., as "political animals") led to behavior that was as absurd as it was horrendous. In May of 1865, for example, while traveling to unite the nation in support of postwar legislation, Johnson met with a group of black Philadelphians concerned about African Americans' postwar civil rights. These were civic leaders who had been granted an audience with the president—they hardly offered examples of black folk as either stupid or lacking in industry. Nevertheless, following this meeting, Johnson opined to the *Philadelphia Press* that the group was seeking federal aid "in order that they may be taken care of in idleness and debauchery" (259–260). Unfortunately, the historical record does not include their response to this libel.

Four months after his comments to the black civic leaders in Philadelphia, Johnson addressed a decommissioned regiment of African American troops from Washington, DC. He "congratulated them on serving with patience and endurance and *exhorted them to be tranquil and peaceful now that the war was ended*" (260, my emphasis). He was not, as one might suppose, referring to any particular instance of black decommissioned soldiers engaging in collective violence, as there were none. Apparently, however, decommissioned *White* soldiers were poised to shed blood in their determination to return the South to explicit white rule (Lemann, *passim*). Rather, Johnson's warped impression of black men's tendencies was clearly on display. Even more dismayingly, Johnson repeated to these black veterans of the nation's bloodiest war the message he had left in Philadelphia: that "freedom" was not a mere idea, neither was it the principle to *live in idleness*; rather, liberty meant a commitment to industry and virtue (260, my emphasis). Again, Johnson's tone-deafness (at best) would be inexplicable if we did not understand the conceptual grid that drove his perceptions and his reactions thereto.

The "laziness" of African Americans is, of course, part of a familiar mythology to anyone socialized in the United States in the last century; it is, though, a strange sort of conception to emerge from our history. While enslaved people reportedly engaged in several sorts of disguised insurrection, including work slowdowns (Aptheker), no reasonable observer could have "learned" from available evidence that black people were more naturally lazy than whites. Black workers were responsible for the vast majority of agricultural and attendant labor—both skilled and unskilled—done in the Southern United States for the 200 years leading up to the Civil War. In large plantations, they engaged in every kind of domestic work in addition to keeping intact families as permitted. This awareness may well contribute to the sense of national identity possessed by many African Americans. Indeed, pride in the knowledge that their work had built this nation was the most prominent of several reasons why freed slaves at the first meeting of the American Colonization Society resolved to *oppose* repatriating to Liberia (Bagwell and Bellows). If Johnson's insupportable convictions regarding the slothful tendencies of African Americans are excused by the widespread acceptance of this trope among whites in the United States, the question becomes how an entire dominant population might be so convinced of a fiction. Johnson is, of course, an *exemplar* of white ignorance, but not its only one.

Anti-black racism and its attendant impact on the reasoning powers of postbellum white Americans was only too clear in the ultimately successful drive to abolish the Freedmen's Bureau well before it could have fulfilled its mission. The Freedmen's Bureau was the federal agency created in order to assist newly emancipated black persons in their transition to freedom—a monumental task, when one considers the number of persons and families (some intact, some geographically separated by the "market") who were left without land, money, or employment by the end of slavery. Further, the Bureau acted to protect the rights of blacks against Southern whites who had, just weeks previously, held these same human beings as property. The local and state political systems, and all legitimate power, was in the hands of white people, most of whom resented the abolition of slavery; without Bureau presence in the South, black people had few resources to enforce their human or civil rights. Nevertheless, for many white Americans, North and South, the Freedmen's Bureau was at best a boondoggle, and at worst a form of theft from "real" Americans (224ff).

Johnson's stubborn ignorance was once again on display during an extraordinary meeting in the spring of 1866 with a group of black leaders, including Frederick Douglass and his son, Lewis. These Black abolition-democrats had requested an audience with the president in order to determine Johnson's position on black suffrage and the Freedmen's Bureau more generally (296). Any clear-eyed observer would, of course, assume from their interest in such a meeting that at least *some* black Americans were appropriately regarded as political agents and thus owed a broad set of human rights; Johnson remained perfectly obtuse to this fact, in a way that suggests there is more at play than merely a "habit" of denying intelligence to black Americans. Johnson, on Du Bois' account, saw formerly enslaved people as *threatening* to poor whites, who had been, he claimed, "opposed both to the slave and his master." He suggested that offering black people the vote in *addition to freedom from slavery* would cause a race war (297–298), as if white men would be moved to violence by the very idea that African Americans might be entitled to democratic participation.

In fact, Johnson may not even have recognized that his views about African-descended people differed from established fact. How else could he have suggested to several of the most accomplished African Americans of his time that black enfranchisement would actually be *antidemocratic*, as it would put white Southerners at the mercy of political changes in which they had had no voice? Johnson, with no apparently awareness of the irony of his position, insisted that *no* people should be subject to material and political changes that result from a vote in which they could not participate (298). In short, Johnson was opposed to allowing a vote on black suffrage because some white men who had betrayed their nation—and would only be indirectly affected by voting rights for African Americans in any case—would not be represented when the decision about the voting rights of African Americans was made.

The irony of Johnson's assertion in the presence of several intelligent, even formidable men—who had long been subject to the decisions of a "democracy" in which they could not participate—is painful. On Mills' account of white ignorance, however, this opacity can be understood: Johnson's conception of humanity as *white* prevented him from perceiving Douglass and the others as human. Formerly enslaved persons, racially marked as these men were, would, for Johnson, belong outside the category of "men." Somehow, the fact that he was indeed discussing abstract principles of democracy with a group of such beings did not change his conviction that *all people* were entitled to political participation, but his discussants were not. As Du Bois repeatedly notes, he simply cannot conceive of these *black* people as human. Of course, Johnson's apparent contradiction is, unfortunately, not easily dismissed as historical artifact; philosophers such as Mills and George Yancy insist that white social practices continue to dehumanize black Americans (and other people of color). "In a form of sociality that is fundamentally structured by race and racism, black people, for example, undergo ontologically truncating traumatic experiences in the face of White others who refuse to recognize their humanity" (Yancy 19).

Again, the significance of Du Bois' analysis cannot be overemphasized in light of the clear historical underpinnings of white epistemic shortcomings in the twenty-first century. Johnson's inability to recognize the humanity of black people even while exchanging views on political theory with those very black people he appears to doubt offers us a crucial indication of the growth of such flimsy belief systems. Further, if it is tempting to suggest that such descriptions of Johnson's worldview are hyperbolic, Du Bois' detailed presentation of Johnson's meeting with Douglass denies such comforting fictions. While no one in the room challenged the president to explain his assumption that black Americans were not fit for democracy, George Downing, a black leader from Rhode Island, attempted to make clear to Johnson the implications of his pronouncements. Agreeing that the majority in a state should never be denied participation in major political decisions, he suggested that Johnson consider the state of South Carolina, where the *majority* of the inhabitants had always been denied political participation, because they *were not white*. Du Bois reports his response as follows:

> [Johnson] could not touch the question as to whether it was right to prevent a majority in South Carolina from ruling because, *to his mind, no number of Negroes could outweigh the will of Whites*. He stumbled on *without mentioning this suppressed minor premise* and said 'It is a fundamental tenet of my creed that the will of the people must be obeyed. Is there anything wrong or unfair in that?' (298, my emphasis)

Du Bois suggests that Downing chose at this point not to pursue the question.

The depth and breadth of white supremacy in American history, and Johnson's particular and sometimes awkward exercise of this ideology, suggest that Johnson's "conceptual grid" was more complex than any simple explanation can capture. For example, Du Bois notes that Johnson's Whites-only democracy relies upon an implicit premise—namely, that "no number of Negroes could outweigh the will of whites." This premise clearly contradicts democratic principles and should therefore doom his position, but Johnson appears unable either to explicitly recognize it *or* deny it. For Du Bois, this strange dual incapacity grounds Johnson's ultimate privileging of former Confederates over previously enslaved people. Because the subhumanity of African Americans went without saying, he did not *need* explicitly to deny that black Americans were proper members of the state, any more than he would feel it necessary to deny the right of horses to vote.

Johnson made at least one other claim during this meeting that sheds significant light on his warped perceptions: he insisted that extending the vote to African American men would result in a race war (298). In response, Douglass suggested that, in fact, the only way to avoid a race war would be to grant suffrage to the freed slaves. Johnson apparently replied that those who were not wanted should simply leave the region. In suggesting that African Americans' best strategy to avoid violence would be to leave the South (and perhaps the nation altogether), Johnson again displays his confused and even contradictory conception of the status of black Americans. Surely, he does not, or cannot, conceive of black Americans as fully human beings. Johnson-as-democrat would have to admit that *human beings* in a democratic state are not required to flee a threat of violence, but have the right to call upon the state for protection.

And yet, even if Johnson could not see African Americans as fully human, he apparently did not see them strictly as "brutes." In fact, his suggestion that they "emigrate" makes clear that he was aware that they were more than chattel. Livestock could neither engage in "racial warfare" with human beings nor choose to emigrate. It seems clear that most white slave owners did not, in fact, mistake the people whom they enslaved for livestock. Enslaved persons were regularly given complex responsibilities on the farm and in the house that would never be assigned to nonhuman animals. Moreover, to my knowledge, nonhuman animals have not been required to *nurse* white babies as many African American women were. Johnson's paradoxical conception of black Americans was thus not idiosyncratic to him, but common to many white Americans. Coherent with Du Bois' account of Johnson's perceptual failures is Charles Mills' contention that white epistemic practices categorize people of color as "humanoid entities," who have a lesser set of rights than humans (*Racial Contract* 56).

Johnson's misperceptions regarding African Americans show up again during his third annual message to Congress in December of 1867, nearly two years after his disastrous meeting with Douglass in February of 1866. Here, Du Bois remarks, "all masking of the Negro problem is removed," as Johnson explicitly attributed the 90-year survival of democracy in North America to "the glory of white men" and, in support of his proposition, he notes that ". . . in the progress of nations, Negroes have shown less capacity for government than any other race of people" (341). Johnson regretfully noted the "constant tendency to relapse into barbarism" that made African-descended people unsuited to democracy. In fact, Black people were so physically distinct that "the great difference between the two races in physical, mental and moral characteristics will prevent an amalgamation or fusion of them together in one homogeneous mass" (342).

Du Bois, with typical decorum, fails to comment on Johnson's contention. Nevertheless, the evidence that interracial "unions" could bear fruit and, further, that these offspring themselves were fertile was everywhere present in the American South. Thus, Johnson's transubstantiation and the moral catastrophe of Reconstruction's collapse present us with a conundrum in need of explanation: not only do white Americans fail properly to perceive African Americans as fully human, but they are resistant to bountiful evidence to the contrary. For Du Bois, as for Mills, the explanation of this phenomenon is neither simple hostility nor a lack of *will* to respect blacks' equality or even bare humanity. In the following section, I briefly focus on the persistence of white ignorance.

The Tenacity of White Epistemic Incapacity

In *The Souls of Black Folk* Du Bois had written, "most Americans answer all queries regarding the Negro *a priori*, . . . the least that human courtesy can do is to listen to the evidence" (431). The "American" misperception of black folk thrives, in part, because the epistemic norms demanded by a white supremacist regime does not encourage, let alone require, that white people make use of the available evidence regarding black humanity. In *Black Reconstruction*, he notes that Edwin Ruffin, a typical Southern oligarch, "jumped at conclusions [about enslaved people] instead of testing them by careful research" (55). Oligarchs and others who adhered to the dominant worldview rarely needed to defend themselves; they simply demanded compliance with their knowledge claims and resulting judgments. Like three-year-old children, they could (metaphorically) cover their ears and chant when confronted with facts they could not bear; unlike such children, they were rarely held to account for their ignorance or its results. This kind of epistemic privilege makes possible the absurdity of Andrew Johnson's insistence that people of African descent were incapable of deliberation during a conversation with African Americans who were, it seems safe to assume, as least his intellectual equals.

Du Bois' attribution of white epistemological impenetrability to Johnson (and other whites) anticipates work done by philosophers like Mills and others to examine not simply what whites do not know about their own white supremacy but ways in which *they are encouraged not to know*. Marilyn Frye's concept of "whiteliness," the elevated sense of entitlement that white people feel about their own judgments about race is particularly useful here. Frye is cautiously optimistic that "whiteliness" is not a *necessary* condition of white people, but its deconstruction requires introspection as well as difficult work with people of color—which is, of course, endangered precisely because of white persons' whiteliness. As noted above, Mills explains that interests shape our perceptions, "influencing what and how we see, what we and society choose to remember, whose testimony is solicited and whose is not, and which facts and frameworks are sought out and accepted" ("White Ignorance" 24).

Repeatedly throughout *Black Reconstruction*, Du Bois notes that what white Americans actually saw, heard, and remembered as *fact*—the presumptions in light of which they comported themselves daily—were inextricably bound up with their interest in white supremacy.

> It is nonsense to say that the South knew nothing about the capabilities of the Negro race. Southerners knew Negroes far better than Northerners. There was not a single Negro slave owner who did not know dozens of Negroes just as capable of learning and efficiency as the mass of poor White people around and about, and some quite as capable as the average slaveholder. They had continually in the course of the history of slavery recognized such men. Here and there teachers and preachers to White folks as well as colored folks had arisen (275).

Du Bois makes clear that Johnson and other Southern whites had access to sufficient evidence of the intelligence of enslaved persons to know or at least *believe in* their intelligence. Thus, not only does Johnson's strange belief in the sub-humanity of black people fly in the face of available evidence, it appears to be highly resistant to *repeated* demonstrations of its inaccuracy.

Johnson, in particular, was exposed to ample evidence of the humanity of black people. As noted above, he had owned eight slaves (242), a small enough number to ensure that Johnson would have had direct contact with those he nominally owned. In addition to prolonged contact with enslaved people, Johnson had had, as vice president, daily interactions with individuals like Charles Sumner and Thaddeus Stevens—white men who were committed to black equality and must have offered him plentiful examples of black humanity. Nevertheless, because of the twisted cognitive norms that allowed white Americans to maintain their sense of superiority despite clear evidence of their own brutality, Johnson would never acknowledge black equality. In fact, 20 pages prior to the passage quoted above, Du Bois notes that "Johnson had little knowledge of Negroes . . . [and] accepted most of the current Southern patterns" (259).

In direct contradiction of all available evidence, Johnson attempted to justify his gutting of federal assistance to black Southerners by insisting that the freedmen were no worse off than poor white workers. "His labor is in demand," Johnson opined, "and [the former slave] can change his dwelling place if one community or state does not please him" (276). Du Bois declares this "an astonishing pronouncement. It was the "American Assumption," of the possibility of labor's achieving wealth, applied with a vengeance to landless slaves under caste conditions, and, for Du Bois, the very strength of its logic was the weakness of its common sense" (277). Of course, Johnson, following white cognitive norms, was precisely able to ignore both common sense, and the reality that black workers who attempted to negotiate wages or working conditions would more likely face violence than a seat at the negotiation table. And because his epistemic context would not hold him accountable for such pronouncements, the question of his epistemic license in making the claim was effectively moot.

Conclusion

In *Black Reconstruction*, Du Bois offers a wealth of material to demonstrate the epistemic and moral failure of white Americans in the post–Civil War era. In sum, he argues, white America remains doubtful and finally apathetic regarding the humanity of African Americans.

> For a brief period—for the seven mystic years that stretched between Johnson's 'Swing Round the Circle' to the Panic of 1873, the majority of thinking Americans of the North believed in the equal manhood of Negroes. [W]hile after long years the American world recovered in most matters, *it has never yet quite understood why it could ever have thought that the black men were altogether human*. (319–320, my emphasis)

Apparently, Johnson's transubstantiation was not only rapid and complete, but it doomed the epistemic capacities of generations of white Americans who followed. Du Bois' grim despair here may have culminated in his decision in 1961 to emigrate to Ghana on the invitation President Kwame Nkrumah in 1961, where he died two years later at the age of 93 (D. Lewis 570).

Even now, white Americans are exposed to information about significant racial disparities in the criminal justice system and other key U.S. institutions on at least an annual basis, and yet apparently believe that these institutions are *fair enough*, for now. This state of affairs is perfectly captured in James Baldwin's observation that white people are "basically confused, bewildered, pathologically fearful beings, in need of a pitying love . . . from the very [B]lacks who have suffered so grievously because of them" (quoted in Spelman 119). Confusion, fear, and needing pity are not desirable states, and so white ignorance is clearly harmful to whites. Unfortunately, the harm is not limited to white people. If there is to be a change, certainly white folk must show a greater willingness to read the insightful, if unflattering, portraits of whiteness found in the work of thinkers such as Du Bois, and those who now carry that work on. Perhaps the first step is to recognize that "ownership of the earth, forever and ever, amen!" (Du Bois, 1920) is neither our right as White people nor even a privilege to be valued; it is only an inexcusable presumption we must commit to unmake.

Acknowledgments

Recognition is given to the organizers of the February 2013 Wings of Atlanta conference at Clark Atlanta University, especially Dr. Stephanie Y. Evans, and the pioneering African American Studies scholars whose work on Du Bois over long decades was made public. I also thank all of those who have contributed to this paper, including Dr. Darlene Clark Hine for the idea, and my colleague Dr. Nancy Daukas for a read-through at a crucial moment. Thanks also go to those colleagues who shared my conference panel: Dr. Derek Catsam, Dr. Colin Fitzgerald, Ms. Alicia Fontenette, Ms. Cassandra Hawkins-Wilson, Dr. Tom Reifer, and our chair, Dr. William Boone. This collection of essays should speak to the value of the conference in producing rigorous and intriguing scholarship, but it cannot replicate the experience of being at the conference itself. The gathering in one place—and in that particular place—of so many scholars knowledgeable about Du Bois' work and committed to sharing his legacy resulted in four days of scholarly satisfaction that is exceedingly rare.

Works Cited

1. Aptheker, Herbert, *American Negro Slave Revolts*, New York: Columbia University Press, 1943. Print.
2. Arnesen, Eric, "Whiteness and the Historians' Imagination", *International Labor and Working-Class History* Vol. 60, October 2001, pp. 3–32. Print.
3. Bagwell, Orlando, and Bellows, Susan, *Africans in America*, Boston: WGBH, 1998/2006. DVD.
4. Bonilla-Silva, Eduardo, *White Supremacy and Racism in the Post-Civil Rights Era*, Boulder: Lynne Rienner Publishers, 2001. Print.

5. Bureau of Labor Statistics, "News Release", 2012. Web. 18 July 2012.
6. Censky, Annalyn, "Black Unemployment Highest in 27 Years", *CNN Money*, 2011. Web. 31 July 2013.
7. Centers for Disease Control, "QuickStats: Infant Mortality Rates, by Race and Hispanic Ethnicity of Mother—United States, 2000, 2005, and 2009", 2013. Web. 31 July 2013.
8. Delgado, Richard, and Stefancic, Jean, *Critical Whiteness Studies: Looking Behind the Mirror*, Philadelphia: Temple University Press, 1997. Print.
7. Du Bois, W.E.B., *Black Reconstruction in American 1860–1880*, New York: The Free Press, 1935/1998. Print.
8. Du Bois, W.E.B., *Dusk of Dawn* in Huggins, N., ed. *Du Bois: Writings*, United States: Library of America, 1940/1986. Print.
9. Du Bois, W.E.B., *The Souls of Black Folk* in Du Bois, *Writings*, pp. 357–548, 1903/1986. Print. J1.1f.
10. Du Bois, W.E.B., "The Souls of White Folk", in *Darkwater: Voices from Within the Veil*, New York: Schocken, 1920/1999. Print.
11. Du Bois, W.E.B., *Writings*, ed. Nathan Huggins, New York: Library of America, 1986. Print.
12. Frederickson, George, *White Supremacy: A Comparative Study of American and South African History*, Oxford University Press, 1982. Print.
13. Frye, Marilyn, "White Woman Feminist", *Feminist Reprise*, 2011. Web. 30 May 2014.
14. Gilmore, Glenda, *Gender and Jim Crow: Women and the Politics of White Supremacy in North Carolina 1896–1920*, Chapel Hill: UNC Press, 1996. Print.
15. Hancock, A., "W.E.B. Du Bois: Intellectual Forefather of Intersectionality?" *SOULS: A Critical Journal of Black Politics, Culture and Society*, Taylor and Francis. Vol. 7: 3–4, 2005; pp. 74–84. Print.
16. Hoagland, Sarah Lucia, "Denying Relationality", in Sullivan and Tuana, *Epistemologies of Ignorance*, Buffalo: SUNY Press, 2007. Print.
17. Lemann, Nicholas, *Redemption*, New York: Farrar, Strous & Giroux, 2006. Print.
18. Lewis, Amanda E., "What Group?" Studying Whites and Whiteness in the Era of "Color-Blindness", *Sociological Theory*, December 2004, Vol. 22, Issue 4, pp. 623–646. Print.
19. Lewis, David Levering, *W.E.B. Du Bois: The Fight For Equality and the American Century 1919–1963*, New York: Henry Holt & Co., 2000. Print.
20. Lopez, Ian Haney, *White by law: The Legal Construction of Race*, New York: NYU Press, 1996. Print.
21. Mills, Charles, *The Racial Contract*, Ithaca: Cornell University Press, 1997. Print.
22. Mills, Charles, "White Ignorance", in Nancy Tuana, *Epistemologies of Ignorance*, Buffalo: SUNY Press, 2007. Print.
23. Owen, David S., "Whiteness in Du Bois' *The Souls of Black Folk*" *Philosophia Africana*, 2007 Vol. 10 Issue 2, p. 107. Print.
24. Painter, Nell Irvin, *The History of White People*, New York: W.W. Norton & Co., 2010. Print Plessy v. Ferguson, 163 U.S. 537 (1896). Print.
25. Porter, Eric, *The Problem of the Future World*, Durham: Duke University Press, 2010. Print.
26. Rabaka, Reiland, "The Souls of White Folk: W.E.B. Du Bois' Critique of White Supremacy and Contributions to Critical White Studies", *Journal of African American Studies* 2007 Vol. 11, Issue 1, pp. 1–15. Print.
27. Roediger, David, *The Wages of Whiteness: Race and the Making of the American Working Class*, New York: Verso, 1999. Print.
28. Shaw, Stephanie J., *W.E.B. Du Bois and The Souls of Black Folk*, Chapel Hill: University of North Carolina Press, 2103. Print.
29. Shuford, John, "Four Du Boisian contributions to Critical Race Theory", *The Transactions of the Charles S. Peirce Sodety* Vol. 37, Summer 2001. Print.
30. Spelman, Elizabeth V., "Managing Ignorance," in Sullivan and Tuana, eds., *Race and the Epistemologies of Ignorance*, Albany: SUNY Press, 2007. Print.
31. Stewart, David O., *Impeached: the Trial of President Andrew Johnson and the Fight for Lincoln's Legacy*, New York: Simon and Schuster, 2009. Print.
32. Sullivan, Shannon, "Remembering the Gift: W.E.B. Du Bois on the Unconscious and Economic Operations of Racism", *Transactions of the Charles S. Peirce Society* Vol. 39, No. 2, Spring 2003. Print.
33. Sullivan, Shannon, and Nancy Tuana, eds., *Race and Epistemologies of Ignorance*, Albany: SUNY Press, 2007. Print.

34. Taylor, Paul (2007) "Race Problems, Unknown Publics", in Sullivan and Tuana, eds., *Race and the Epistemologies of Ignorance*, pp. 135–151. Print.
35. *The Purdue OWL*. Purdue U Writing Lab, 2010. Web. 24 July 2014.
36. Winant, Howard, Review: Eric Porter, "The Problem of the Future World: W.E.B. Du Bois and the Race Concept at Midcentury," *Ethnic and Racial Studies*, 2001. 01:10.1080/01419870.2011.607777. Web. 27 December 2013.
37. Yancy, George, *Look, a White!: Philosophical Essays on Whiteness*, Philadelphia: Temple University Press, 2012. Print.

LISA J. MCLEOD is an associate professor of Philosophy at Guilford College. She has published much scholarly work on understanding racism.

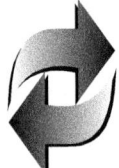

Adam Fairclough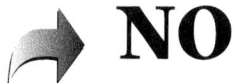

Was the Grant of Black Suffrage a Political Error? Reconsidering the Views of John W. Burgess, William A. Dunning, and Eric Foner on Congressional Reconstruction

... the so-called "Dunning school." ... presented a relentlessly negative assessment of Congressional Reconstruction. All agreed that black suffrage had been a political blunder and that the Republican state governments in the South that rested upon black votes had been corrupt, extravagant, unrepresentative, and oppressive. . . sympathies. . . lay with the white Southerners who . . . used legal opposition and extralegal violence to oust the Republicans from state power. Although "Dunningite" historians did not necessarily endorse those extralegal methods, they did tend to palliate them. From start to finish, they argued, . . . "Radical Reconstruction"—lacked political wisdom and legitimacy.[1]

From the perspective of present-day historians, however, the racism of the "Dunningites," sometimes implied but often explicit, vitiated their interpretation of Reconstruction. "Dunningite" historians contended that the enfranchised freedmen were unfit to exercise political responsibility and had been putty in the hands of "carpetbaggers," unscrupulous northern interlopers who headed the Republican Party in the former Confederacy. In Texas, wrote Charles W. Ramsdell, "the most unprincipled adventurers that ever disgraced a state" manipulated "the child-like Negro." The historian . . . J. G. de R. Hamilton, emphasized "the dense ignorance of the negroes," many of whom "were vicious and idle." Dunning himself argued that Congressional Reconstruction arrayed "a mass of barbarous freedmen" against "all the forces that made for civilization." Placed under the political control of "ignorant barbarians," wrote John W. Burgess, Dunning's mentor, whites in the South suffered "terrible degradation" inflicted by men who were "tyrannic, corrupt, mean, and vulgar." . . . these historians utilized racist stereotypes and neglected black sources.[2]

In his magnum opus, *Black Reconstruction* (1935), W. E. B. Du Bois complained that the "Dunningite" studies . . . displayed "endless sympathy for the white South . . . [and] ridicule, contempt or silence for the Negro."[3] Refusing to take the former slaves seriously as political actors, they depicted blacks as "ignorant and silly." Du Bois's indictment—at the time a minority view—is now widely accepted. Many present-day historians of Reconstruction dismiss the work of the "Dunning school" as worthless. Michael W. Fitzgerald, for example, contends that its only real value is to "highlight the racist enormities of early twentieth century historians." In Eric Foner's damning judgment, the "Dunningite" historians brought "everlasting shame" to the historical profession.[4]

Before dismissing the "Dunningites" as beyond the pale, however, two questions should be considered. First, must one condemn historians writing a 100 years ago for holding views that are, by our standards, morally abhorrent? The answer must be—if such views reflected the thinking of their time—certainly not. As evolutionary biologist Richard Dawkins has pointed out, it is a gross historical fallacy "to view the writings of one century through the politically tinted glasses of another." . . . the racialist views of John W. Burgess reflected commonplace assumptions among white Americans and Europeans in the age of high imperialism. Placing human races in a hierarchy is something "educated moderns never do," notes Dawkins, "but equivalent Victorians always did." . . . New evidence, new values, and new approaches promote constant questioning of older accounts. As Foner acknowledges, "our understanding of history is constantly changing. There is nothing unusual in the fact that each generation rewrites history to meet its own needs."[5]

Fairclough, Adam. "Was the Grant of Black Suffrage a Political Error? Reconsidering the Views of John W. Burgess, William A. Dunning, and Eric Foner on Congressional Reconstruction," *Journal of the Historical Society, pages 155–188*. Copyright ©2012 The Historical Society and Wiley Periodicals, Inc. Used with permission of Blackwell Publishing Ltd.

A second, more substantive, consideration arises from the assumption that the racism of the "Dunning school" historians renders their entire *oeuvre* valueless. True, a presumption of black incapacity dissuaded these scholars from seriously studying black political behavior. But did this racial bias invalidate their discussions of constitutional issues, legal questions, economic matters, congressional politics, and other topics? Did their racism so blind "Dunningite" historians that they had *nothing* useful to say about Reconstruction? . . .

Du Bois himself, be it noted, tempered his condemnation of the "Dunning school" with occasional praise. Burgess, he conceded, was "more than fair" on matters of law. Dunning's statements, he admitted, were "often judicious." Garner's study of Mississippi, he acknowledged, treated "the Negro as an integral part of the scene and . . . as a human being." Du Bois recognized that John G. Ficklen and Walter L. Fleming, writing on Louisiana and Alabama, respectively, displayed "a certain fairness and sense of historic honesty." . . . Even the studies that Du Bois dismissed as "thoroughly bad" contain passages in which professionalism overcomes bias. Mildred Thompson, in her study of Georgia, gives an excellent analysis of postwar southern agriculture, describing the impact of emancipation on the plantation system and the reasons for the emergence of sharecropping. And, despite her inclination to play down the significance of the Ku Klux Klan, she cites chapter and verse to illustrate that organization's racism, violence, and political intent. Ella Lonn's study of Louisiana gives a finely grained account of politics at the state level and, especially, the factional battles within the Republican Party. Despite her hostility to the Republicans, she scrupulously documents the extent of Democratic frauds in the 1872 election. Ramsdell's work on Texas provides a vivid picture of the violence and confusion that prevailed in that state, and he supplies copious evidence that many whites accepted the end of slavery with the greatest reluctance, often treating blacks cruelly and sometimes trying to keep them in bondage. Despite their bias, the "Dunningites" got many things right.[6]

The argument of this essay . . . suggests that the "Dunningite" historians identified one of the basic reasons for the failure of Congressional Reconstruction: the policy of black suffrage. Enfranchisement of the freedmen, the central plank in the Congressional plan, evoked implacable opposition from the masses of southern whites, and support for the policy in the North proved too shallow to sustain it. The Republican Party legislated civil and political equality for black Southerners but failed to create the national institutions to enforce those rights. "Ideally," wrote Mildred Thompson, "it may have been a humane and civilizing act to protect the weaker race with the power of the ballot, but practically, when enfranchisement was enforced against the will of the white people, and contrary to their profound sense of right and fitness, the new power left the freedmen with but little more actual freedom in 1872 than they had enjoyed in 1866."[7]

This conclusion directly contradicts more positive assessments of Congressional Reconstruction that emphasize the empowerment of blacks, the achievements of the South's "black-and-tan" governments, and the potential of Congressional Reconstruction to have succeeded. For example, in his influential 1988 study, *Reconstruction: America's Unfinished Revolution*, Eric Foner argued that Congressional Reconstruction should be judged by its intentions and achievements, not solely by its failures. He rejects the notion that black suffrage was misguided or self-defeating. Rather, he describes Congressional Reconstruction as a magnificent expression of American idealism that, but for contingent factors, might have succeeded. This essay contends that . . . black suffrage was a political error whose failure was foreordained, and the damaging consequences of that error far outweighed any lasting benefits.

John W. Burgess (1844–1933), Dunning's mentor at Columbia University, published the first critique of Reconstruction . . . his study, *Reconstruction and the Constitution, 1866–1876* (1902), raises the question of whether elements of sound scholarship can coexist with elements of racism in its most direct form. Unlike Dunning, Burgess frankly avowed a belief in the superiority of the white "race." A convinced imperialist, he dismissed the "political equality of man" as a chimera.[8]

Frequently damned but rarely read, Burgess's *Reconstruction and the Constitution* presents a surprisingly "modern" analysis of the political struggle that led to Congressional Reconstruction.[9] In fact, it bears little resemblance to the so-called "Dunningite" portrayal of a courageous President Andrew Johnson defending the Constitution, and fighting to implement Lincoln's plan for a speedy, magnanimous reunion, against the onslaught of vengeful Radicals.[10] According to Burgess, Johnson clung to a fallacious view that the Confederate states had never been "out" of the Union, simplistically contending that they could resume their normal status as soon as the rebellion had ceased. Both Johnson and Lincoln, he complained, approached the question of Reconstruction from the false theory that the states were indestructible, . . . that denied Congress any significant role in shaping the postwar settlement. Yet Burgess recognized that Lincoln had been much more flexible than Johnson, and had a "cautious habit of leaving open a way of escape out of any position when necessity or prudence might require its abandonment." It was Johnson's dogmatism regarding constitutional matters, as well as his lack of everyday political skill, that caused the Republican Party to coalesce around its own plan of Reconstruction.[11]

On constitutional questions, Burgess more often agreed with Thaddeus Stevens and Charles Sumner than with Andrew Johnson.[12] He never suggested that Congressional Reconstruction was driven by revenge or partisan advantage. Thaddeus Stevens's "undoubted personal rancor" toward Johnson, Burgess acknowledged, was an understandable result of the president's public abuse of him as a traitor.[13] Rather than condemning the Radicals, Burgess praised the Republican leaders who crafted Congressional Reconstruction as "men of as rugged moral and intellectual power as Grant [and] Sherman."[14] Burgess, like Dunning, saw that Republican measures, far from being rammed through Congress by vindictive Radicals, represented compromises between the Radical and conservative wings of the party. The Republicans in Congress were, to a large extent, reacting rather than initiating, and how far they went in the matter of legislation "depended largely upon the moderation of the President, and the sincerity of the [white] people of the South."[15]

... Burgess, like later "revisionists," castigated Johnson and the former Confederates for their incautious extremism. The "Black Codes" enacted by southern legislatures in 1865–1866 persuaded Republicans "that the freedom of the Negro had not yet been sufficiently guaranteed," and that the state governments set up under Johnson's authority could not be trusted. Burgess noted the resemblance of Mississippi's vagrancy law to the state's old slave code. "Almost every act, word, or gesture of the Negro, not consonant with good taste and good manners, as well as good morals, was made a crime or misdemeanor, for which he could be fined ... and then consigned to a condition almost of slavery for an indefinite time, if he could not pay the fine." The election to Congress of former Confederate leaders increased the Republicans' doubts about Johnson's policies, and with good reason. The South's "arrogant demands for the immediate admission to seats in Congress of the very men who had led the rebellion" helped persuade the governing party that it must legislate to prevent "the work of four years of terrible sacrifice [from] being undone." When Congress sought information about conditions in the South, it naturally placed more credence upon a pessimistic report by Carl Schurz than an optimistic one by General U. S. Grant. Apart from having spent more time in the South than Grant, Schurz was "a keener observer ... and a much better reasoner." The result was the passage by Congress of the Freedmen's Bureau Bill and the Civil Rights Bill, both of which Johnson vetoed.[16]

Burgess deemed Johnson's vetoes politically unwise and, in the case of the Civil Rights Bill, a "monumental blunder." An expansion of national power, Burgess insisted, was the logical consequence of the Civil War and emancipation. The Thirteenth Amendment implied that the central government had ample authority to "define and protect civil equality within the States." Indeed, Burgess argued that a strong federal government was the *only* reliable guarantor of civil liberty and legal equality. Congress responded to Johnson's veto by enacting the Fourteenth Amendment. Although this measure clearly served the political interests of the Republican Party in tying congressional representation to suffrage, Burgess considered it justified in terms of "prudence and patriotism." He denied that the temporary disqualification from office of high-ranking ex-confederates was harsh or vindictive. "It is difficult to see how the Confederate leaders could have suffered less, and have been rebuked at all for their acts." Johnson's recommendation that the southern states should reject the amendment was an act of folly that played into the hands of his Republican critics.[17]

... "Logically, morally, and legally," Burgess wrote, Congress was justified in brushing aside the state governments established by President Johnson and "beginning the work itself from the bottom up." It had the right and the duty to protect the freedmen and establish loyal civil governments in the South. When, in 1867, Congress declared the Johnson governments void and subjected the former Confederacy to direct federal control using the Army as its instrument, it acted within its competence. In fact, he argued, "it ought to have done so in 1865."[18]

Dunning, too, was no "Dunningite"—in 1897 at least—when he described Congressional Reconstruction, without irony, as "one of the most remarkable achievements in the history of government." It was as impressive in political and administrative terms as the subjugation of the Confederate armies had been in military terms. "The obstacles to success were as great for the one set of men as for the other. In the path of reconstruction lay a hostile white population in the South, a hostile executive at Washington, a doubtful if not decidedly hostile Supreme Court, a divided Northern sentiment in respect to negro suffrage and an active and skillfully directed Democratic Party. Yet the process as laid out in 1867 was carried through to its completion." Like Burgess, Dunning dismissed the charge that Congressional Reconstruction violated the Constitution. Abnormal circumstances justified drastic measures. "The methods were well adapted to the end, and the end was a huge social and political revolution under the forms of law."[19]

There is another resemblance between these arguments and those advanced by post-1960 "revisionists."

Burgess argued that Congress made it too easy for the new civil governments of the South to escape direct rule and regain their position as states within the Union. Instead of rushing the process, he argued, Congress ought to have kept the ex-rebel states in territorial status for as long as was necessary. But too many Republicans were in thrall to the "phantom of the 'indestructible State'" to approve a long period of federal rule. The Republicans decided that black suffrage would facilitate a swift termination of military rule and constitute a guarantee of loyalty on the part of the readmitted states.[20] This turned out to be a fatal miscalculation. The period of probation was far too short—by 1868 seven former Confederate states had regained statehood within the Union and by 1870 all had—to ensure stable governments that could protect the civil rights of all citizens. The establishment of Republican state governments sustained by black suffrage, far from cementing loyalty and ensuring order, alienated the mass of southern whites, and produced chaos.[21]

At this point, Burgess and Dunning veer sharply from modern views. In 1897, Dunning had questioned the wisdom of black suffrage by noting that "To stand the social pyramid on its apex was not the surest way to restore the shattered equilibrium in the South." Ten years later—by which time most of the ex-confederate states had disfranchised black voters—he condemned Republican rule in the South as a "mere travesty of civilized government." Burgess, for his part, damned black suffrage as "one of the 'blundercrimes' of the century." The congressional plan of Reconstruction subjected the South to "a period of darkness . . . blacker and more hopeless than the worst experiences of the war." Small wonder, he concluded, that white Southerners resorted to fraud, intimidation, and violence, and that the "conscience of the nation" revolted against the "hideous situation in the South" and the "everlasting 'waving of the bloody shirt.'" The restoration of white rule in the South, Burgess wrote, was as natural as it was inevitable, for "it is the white man's mission, his duty and his right, to hold the reins of political power in his own hands."[22]

Such views offend modern historians. Nevertheless, the fact remains that black suffrage failed to yield the intended results. It failed to produce a law-abiding South; failed to protect the black population; failed to produce a viable Republican Party in the South; and failed to persuade the North that the defense of black rights merited the costs of incessant intervention. Above all, black suffrage evoked bitter hostility from white Southerners, the majority of whom were never reconciled to blacks voting and holding office. Congressional Republicans had deemed black suffrage "protection" for the freedmen and for white Unionists: a cheap alternative to a long military occupation. But as an attempt to restore law and order in the former Confederacy, thereby safeguarding the freedmen, it backfired utterly.[23]

On this point, then, Burgess, Dunning, and the post-1960 "revisionists" agree. Unyielding white opposition to black suffrage proved the Achilles' heel of Congressional Reconstruction. "The [Republican] party and its governments faced a crisis of legitimacy," writes Eric Foner. "Ordinarily, political parties take for granted the authority of the government and the integrity of their foes. Reconstruction's opponents, however, viewed the new regimes as alien impositions, and their black constituency as not entitled to a permanent role in the body politic." Black suffrage "infuriated most of the white population," agrees Michael Fitzgerald. "Seldom have so large a number of citizens in a democracy been so antagonized by those in power."[24] As Michael Perman puts it, "The Republican party was so stigmatized that any means were deemed acceptable to defeat it." Even when white Democrats courted black voters and sought tactical alliances with dissident Republicans, they never lost sight of their larger goal of establishing some new form of white supremacy. And even as they distanced themselves from the discredited Ku Klux Klan, after 1872 Democrats reverted to violence and intimidation in the form of White Leagues, "rifle clubs," and Red Shirts. Democratic promises in 1876 to respect the civil and political rights of blacks were insincere. Once they ousted the Republican Party from state power, the Democrats used fraud, intimidation, violence, and legislation to erode those rights.[25]

It can be argued, therefore, that less separates the revisionists from the views of Burgess and the "Dunning school" than meets the eye. Whether one sympathized with the black Republicans or with the white Democrats, the latter's opposition to black suffrage was a reality. Dunning, although hesitant to endorse the racism of the Democrats, made the basic, essential point: the whites' "pride in their race" and dislike and fear of blacks was a hard fact. "Whether or not this feeling and spirit were abstractly preferable to those which animated the northern idealist who preached equality, the fact that such feeling and spirit were at work must be taken squarely into account by the historian."[26] Like . . . groups that displayed similar prejudices and political stubbornness, the ex-confederates tenaciously resisted any threat to their social status, economic position, and political dominance.

Here is Burgess on the Ku Klux Klan:

> After the Reconstruction Acts were passed and put into operation . . . this organization spread all over the South. . . . As it extended, its methods became more lawless and violent. Its mem-

bers whipped, plundered, burned, abducted, imprisoned, tortured and murdered, for the prime purpose of keeping the negroes from exercising suffrage and holding office. They were protected by many respectable people who would not have participated personally in its nefarious work. And they had confederates everywhere, who, upon the witness box, would perjure themselves to prevent their conviction and punishment.... The respectable people of the South tried to make it appear that these lawless bands were simply freebooters, such as generally infest a country . . . after a period of war and had no political meaning or purpose whatsoever, and it was probably true that the Klan never went beyond county organization, any wider bond . . . being rather the moral bond of common purpose; but it cannot be well questioned now that they had one purpose at least in common, and that that was a chief purpose with them all, viz., to terrorize the negro out of the exercise of his newly-granted privileges of suffrage and office-holding, and to keep him in his place as a menial.[27]

It would be hard to improve upon this analysis.

There is a world of difference, of course, between explaining violent white resistance as a response to a "travesty of civilized government," and blaming that resistance on a bigoted refusal by whites to tolerate black suffrage under any circumstances. One view sympathizes with the white Southerners; the other deplores their racism. If, however, the end result were foreordained—political equality between the races being unenforceable—then the enactment of black suffrage could indeed be judged "reckless." And on this point, most post-1960 "revisionists" agree: the factors militating against the success of Congressional Reconstruction were overwhelming. As Perman argued in 1973, by rejecting Radical demands for the destruction, as a class, of the former slaveholders, the moderate Republicans crippled Congressional Reconstruction at the outset. The plan, as implemented, created "confusion, frustration, and antagonism," and was "bound to end in disaster sooner rather than later."[28]

An anthology of state studies published in 1980 expressed what amounted to a consensus among historians of Reconstruction. In the opinion of Jerrel Shofner, "Without basic changes in the racial attitudes of nearly all southern whites—attitudes which they shared with most northern whites—there was scant likelihood that any solution to postwar problems in the United States could have been found." According to Joe Gray Taylor, "Radical Reconstruction probably had no chance of success anywhere in the South." Southern Republicans, wrote Otto Olsen, "faced insurmountable internal obstacles and were dependent . . . on an unreliable and severely handicapped external force" (i.e., the federal government). A ¼ of a century later, Lawrence Powell and Michael Fitzgerald came to the same conclusion. In order to succeed, writes Powell, Congressional Reconstruction would have required the sustained application of federal power over "several generations." But the national leaders of the Republican Party demanded that Republicans in the South "implement their top-down blueprint within the constraints of American federalism." Then, adds Powell, those leaders expected their southern allies to sink or swim—they "cut them loose." According to Fitzgerald, "the prospects for a positive outcome through the electoral process were slim, given the size, wealth, and resources of the Southern opposition."[29]

Foner disputes this pessimistic consensus. In *Reconstruction: The Unfinished Revolution* and in other writings, he argues that black suffrage was a policy worth trying. Its failure was by no means foreordained: contingent factors, many of them unforeseen and unforeseeable, influenced the course of events; given different contingencies, the outcome might have been different. "One can, I think, imagine alternative scenarios and modest successes: the Republican Party establishing itself as a permanent fixture on the Southern landscape, the North summoning the resolve to insist that the Constitution must be respected." Even after 1877, Foner asserts, "the experiences of Readjuster Virginia and Populist-Republican North Carolina" showed that "Redemption did not entirely foreclose the possibilities of biracial politics."[30]

This optimistic might-have-been, however, is belied by the evidence that Foner marshals in the 600 deeply researched pages of *Reconstruction*. In persuasive detail, *Reconstruction* documents the virulent, unrelenting opposition of southern whites to black suffrage, and their ability to count on the solid support of northern Democrats; the suicidal factionalism of the southern Republicans; the rapid ebbing of the national party's enthusiasm for intervention in the South; the woeful inadequacy of the federal government's efforts to ensure free and fair elections; the thin, ineffective federal military presence in the South; and the Supreme Court decisions that gutted the Fourteenth and Fifteenth Amendments. As Foner confesses, in imagining a successful outcome "we enter the realm of the purely speculative. What remains certain is that Reconstruction failed."[31]

The end of Reconstruction, of course, did not immediately extinguish black political influence and plunge African Americans into what Rayford Logan called "the nadir." As C. Vann Woodward pointed out many decades ago, and as other scholars subsequently documented, race relations remained somewhat fluid after 1877—for between 15 and 30 years, depending upon the state. Indeed, in parts of the South, blacks demonstrated great persistence in utilizing the ballot to improve public schools, gain jobs as teachers and city employees, and bring state-supported colleges into being.[32]

Yet there were sharp limits to what biracial politics could secure for blacks. In the two states where black voters helped oust the Democrats from power after Reconstruction, Readjuster Virginia in 1879–1883 and Populist-Republican North Carolina in 1894–1898, the promise of change proved short-lived. Democrats again resorted to fraud, intimidation, and violence to crush their opponents. In the rest of the South "the black vote had become, . . . quite minimal," writes Michael Perman. . . . many of the gains secured . . . disappeared. In the field of education, blacks remained dependent upon northern philanthropy, and their own initiative, for schools above the elementary level. In the rural South, where the great majority of blacks lived, the only good schools were private ones.[33]

In searching for a silver lining, Foner cites the "enduring accomplishments" of Congressional Reconstruction. These included the "autonomous black family and a network of religious and social institutions." Moreover, Reconstruction "pioneered civil rights legislation"; although "largely unenforced," these laws "established for the first time at the state level a standard of equal citizenship." After conceding that the consequences of Reconstruction's demise were damaging for blacks, Foner counters that they would have been much worse had the policy never been essayed. Former slaveholders failed to impose a coercive system of gang labor under strict white supervision. . . .

None of these advances, however, required black suffrage, the rock upon which Congressional Reconstruction foundered. Blacks formed family units and organized churches on their own initiative in the wake of emancipation, with little resistance from—and sometimes with the assistance of—their former masters. Similarly, blacks rejected gang labor very soon after emancipation, engaging in a tug-of-war with white landlords that, after a series of experiments, resulted in sharecropping, a system fairly well established by the time Congressional Reconstruction enfranchised the freedmen. Certainly, their hand was strengthened by the intervention of the Freedman's Bureau and the actions of U.S. military commanders, both of which restrained the power of white landlords and inhibited the enforcement of the oppressive Black Codes. . . . It does not follow, however, that equality of citizenship required black suffrage. It was the Civil Rights Act and the Fourteenth Amendment, not the enfranchising clauses of Military Reconstruction, that established the principle of equal citizenship and equality before the law. When, after 1900, the federal government prosecuted peonage in the South, it based its actions on the Thirteenth Amendment's prohibition of "involuntary servitude." In short, by attributing all these advances to "Reconstruction"—meaning Congressional Reconstruction—Foner elides the distinction between emancipation, civil rights, and suffrage.

Foner finds crumbs of comfort in the fact that, despite the undermining of Congressional Reconstruction, the Fourteenth and Fifteenth Amendments remained in the text of the Constitution. Although the Democratic Party had effectively nullified these amendments by the 1900s, he contends that its failure to formally repeal them constituted a residual gain for blacks. "While flagrantly violated" after 1877, he writes, the Reconstruction amendments "planted the seeds of future struggle and left intact a vehicle for future federal intervention in southern affairs." They were "sleeping giants," to be "awakened by the efforts of a subsequent generation."[34]

To regard the Reconstruction amendments as crucial to the success of the civil rights movement, however, is to attribute extraordinary power to legal forms. In no other nation have far-reaching political changes in the second half of the twentieth century depended upon an organic law enacted almost a century earlier. It took 100 years to make civil and political equality a reality in the South—counting from 1866–1870 to 1964–1970—and during the intervening decades the Fourteenth and Fifteenth Amendments were virtual dead letters as far as black Southerners were concerned. Indeed, the evisceration of these amendments by the Supreme Court inhibited the federal government's willingness and ability to intervene in the South on behalf of blacks. Whenever the Eisenhower, Kennedy, and Johnson administrations did so, they were responding to inescapable political pressures. To be sure, the NAACP based its legal strategy upon constitutional grounds. . . . But its numerous courtroom victories were substantively hollow until, from the 1940s on, economic and intellectual changes, as well as world events, propelled political change.[35] The civil rights movement that arose in the 1950s mobilized moral rather than constitutional arguments—nonviolent direct action transcended legalism. Through nonviolent direct action, blacks changed the facts on the ground and made white supremacy unworkable. Then the law caught up.

The same political pressure that made radical change unavoidable impelled the Supreme Court to find constitutional pretexts for accommodating that change. "Judges and lawyers do not 'discover' law," writes Christopher Waldrep. "They make it." In *Brown v. Board of Education*, for example, the Supreme Court first decided to rule against segregated public schools and then, ignoring history and discarding precedent, found a constitutional justification to do so.[36] It did the same in the sit-in cases. The notion that the civil rights revolution depended upon the constitutional legacy of Reconstruction puts the cart before the horse. As Michael Lind has argued, to describe the civil rights movement as the fulfillment of . . . misleading. "Like many successful revolutions, the civil rights revolution was disguised as a restoration. But in reality it was part of a global process of overturning white supremacy that occurred simultaneously throughout the world in the decades following World War II." In 1950, . . . India became the world's largest democracy. The period of black disfranchisement in America actually coincided fairly accurately with the period of European colonial rule in Africa. In 1957, the year Congress passed the first civil rights law since 1875. . . . In short, the notion that the constitutional legacy of Congressional Reconstruction conferred a particular advantage on black Americans in their fight for suffrage is questionable. It turned out to be no greater practical advantage than to be ruled as colonial subjects in Britain's empire. As Justice Robert H. Jackson put it in 1954, "present-day conditions" made a Supreme Court decision overturning *Plessy v. Ferguson* unavoidable.[37]

Most historians offer a bleak assessment of what Congressional Reconstruction achieved. In his 1961 synthesis, *Reconstruction: After the Civil War*, John Hope Franklin emphasized blacks' political powerlessness and physical vulnerability. "The great mass of [blacks] remained impoverished, with only their labor to sell under conditions peculiarly disadvantageous to them. . . . In the towns and cities they were barred from employment in the new industries that were arising." In Louisiana, writes Joe Gray Taylor, the state's civil rights law was largely ignored in New Orleans and wholly ignored outside it. The Civil Rights Act passed by Congress in 1875 was a "dead letter from the moment of its enactment, and Southerners boasted that . . . it could not be enforced anywhere in the South." Far from establishing an important principle, civil rights laws, through their ineffectiveness, fostered a belief among the nation's white leaders that the prejudices of whites in the South were immutable. "Legislation is powerless to eradicate racial instincts," the Supreme Court declared in 1896, "and the attempt to do so can only result in accentuating the difficulties of the present situation." The conviction that race relations could not be changed by statute became a new orthodoxy that discouraged federal intervention for decades to come. As sociologist William Graham Sumner put it in 1906: "It is not at all what the humanitarian hoped and expected," but "legislation cannot make mores."[38]

Even if we take into account the fact that blacks continued to wield some political influence after 1877, the end of Reconstruction pointed to the same outcome: segregation, lack of "due process," and exposure to extralegal violence. "In terms of political tolerance and black rights," William C. Harris concludes, Mississippi "reverted to a situation hardly better than the one existing in 1865." In Louisiana, writes Joe Gray Taylor, blacks' civil rights and voting rights "disappeared as if they had never been." In material terms, he adds, most blacks may even have been worse off "insofar as food, clothing, and shelter were concerned." Under the rule of the Democrats, laws so restricted "free labor" as to reduce blacks, in the words of George Rable, "to a condition more resembling serfdom than freedom." Michael Perman described the post-Reconstruction labor system as "coercive" and "oppressive." At its not uncommon harshest, that system held blacks in peonage, a form of "involuntary servitude" no better—often worse—than slavery. In the sugar parishes of Louisiana, where black political power outlasted Reconstruction, a drastic leveling down took pace. "Sugar workers became a rural proletariat," writes John C. Rodrigue, "living within a larger South characterized by a deplorable lack of educational opportunities, economic underdevelopment, and discrimination in all forms of life." A burgeoning convict labor system subjected black prisoners, many of them arrested on petty or trumped-up charges, to work regimes of extreme brutality. No doubt the Black Codes would have been worse. Yet by 1900, important elements of the Black Codes had become embedded in the formal and informal structures of southern race relations.[39]

"The North won the battles but the South dictated the peace terms," William Barney contends. "The white South . . . lost the conventional war for secession," agrees Joe Gray Taylor, "but with northern allies it . . . won the political and guerilla war of Reconstruction." Richard Zuczek makes an obvious but necessary point when it comes to weighing what blacks gained from Congressional Reconstruction. "Although the South's losses—the changes, in effect—were significant, to focus on these is to examine the issue in reverse." White Southerners initiated the Civil War to protect their white supremacist slave society. Although they lost the military struggle for independence, they succeeded in recreating "a white supremacist society with a reasonable degree of autonomy." Moreover, this counterrevolution "guided the South for the next hundred years." No wonder Confederate nationalism did not survive as a political force: ex-confederates achieved most of what they wanted *within* the United States.[40]

Foner, however, refuses to see black suffrage as an ill-thought-out political expedient that thrust blacks into a cauldron of violence. Rather, he depicts it as part of an ongoing struggle for freedom that defines the essential meaning of American history. "Freedom," he argues, has been "fundamental to Americans' sense of themselves"; this idea "anchors the American sense of exceptional national identity." During Reconstruction, he wrote, "Americans made their first attempt to live up to the noble professions of their political creed—something few societies have ever done."[41] Foner's notion of American exceptionalism, however, exaggerates the nation's historical commitment to universal suffrage and underestimates its "democratic deficit."[42] As Alexander Keyssar has written, a comparative study of democratization reveals that the United States "was not an exceptional example of democratic destiny and idealism."[43] Foner's emphasis upon "freedom" also predisposes him to assume that the fight is always worth the cost. To concede that blacks struggled for freedom and suffered an unmitigated defeat would be too bleak a conclusion—hence his description of Reconstruction as an "unfinished revolution" rather than a failed one.

Foner's treatment of African Americans reinforces his overoptimistic reading of Reconstruction's legacy. In this case, it is a matter of pushing a good argument too far. In placing blacks at the center of his narrative, stressing that they were "active agents" rather than "passive victims," Foner followed a scholarly trend that has greatly expanded our knowledge of how blacks perceived and acted upon their freedom. With others, he has demolished the "Dunningite" notion of ignorant freedmen being led astray by conscienceless "carpetbaggers." Moreover, Foner's effort to identify and quantify black officeholders throughout the South has helped to fill an enormous gap in our knowledge of Reconstruction.[44]

In emphasizing black initiative, however, Foner implies that black demands constituted the *primary* cause of Congressional Reconstruction. "Prodded by the demands of four million men and women just emerging from slavery," he writes in *Reconstruction*, Americans attempted to make racial equality real. The enactment of black suffrage, he explains elsewhere, was impelled by "demands by former slaves for the right to vote, the Radicals' commitment to the ideas of equality, widespread disgust with Johnson's policies, the desire to fortify the Republican Party in the South, and the determination to keep ex-confederates from office." Given historians' penchant for ranking causes, this list implies that black demands for the franchise constituted the *leading* reason for black suffrage. This claim, advanced by no other historian (to this author's knowledge), obscures an important reason for Congressional Reconstruction's failure.[45] Black demands for the ballot played such a *small* part in Congress's deliberations that, even as loyal Republican voters, blacks did not constitute a strong enough force for the maintenance of their political rights. True, Republican administrations did not completely abandon efforts to protect black voting rights after 1877. But those efforts proved ineffectual, and after 1894 they ceased altogether. If we consider the amount of moral, legal, political, and economic power mobilized by the civil rights movement in its campaign to re-enfranchise black Southerners, we can appreciate the relative weakness of the freedpeople's position after emancipation.[46]

A second consequence of Foner's emphasis upon black initiative, especially black labor militancy, is to undercut his argument for a potentially successful outcome for Congressional Reconstruction. Emancipation produced a class conflict between freedpeople and former slaveowners, now laborers and landlords. Blacks expected to receive land, resisted signing contracts with white landowners, and occasionally struck for higher wages. Congressional Reconstruction exacerbated this class conflict. It superimposed a political struggle between black and white; it encouraged black laborers to press for higher wages; and it enabled Republican legislatures to use the tax laws "to force land onto the market and stimulate the breakup of the plantation system." While wholly sympathetic to the freedpeople's economic aspirations, Foner admits that the class interests of laborers and landlords were "irreconcilable," and that this incompatibility was a "recipe for continuing conflict." Given this clash of interests, it is hard to see how the former slaveholders could have reacted to Congressional Reconstruction in any other way than they did: by fighting it tooth and nail. Congressional Reconstruction not only threatened their social status and political power but also threatened their very existence as a class. Fortunately for the landlords, the Republican Party's refusal to mandate large-scale land redistribution, its commitment to a laissez-faire conception of "free labor," and its preference for what Lawrence Powell labels "states-rights federalism" made this a class struggle they were very likely to win.[47]

If the odds against Congressional Reconstruction were overwhelming, should the Republicans have made black suffrage their central policy? The only possible justification for adopting a plan that yielded disastrous results is that the Republicans could not have foreseen the violent white response. . . . "No one imagined the terrorist resistance to come." Charles Sumner, overjoyed that his party had enfranchised the ex-slaves, believed that the ballot would provide effective deterrence against white oppression. "The right of suffrage once given can never be taken away," he exulted. "It will be immortal."[48]

Such wishful thinking was natural and understandable. Nevertheless, the Republicans had evidence at their disposal suggesting that black suffrage, if accompanied by the rapid termination of military rule, would expose black and white Republicans to violent reprisals. A steady flow of reports and letters from Freedmen's Bureau officials, army commanders, northern migrants, and former wartime Unionists warned that the removal of troops would embolden ex-confederates to further acts of aggression. Ex-confederates, moreover, made no secret of how they would respond to what they deemed harsh or dishonorable peace terms. Even at the moment of surrender, Edmund Kirby Smith and other Confederate commanders warned that anything less than generous terms would cause violent disturbances.[49] If humiliating oaths that required admissions of guilt were required of returning Confederate soldiers, a Louisianan wrote General Banks, "or if the right of franchise is denied them, they will become so embittered that the most dangerous consequences will ensue—murder, robbery, arson, and the destruction of levees will be an every-day occurrence."[50]

When the Republican Party turned to black suffrage, southern newspapers filled their pages with "darkey" jokes, complaints about black idleness and immorality, bitter denunciations of "radicalism," and dire predictions of racial strife.[51] After the New Orleans riot, the newspapers of the South unanimously blamed the victims and applauded the attackers for a job well done. The riot was a "salutary warning," opined one, that whites would "never submit to be ruled and made strangers in their home by Northern emissaries, a few mischievous southern men and their Negro allies."[52] In 1868, with black suffrage a *fait accompli*, some whites attempted to influence the way blacks voted by treating them to barbecues and posing as their "friends." But when blacks voted solidly Republican, whites had their worst fears confirmed. Refusing to be reconciled to Congressional Reconstruction, their thoughts again turned to violence.[53]

In *The Lost Cause Regained* (1868), a sequel to his bestselling *The Lost Cause*, a heroic history of the Confederacy, newspaper editor Edward A. Pollard sketched the following scenario:

> The South is incapable of the *grand duello* of the past, but not incapable of the fierce and desultory rebellion of mobile columns and raids; incapable of a war of calculation, but not incapable of a war of vengeance. . . . Such vengeful rebellions, spread over the whole space of the country . . . have sometimes, as we are assured by history, been more difficult to quell than regular wars. . . . Let Congress beware of too much experiment on the temper of the South, for a rebellion may yet be kindled there.[54]

By the time these words were in print, the Ku Klux Klan and the Knights of the White Camellia were already active. Governor Henry Warmoth of Louisiana, who had received a death threat, dispatched an emissary to Washington to procure arms. He pleaded for an increased military presence in his state.[55] As Dunning noted, "The actual working of the reconstructed governments during the first few weeks of their existence . . . suggested, if it had not clearly revealed, the inability of those governments to stand alone."[56]

The Republicans could have foreseen the escalating violence, and some did. Thaddeus Stevens and other Radicals argued that it would be folly to impose black suffrage and then quickly concede home rule. They warned that the former slaveholders would regain political supremacy unless checked by federal power and restrained by . . . "a healthy and intelligent public opinion." They therefore envisaged Reconstruction as a long-term project during which Congress would hold the former Confederates to strict terms, a long period of direct federal rule to reshape southern society. Congress would govern the ex-Confederacy as territories, only restoring their rights as states when, to quote the Union General and postwar Congressman Benjamin Butler, "all possibilities of a race war or race dissensions between white and black" had ceased, "the negro had learned how to be a citizen, and the white man how to be a loyal one."[57]

This was the road not taken. As ex-slaves received the vote and former Confederate leaders were temporarily disfranchised, Congress ruled the ex-Confederacy through the Army. If Congressional Reconstruction had democratic ends, its imposition through military means bred charges of tyranny that were not assuaged by the swift termination of military rule—which moderate Republicans had demanded in return for the passage of black suffrage. Troops in the South were soon demobilized and withdrawn. By 1869, only 11,200 blue-clad soldiers remained, a third of whom were policing the Texas frontier.[58] This skeleton force, notes William Barney, was large enough "to be an irritant to southern whites, and a reminder of their defeat, but far too small to constitute an effective army of occupation." As Dunning observed, the outbreaks of racial violence "were almost invariably at points beyond the ready reach of the soldiery. Detachments were always sent to the scene with promptness, but never reached it until the trouble was over."⁵⁹

Although the failure of Congressional Reconstruction had many causes, numerous historians . . . have argued that the terms of its enactment made the prospect of success faint. "By propelling the states into quick restoration," wrote Benedict, "the Reconstruction Acts prevented the slow maturation of healthy public opinion and democratic capabilities that radicals had hoped to nurture in the South through territorialization." The root problem was the Republicans' reluctance to exercise national power in a positive sense. Rather than act directly to enforce civil order in the South, they assumed that state governments, if controlled by Republicans, could do the job. As Barney put it, the Republicans failed to "conceive of a philosophy of national power capable of administering the vast social and economic changes wrought by the war."⁶⁰

This was precisely the argument that Burgess made in 1902. The Republicans, he complained, were too much in thrall to the theory of states' rights to assert and maintain the necessary application of national power. Instead of utilizing black suffrage as a means of quickly ending direct federal rule, Congress should have kept the ex-confederate states under Territorial civil government "until the spirit of loyalty to the nation was established and the principle and practice of civil equality among all citizens was made thoroughly secure"—in other words, for as long as necessary. Moreover, under a Territorial system "Congress could have established a system of free schools." Above all, Congress ought to have brought about, by constitutional amendment or other means, the "nationalization of civil liberty, and its protection by the United States courts." Such a program, *without* black suffrage, might have pacified the South and anchored the rights of the freedmen.⁶¹

In 1870, . . . the Republican Party rejected proposals for federal funding of public education, a decision that, in the opinion of Senator George F. Hoar of Massachusetts, fatally compromised its policy of black suffrage.

Moreover, having endowed black men with the franchise and engineered the election of Republican state governments, Congress failed to create federal machinery to ensure free and fair elections, mistakenly believing that the states would be able to maintain the new dispensation. When white terrorism revealed these governments' vulnerability, Congress responded with the Enforcement Acts (1870–1871) in an attempt to break up the Ku Klux Klan and ensure free and fair elections. Although these measures suppressed the Klan, they failed to dissuade whites that violence and intimidation did not pay. The consistent application of the Enforcement Acts and the exemplary punishment of a few ringleaders might have had some deterrent effect. But federal authorities prosecuted only a fraction of the potential cases, and those convicted received very light sentences and were often released from prison early. Even selective enforcement, Foner concedes, "placed an unprecedented—and unrealistic—burden . . . on the federal courts." Dunning made the same point in 1907, noting that efficient enforcement would have required "at least a threefold increase" in the number of federal courts in the South. By 1874—the year that Justice Joseph P. Bradley threw out the convictions in *U.S. v. Cruikshank*, the Colfax massacre case—the conviction rate had fallen to 10.5 percent of cases prosecuted. Bradley's ruling, affirmed by the Supreme Court in 1876, made it virtually impossible to convict anyone for politically motivated racial violence.⁶²

Praising Congressional Reconstruction as a shining example of American democratic idealism, Foner describes the grant of black suffrage as "unique," "stunning," and "remarkable." As a "massive experiment in interracial democracy," it was "without precedent in the history of this or any other country that abolished slavery in the nineteenth century." More significant than its failure was the fact that "it was attempted at all."⁶³

Other historians, "revisionists" as well as "Dunningites," have been less impressed by Congressional Reconstruction. "On the issue of Negro equality," wrote C. Vann Woodward, "the [Republican] party remained divided, hesitant, and unsure of its purpose." Well aware that most of their white constituents feared and disliked blacks, and did not wish to enfranchise them, the Republicans forced black suffrage upon the South while reserving "the question of suffrage in all the loyal States to the people of those States." Even when framing the Fifteenth Amendment, which forbade suffrage restriction on the grounds of race or color, the Republicans refused to make a positive commitment to universal suffrage, well aware that northern states such as Massachusetts employed property and educational tests to narrow the electorate. The Republicans also "turned down [Thaddeus] Stevens' proposal to assure an economic foundation for Negro equality and Sumner's resolution to give the Negro equal opportunity in schools, in homesteads, and full civil rights."⁶⁴

None of this is to deny that a desire to protect the freedmen from neo-Confederate aggression informed Congressional Reconstruction. Yet Sumner and other Radicals recognized that their "moderate" colleagues could only be induced to support black suffrage through fear that without it, loyal governments in the South could not be organized. . . . The speed with which the Republican

Party abandoned the cause of democratization—first the liberal reformers and then the national party—confirmed the weakness of its commitment to universal suffrage. The Republicans' fear of neo-Confederate aggression rapidly faded, and the Republican consensus over Reconstruction started to splinter very soon after Grant's inauguration in 1869. "Many liberal reformers retreated from democratic principles altogether," writes Foner, "advocating educational and property qualifications for voting." Some Radicals, too, concluded that Congressional Reconstruction was a failure. The hasty readmission of the southern states, wrote George W. Julian in 1883, had produced "the horrors of carpet-bag government, Ku Klux outrages, and a system of pro-consular government as inconsistent with the rights of those states as it has been disgraceful to the very idea of free government and fatal to the best interests of the colored race."[65]

Historians have long debated the motives behind Congressional Reconstruction and the argument will, by its very nature, remain unresolved. Ultimately, however, the terms in which the argument is usually presented—idealism versus partisanship, sincerity versus hypocrisy—may obscure rather than explain the failure of Congressional Reconstruction. Pure motives are no guarantee of success, and shallow opportunism is no predictor of failure. Even if one concedes Foner's emphasis upon Republican idealism, the question remains: Was the grant of black suffrage a mistake? If a policy is based on faulty political assumptions, good intentions may pave a road to hell. Universal suffrage was never likely to work in the premodern, preindustrial South, especially when a black rural proletariat displaced their white landlords from political power. The only precedent for such a policy was the institution of universal suffrage during the French Revolution: not a happy example. The slogan "the bottom rail's on top" may appeal to historians who sympathize with the freed people, but it exemplified a key problem with Congressional Reconstruction: black suffrage drove the white landowning class to fight for its social and economic position by effecting a counterrevolution.[66]

Congressional Reconstruction was indeed remarkable. It would be hard to think of a more poorly designed program for pacifying the South and turning ex-slaves into citizens. It embodied two of the very things that Lincoln had opposed as unwise: black suffrage imposed by the federal government, and the domination of southern politics by northern migrants. "What ifs" are treacherous, but it is hard to imagine that blacks, the South, and the nation would have been worse off under a program that stopped short of black suffrage, or which entailed partial black suffrage, coupled with a federal commitment to public education and the vigorous enforcement of law and order. The white reaction against black suffrage created the Solid South and, in Burgess's words, "extinguished every sense of culpability" in the minds of the ex-confederates. Worse yet, whites in the North came to accept Democratic arguments that black suffrage had been a mistake and that federal intervention in southern race relations would always backfire. As Justice Robert Jackson noted in weighing the *Brown* cases, the memory of Reconstruction, and the "lessons" learned from it, had sustained segregation by emphasizing "the deep humiliation of carpetbag government imposed by conquest." The ironic result of enacting black suffrage in 1867–1868 was to delay the democratization of the South until 1965.[67]

In judging our professional predecessors, we must acknowledge that our own interpretations of the past will be revised and perhaps rejected. As Churchill put it: "In one phase men seem to have been right, in another they seem to have been wrong. Then again, a few years later, when the perspective of time has lengthened, all stands in a different setting. There is a new proportion. There is another scale of values." The same question that we direct against the "Dunning school" will in all likelihood be directed against us: "How on earth could they possibly have believed *that*?" . . . If one reads them with an open mind, treating them as individuals rather than a "school," he will find that they often rose above their limitations. One thing in particular they got right. The enactment of black suffrage proved one of the greatest legislative missteps in the nation's history. As Burgess wrote, "It is simply astounding that [Congress] made such a mess of it in 1867."[68]

Notes

1. I retain scare quotes for "Dunning school" and "Dunningite" because these terms wrongly attribute the views of Dunning's students to Dunning himself; fail to distinguish between the views of Dunning and John W. Burgess, Dunning's mentor; and misleadingly include popular, non-academic works such as Claude Bowers, *The Tragic Era: The Revolution after Lincoln* (New York: Blue Ribbon Books, 1929).

2. Charles W. Ramsdell, *Reconstruction in Texas* (New York: Columbia University Press, 1910), 49, 318; J. G. de Roulhac Hamilton, *Reconstruction in North Carolina* (Raleigh: privately published, 1906), 215; William Archibald Dunning, *Reconstruction, Political and Economic, 1865–1877* (New York: Harper and Brothers, 1907), 212; John W. Burgess, *Reconstruction and the Constitution, 1866–1876* (New York: Charles Scribner's Sons, 1902), 246, 252.

For a scathing critique of the "Dunning school," see John Hope Franklin, "Mirror for Americans: A Century of Reconstruction History," *American Historical Review* 85:1 (February 1980): 3–4, 6–10.

3. W. E. B. Du Bois, *Black Reconstruction in America, 1860–1880* (1935; reprint, New York: Atheneum, 1969), 718–720.

4. Michael W. Fitzgerald, *Splendid Failure: Postwar Reconstruction in the American South* (Chicago: Ivan R. Dee, 2007), 213; Eric Foner, *Reconstruction: America's Unfinished Revolution, 1863–1877* (New York: Harper & Row, 1988), 609.

5. Richard Dawkins, *A Devil's Chaplain: Reflections on Hope, Lies, Science, and Love* (Boston: Houghton Mifflin, 2003), 66; Eric Foner, *Give Me Liberty!: An American History*, 2 vols. (New York: Norton, Seagull ed., 2006), 2:xxii; Wilfred M. McClay, "John W. Burgess and the Search for Cohesion in American Political Thought," *Polity* 26:1 (1993): 53–63.

6. Du Bois, *Black Reconstruction*, 719–720; C. Mildred Thompson, *Reconstruction in Georgia, Economic, Social, and Political, 1865–1872* (New York: Columbia University Press, 1915), 52–94, 279–298, 361–394; Ella Lonn, *Reconstruction in Louisiana after 1868* (New York: G. P. Putnam's, 1918), 73–180; Ramsdell, *Reconstruction in Texas*, 44–51, 66–70.

7. Thompson, *Reconstruction in Georgia*, 394.

8. Phillip R. Muller, "Look Back Without Anger: A Reappraisal of William A. Dunning," *Journal of American History* 61:2 (September 1974): 325–338; Burgess, *Reconstruction and the Constitution*, ix, 245, 298. In *Reconstruction, Political and Economic*, Dunning acknowledged his debt to popular historian James Ford Rhodes, who had just completed a two-volume account of Reconstruction in his multivolume *History of the United States from the Compromise of 1850* (New York: Macmillan, 1906). Dunning's 1907 synthesis, although not entirely without merit, was a potboiler in which Dunning took little interest and for which he did little research. Most of what is valuable in Dunning's work can be found in his earlier essays, some of which were published in *Essays on the Civil War and Reconstruction and Related Topics* (New York: Macmillan, 1897).

9. In reviewing a version of this article, three leading historians of Reconstruction admitted that they had never read Burgess with any care.

10. For the caricature version of the "Dunning school," see Eric Foner, "Reconstruction Revisited," *Reviews in American History* 10:4 (December 1982): 82; Foner, *Reconstruction*, xix.

11. Burgess, *Reconstruction and the Constitution*, 9, 12, 18, 36–41.

12. Ibid., 42–43, 61, 81, 116.

13. Ibid., 67.

14. Dunning, *Essays on the Civil War and Reconstruction*, 248.

15. Burgess, *Reconstruction and the Constitution*, 61.

16. Ibid., 53, 72–73, 63–64.

17. Ibid., 65–78.

18. Ibid., 111.

19. Dunning, *Essays on the Civil War and Reconstruction*, 248, 250.

20. James G. Blaine, *Twenty Years of Congress; From Lincoln to Garfield*, 2 vols. (Norwich, CT: Henry Hill Publishing Company, 1886), 2:264.

21. Burgess, *Reconstruction and the Constitution*, 111.

22. Dunning, *Essays on the Civil War and Reconstruction*, 250; Dunning, *Reconstruction, Political and Economic*, 204; Burgess, *Reconstruction and the Constitution*, ix, 245–246, 252, 263.

23. Charles Sumner to the Duchess of Argyll, April 3, 1866, in Beverly Wilson Palmer, ed., *The Selected Letters of Charles Sumner*, 2 vols. (Boston: Northeastern University Press, 1990), 2:359.

24. Foner, *Reconstruction*, 346; Fitzgerald, *Splendid Failure*, 97.

25. Michael Perman, *Struggle for Mastery: Disfranchisement in the South, 1888–1908* (Chapel Hill: University of North Carolina Press, 2010), 10–22.

26. Dunning, *Reconstruction, Political and Economic*, 213.

27. Burgess, *Reconstruction and the Constitution*, 251–252.

28. Michael Perman, *Reunion Without Compromise: The South and Reconstruction, 1865–1868* (Cambridge: Cambridge University Press, 1973), 346–347.

29. Otto H. Olsen, ed., *Reconstruction and Redemption in the South* (Baton Rouge: Louisiana State University Press, 1980), 42, 197, 202; Lawrence N. Powell, "Centralization and its Discontents in Reconstruction Louisiana," *Studies in American Political Development* 20 (Fall 2006): 131; Fitzgerald, *Splendid Failure*, 96–97.

30. Foner, *Reconstruction*, 603–604.

31. *Loc. cit.*

32. C. Vann Woodward, *The Strange Career of Jim Crow* (London: Oxford University Press, 1966), 31–65. On biracial politics between the end of Reconstruction and disfranchisement, see, for example, J. Morgan Kousser, *The Shaping of Southern Politics: Suffrage Restriction and the Establishment of the One-Party South, 1880–1910* (New Haven: Yale University Press, 1974); Eric Anderson, *Race and Politics in North Carolina, 1872–1901: The Black Second* (Baton Rouge: Louisiana State University Press, 1981); Howard N. Rabinowitz, *Race Relations in the Urban South, 1865–1890* (Athens: University of Georgia Press, 1996); *Before Jim Crow: The Politics of Race in Postemancipation Virginia* (Chapel Hill: University of North Carolina Press, 2000); Michael Fitzgerald, *Urban Emancipation: Popular Politics in Reconstruction Mobile, 1860–1890* (Baton Rouge: Louisiana State University Press, 2001); Steven Hahn, *A Nation Under Our Feet: Black Political Struggles in the Rural South from Slavery to the Great Migration* (Cambridge: Harvard University Press, 2003).

33. Perman, *Struggle for Mastery*, 25. On the condition of black schools, see Adam Fairclough, *A Class of Their Own: Black Teachers in the Segregated South* (Cambridge: Belknap Press, 2007).

34. Eric Foner, *Nothing But Freedom: Emancipation and Its Legacy* (Baton Rouge: Louisiana State University Press, 1983), 73; Eric Foner, "The Civil War and the Idea of Freedom," *Art Institute of Chicago Museum Studies* 27:1 (2001): 25.

35. For the influence of social and political context in determining Supreme Court decisions and the effectiveness of those decisions in promoting change, see Michael J. Klarman, *From Jim Crow to Civil Rights: The Supreme Court and the Struggle for Racial Equality* (New York: Oxford University Press, 2004).

36. In drafting the 1964 Civil Rights Act, a measure forced upon it by the explosion of street protests sweeping the South, the Kennedy administration considered the Fourteenth Amendment such a weak reed that it initially looked to the Commerce clause as a constitutional basis for banning segregated public accommodations.

37. Christopher Waldrep, *Roots of Disorder: Race and Criminal Justice in the American South, 1817–1880* (Urbana: University of Illinois Press, 1998), 171; Michael Lind, *What Lincoln Believed: The Values and Convictions of America's Greatest President* (New York: Anchor Books, 2006), 251; "Memorandum by Mr. Justice Jackson," 1 March 15, 1954, pp. 20–22, copy provided to author by Michael J. Klarman.

38. John Hope Franklin, *Reconstruction: After the Civil War* (Chicago: University of Chicago Press, 1961), 219, 221; Joe Gray Taylor, *Louisiana Reconstructed, 1863–1877* (Baton Rouge: Louisiana State University Press, 1974), 259; Joe Gray Taylor, "Louisiana: An Impossible Task," in Olsen, ed., *Reconstruction and Redemption in the South*, 213; *Plessy v. Ferguson* 163 U.S. 557 (1896), at 251, http://www.law.cornell.edu/supct/html/historics/USSC_CR_0163_0537_ZO.html; William Graham Sumner, *Folkways: A Study of the Sociological Importance of Usages, Manners, Customs, Mores, and Morals* (Boston: Ginn & Company, 1906), 78–79. On the influence of Sumner on American social science, see Gunnar Myrdal, *An American Dilemma: The Negro Problem and Modern Democracy* (New York: Harper & Bros., 1944), 1048–1057; James W. Prothro, "Stateways v. Folkways Revisited: An Error in Prediction," *Journal of Politics* 34:2 (May 1972): 352–353.

39. William C. Harris, "Mississippi: Republican Factionalism and Mismanagement," in Olsen, ed., *Reconstruction and Redemption in the South*, 108; Taylor, "Louisiana: An Impossible Task," 215; George C. Rable, *But There Was No Peace: The Role of Violence in the Politics of Reconstruction* (Athens: University of Georgia Press, 2007), 185; Michael Perman, *The Road to Redemption: Southern Politics, 1869–1879* (Chapel Hill: University of North Carolina Press, 1984), 260–262; Pete Daniel, *The Shadow of Slavery: Peonage in the South, 1901–1969* (Urbana: University of Illinois Press, 1990); William Cohen, *At Freedom's Edge: Black Mobility and the Southern Quest for Racial Control, 1861–1915* (Baton Rouge: Louisiana State University Press, 1991); John C. Rodrigue, *Reconstruction in the Cane Fields: From Slavery to Free Labor in Louisiana's Sugar Parishes, 1862–1880* (Baton Rouge: Louisiana State University Press, 2001), 190; Douglas A. Blackmon, *Slavery by Another Name: The Re-enslavement of Black Americans from the Civil War to World War II* (New York: Doubleday, 2008). See also Jeffrey R. Kerr-Ritchie, *Freedpeople in the Tobacco South: Virginia, 1860–1900* (Chapel Hill: University of North Carolina Press, 1989); Mary Ellen Curtin, *Black Prisoners and Their World: Alabama, 1865–1900* (Charlottesville: University of Virginia Press, 2000).

40. William L. Barney, *Flawed Victory: A New Perspective on the Civil War* (New York: Praeger, 1975), 194; Taylor, "Louisiana: An Impossible Task," 230; Richard Zuczek, *State of Rebellion: Reconstruction in South Carolina* (Columbia: University of South Carolina Press, 1996), 208–209. See also Anne Sarah Rubin, *A Shattered Nation: The Rise and Fall of the Confederacy, 1861–1869* (Chapel Hill: University of North Carolina Press, 2005).

41. Foner, "The Civil War and the Idea of Freedom," 8; Eric Foner, "American Freedom in a Global Age," *American Historical Review* 106:1 (February 2001): 4–6; Eric Foner, "American Freedom in the Age of Emancipation," *Journal of American History* 81:2 (September 1994): 436; Foner, *Reconstruction*, xxvii.

42. Congress has never made the right to vote an affirmative national right. As a result, many states have imposed complicated registration and voter identification requirements. The United States is the only democracy to disfranchise ex-prisoners on a large scale. In addition, voter turnout in the United States has long been significantly lower than that of most other democracies. It could also be argued that the power of the Supreme Court to overturn federal legislation, as well as the constitution and operation of the Senate, further weakens the democratic principle.

43. Alexander Keyssar, *The Right to Vote: The Contested History of Democracy in the United States* (New York: Basic Books, 2000), xxiii.

44. Foner, *Reconstruction*, xxiv–xxv; idem, *Freedom's Lawmakers: A Directory of Black Officeholders during Reconstruction* (Baton Rouge: Louisiana State University Press, 1996). For the scholarly trend, see Roberta Sue Alexander, "Presidential Reconstruction: Ideology and Change," in Eric Anderson and Alfred A. Moss, eds., *The Facts of Reconstruction: Essays in Honor of John Hope Franklin* (Baton Rouge: Louisiana State University Press, 1991), 44–49.

45. See also Hahn, *A Nation Under Our Feet,* 159, 163. Although Hahn emphasizes the role of "African-American agitation" in the enactment of Congressional Reconstruction, he does not assign it priority as a cause of black suffrage.

46. Foner, *Reconstruction*, xxvii; Foner, *Give Me Liberty!*, 2:493; Stanley P. Hirshon, *Farewell to the Bloody Shirt: Northern Republicans and the Southern Negro, 1877–1893* (Chicago: Quadrangle, 1962); Robert M. Goldman, *"A Free Ballot and a Fair Count": The Department of Justice and the Enforcement of Voting Rights in the South, 1877–1893* (New York: Garland Pub., 1990); Xi Wang, *The Trial of Democracy: Black Suffrage and Northern Republicans, 1860–1910* (Athens: University of Georgia Press, 1997).

47. Foner, *Nothing But Freedom*, 69, 82; Powell, "Centralization and its Discontents in Reconstruction Louisiana," 106–107.

48. Fitzgerald, *Splendid Failure*, 72; Sumner to Theodore Tilton, April 18, 1867, *Selected Letters of Charles Sumner*, 2:394.

49. Edmund Kirby Smith, "Memorandum for Colonel Sprague," May 15, 1865, in *The War of the Rebellion: a Compilation of the Official Records of the Union and Confederate Armies: Series I, Vol. 48, Part I* (Washington, DC: Government Printing Office, 1891), 191; Edmund Kirby Smith to Sprague, May 30, 1865, ibid., 198–199.

50. F. L. Claiborne to Nathaniel P. Banks, May 22, 1865, ibid., *Series 1, Vol. 48, Part II*, 220.

51. Dunning, *Reconstruction, Political and Economic*, 83–84, 117; Dan Carter, *When the War Was Over: The Failure of Self-Reconstruction in the South, 1865–1867* (Baton Rouge: Louisiana State University Press, 1985), 244–245, 261–275.

52. Carter, *When the War Was Over*, 252.

53. Dunning, *Reconstruction, Political and Economic*, 114–115; Lonn, *Reconstruction in Louisiana After 1868*, 14–15; 41st Cong., 2d Session, House Mis. Doc. 154, part 2, *Louisiana Contested Elections* (Washington, DC: Government Printing Office, 1870), 54, 100, 164–165.

54. Edward A. Pollard, *The Lost Cause Regained* (New York: E. W. Carleton & Co., 1868), 152–153.

55. Francis W. Binning, "Henry Clay Warmoth and Louisiana Reconstruction," PhD dissertation, University of North Carolina at Chapel Hill, 1968, 118–119, 146–147. Major General Joseph Mower warned that "serious trouble may be reasonably anticipated at the coming election [in Louisiana]. . . . I consider the number of troops in my command too few to meet the responsibilities of the service required": Mower to Gen. G. L. Hartsuff, September 15, 1868, box 4, Letters Received, Fifth Military District, Department of the Gulf, RG393, Records of U.S. Army Continental Commands, National Archives. For the dangerously unstable

situation in Louisiana in 1868, see also Joseph G. Dawson III, *Army Generals and Reconstruction, Louisiana, 1862–1877* (Baton Rouge: Louisiana State University Press, 1982), 81–92.

56. Dunning, *Essays on the Civil War and Reconstruction*, 228.
57. George W. Julian, *Political Recollections, 1840 to 1872* (1883; reprint, Miami: Mnemosyne, 1969); Benjamin F. Butler, *Butler's Book: A Review of His Legal, Political, and Military Career* (Boston: A. M. Thayer & Co., 1892), 960.
58. Harold M. Hyman and William M. Wieck, *Equal Justice Under Law: Constitutional Development, 1835–1875* (New York: Harper & Row, 1982), 444–452; Richard M. Valelly, *The Two Reconstructions: The Struggle for Black Enfranchisement* (Chicago: University of Chicago Press, 2004), 95.
59. Barney, *Flawed Victory*, 188; Dunning, *Reconstruction, Political and Economic*, 271.
60. W. R. Brock, *An American Crisis: Congress and Reconstruction, 1865–1867* (New York: Harper Torchbooks, 1963), 268, 274; Powell, "Centralization and its Discontents in Reconstruction Louisiana," 106–107, 131; Michael Les Benedict, *A Compromise of Principle: Congressional Republicans and Reconstruction, 1863–1869* (New York: W. W. Norton, 1974), 243; Hyman and Wieck, *Equal Justice Under Law*, 444, 462, 509–512; Barney, *Flawed Victory*, 185.
61. Burgess, *Reconstruction and the Constitution*, 111, 134–135.
62. George F. Hoar, *Autobiography of Seventy Years*, 2 vols. (New York: Charles Scribner's Sons, 1906), 1:255–258; Blaine, *Twenty Years of Congress*, 2:42; Zuczek, *State of Rebellion*, 96–108; J. Michael Martinez, *Carpetbaggers, Cavalry, and the Ku Klux Klan: Exposing the Invisible Empire During Reconstruction* (Lanham, MD: Rowman & Littlefield, 2007), 186–187; Foner, *Reconstruction*, 245; Dunning, *Reconstruction, Political and Economic*, 270–271; Hyman and Wieck, *Equal Justice Under Law*, 473–488; Charles Lane, *The Day Freedom Died: The Colfax Massacre, the Supreme Court, and the Betrayal of Reconstruction* (New York: Henry Holt, 2008), 205–214, 244–247, 251–252; J. R. Beckwith to George H. Williams, October 21, 1874, Letters Received by the Department of Justice from the State of Louisiana, 1871–1884, M940, RG 60, reel 2, National Archives.
63. Foner, "The Civil War and the Idea of Freedom," 25; Foner, "American Freedom in the Age of Emancipation," 436; Foner, "American Freedom in a Global Age," 4–6; Foner, *Reconstruction*, xxvii.
64. C. Vann Woodward, "Seeds of Failure in Radical Race Policy," *Proceedings of the American Philosophical Society* 110:1 (February 18, 1966), 3–7; Keyssar, *The Right to Vote*, xxiii.
65. Sumner to Bright, May 27, 1867, *Selected Letters of Charles Sumner*, 398; Foner, *Reconstruction*, 492; Julian, *Political Recollections*.
66. Seymour Martin Lipset, *Political Man: The Social Bases of Politics* (Baltimore: Johns Hopkins University Press, 1981), 469. For the development of American democracy in the international context of democratization, see also Walter D. Burnham, "The Appearance and Disappearance of the American Voter," in Richard Rose, ed., *Electoral Participation: A Comparative Perspective* (Beverly Hills: Sage, 1980), 35–73; Arend Lijphart, *Patterns of Democracy: Government Forms and Performance in Thirty-Six Countries* (New Haven: Yale University Press, 1999), 2–15, 52, 143–144; S. N. Eisenstadt, *Paradoxes of Democracy: Fragility, Continuity, and Change* (Washington, DC: Woodrow Wilson Center Press, 1999), 16–19; Teri L. Caraway, "Democratization: Class, Gender, Race, and the Extension of the Suffrage," *Comparative Politics* 36:4 (July 2004): 447; Daron Acemoglu and James A. Robinson, *Economic Origins of Dictatorship and Democracy* (Cambridge: Cambridge University Press, 2006), 63–68, 270–271; Rosemary O'Kane, *Paths to Democracy: Revolution and Totalitarianism* (London: Routledge, 2004), 42–85; John Dunn, *Democracy: A History* (New York: Atlantic Monthly Press, 2005), 72, 91–117, 153–154; Lind, *What Lincoln Believed*, 299–308.
67. Lincoln to George F. Shepley, November 21, 1862; Lincoln to Nathaniel N. Banks, March 13, 1864; Lincoln to Lyman Trumbull, January 9, 1865, all in Abraham Lincoln Papers at the Library of Congress, digital version; Lincoln, "Last Public Address," April 11, 1865, in Roy P. Basler, ed., *Collected Works of Abraham Lincoln*, digital version (Abraham Lincoln Association, 1953), 401–403; John Hay, *Letters of John Hay and Extracts from Diary*, 3 vols. (Washington, DC: Printed but not Published, 1908), 3:250–252; Benedict, *A Compromise of Principle*, 90–92;

William C. Harris, *With Charity for All: Lincoln and the Reconstruction of the Union* (Lexington: University Press of Kentucky, 1996), 232–260; Burgess, *Reconstruction and the Constitution*, 296–298; Keyssar, *Right to Vote*, xviii, 111–116; Jackson memo, 3.

68. David Reynolds, *In Command of History: Churchill Fighting and Writing the Second World War* (New York: Random House, 2005), 37; Burgess, *Reconstruction and the Constitution*, 111. Cf. Woodward, "Seeds of Failure in Radical Race Policy," 5: "It was on the whole a sorry performance."

ADAM FAIRCLOUGH is a Professor Emeritus of American History at the Leiden University Institute for History. He served as the Raymond and Beverly Sackler chair from 2005 to 2016. Dr. Fairclough expertise lies in the Black Civil Rights Movement in the United States.

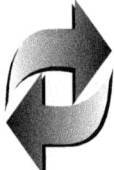

EXPLORING THE ISSUE

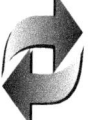

Did Reconstruction Fail as a Result of Racism?

Critical Thinking and Reflection

1. Reflect on W. E. B. Du Bois' statement: "When [Johnson] asked that plantations be divided in the South and lands opened in the West, he had in mind White men, who would thus become rich or at least richer. But for Negroes, he had nothing of the sort in mind, except the bare possibility that, if given freedom, they might continue to exist and not die out."
2. Reflect on Adam Fairclough's assertion that "historians have long debated the motives behind Congressional Reconstruction and the argument will, by its very nature, remain unresolved." Do you agree or disagree? Why or why not?
3. Comment on the notion that most historians agree that "without basic changes in the racial attitudes of nearly all southern whites—attitudes which they shared with most northern whites—there was scant likelihood that any solution to postwar problems in the United States could be found." Do you agree or disagree? Why or why not?
4. Why did Republicans believe that the "ballot would provide effective deterrence against White oppression"?
5. Comment on the "American Assumption" (noted in McLeod's analysis) that hard work will lead to the achievement of wealth.

Is There Common Ground?

Racism in the Reconstruction era is a common thread between the two articles. While both articles address the centrality of racism, their conclusions for its role in Reconstruction differ. McLeod argues that Andrew Johnson's racist views of blacks limited his willingness to see the possibilities for a post–Civil War United States in which blacks would be on equal ground with whites. Fairclough, in his reexamination of histories on Reconstruction, notes that racism was very much part of the Reconstruction era, but was not the reason for its failure. Failure, to Fairclough, rests with Congress, which enacted policies that were not given enough support from the government thus allowing state governments that were adamantly opposed to freedom for blacks to limit rights of African Americans in law and through the social structures of the South.

Perhaps we are still in a period of Reconstruction since we are, without question, dealing with the implications of the civic war and the ideologies that led to current social relations and social relations of production. This legacy is alive and well within all parts of the country, perhaps even more insidiously outside the South where it often lives beneath surface-level interactions. In our opinion, if we are to move beyond this legacy, we must begin by providing reparations for African Americans, as well as a living wage and basic social welfare for all US citizens.

Additional Resources

Fitzgerald, Michael W. *Splendid failure: postwar reconstruction in the American South*. Chicago: Ivan R. Dee, 2007.

Foner, Eric. *Reconstruction: America's Unfinished Revolution, 1863–1877*. New American Nation Series. Vol. 9. New York: Harper & Row, 1988.

Guelzo, Allen C. *Reconstruction: A Concise History*. New York: Oxford University Press, 2018.

Langguth, A. J. *After Lincoln: How the North Won the Civil War and Lost the Peace*. New York: Simon and Schuster, 2015.

Paludan, Phillip S. "Law and the Failure of Reconstruction: The Case of Thomas Cooley." *Journal of the History of Ideas* 33.4 (1972): 597–614.

Richardson, Heather Cox. *The Death of Reconstruction: Race, Labor, and Politics in the Post-Civil War North*. Cambridge: Harvard University Press, 2009.

Upchurch, Thomas Adams. *Legislating Racism: The Billion Dollar Congress and the Birth of Jim Crow*. Lexington: University Press of Kentucky, 2015.

Internet References...

America's Reconstruction: People and Politics after the Civil War: From Slave Labor to Free Labor

http://www.digitalhistory.uh.edu/exhibits/reconstruction/section3/section3_intro.html.

Foner, Eric. "The New View of Reconstruction." *American Heritage*. October/November 1983

https://www.americanheritage.com/content/new-view-reconstruction

Gordon-Reed, Annette. "What If Reconstruction Hadn't Failed?" *The Atlantic*. October 26, 2015

https://www.theatlantic.com/politics/archive/2015/10/what-if-reconstruction-hadnt-failed/412219/

Loewen, James W. "Five Myths about Reconstruction." *The Washington Post*. January 21, 2016

https://www.washingtonpost.com/opinions/five-myths-about-reconstruction/2016/01/21/0719b324-bfc5-11e5-83d4-42e3bceea902_story.html?utm_term=.7bd34f063813

National Archives: Civil War and Reconstruction (1850–1877)

https://www.archives.gov/education/lessons/civil-war-reconstruction.html

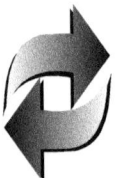